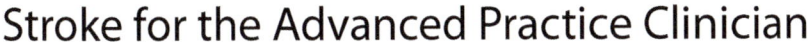

Stroke for the Advanced Practice Clinician

Hardik P. Amin

Editor

Stroke for the Advanced Practice Clinician

A Clinically Focused Guide for Acute, Inpatient, and Outpatient Care

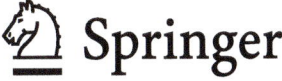 Springer

Editor
Hardik P. Amin
Neurology
Hartford Hospital
Hartford, CT, USA

ISBN 978-3-031-66288-1   ISBN 978-3-031-66289-8   (eBook)
https://doi.org/10.1007/978-3-031-66289-8

This Springer imprint is published by the registered company Springer Nature Switzerland AG
The registered company address is: Gewerbestrasse 11, 6330 Cham, Switzerland

If disposing of this product, please recycle the paper.

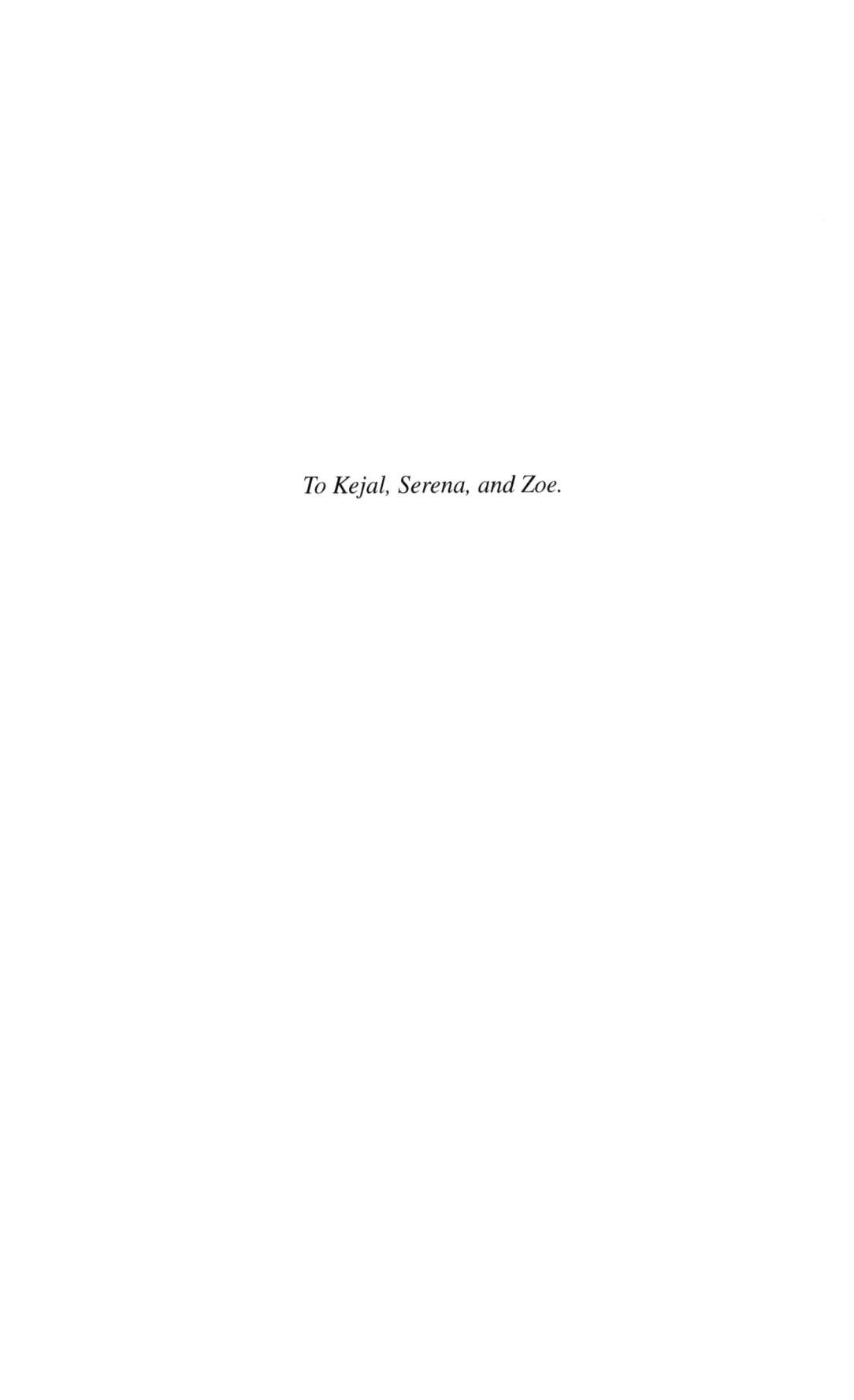

To Kejal, Serena, and Zoe.

Foreword

Advanced practice clinicians (APRNs, PAs) have played a vital role in the care of patients with cerebrovascular disease over the last several decades. They have assisted their neurosurgical colleagues in the operating room and procedural suites as well as during the immediate post-procedure period. They have worked alongside residents, fellows, and attending physicians in the neuro-intensive care units caring for complex neurological patients with life-threatening brain injuries. They have been active participants in the field with paramedics and colleagues in mobile stroke units, as part of telestroke teams and as first responders and part of stroke code teams in the hyper-acute phase of stroke care. They have taken the lead role in the transitions of care for patients and families after hospital discharge. They advocate for a comprehensive secondary stroke prevention approach in the clinics and communicate with primary care providers in the community. They are experts in promoting many of the evidence-based practice metrics that meet the requirements for stroke certification status across organizations.

As such, this comprehensive and practical textbook geared for the clinical APCs is long overdue. Dr. Amin and colleagues have collaborated on a broad scope of topics across the stroke care continuum, from the hyper-acute treatment phase to the inpatient course and through the outpatient recovery phase, and offer valuable and practical recommendations to support clinicians who care for the more than 800,000 patients and families in the USA that survive after stroke. This textbook reflects the collaboration and expertise among the clinicians who work at the bedside and who study the many unanswered questions to improve the quality of care for stroke survivors and caregivers in our communities.

Yale New Haven Hospital   Karin V. Nyström,
New Haven, CT, USA

Preface

The idea for this book came from conversations with my stroke APRN colleagues at Yale New Haven Hospital addressing the resources available for continuing education. They shared that the recommended textbooks are geared more toward medical students and residents, with a heavy emphasis on basic science and pathophysiology, which often overshadows the clinical aspects. Journals are a great resource for guidelines, but articles are frequently too specific, written for experts in the field, and include complex statistics. This book is meant to be more clinically focused and written such that any interested advanced practice clinician, regardless of experience, can appreciate and get up-to-date information on the entire continuum of stroke care. Importantly, this book includes many topics outside the medical model of care, including aspects of stroke recovery, caregiver issues, stroke center certification, and patient-oriented outcomes. To that end, most chapters are co-written by experienced APCs and expert stroke physicians to ensure readability and accuracy.

Given its size, this book is certainly not meant to be read cover to cover in one sitting. Rather, we hope that you will use it as an ongoing reference when you care for stroke patients as a supplement to teaching rounds, podcasts, conferences, and other learning opportunities. We think that this book will be a useful supplement to all APCs who care for stroke patients, including those who practice outside neurology.

I would like to express my deepest gratitude to our team of almost 70 co-authors from across the USA! It is not easy to simplify complex topics to make them more broadly accessible, but they were up to the task. I also wish to thank Swathiga Karthikeyan and Gregory Sutorius from Springer, USA, for shepherding the book along its long and windy road to publication. Finally, I would like to acknowledge my colleagues, friends, and family who have provided much encouragement during this journey.

Hartford, CT, USA   Hardik P. Amin

Contents

Contributors

Mohammed W. Al-Dulaimi, MD Neuro Critical Care, Inova Fairfax Hospital, Falls Church, VA, USA

Emily Alston, APRN University of Utah, Salt Lake City, UT, USA

Hardik P. Amin Neurology, Hartford Hospital, Hartford, CT, USA

Abdalla A. Ammar, PharmD, BCCCP, BCPS New York Presbyterian Hospital, New York, NY, USA

Jane Anderson, PhD, RN, FNP-BC Baylor College of Medicine, Houston, TX, USA

Sue Ashcraft, APRN Novant Health, Charlotte, NC, USA

Jennifer Bajek, MPAS, PA-C VA National Telestroke Program, Palo Alto VA Medical Center, Palo Alto, CA, USA

Kathryn Bard, PA-C University of Minnesota, Minneapolis, MN, USA

Rachel Beekman, MD Yale School of Medicine, New Haven, CT, USA

Lauren A. Beslow, MD, MSCE, FAHA Division of Neurology, Children's Hospital of Philadelphia, Philadelphia, PA, USA

Departments of Neurology and Pediatrics, Perelman School of Medicine at the University of Pennsylvania, Philadelphia, PA, USA

Jeremy Bingham, NP Vanderbilt University Medical Center, Nashville, TN, USA

Sharon Bottomley, APRN Veterans Affairs Medical Center, West Haven, CT, USA

Daniel C. Brooks, MD Providence Specialty Medical Group, Santa Monica, CA, USA

Yee Kuang Cheng, MD St. Luke's Medical Center, Boise, ID, USA

Lee Chung, MD University of Utah, Salt Lake City, UT, USA

Carrie Crowder, PA VA National Telestroke Program, Palo Alto VA Medical Center, Palo Alto, CA, USA

Adam S. De Havenon, MD, MSCI Yale School of Medicine, New Haven, CT, USA

Jennifer L. Dearborn-Tomazos, MD, MPH Department of Neurology, Beth Israel Deaconess Medical Center, Harvard Medical School, Boston, MA, USA

Carolin Dohle, MD, MPH Neurology, Neurorehabilitation, Westchester Medical Center, Valhalla, NY, USA

Amberlea Elliott, APRN-CNS Mercy Hospital, Oklahoma City, OK, USA

Safa Hakim Elnazer, MD Yale School of Medicine, New Haven, CT, USA

Pue Farooque, DO NYU Grossman School of Medicine, New York, NY, USA

Julia Gray, MSN, AGACNP-BC, NVRN-BC University of Alabama, Birmingham, AL, USA

Mary Ann Harmon, APRN Yale New Haven Hospital, New Haven, CT, USA

Ryan Hebert, MD Yale School of Medicine, New Haven, CT, USA

Andrew Huffer, MD University of Washington, Seattle, WA, USA

Adam S. Jasne, MD Yale School of Medicine, New Haven, CT, USA

Rebecca Karb, MD, PhD Warren Alpert School of Medicine, Providence, RI, USA

Jessica Kaslow, APRN, MSN Yale School of Medicine, New Haven, CT, USA

Kiffon Keigher, MSN, RN Advocate Health Care, Downers Grove, IL, USA

Walter N. Kernan, MD Yale School of Medicine, New Haven, CT, USA

Deborah Kerrigan, MD, MA Vanderbilt University Medical Center, Nashville, TN, USA

Natalie Le-Blanc, PA-C Yale School of Medicine, New Haven, CT, USA

Kun He Lee, MD Temple Health, Philadelphia, PA, USA

Michael Levien, APRN Yale New Haven Hospital, New Haven, CT, USA

Allison Lewandowski, PA-C Department of Anesthesia, Beth Israel Deaconess Medical Center, Boston, MA, USA

Naomi Lowe, PA-C Yale School of Medicine, New Haven, CT, USA

Michael Lyerly, MD, MSPH University of Alabama, Birmingham, AL, USA

Razaz Mageid, MD Beth Israel Lahey Health, Burlington, MA, USA

Ajay Malhotra, MBBS, MD, MMM Yale School of Medicine, New Haven, CT, USA

Margy McCullough-Hicks, MD University of Minnesota Medical School, Minneapolis, MN, USA

Caitlin McElroy-Cox, APRN Yale School of Medicine, New Haven, CT, USA

William S. Musser, MD VA National Telestroke Program, Palo Alto VA Medical Center, Palo Alto, CA, USA

VA National Telestroke Program, Palo Alto VA Medical Center, Palo Alto, California, CA, USA

Karin V. Nyström, MSN, APRN, FAHA Yale New Haven Hospital, New Haven, CT, USA

Ryan L. Orie, PA-C University of Pittsburgh Medical Center, Pittsburgh, PA, USA

Kent A. Owusu, PharmD, BCCCP, BCPS Yale New Haven Hospital, New Haven, CT, USA

Gino Paolucci, DNP, ACNP-BC, ANVP-BC Rhode Island Hospital, Providence, RI, USA

Akash Patel, MD Yale School of Medicine, New Haven, CT, USA

Darshna Patel, MSN, APRN, FNP-C University of Alabama, Birmingham, AL, USA

Teng J. Peng, MD University of Florida School of Medicine, Gainesville, FL, USA

Trista Pennington, PA-C Bridgeport Hospital, Bridgeport, CT, USA

Jennifer Picagli, APRN, MSN Yale New Haven Hospital, New Haven, CT, USA

Amber Robinson, APRN, MSN Yale New Haven Hospital, New Haven, CT, USA

Samantha Salas, APRN Stanford Health, Stanford, CA, USA

Richa Sharma, MD, MPH Yale School of Medicine, New Haven, CT, USA

Jason Sico, MD, MHS, FAHA, FAAN Yale School of Medicine, New Haven, CT, USA

Karan Tarasaria, MD Hartford HealthCare, Hartford, CT, USA

Neeharika Thottempudi, MD Carson Tahoe Health, Carson City, NV, USA

Natalie L. Ullman, MD, MPH Division of Neurology, Children's Hospital of Philadelphia, Philadelphia, PA, USA

Department of Neurology, The Hospital of the University of Pennsylvania, Philadelphia, PA, USA

Nicole Veltri, MSN, APRN Yale New Haven Hospital, New Haven, CT, USA

Divya Viswanathan, PA-C Westchester Medical Center, Valhalla, NY, USA

Darren Volpe, MD Yale School of Medicine, New Haven, CT, USA

Kathleen E. Walsh, CRNP, MSN Division of Neurology, Children's Hospital of Philadelphia, Philadelphia, PA, USA

Susan Wilson, DNP, RN, MSN University of North Carolina School of Medicine, Chapel Hill, NC, USA

Deonna Wissler, APRN University of Arkansas for Medical Sciences, Little Rock, AR, USA

Islam Zaydan, MD University of Pittsburgh Medical Center, Pittsburgh, PA, USA

Stroke Epidemiology

Michael Levien, Safa Hakim Elnazer, and Richa Sharma

Definition of Stroke

A stroke is an injury to the brain due to ischemia or hemorrhage [1]. Cerebral ischemia occurs when the blood supply to an area of the brain is reduced or interrupted, depriving it of oxygen and nutrients. Ischemic strokes account for 80–90% of all strokes [2]. Cerebral hemorrhage occurs when an artery bursts, leading to bleeding into brain tissue. Cerebral hemorrhage accounts for 10–20% of all strokes but is associated with higher morbidity and mortality. While there are clinically silent strokes that are only seen on imaging without symptoms, this chapter on stroke epidemiology focuses on clinically evident strokes that lead to a functional deficit.

Ischemic stroke is caused by thrombosis, embolism, or hypoperfusion [3]. Thrombosis can result from disease or injury to the arterial wall from atherosclerosis related to cardiovascular risk factors, dissection, or inflammation. A thrombus develops *at the site* of blood vessel injury. The thrombus can "clog" the vessel and impair blood flow downstream (hypoperfusion) or can embolize, whereby a piece of the thrombus dislodges and travels downstream to occlude a more distal vessel (sometimes called artery-to-artery embolism). Other sources of embolism include fat particles from bone fractures, atherosclerosis from plaque rupture, air from vessel puncture, amniotic fluid after pregnancy, and fibrous cartilage from vertebral disc injury [4]. Cerebral hypoperfusion happens when there is a reduction in the blood flow to the brain due to various triggers such as hypotension, sepsis, or

M. Levien
Yale New Haven Hospital, New Haven, CT, USA
e-mail: michael.levien@yale.edu

S. H. Elnazer · R. Sharma (✉)
Yale School of Medicine, New Haven, CT, USA
e-mail: safa.abdelhakim@yale.edu; richa.sharma@yale.edu

cardiac arrest. Intracerebral hemorrhage occurs following chronic arteriolar injury from hypertension, vascular malformations, or amyloid deposition that weakens vessel walls [5].

Burden of Stroke Globally and in the United States

Approximately 795,000 patients will experience a new or recurrent (second, third, or more) stroke in the United States each year. In 2018, the United States had approximately 7.6 million stroke survivors; by 2030, that number is expected to rise to over 10 million. Worldwide, stroke is the second leading cause of death, the third leading cause of disability, and a major cause of dementia [6]. The Framingham study demonstrated that nearly 26% of survivors maintain disability in activities of daily living following stroke [7]. Mobility decreases in nearly 50% of survivors due to hemiparesis. In developed countries, stroke is the third largest contributor to disability [8]. In 2019 and 2020, stroke was the fifth leading cause of death in the United States, following heart disease, cancer, COVID-19, and unintentional injuries [9]. A recent study by the World Stroke Organization reported that worldwide stroke-related deaths could reach ten million by 2050, with lower- to middle-income countries seeing the sharpest rise in stroke-related mortality [10]. Stroke incidence and stroke-related deaths have remained largely stable in high-income countries, however (Fig. 1.1).

Stroke also bears a heavy economic toll on patients, families, and society. In 2017–2018, the annual cost of stroke care in the United States was $52.8 billion (medical care, rehabilitation, lost earnings) [8]. However, this is likely an underestimate since "informal care" and its ramifications, such as a caregiver's reduced

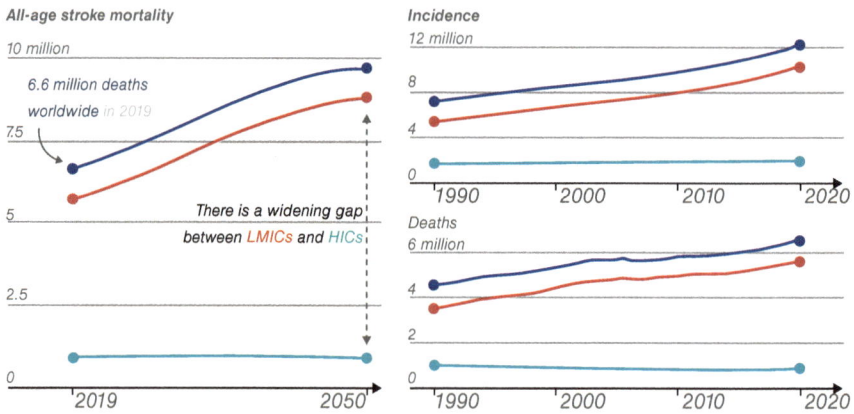

Fig. 1.1 Projected stroke mortality by 2050 (left). Incidence of stroke worldwide (right upper), and stroke-related deaths worldwide (right lower) between 1990 and 2020. Blue line: Global, Orange line: Low-middle income countries, Aqua line: High-income countries. Source: Feigin VL, Owolabi, MO, Lancet Neurol 2023

hours and lost wages, were likely not captured in its entirety. In one study of individuals 65 and older, the annual economic cost of "informal care" of stroke patients totaled $14.2 billion [11].

The Stroke Belt in the United States

Stroke is endemic throughout the United States. However, as demonstrated in a map generated by the CDC (Fig. 1.2), certain regions have inordinately high stroke rates [12]. The highest stroke and stroke-related mortality rates are in the American Southeastern states: Alabama, Arkansas, Georgia, Kentucky, Louisiana, Missouri, South Carolina, and Tennessee, and this area is referred to as the "stroke belt" [12]. The likelihood of death following a stroke is 30% higher in the stroke belt than in the rest of the nation. Even within this region, disparities exist in the burden of stroke and stroke-related mortality among counties [13]. Demographic characteristics of people living in counties with the highest stroke burden include higher proportions of African American residents, higher unemployment rates, lower median income, less educational attainment, and lower health insurance enrollment rates.

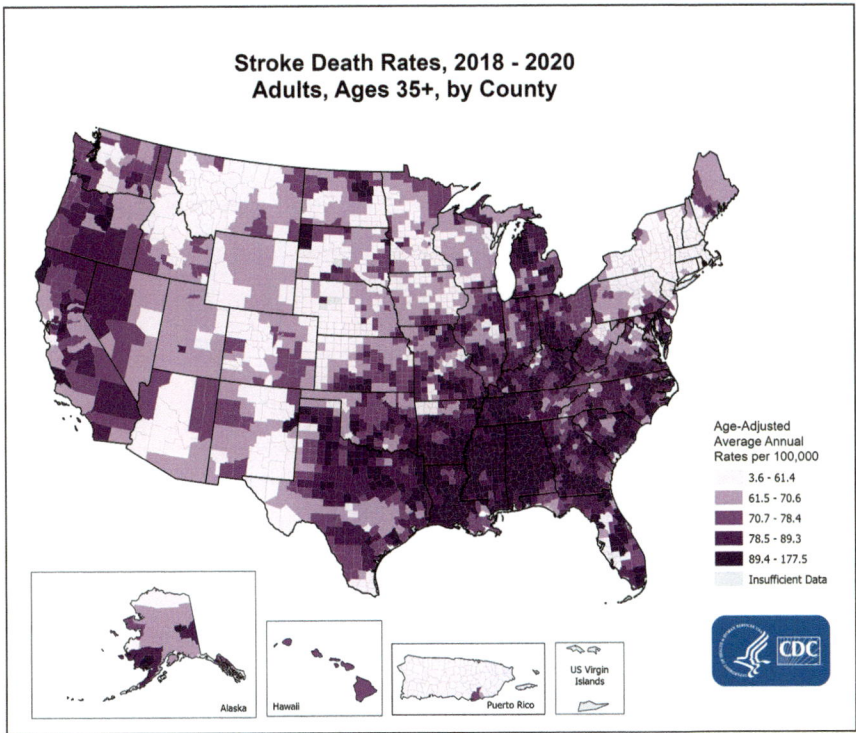

Fig. 1.2 Stroke mortality in the United States. Note the darker shades in the southeastern United States, termed the "stroke belt." Source: CDC.gov

Within these regions, the prevalence of common stroke risk factors such as hypertension, diabetes, and obesity tend to be higher [14, 15], potentially driving higher stroke rates in these communities.

Current and Future Trends in Stroke Epidemiology

Emerging trends in vascular risk factors in the United States forecast potential shifts in the epidemiology of stroke in the future.

The Atherosclerosis Risk in Communities, or ARIC, study demonstrated that stroke incidence rates have decreased by 32% in adults ≥65 [16]. A large percentage of this decrease may be due to improved treatment of cardiovascular risk factors [17]. Encouraging trends are also evident in certain aspects of stroke epidemiology, including decreased overall stroke-related mortality and improved functional outcomes after stroke. These trends have been driven by improvements in systems of acute stroke care [18], including endovascular thrombectomy [19], improved understanding and treatment of traditional and novel risk factors [20], and the development of technologies that enhance rehabilitation.

As the population ages, however, we can expect a sharp rise in the number of adults older than 65 (Fig. 1.3) [21]. Older adults are more likely to have stroke risk factors that accrue with age, such as atrial fibrillation and malignancy. The prevalence of atrial fibrillation in patients ≥80 is about 10%. The annual number of new

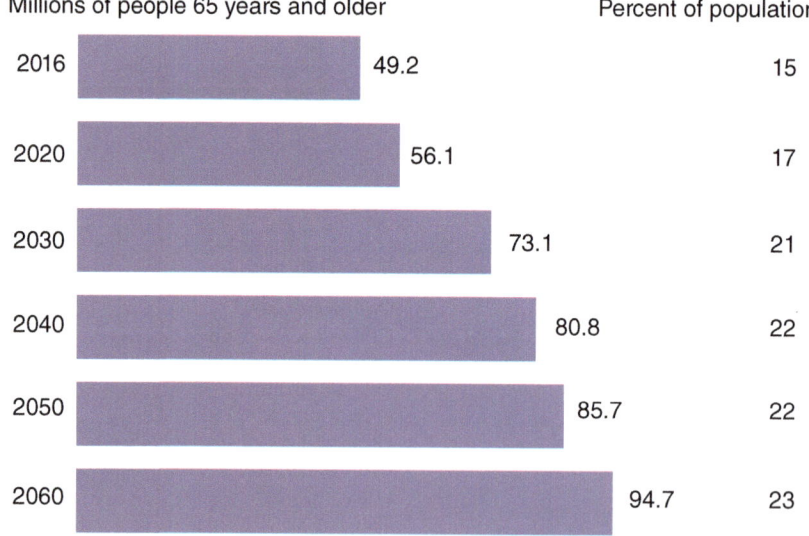

Fig. 1.3 By 2060, nearly one in four Americans is projected to be an older adult [21]. Source: U.S. Census Bureau, 2017 National Population Projections

cancer cases has risen from 1.3 million in 1999 to 1.75 million in 2019 [22]. Thus, a higher incidence and prevalence of stroke in the aging United States population may change the distribution of stroke etiology. Additionally, due to rising rates of risk factors such as hypertension [23], diabetes [24], and obesity in younger Americans, the rates of stroke in the young are *increasing*. Hospitalizations for acute ischemic stroke almost doubled for males 18–44 years of age from 1995 to 2011 [25]. The impact of steeply rising rates of drug abuse is also associated with increased rates of infective endocarditis, another risk factor for stroke at any age [26]. Increasing rates of diabetes, obesity, and physical inactivity may contribute to the rising incidence of pancreatic, breast, and colorectal cancer, all of which are associated with hypercoagulability of malignancy.

Global phenomena have also been implicated as emerging stroke risk factors contributing to inflammation, vascular damage, and autonomic and hemostatic disturbances [27]. Air pollution is estimated to be responsible for more than one-eighth of stroke deaths [28]. For instance, particulate matter in polluted air has been associated with atherosclerosis of the carotid artery and increased blood pressure, and elevated ambient nitrous oxide and carbon monoxide are associated with increased plasma fibrinogen levels, promoting the formation of blood clots. Acute ischemic stroke is a known neurological complication of COVID-19, partly due to the interaction between traditional vascular risk factors and endotheliopathy and coagulopathy from the disease [29, 30]. One small case series of men aged younger than 50 and diagnosed with asymptomatic COVID found that the risk of stroke more than doubled compared to a matched cohort [31].

Disparities in Stroke Incidence, Treatment, and Outcomes

Health disparity is a health and medical outcome discrepancy linked to social, economic, and environmental disadvantages. This topic is discussed in more depth in a subsequent chapter. Disparities in health outcomes have been historically demonstrated by race, ethnicity, religion, socioeconomic status, sex, age, mental health, cognitive function, physical disability, sexual orientation, gender identity, and geographic location. In terms of stroke incidence, despite an overall decrease in stroke incidence among Whites, stroke incidence among Blacks has not changed [32]. Studies have also shown that Black individuals have a higher risk of recurrent strokes than non-Hispanic Whites.

There are disparities in the burden of stroke-related disability and mortality as well. Female sex and young age are associated with delays in the administration of thrombolytic therapy, possibly due to higher suspicion of stroke mimics. Black individuals are also less likely than Whites to present within 3 h of acute symptom onset [33]. Studies have demonstrated that delayed thrombolytic therapy is associated with higher mortality, symptomatic intracranial hemorrhage, and lower rates of functional independence, as well as discharge to home after an acute ischemic stroke [34]. Blacks are one-third less likely than Whites to receive thrombolytic therapy, and Black stroke survivors tend to achieve worse functional outcomes than

White patients [35]. Black patients are less likely than White patients to report independence in activities of daily living 1 year after stroke [36]. Factors contributing to disparities in stroke outcomes include limitations with doctor–patient communication, distrust of the medical community, ambulance and medical costs, and lack of awareness of stroke warning signs [37–39].

Key Points

- Strokes are a significant cause of death, disability, and healthcare expenditure worldwide.
- The southeastern United States is known as the "stroke belt" due to the highest risk of stroke-associated death.
- Overall, stroke incidence and mortality rates have been decreasing over time. However, certain stroke risk factors have been increasing in prevalence recently and are of concern.
- Disparities in stroke outcomes currently exist and are related to sex, race, socio-economic status, age, and religion.

Summary of Key Epidemiologic Studies

The Framingham Heart Study, initiated in 1948, follows a cohort of participants and their offspring in Framingham, Massachusetts. Nearly 43% of stroke survivors in this cohort who were elderly had moderate to severe deficits [7].

The Atherosclerosis Risk in Communities Study, which began in 1987, is an epidemiologic study performed prospectively in four communities in the United States. The study found that stroke incidence rates among older adults decreased from 1987 to 2011 [16].

References

1. Caplan LR. Caplan's stroke: a clinical approach. 4th ed. Cambridge: Cambridge University Press; 2017. p. 22.
2. Benjamin EJ, Virani SS, Callaway CW, et al. Heart Disease and Stroke Statistics-2018 Update: A Report From the American Heart Association [published correction appears in Circulation. 2018;137(12):e493]. Circulation. 2018;137(12):e67–e492. https://doi.org/10.1161/CIR.0000000000000558.
3. Ay H, Furie KL, Singhal A, Smith WS, Sorensen AG, Koroshetz WJ. An evidence-based causative classification system for acute ischemic stroke. Ann Neurol. 2005;58(5):688–97. https://doi.org/10.1002/ana.20617.
4. Caplan LR. Brain embolism, revisited. Neurology. 1993;43(7):1281–7. https://doi.org/10.1212/wnl.43.7.1281.
5. About Stroke. Centers for Disease Control and Prevention. https://www.cdc.gov/stroke/about.htm. Published November 2, 2022. Accessed 10 Nov 2022.
6. GBD 2019 Stroke Collaborators. Global, regional, and national burden of stroke and its risk factors, 1990–2019: a systematic analysis for the Global Burden of Disease Study 2019, Lancet Neurol. 2021;20(10):795–820. https://doi.org/10.1016/S1474-4422(21)00252-0.

7. Kelly-Hayes M, Beiser A, Kase CS, Scaramucci A, D'Agostino RB, Wolf PA. The influence of gender and age on disability following ischemic stroke: The Framingham study. J Stroke Cerebrovasc Dis. 2003;12(3):119–26. https://doi.org/10.1016/S1052-3057(03)00042-9.

8. Tsao CW, Aday AW, Almarzooq ZI, et al. Heart disease and stroke Statistics-2022 update: a report from the American Heart Association [published correction appears in Circulation. 2022 Sep 6;146(10):e141]. Circulation. 2022;145(8):e153–639. https://doi.org/10.1161/CIR.0000000000001052.

9. Mortality in the United States. Centers for Disease Control and Prevention. 2020. https://www.cdc.gov/nchs/products/databriefs/db427.htm. Published December 2021. Accessed 1 Jan 2023.

10. Feigin V, Owolabi M, on behalf of the World Stroke Organization. Pragmatic solutions to reduce the global burden of stroke: a world stroke organization-lancet neurology commission. Lancet Neurol. 2023;22(12):1160–206.

11. Joo H, Dunet DO, Fang J, Wang G. Cost of informal caregiving associated with stroke among the elderly in the United States. Neurology. 2014;83(20):1831–7. https://doi.org/10.1212/WNL.0000000000000986.

12. Stroke Death Rates. National Center for Health Statistics and National Vital Statistics System. https://www.cdc.gov/dhdsp/maps/pdfs/stroke_all.pdf. Accessed 1 Jan 2023.

13. Mullen MT, Judd S, Howard VJ, et al. Disparities in evaluation at certified primary stroke centers: Reasons for geographic and racial differences in stroke. Stroke. 2013;44(7):1930–5. https://doi.org/10.1161/STROKEAHA.111.000162.

14. Karp DN, Wolff CS, Wiebe DJ, Branas CC, Carr BG, Mullen MT. Reassessing the stroke belt: Using small area spatial statistics to identify clusters of high stroke mortality in the United States. Stroke. 2016;47(7):1939–42. https://doi.org/10.1161/STROKEAHA.116.012997.

15. Otite FO, Liaw N, Khandelwal P, et al. Increasing prevalence of vascular risk factors in patients with stroke: A call to action. Neurology. 2017;89(19):1985–94. https://doi.org/10.1212/WNL.0000000000004617.

16. Koton S, Sang Y, Schneider ALC, Rosamond WD, Gottesman RF, Coresh J. Trends in stroke incidence rates in older US adults: an update from the atherosclerosis risk in communities (ARIC) cohort study. JAMA Neurol. 2020;77(1):109–13. https://doi.org/10.1001/jamaneurol.2019.3258.

17. Vangen-Lønne AM, Wilsgaard T, Johnsen SH, Løchen ML, Njølstad I, Mathiesen EB. Declining incidence of ischemic stroke: what is the impact of changing risk factors? The Tromsø study 1995 to 2012. Stroke. 2017;48(3):544–50. https://doi.org/10.1161/STROKEAHA.116.014377.

18. National Institute of Neurological Disorders and Stroke rt-PA Stroke Study Group. Tissue plasminogen activator for acute ischemic stroke. N Engl J Med. 1995;333(24):1581–7. https://doi.org/10.1056/NEJM199512143332401.

19. Goyal M, Menon BK, van Zwam WH, et al. Endovascular thrombectomy after large-vessel ischaemic stroke: a meta-analysis of individual patient data from five randomised trials. Lancet. 2016;387(10029):1723–31. https://doi.org/10.1016/S0140-6736(16)00163-X.

20. Timaran CH, Mantese VA, Malas M, et al. Differential outcomes of carotid stenting and endarterectomy performed exclusively by vascular surgeons in the carotid revascularization endarterectomy versus stenting trial (CREST). J Vasc Surg. 2013;57(2):303–8. https://doi.org/10.1016/j.jvs.2012.09.014.

21. Mitchell GW. The silver tsunami. Physician Exec. 2014;40(4):34–8.

22. Annual Report to the Nation 2022: Overall Cancer Statistics. Surveillance, Epidemiology, and End Results Program. National Cancer Institute. https://seer.cancer.gov/report_to_nation/statistics.html. Accessed 10 Nov 2022.

23. Kearney PM, Whelton M, Reynolds K, Muntner P, Whelton PK, He J. Global burden of hypertension: analysis of worldwide data. Lancet. 2005;365(9455):217–23. https://doi.org/10.1016/S0140-6736(05)17741-1.

24. Lawrence JM, Divers J, Isom S, et al. Trends in prevalence of type 1 and type 2 diabetes in children and adolescents in the U.S., 2001–2017 [published correction appears in JAMA. 2021 Oct 5;326(13):1331]. JAMA. 2021;326(8):717–27. https://doi.org/10.1001/jama.2021.11165.

25. George MG, Tong X, Bowman BA. Prevalence of cardiovascular risk factors and strokes in younger adults. JAMA Neurol. 2017;74(6):695–703. https://doi.org/10.1001/jamaneurol.2017.0020.
26. Merkler AE, Chu SY, Lerario MP, Navi BB, Kamel H. Temporal relationship between infective endocarditis and stroke. Neurology. 2015;85(6):512–6. https://doi.org/10.1212/WNL.0000000000001835.
27. Wellenius GA, Burger MR, Coull BA, et al. Ambient air pollution and the risk of acute ischemic stroke. Arch Intern Med. 2012;172(3):229–34. https://doi.org/10.1001/archinternmed.2011.732.
28. Verhoeven JI, Allach Y, Vaartjes ICH, Klijn CJM, de Leeuw FE. Ambient air pollution and the risk of ischaemic and haemorrhagic stroke. Lancet Planet Health. 2021;5(8):e542–52. https://doi.org/10.1016/S2542-5196(21)00145-5.
29. Mbonde AA, O'Carroll CB, Grill MF, Zhang N, Butterfield R, Demaerschalk BM. Stroke features, risk factors, and pathophysiology in SARS-CoV-2-infected patients. Mayo Clin Proc Innov Qual Outcomes. 2022;6(2):156–65. https://doi.org/10.1016/j.mayocpiqo.2022.01.003.
30. McAlpine LS, Zubair AS, Maran I, et al. Ischemic stroke, inflammation, and endotheliopathy in COVID-19 patients. Stroke. 2021;52(6):e233–8. https://doi.org/10.1161/STROKEAHA.120.031971.
31. Tu TM, Seet CYH, Koh JS, et al. Acute ischemic stroke during the convalescent phase of asymptomatic COVID-2019 infection in men. JAMA Netw Open. 2021;4(4):e217498. Published 2021 Apr 1. https://doi.org/10.1001/jamanetworkopen.2021.7498.
32. Kleindorfer DO, Khoury J, Moomaw CJ, et al. Stroke incidence is decreasing in whites but not in blacks: a population-based estimate of temporal trends in stroke incidence from the Greater Cincinnati/Northern Kentucky Stroke Study. Stroke. 2010;41(7):1326–31. https://doi.org/10.1161/STROKEAHA.109.575043.
33. Hsia AW, Edwards DF, Morgenstern LB, et al. Racial disparities in tissue plasminogen activator treatment rate for stroke: a population-based study. Stroke. 2011;42(8):2217–21. https://doi.org/10.1161/STROKEAHA.111.613828.
34. Ellis C, Hyacinth HI, Beckett J, et al. Racial/ethnic differences in poststroke rehabilitation outcomes. Stroke Res Treat. 2014;2014:950746. https://doi.org/10.1155/2014/950746.
35. Ikeme S, Kottenmeier E, Uzochukwu G, Brinjikji W. Evidence-based disparities in stroke care metrics and outcomes in the United States: a systematic review. Stroke. 2022;53(3):670–9. https://doi.org/10.1161/STROKEAHA.121.036263.
36. Ellis C, Boan AD, Turan TN, Ozark S, Bachman D, Lackland DT. Racial differences in poststroke rehabilitation utilization and functional outcomes. Arch Phys Med Rehabil. 2015;96(1):84–90. https://doi.org/10.1016/j.apmr.2014.08.018.
37. Lacy CRSD-C, Bueno M, Kostis. Delay in presentation and evaluation for acute stroke. Stroke. 2001;32:63–9.
38. Skolarus LMJ, Zimmerman M, Bailey S, Fowlkes S, Brown D, Lisabeth L, Greenberg E, Morgenstern L. Individual and community determinants of calling 911 for stroke among African Americans in an Urban Community. Circ Cardiovasc Qual Outcomes. 2013;6:278–83.
39. Biederman DJSH, Bibeau DL, Chase CM, Spann LI, Romanchuck R, Aronson RE, Schulz MR, Tiberia-Galka A. Ethnic and racial differences of baseline stroke knowledge in a "stroke belt" community. SAGE J. 2012;13:63–70.

Cerebrovascular Anatomy

2

Jennifer Bajek, Islam Zaydan, and Hardik P. Amin

Introduction

The central nervous system includes the brain and spinal cord. The brain is composed of three major parts: the cerebrum or cortex (top part), cerebellum, and brainstem, which can all be divided into a left and right side. The cerebrum is divided into two hemispheres—left and right, each further divided into the deeper subcortical structures and four major lobes: frontal, parietal, temporal, and occipital. On the outer surface of the brain are small bulges and crevasses called gyri and sulci. The basal ganglia are the deeper structures of each hemisphere and include the caudate, putamen, internal capsule, and thalamus. The cerebellum sits under the cortex behind the brainstem. The brainstem connects the cortex and cerebellum with the spinal cord.

The fundamental pathways controlling body functions begin in the cortex and travel through the basal ganglia, down the brainstem, into the spinal cord, and their respective areas.

J. Bajek
Veterans Affairs Medical Center, Palo Alto, CT, USA
e-mail: j.bajek@chatham.edu

I. Zaydan (✉)
University of Pittsburgh Medical Center, Pittsburgh, PA, USA
e-mail: islam.zaydan@va.gov

H. P. Amin
Hartford Hospital, Hartford, CT, USA
e-mail: hardik.amin@hhchealth.org

Motor Function

Movement is controlled by the primary motor cortex which gives rise to the cortico-spinal tract (CST). These fibers originate in the motor cortex located in the precentral gyrus in the frontal lobe, then travel down through the basal ganglia into the medial brainstem toward the medulla, where they form visible ridges called the "pyramids." At the base of the pyramids in the medulla, the fibers cross, or decussate, to the other side and travel down the spinal cord to move the arm and leg on that side. Since the CST fibers cross over (decussate) to the opposite side of the brain in the medulla, the CST therefore controls contralateral body movement. A lesion of the CST anywhere between the motor cortex and the pyramidal decussation, therefore, will lead to contralateral hemiparesis (or weakness on the opposite side). A lesion in the spinal cord will lead to ipsilateral (same side) weakness. Figure 2.1 depicts the motor "homunculus" in the motor cortex, which can predict what part of the body will be affected based on the location of the injury.

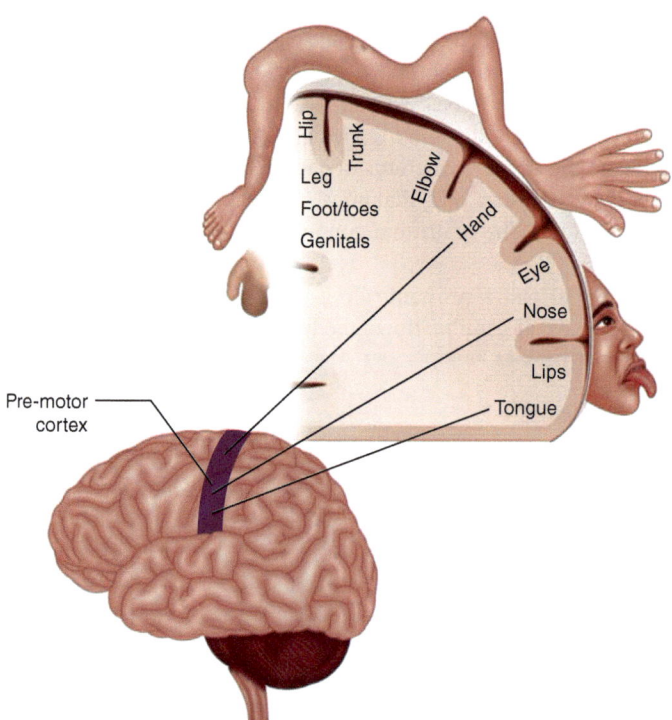

Fig. 2.1 Homunculus. It looks like an upside-down man, with the leg bending over the top of the cortex. The leg territory is mostly supplied by the anterior cerebral artery, whereas the face and arm are mostly supplied by the middle cerebral artery. The Pre-motor cortex, located just anterior to the primary motor cortex, plans and organizes movements prior to activation of the primary motor cortex

Sensation

Sensation is interpreted by the primary sensory cortex, located in the postcentral gyrus of the parietal lobe. Sensory input is received by nerve endings in the skin and then transmitted towards the brain through the spinothalamic and dorsal column pathways, up the spinal cord and brainstem, and finally reaches the sensory cortex via the thalamus. The direction of the sensory pathways is opposite to the motor pathway, which moves in a top-down direction.

The sensory modalities (soft touch, pain, temperature, vibration, and proprioception) are processed in the central nervous system to help the individual respond to the stimulus (e.g., recoil from a painful stimulus). The fibers responsible for interpreting vibration, fine touch, and proprioception are known as the Medial Lemniscal pathway. These fibers run up the spinal cord on the same side of the body as the stimulus but cross over to the opposite side at the medulla. From there, they travel upward to the thalamus and eventually to the sensory cortex. The fibers for pain and temperature are called the Spinothalamic pathway, which cross over at the same level of the sensory input in the spinal cord, travels upward toward the thalamus, and, finally, the sensory cortex. Therefore, a stroke involving the sensory cortex or thalamus will lead to sensory loss on the contralateral side, not because of damage to the primary receptors in the skin but due to injury of the processing centers in the brain.

Dermatomes are specific areas on the skin surface that correlate to specific spinal cord levels. Sensory loss in a specific dermatome can help pinpoint a lesion at a specific spinal cord level or peripheral nerve, which is unlikely to be due to a stroke. Sensory loss in a broader distribution, such as face, arm, and leg, points to a brain lesion such as a stroke. Since dermatomes are not as significant in a stroke exam, we will not include a diagram, which can be found elsewhere.

Language and Speech

Language is a system of spoken and written communication, including grammar, social context, and meaning of words. Speech is actual verbal communication. For most people, the left hemisphere is "dominant" and thus responsible for language and speech. Disorders of speech and language are called aphasia.

Broca's area, located in the inferior frontal lobe of the dominant hemisphere, controls speech production. Wernicke's area involves language comprehension and is in the dominant superior temporal lobe. Lesions in these locations will lead to aphasia, which is covered in greater depth in another chapter.

Vision

Light and color enter through the retinas in the eyes. The visual input from the retina travels through the optic nerve behind each eye. Each optic nerve contains fibers that will eventually end in either the left or right occipital lobe, demonstrated by the red and blue lines in Fig. 2.2. The optic nerves first converge at the optic chiasm. From the chiasm, optic tracts eventually turn into optic radiations that transmit signals from the right half of both eyes to the left occipital lobe and from the left half of both eyes to the right occipital lobe (Fig. 2.2). The primary visual cortex is in the occipital lobes. Each occipital lobe processes visual information brought in by the contralateral hemifield of *both eyes*. Optic radiations send information from the top or bottom half of their hemifield. Lesions along the optic radiations, therefore, can cause a type of visual field defect called quadrantanopsia. This results in the loss of a quarter of the visual field in both eyes, usually in a pie wedge shape, either in the upper or lower quadrant. Lesions in an occipital lobe will produce a complete homonymous hemianopia (missing the same half of the visual field from both eyes), since it processes information from both optic radiations. Occlusion of the retinal artery, on the other hand, will produce complete vision loss in one eye.

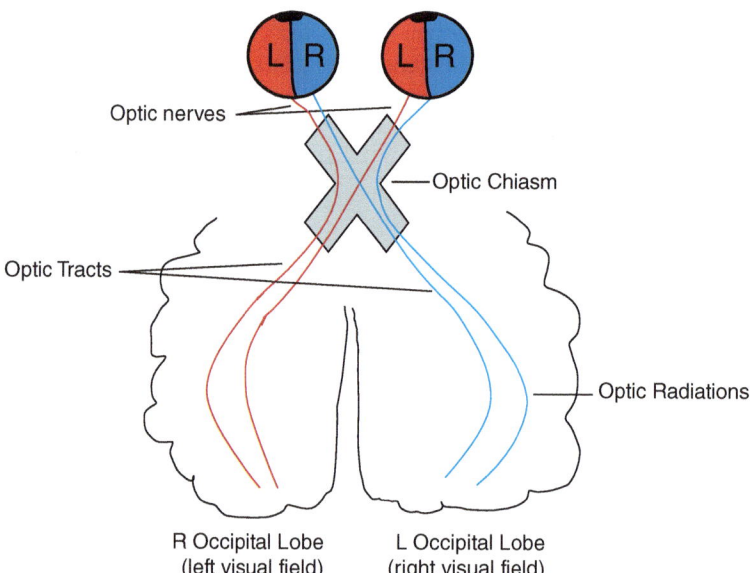

Fig. 2.2 Visual pathway

Coordination

The cerebellum is located under the cortex and behind the brainstem (see the vascular anatomy section for images). It comprises two hemispheres, the right and left, and sits behind the fourth ventricle. Each cerebellar hemisphere controls the coordination and planning of the ipsilateral arm and leg movements. Therefore, lesions in a cerebellar hemisphere will lead to dyscoordination (dysmetria) of the same side. A large cerebellar stroke or mass lesion can compress the fourth ventricle, preventing the outflow of cerebrospinal fluid and leading to hydrocephalus.

The Brainstem

The brainstem consists of the midbrain, pons, and medulla and extends down to form the spinal cord. Just above the brainstem rest the thalami (one on each hemisphere). Most cranial nerves, except Olfactory (CN I) and Optic (CN II), come from the brainstem. See Table 2.1 for the origins of the cranial nerve nuclei and respective functions (all functions are ipsilateral except for CN IV).

Table 2.1 Cranial nerves

Location	Cranial nerve	Function
Olfactory bulb (forebrain)	CN I (Olfactory)	Olfaction
Retina	CN II (Optic)	Vision
Midbrain	CN III (Oculomotor)	Extraocular muscles, pupillary constriction
	CN IV (Trochlear)	Extraocular muscle (superior oblique) that moves the eye down and inward
Pons	CN V (Trigeminal)	Facial sensation
	CN VI (Abducens)	Extraocular muscle (lateral rectus) that moves eyes laterally outward
	CN VII (Facial)	Muscles of facial expression, taste, eye tearing, and saliva production
	CN VIII (Vestibulocochlear)	Hearing
Medulla	CN IX (Glossopharyngeal)	Taste, sensation from the pharynx (gag reflex)
	CN X (Vagus)	Swallowing, larynx (voice box), parasympathetic innervation of the heart, lungs, and digestive tract
	CN XI (Spinal accessory)	Neck and shoulder movement and sensation
	CN XII (Hypoglossal)	Tongue movement

The Rule of 4

Let's work on a framework for localizing brainstem lesions using cranial nerve deficits and other exam findings. One common method is to remember the "Rule of 4." This rule identifies four structures that are in the medial brainstem (that start with "m") and four structures that are in the lateral brainstem (that begin with "S," for side) (Table 2.2). When you're comfortable with the Rule of 4, match up the structures with their respective blood vessels (coming up), and you'll be a brainstem pro! Figure 2.3 illustrates all pathways and cranial nerves combined with their vascular supply.

- **Medial Lemniscus**: Located in the medial medulla and plays a role in contralateral proprioception and vibration sense.
- **Medial Longitudinal Fasciculus:** Ascends along the medial pons and midbrain and plays a role in coordinating eye movements.
- **Motor (Corticospinal) Tract**: Originates in the motor cortex, travels down the medial brainstem, and decussates (crosses over) in the medulla to innervate the *contralateral* side of the body.
- **Motor Nuclei:** See above for functions related to these cranial nerves.
- **Spinothalamic Tract:** Brings pain and temperature sense from nerve endings in the skin, crossing immediately at the same spinal cord level, and travels up towards the lateral brainstem to the thalamus and eventually the primary sensory cortex.
- **Sympathetic Pathway:** Forms in the hypothalamus and travels down the lateral brainstem, exits the CNS in the upper thoracic cord, then travels in the superior cervical ganglion and eventually with the internal and external carotid arteries. Plays a role in "flight or fight" responses. Lesions in the sympathetic pathway can lead to Horner Syndrome, where a pupil on the ipsilateral side will not dilate in the dark like the other eye (miosis), ipsilateral eyelid droop (ptosis), and the lack of sweating on the ipsilateral face (anhidrosis).
- **Sensory nucleus of CN V (Trigeminal):** Ipsilateral sensation to the face, starts in the Pons and extends into the upper cervical spinal cord.
- **Spinocerebellar Tract:** Conveys information about limb movements to the ipsilateral cerebellar hemisphere. Lesions can lead to gait ataxia.

Table 2.2 Rule of 4s. The functions of each structure are described ahead

Medial	Lateral
• Medial lemniscus	• Spinothalamic tract
• Medial longitudinal Fasiculus	• Sympathetic pathway
• Motor (corticospinal) tract	• Sensory nucleus of CN V
• Motor nuclei of CN III, IV, VI, XII	• Spinocerebellar tract

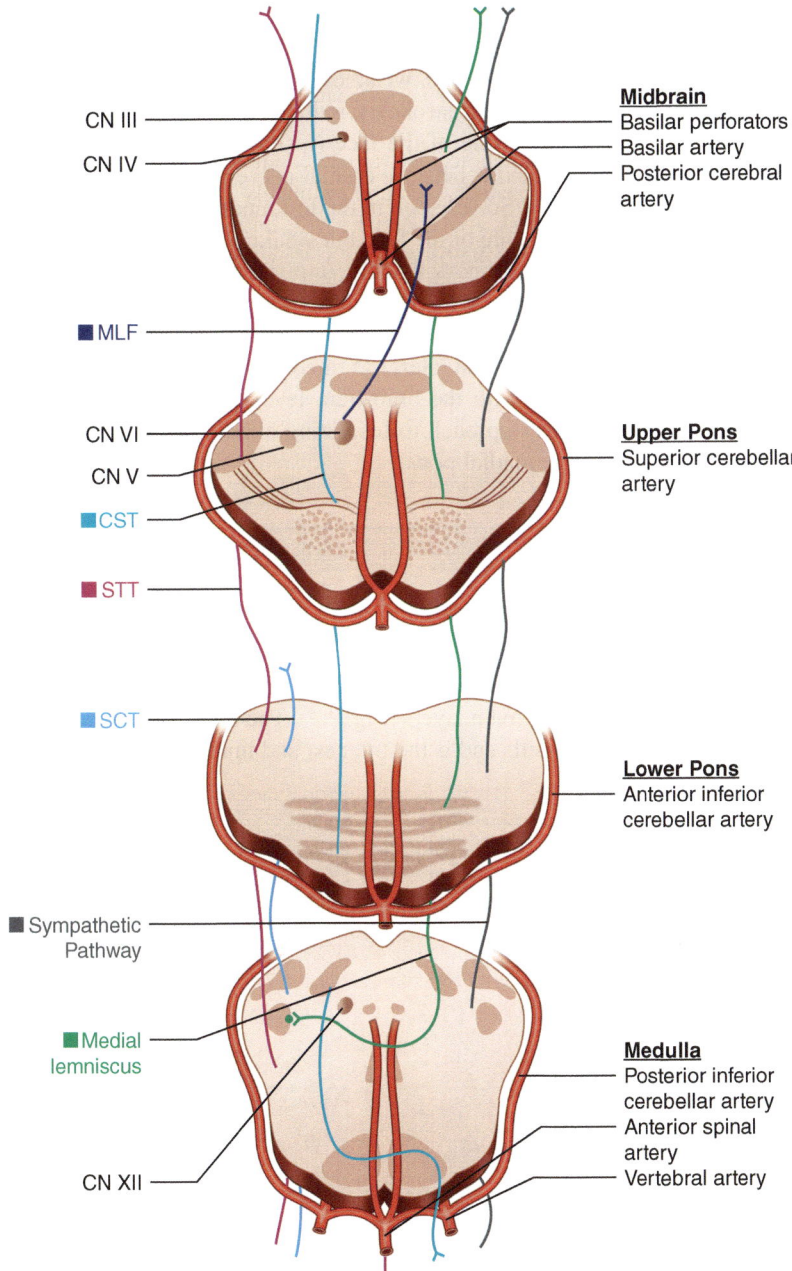

Fig. 2.3 Rule of 4 brainstem structures, pathways, and vasculature. *CN* cranial nerve, *MLF* medial longitudinal fasiculus, *CST* corticospinal tract, *STT* spinothalamic tract, *SCT* spinocerebellar tract

A key difference between brainstem strokes and cortical strokes in the hemispheres is that brainstem strokes may have "crossed signs." When a stroke occurs in the motor cortex of the frontal lobe, weakness of the face, arm, and leg will all be on one side (contralateral to the stroke). On the other hand, a brainstem stroke can lead to weakness on one side of the face (ipsilateral to the stroke) and the opposite side of the body. That is because cranial nerve palsies are ipsilateral for all except CN IV (trochlear). So, a lesion in the left medial pons may lead to cranial neuropathies on the left side of the face but weakness on the right side of the body. Crossed signs with weakness usually imply a medial brainstem stroke. Using the Rule of 4s, numbness to pain/temperature with ataxia suggests the lesion may be in the lateral brainstem. For suspected brainstem strokes, after determining laterality (right vs. left) and lateral vs. medial based the Rule of 4, matching up cranial neuropathies with the brainstem level of their nuclei (midbrain, pons, medulla) is a reliable approach to localizing exact brainstem lesions (i.e., left lateral medulla or right medial pons).

Blood Vessels

Arteries

Arteries bring oxygenated blood and nutrients to the brain (like clean water pipes to a house) and comprises three main layers (Fig. 2.4). The tunica intima consists of a single layer of endothelial cells and is the thinnest and innermost layer. The tunica

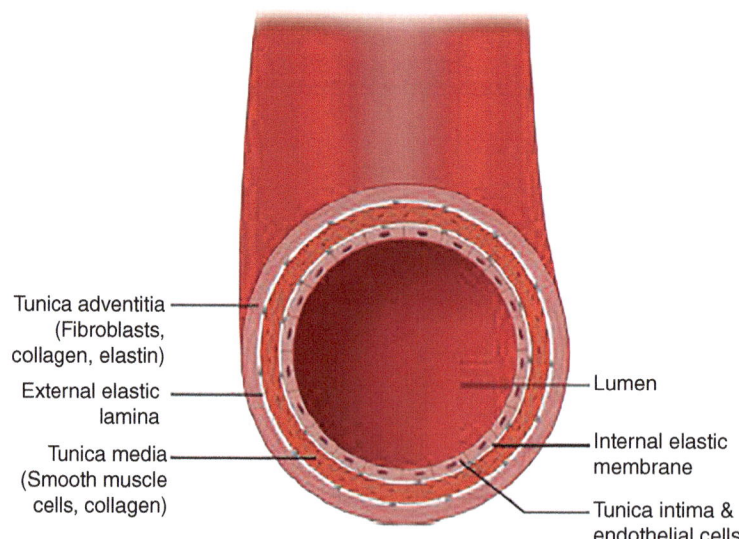

Fig. 2.4 Blood vessel structure. Source: Vascular Neurology Board Review

media is the middle layer and consists of several layers of smooth muscle cells that modulate the vessel's tone, or diameter, in response to blood pressure changes. The tunica adventitia is the outermost layer and consists of connective tissue, nerve endings, and blood vessels called *vasa vasorum* (tiny blood vessels that supply nutrients to the walls of larger blood vessels).

The aorta is the first and largest artery originating from the heart, from which all subsequent vessels originate (Fig. 2.5). The brachiocephalic (innominate) artery is the first branch of the aortic arch and bifurcates into the right common carotid and right subclavian artery. The left common carotid artery is often the next branch of the aortic arch (notice it does not share a branch with the subclavian on the left, in most cases). The left subclavian artery is the last branch of the aortic arch and further divides into the left vertebral artery, internal thoracic artery, thyrocervical trunk, and dorsal scapular artery.

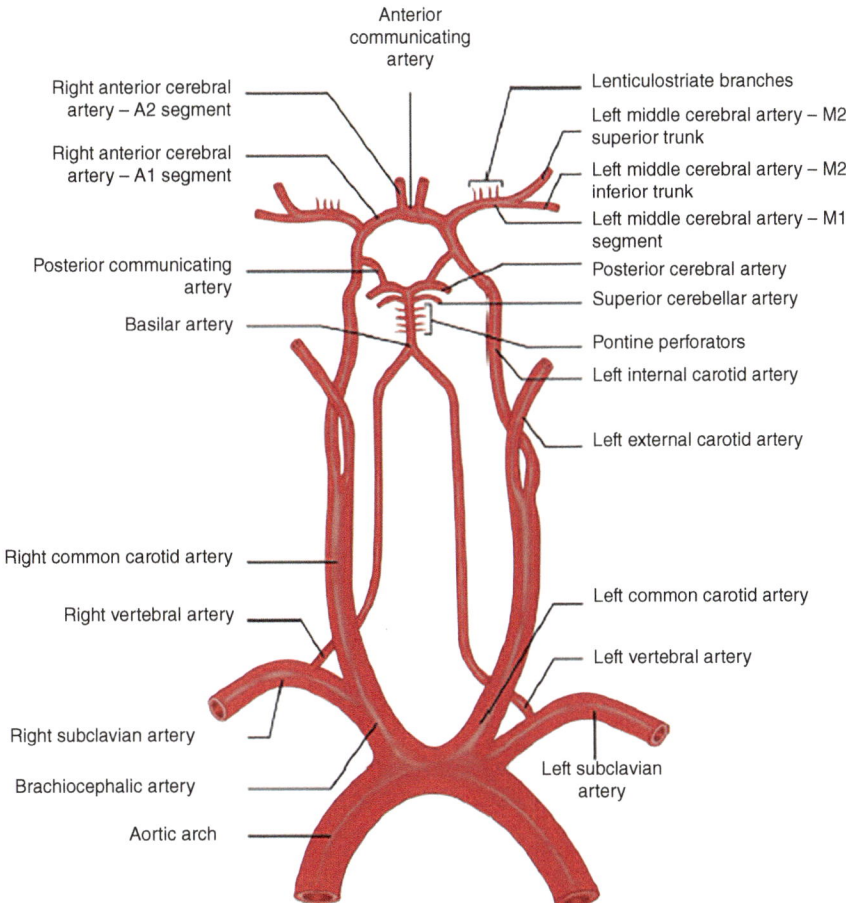

Fig. 2.5 Cerebral vasculature. Source: Vascular Neurology Board Review

- **The Common Carotid artery (CCA)** will bifurcate into the internal and external carotid arteries at the C4 vertebral level (about the level of the jaw). The proximal ICA has a bulge, often called the carotid bulb or sinus. The carotid sinus acts as a pressure receptor for regulating blood pressure in the cerebral arteries. External pressure to the carotid sinus leads to slowed heart rate and can lead to syncope in some patients.
- **The External Carotid artery (ECA)** supplies the muscles of the face and scalp. It gives off multiple branches in the neck (unlike the ICA, which has no branches until it reaches the brain). The most important branch of the ECA for stroke-related purposes is the superficial temporal artery, which can become inflamed in giant cell arteritis.
- **The Internal Carotid Artery (ICA)** supplies the anterior portion of the brain (frontal, parietal, and superior temporal lobes, Fig. 2.5). In the neck, the ICA is usually positioned posteriorly and laterally to the external carotid artery, which makes it more accessible for endarterectomy but also more vulnerable to dissections. The following are the segments of the ICA that are most referred to, listed from the bottom to the top (Fig. 2.6).

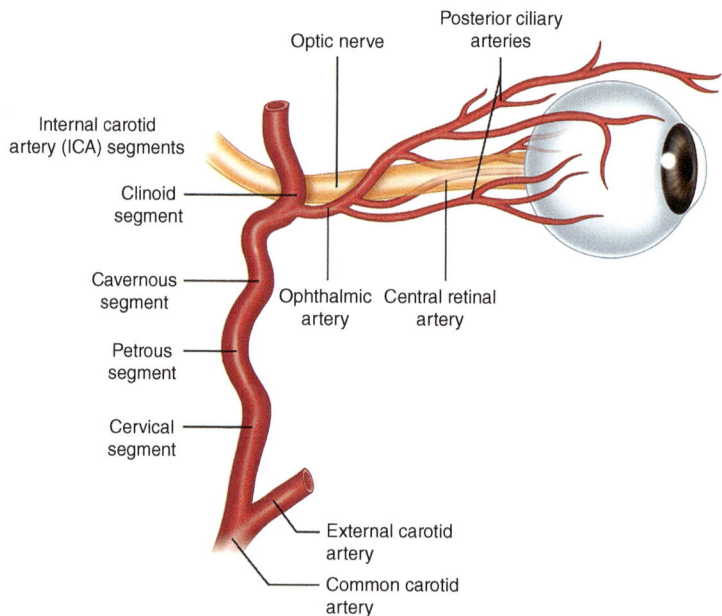

Fig. 2.6 ICA branches. Source: Vascular Neurology Board Review. **Image not drawn to scale. The eye is larger relative to the ICA only to demonstrate the smaller branches of the Ophthalmic Artery**

- Cervical segment: This segment begins at the carotid bifurcation and extends between the carotid bulb and the carotid canal within the petrous bone. Atherosclerosis commonly occurs where the ICA originates from the bifurcation. This segment is where endarterectomy and stenting are performed.
- Petrous segment: Starts at the base of the skull to the apex of the petrous bone.
- Cavernous segment: Travels within the cavernous sinus with the abducens nerve, ending by piercing the dura. It is close to multiple cranial nerves and the sympathetic trunk.
- Supraclinoid segment: Final segment that gives off the ophthalmic artery, posterior communicating artery, anterior choroidal artery, and eventually bifurcates at the "terminus" into the ACA and MCA.
- The **Ophthalmic artery** is the primary source of blood supply to the globe, orbit, and frontal scalp. It gives off the retinal artery, which then has smaller distal branches. Central retinal artery occlusion (CRAO) or branch retinal artery occlusion (BRAO) leads to complete or partial vision loss, respectively, in the ipsilateral eye.

The Anterior Cerebral Artery (ACA) is one of the two terminal branches of the ICA and supplies the medial frontal and parietal lobes. Notice on the homunculus that this territory predominantly controls the leg, foot, and bladder. The main segments are the A1 and A2, with the transition demarcated by the anterior communicating artery.

- **The Middle Cerebral Artery (MCA)** is the main branch of the internal carotid artery. It supplies most of the cortex, including the medial frontal, parietal, and anterior temporal lobes (Fig. 2.7). From proximally to distally, the segments are numbered M1, M2, M3, and M4, with the M4 segments being the smallest and most distal.
  - M 1: Extends from the ICA terminus, courses laterally. The most common location of large vessel occlusions. The main branches are the lenticulostriate arteries that supply the basal ganglia and internal capsule.
  - M 2: The M1 segment then bifurcates into two M2 segments: superior M2 and inferior M2. Superior trunk: Supplies frontal and parietal lobes. Occlusion can lead to contralateral hemiplegia, hemi hypesthesia, expressive aphasia, gaze deviation, and neglect. Inferior trunk: Supplies inferior frontal and superior temporal lobes. Occlusion leads to receptive aphasia and usually no weakness.
  - M3/4: More distal branches with smaller perfusion areas are typically not amenable to thrombectomy.

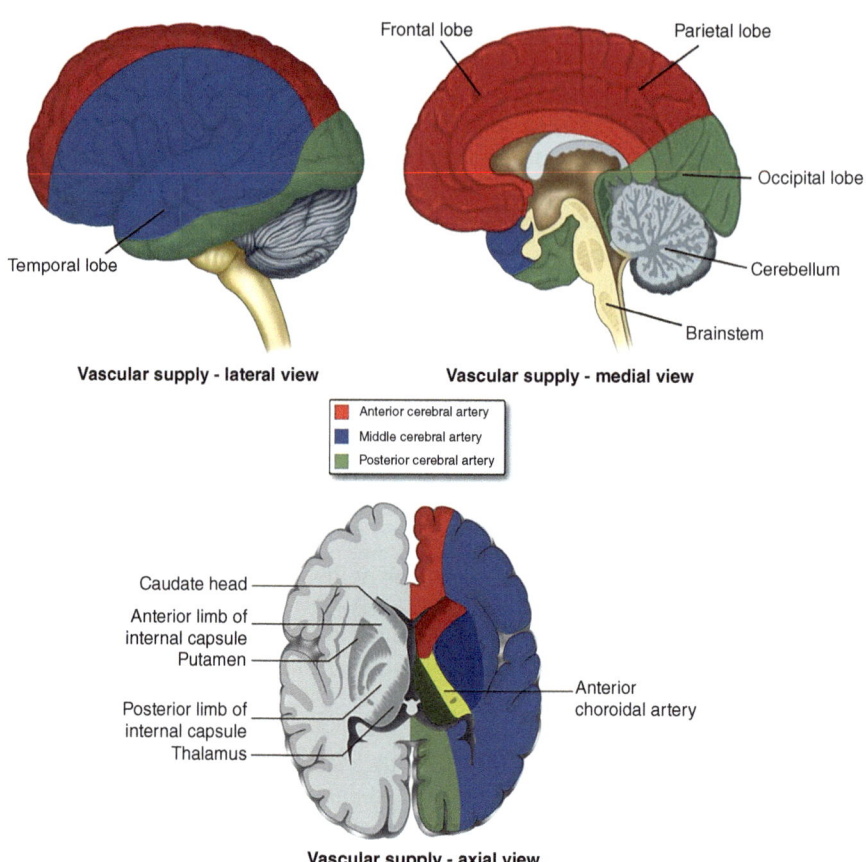

Fig. 2.7 Vascular supply of the brain

- **The Circle of Willis** is the equivalent of a traffic circle at the base of the brain that functions as an anastomosis (connection) between anterior and posterior circulations (Fig. 2.8). These connections allow hypoperfused areas to draw blood from other sources in the event of vascular disease and stenosis, mainly via the ACOM and PCOM vessels. A complete circle of Willis is only seen in about 25% of the population, and most people will have one or more missing communicating vessels!

Fig. 2.8 The (traffic) Circle of Willis. *ICA* internal carotid artery, *MCA* middle cerebral artery, *A1* anterior cerebral artery, A1 segment, *ACOM* anterior communicating artery, *A1* anterior cerebral artery, A2 segment, *PCA* posterior cerebral artery, *PCOM* posterior communicating artery. White arrows indicate the direction of blood flow in normal circumstances

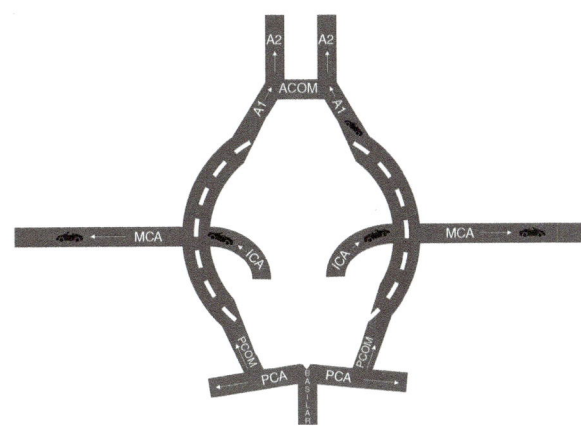

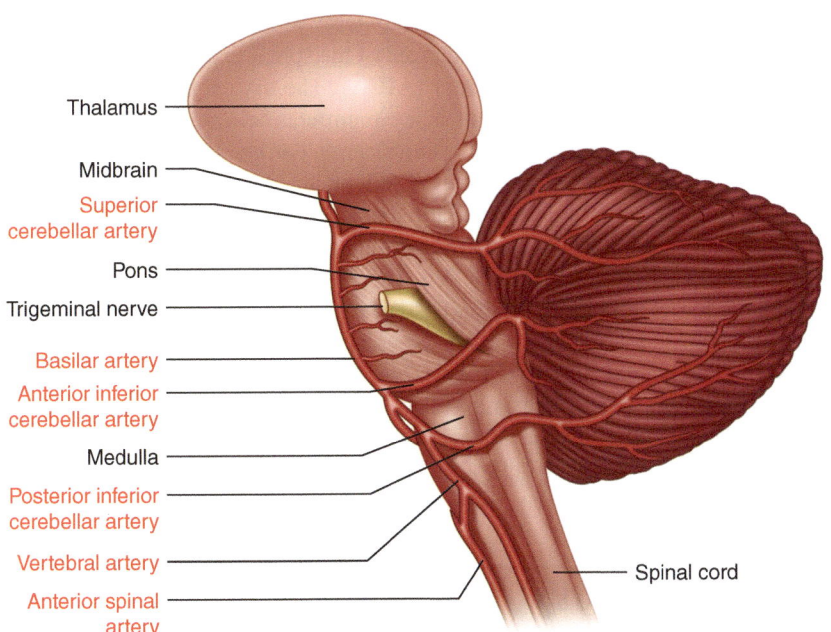

Fig. 2.9 Brainstem vasculature, sagittal view

Posterior Circulation Vasculature

The posterior circulation (Fig. 2.9) starts with the vertebral arteries, which come off their respective subclavian arteries. The vertebral arteries travel toward the brain through the transverse foramina of the C6-C2 spinal levels. The two vertebral arteries then join to form the basilar artery at the pontomedullary junction, or where the medulla turns into the pons. The basilar artery is a crucial vessel that supplies the pons and midbrain. Coming off the vertebral and basilar arteries are two types of branches. The first group of branches are the paired *circumferential* vessels, which wrap around and supply blood to the left and right lateral portions of the brainstem structures and cerebellum. Most are unnamed, but a handful are named and supply important territories. The other group of branches are the medial *perforators* that pierce the middle and supply the medial portions of the brainstem. We will review the main circumferential and perforator vessels, starting from the bottom and going up. Each vessel described below, except the anterior spinal and basilar perforator vessels, has a right and left sided branch.

- **Posterior Inferior Cerebellar Artery (PICA):** Circumferential vessels (left and right) that come off each vertebral artery just before the basilar artery forms. They wrap around the left and right side of the medulla and supply the lateral portions. Occlusion will lead to the famous Wallenberg syndrome.
- **Anterior spinal artery:** Two branches form from the medial portions of the vertebral artery, coursing downward and quickly joining to form the single anterior spinal artery that runs down the front of the spinal cord.
- **Anterior inferior cerebellar artery (AICA):** The first large branches (left and right) of the basilar artery. AICA is a circumferential artery that supplies the inferior lateral pons, anterior and inferior cerebellar hemispheres, and the inner ear. Ipsilateral sudden hearing loss is seen with an AICA occlusion.
- **Basilar perforators:** Small penetrating arteries (not circumferential) from the basilar artery that supply the middle portion of the pons and midbrain.
- **Superior cerebellar artery (SCA):** This is the next circumferential artery pair that comes off the tip of the basilar, supplying the superior lateral pons, medial cerebellar hemispheres, and cerebellar peduncles.
- **Posterior cerebral artery (PCA):** The last circumferential vessel pair also coming off the tip of the basilar. The PCOM separates the P1 and P2 segments. The P1 supplies the midbrain and thalamus via the thalamic perforators. The P2 segment wraps around the midbrain and heads toward the occipital lobe.

The Blood-Brain Barrier

To fully understand arterial blood flow, it is important to understand the blood-brain barrier (BBB), unique to the vessels that supply the central nervous system. The BBB is a layer of endothelial cells connected by tight junctions that facilitates the transport of physiologically important molecules and substances between blood and brain. Other suggested functions include protecting the brain from toxins in the blood and preventing the leakage of neurotransmitters into the general circulation.

Injury to the blood-brain barrier is often noted after stroke, trauma, inflammation, and radiation. It shows up on MRI as "contrast enhancement," where the injected contrast is leaking out of the vessels into the brain tissue. Breakdown of the blood-brain barrier also leads to hemorrhagic conversion of ischemic stroke, where small amounts of blood leak into an ischemic stroke bed.

Cerebral Blood Flow and Autoregulation

Due to the high metabolic demands of the brain, the average cerebral blood flow in healthy adults is around 50 mL/100 g/min. The cerebral blood flow has an unequal distribution along the brain, with the highest flow in the cerebral and cerebellar cortex.

Cerebral autoregulation is a complicated concept, but we will try to simplify it to its main points. Other resources go into it in much more detail. In essence, cerebral blood vessels can dilate or constrict in response to changes in blood pressure to maintain necessary and adequate blood flow. Autoregulation prevents neurological symptoms during blood pressure fluctuations, but only within a specific range (or threshold) of blood pressure or mean arterial pressures (MAP). Bad things will happen if the MAP drops below the lower limit threshold (ischemic stroke) or goes above the upper limit (hemorrhage, edema).

Venous System

Recall that arteries supply oxygenated blood to the brain. Veins drain deoxygenated blood in the opposite direction, away from the brain (like a septic system from a house), and return it to the heart. Occlusion of a vein or sinus at any point leads to an outflow obstruction. This can lead to edema or hemorrhage, but not as quickly as an arterial occlusion since it is a slower process (you'll notice immediately if the water is shut off, but it will take a while for a clogged sink to overflow).

Let's quickly go over the major veins we must keep in mind (Fig. 2.10).

The **Superior Sagittal Sinus (one)**: Travels along the top of the brain in the longitudinal cerebral fissure and collects blood from cortical veins. It also drains cerebrospinal fluid (CSF) in addition to blood. Thrombosis therefore leads to impaired CSF drainage and hydrocephalus. The Straight Sinus and Superior Sagittal Sinus combine at the back of the head to form the Confluence of the Sinuses (also known as the Torcula).

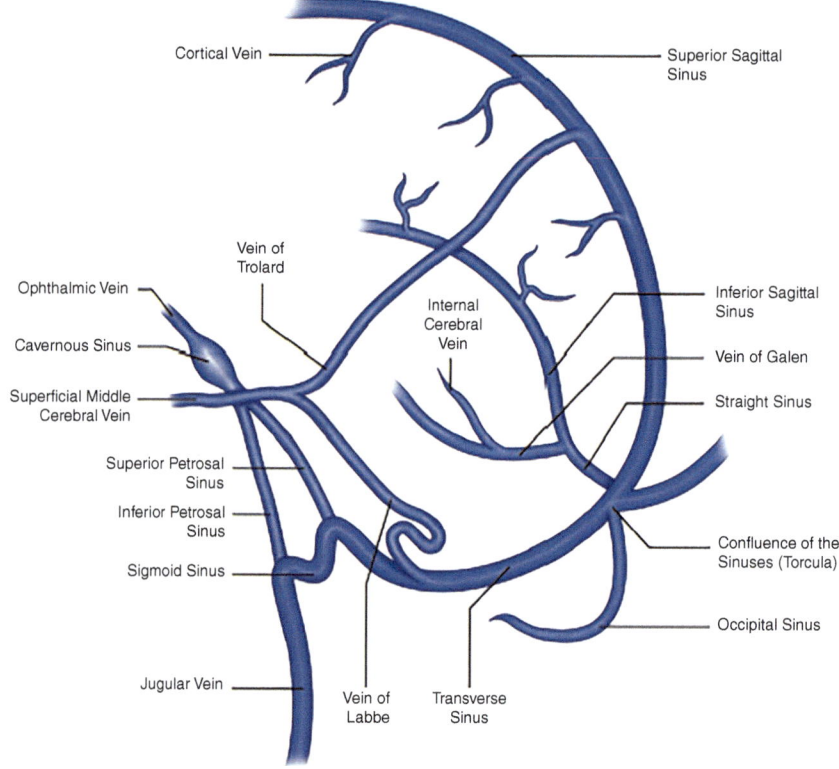

Fig. 2.10 Cerebral venous system. Source: Vascular Neurology Board Review

The **Inferior Sagittal Sinus (one)** drains blood from the deep portions of the brain and is joined by the great cerebral vein of Galen to form the straight sinus.

The **Cavernous sinuses (two)** drain multiple veins, including the ophthalmic vein from each eye, and empty into their respective internal jugular veins. They also carry the internal carotid artery and cranial nerves to the eye and can be a source of entry from eye and facial infections.

The **Transverse sinuses (two)** run laterally from the confluence and turn into the sigmoid sinuses on both sides.

The **Sigmoid sinuses (two)** then become the jugular veins, which drain into the superior vena cava.

Clinical Pearls
- Arteries supply oxygenated blood to the brain, and veins drain deoxygenated blood back to the heart.
- The anterior circulation is composed of the ICA, MCA, ACA, and ACOM arteries.
- The posterior circulation is composed of the vertebral, basilar, PCA, and PCOM arteries.
- The brainstem is fed by circumferential vessels that "hug" and supply the left and right lateral portions, and medial perforators that supply the medial portions.
- The anterior and posterior circulations are connected by the Circle of Willis.
- Cortical veins drain into larger sinuses that drain into the jugular veins.

Further Reading

Ashby JW. Endothelial control of cerebral blood flow. Am J Pathol. 2021;191(11):1906–16.
Blumenfeld H. Neuroanatomy through Clinical Cases. Oxford University Press; 3rd edition (February 28, 2021)
Barrett KE, Boitano S, Barman SM, Brooks HL (n.d.). Ganong's Review of Medical Physiology, Twenty sixth Edition. McGraw-Hill Education / Medical

Stroke Syndromes

3

Nicole Veltri and Razaz Mageid

Introduction

Now that you have reviewed neuroanatomy, let us focus on common stroke syndromes. There are two types of stroke, hemorrhagic and ischemic, both of which can lead to similar clinical presentations. The two general locations for stroke are the anterior or posterior circulation, and anterior circulation strokes can be further divided as cortical or subcortical based on location. Let's dive in!

Cortical Vs. Subcortical Strokes

Subcortical/Lacunar strokes: Lacunar strokes are small, single lesions ranging from 2 mm to 15 mm in diameter. "Lacunes" account for about a quarter of all strokes and are due to the occlusion of tiny, deep penetrating arteries, which cannot be seen on conventional vessel imaging. Lacunar strokes typically occur in the basal ganglia, thalamus, subcortical white matter, and brainstem, also called the "subcortical structures" (Fig. 3.1). These areas get blood supply from small perforating arteries (lenticulostriates, thalamic, and brainstem perforators) that stem off the larger intracranial parent vessels. Occlusion of these penetrating vessels occurs after long-term exposure to risk factors like hypertension, hyperlipidemia, diabetes, and tobacco use). These strokes are small because these vessels are only responsible for supplying a small area of the brain; therefore, when one vessel goes down, only that tiny area suffers the stroke. Cortical strokes, in contrast, are due to the occlusion of

N. Veltri
Yale New Haven Hospital, New Haven, CT, USA
e-mail: Nicole.veltri@yale.edu

R. Mageid (✉)
Beth Israel Lahey Health, Burlington, MA, USA
e-mail: razaz.h.mageid@lahey.org

Fig. 3.1 73-year-old female with hypertension presenting with sudden onset right-sided weakness and numbness. The degree of weakness is the same in the arm and leg. Found to have a lacunar stroke in the left basal ganglia, likely due to small vessel ischemic disease. Note the smaller size, deep location, and single location of injury. Note that the "right" and "left" sides are flipped on brain imaging, like a mirror image

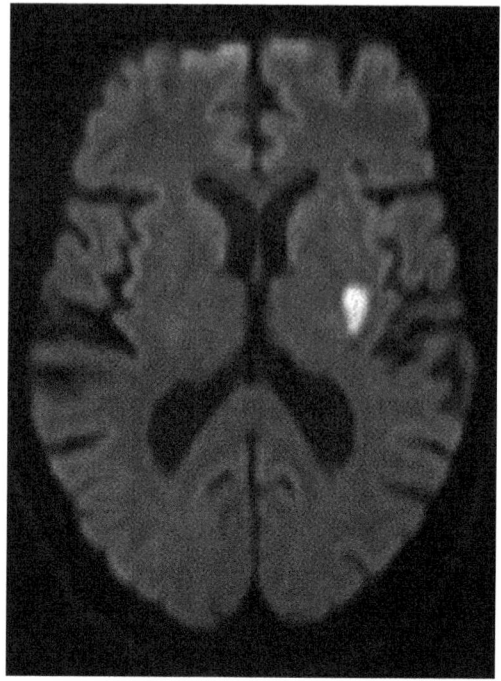

larger vessels that supply bigger territories in the brain. Subcortical structures, while small, are very high-value real estate with important functions. So, a single tiny stroke measuring 10 mm in diameter can still have devastating consequences! Clinically, subcortical strokes typically manifest as weakness, numbness, dysarthria, and coordination problems.

Table 3.1 describes each lacunar syndrome. Lacunar syndromes may present with a "stuttering course" where symptoms wax and wane for hours or days until they become fixed, compared with cortical strokes due to embolism, which tend to have maximum symptoms at onset.

Cortical Strokes: Cortical syndromes involve larger territories in the frontal, parietal, temporal, or occipital lobes (also known as the cortex) and are caused by occlusions in large arteries (ICA, MCA, ACA, basilar, and PCA). These strokes are bigger in diameter, can be multifocal, and often appear as wedge-shaped areas on MRI. The classic signs and symptoms of cortical strokes (in addition to weakness or numbness) include aphasia, apraxia, agnosia, gaze deviation, graphesthesia, stereognosis, and extinction (we will delve into these symptoms in greater detail as we discuss various stroke syndromes). Figure 3.2

Table 3.1 Lacunar syndromes. Note the absence of cortical signs

Lacunar syndromes	Symptoms	Location
Pure motor	Unilateral face, arm, and leg weakness	Contralateral basis pontis, corona radiata, posterior limb of the internal capsule
Pure sensory	Unilateral face, arm, and leg numbness	Contralateral internal capsule and thalamus
Ataxic hemiparesis	Ipsilateral weakness and ataxia (out of proportion to weakness), possible dysarthria, nystagmus, cranial nerve findings	Corona radiata, posterior limb of the internal capsule, pons
Clumsy hand dysarthria	Facial weakness, dysarthria, dysphagia, contralateral hand clumsiness	Contralateral anterior limb/genu of internal capsule, pons
Mixed sensory motor	Unilateral face, arm, and leg weakness and numbness	Contralateral internal capsule, thalamus, pons

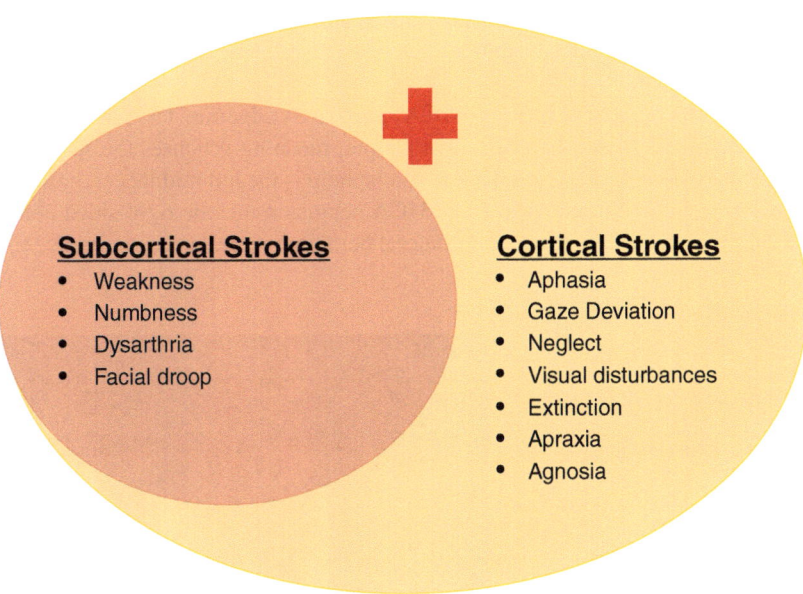

Fig. 3.2 Weakness, sensory loss, facial droop, and dysarthria occur in both cortical and subcortical strokes, whereas cortical symptoms only happen with cortical strokes

compares symptoms from cortical and subcortical strokes. The mechanisms of cortical strokes include cardioembolic from arrhythmia or cardiac thrombus that travel from the heart into the brain, eventually occluding an intracranial artery, or carotid artery atherosclerosis leading to watershed strokes (low blood flow) or plaque rupture and atheroembolism (plaque fragments embolizing downstream and occluding intracranial vessels).

Anterior Circulation Syndromes

Monocular blindness (transient or permanent): The first branch of the ICA is the ophthalmic artery, which continues toward the eye as the central retinal artery. Occlusion here can cause sudden, painless vision *loss* (blackout) in the ipsilateral (same side) eye from damage to the retina. Make sure to distinguish this from blurry vision (impaired acuity), which has a broader differential, and hemianopia which affects both eyes and localizes to the occipital lobe. The key is baseline vision *in one eye* (monocular) that suddenly goes black, like a nightshade being pulled down over the eye. The most common causes are occlusion of the Ophthalmic artery, or its downstream branches leading to Central Retinal Artery Occlusion (CRAO) or Branch Retinal Artery Occlusion (BRAO). Amaurosis Fugax is a fancy-sounding term that means temporary **monocular** vision loss that fully resolves (effectively, a TIA of the eye) from transient occlusion of the retinal artery or its branches.

Anterior Cerebral Artery (ACA) Stroke Syndrome: Occlusion of the anterior cerebral artery (Fig. 3.3) can cause contralateral weakness (leg more than arm), numbness, and incontinence. Abulia (lack of motivation or decisiveness to act) is a common symptom.

Left Middle Cerebral Artery (MCA) Stroke Syndrome: The left hemisphere is the "dominant" hemisphere for most people, meaning it houses the speech centers. The main artery supplying the left hemisphere is the left middle cerebral artery. Exam findings corresponding to a left MCA occlusion include right-sided hemiparesis and sensory loss, aphasia, contralateral hemianopia, and gaze preference to the

Fig. 3.3 A 67-year-old male presents with right leg greater than arm weakness. Found to have new atrial fibrillation and left ACA occlusion on vessel imaging. MRI confirmed left ACA territory infarct

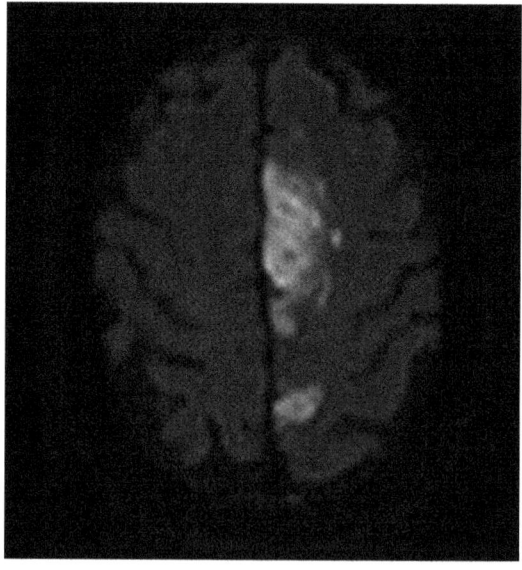

left (ipsilateral). Recall that the right and left frontal eye fields function in the movement of the eyes in the opposite direction, allowing normal midline gaze in normal conditions. A stroke in the left frontal lobe knocks out the left frontal eye fields, leaving the right frontal eye fields to act unopposed and thus pushing both eyes toward the left (Fig. 3.4). Such a forced gaze deviation is typically seen with large strokes from large vessel occlusions.

Aphasia is a cognitive language impairment (cortical symptom) seen with left hemispheric strokes. Dysarthria is slurring of words due to weakness of the oropharyngeal muscles. It is important to understand this distinction! Table 3.2 lists the common types of aphasia. A common term to know is "paraphasic errors," which are substitutions of words or sounds that either sound like or are associated with the intended word.

Additional dominant hemispheric symptoms that may be evident on a more in-depth neurologic examination include apraxia, agraphia, acalculia, right/left confusion, and finger agnosia. This combination of findings is known as Gerstmann Syndrome, which localizes to the dominant (usually left) parietal lobe.

Right Middle Cerebral Artery (MCA) Stroke Syndrome: For most people, the right hemisphere is the nondominant hemisphere. For *some* left-handed patients, however, the right hemisphere is dominant and houses the language areas. The primary vascular supply comes from the right MCA. Exam findings corresponding to a right MCA stroke include left-sided hemiparesis and sensory loss, left-sided hemineglect (inattention to the left side of their world Fig. 3.5), contralateral

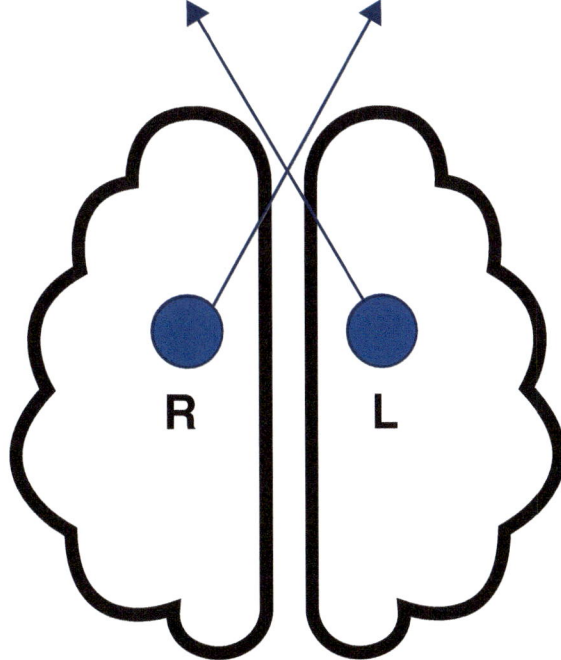

Fig. 3.4 The frontal eye fields control gaze to the opposite direction. A stroke involving the right frontal eye field, therefore, allows the left frontal eye field to push the eyes to the right, causing a gaze deviation "toward the stroke"

Table 3.2 Common aphasias

Types of aphasia	Fluency	Impaired	Preserved
Broca's: Expressive/motor	Nonfluent	Fluency, repetition, naming, writing	Comprehension
Wernicke's: Receptive/sensory	Fluent	Comprehension, repetition, naming, writing	Fluency
Global	Nonfluent	Comprehension, repetition, naming, writing	N/A
Transcortical (motor or sensory) aphasia	Both	Either motor or sensory aphasia depending on the location of injury	Repetition

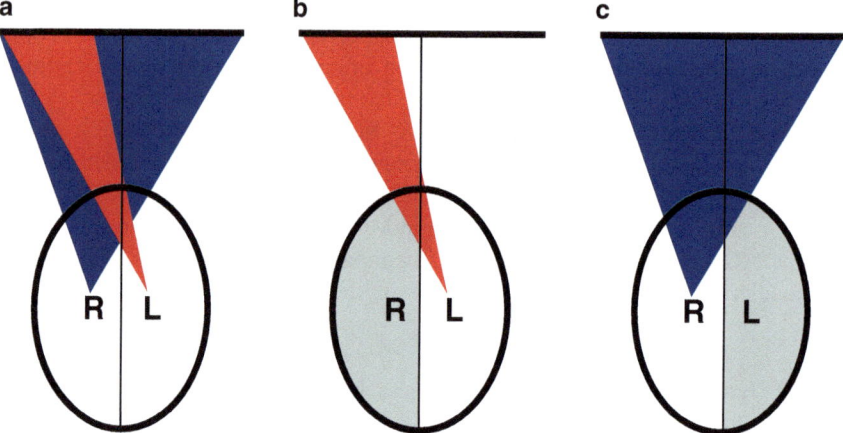

Fig. 3.5 Hemispatial neglect. The right hemisphere attends to both fields, and the left hemisphere primarily attends to the right field. A right hemispheric stroke only leaves the patient attentive to the right field, whereas a left hemispheric stroke typically does not lead to neglect. **Patient a**: normal. **Patient b**: right hemispheric stroke (grayed), with left hemi-field neglect. **Patient c**: left hemispheric stroke, with minimal to no neglect of the right due to the preserved right hemisphere allowing for attention to both fields. Source: Vascular Neurology Board Review

hemianopia, and gaze preference. Additional symptoms seen on a more in-depth neurologic exam can include apraxia (difficulty executing motor tasks despite normal strength), visual agnosia (impaired recognition of objects as they are), prosopagnosia (difficulty recognizing known faces), anosognosia (lack of understanding, interest, or denial of deficits), or asomatognosia (not recognizing the affected side as their own). Patients with asomatognosia may say their weak left arm isn't theirs but someone else's. These symptoms can provide significant additional challenges during rehabilitation. Neglect is inattention to or lack of *awareness* of something, and agnosia is the inability to *recognize* something for what it is.

Horner's syndrome: The sympathetic pathway is an arm of the central nervous system that functions in the "fight or flight" or protective response. A Horner's syndrome results from a lesion to the sympathetic pathway in the head or neck, resulting in the clinical syndrome of ptosis (drooping of the eyelid), miosis (small pupil due to inability to dilate in darker settings), and anhidrosis (lack of sweating). An ICA dissection may lead to headache, neck pain, and Horner's syndrome due to damage to the adjacent sympathetic fibers that travel with the artery.

Posterior Circulation Syndromes

Posterior circulation syndromes involve the thalami, occipital lobes, brainstem, and cerebellum. They can be challenging to identify as they often present with subtle or nonspecific symptoms (dizziness, nausea, vomiting, imbalance). A hallmark feature of brainstem strokes is "crossed signs," where the affected sides of the face and body are opposite. This is because the cranial nerve lesions in the brainstem lead to ipsilateral face symptoms (except CN IV). However, the corticospinal and sensory tracts to the body crossover in the brainstem and go to the contralateral side. In contrast, anterior circulation strokes have ipsilateral face, arm, and leg symptoms. A detailed exam may identify cranial nerve involvement, suggesting a brainstem stroke or dysmetria localizing to the cerebellum. Figure 3.6 lists cranial nerve nuclei at each brainstem location and what would occur if infarcted. Also, Fig. 3.7 is a

Midbrain:
- III- Oculomotor: impaired adduction, supraduction and infraduction of the ipsilateral eye with or without a dilated pupil. The eye is turned out and slightly down.
- IV-Trochlear: eye unable to look down when the eye is looking in towards the nose.

Pons:
- V- Trigeminal: ipsilateral alteration of pain, temperature and light touch on the face
- VI- Abducens: ipsilateral weakness of abduction of the eye.
- VII- Facial: ipsilateral facial weakness.
- VIII- Auditory: ipsilateral deafness

Medulla:
- IX- Glossopharyngeal: ipsilateral loss of pharyngeal sensation.
- X- Vagus: ipsilateral palatal weakness.
- XI- Spinal accessory: ipsilateral weakness of the trapezius and sternocleidomastoid muscles.
- XII- Hypoglossal: ipsilateral weakness of the tongue

Fig. 3.6 Cranial nerve palsies

Fig. 3.7 Rule of 4

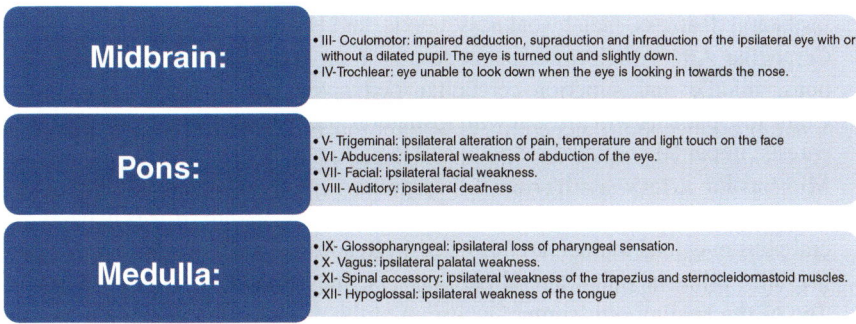

Medial Brainstem:	Lateral Brainstem:
• Medial lemniscus • Motor nucleus of CN III, IV, VI, XII • Medial longitudinal fasiculus • Motor (corticospinal tract)	• Spinothalamic Tract • Sympathetic Tract • Spinocerbellar tract • Sensory Nucleus of CN V

quick reminder of the Rule of 4 structures in the brainstem, covered in the anatomy chapter.

To examine the various stroke syndromes in the posterior circulation, we will start proximally at the vertebral arteries and work our way up to the basilar artery, AICA, SCA, and PCA, which leads to the Circle of Willis.

Medullary syndromes: Lateral medullary syndrome, also known as Wallenberg syndrome, is from occlusion of the posterior inferior cerebellar artery (PICA) or its parent vessel, the vertebral artery, leading to ischemia in the lateral medulla. Symptoms include numbness of the ipsilateral face (spinal trigeminal nucleus), impaired pain and temperature sensation in the contralateral limbs (spinothalamic tract), hoarseness, dysphagia (IX and X), dysarthria, loss of taste, ipsilateral Horner's syndrome (sympathetic pathway), and ataxia (spinocerebellar tract). Note there is no weakness in this syndrome.

A medial medullary stroke caused by distal vertebral, anterior spinal, or lower basilar artery occlusion leads to ipsilateral tongue weakness, contralateral hemiparesis (corticospinal tract), and contralateral loss of vibration and position sense (medial lemniscus).

Pontine Syndromes: The main artery supplying the pons is the basilar artery, with smaller branches including the anterior inferior, superior cerebellar, and medial perforating arteries. The symptoms of a pontine infarct include dysarthria, dysphagia, contralateral hemiparesis (corticobulbar and corticospinal tracts), ipsilateral ocular abduction difficulty (CN VI), horizontal gaze defects (PPRF), ipsilateral facial weakness (CNVII).

- **AICA/SCA:** An Anterior inferior cerebellar artery (AICA) occlusion can lead to ipsilateral deafness, facial weakness, ataxia, and Horner's syndrome. A Superior Cerebellar Artery (SCA) occlusion results in an infarct of the lateral superior pons, middle and superior cerebellar peduncles, and superior cerebellum. Clinically, patients will present with ipsilateral ataxia, dysarthria, conjugate gaze paresis, impaired contralateral pain, and temperature.
- **Mid basilar artery syndrome:** It may present simply as ophthalmoplegia and vertigo or severe weakness and mental status changes. Severe strokes in the bilateral pons may lead to the feared Locked-in Syndrome, which leads to quadriplegia, bilateral facial palsy, lateral gaze paresis, and aphonia.
- **Top of the basilar syndrome:** Occlusion of this vessel, often by embolism, can lead to infarcts of the upper brainstem, bilateral thalami, bilateral occipital lobes, and medial temporal lobes. The clinical presentation may include drowsiness or loss of consciousness (from the involvement of the thalami and reticular activating system in the brainstem), vertical gaze paralysis, and cortical blindness from ischemia to bilateral occipital lobes. Anton's syndrome (cortical blindness) occurs because of bilateral occipital lobe damage, causing visual anosognosia in which patients deny their visual deficits and make up things they see.

PCA: Proximal posterior cerebral artery (PCA) occlusions may result in contralateral homonymous hemianopia (occipital lobe infarction), contralateral sensory loss (from thalamic stroke), or a variety of midbrain syndromes.

Clinical Vignette 1

HPI: 82-year-old woman with no previously diagnosed medical conditions who presented to the ED for left hand and face numbness. She was in her usual state of health until the afternoon prior to presentation, when she initially noticed left face numbness, most prominently around her left lip. She did not appreciate any facial weakness. The next morning, she developed left-hand numbness in addition to her left face numbness. She denied ever having any weakness, visual changes, or speech changes.

Exam: Her blood pressure was 165/86 and glucose 104. She was fully oriented with normal fluent speech, and cranial nerves were intact except for minor numbness in the left corner of the mouth. Strength full throughout. Sensory intact except for resolving numbness of the left hand. No dysmetria was noted on finger-nose-finger testing.

Workup: CTA head and neck were normal. MRI-DWI of the brain demonstrated an acute infarct of the right thalamus (a, white arrow) with corresponding *hypo*intensity on ADC (b, orange arrow) and *hyper*intensity on FLAIR (c, green arrow), consistent with a stroke that was more than 6 h old. Transthoracic Echocardiogram demonstrated EF68%, no thrombus but did show early right-to-left shunt after injection of agitated saline, most likely patent foramen ovale.

Pertinent Labs: LDL 132, Hgb A1C 5.4%

Management: The most likely etiology of her stroke is small vessel disease in the setting of untreated hypertension and hyperlipidemia. She was started on dual antiplatelet therapy with aspirin 81 mg and clopidogrel 75 mg (for 21 days, then aspirin monotherapy), losartan 12.5 mg daily for blood pressure control with a goal of <120/80 over the next few weeks, and rosuvastatin 40 mg daily. Given her age and the deep location of her stroke, the PFO was not felt to be related. Her presentation is called cheiro-oral syndrome.

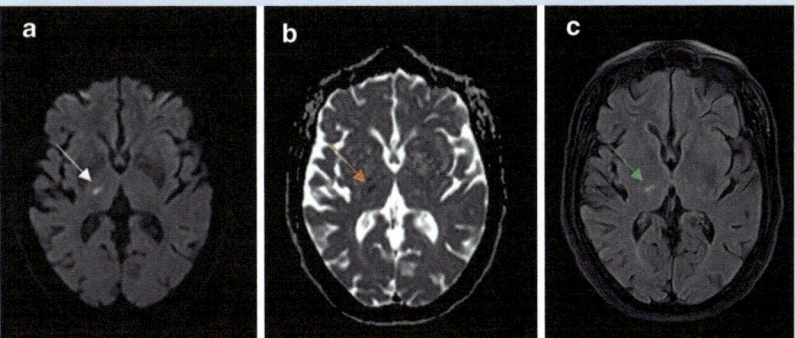

Case contributed by Dr. Barbara Gordon-Kundu

Clinical Vignette 2

Alexia without agraphia. Patients with right homonymous hemianopia can only see through their left hemifield (R occipital lobe). Due to the stroke in the splenium, information from the right occipital lobe cannot cross over to the language and comprehension centers in the left frontal lobe, leading to alexia. The speech and comprehension centers and motor cortex in the left hemisphere are intact, sparing the ability to write, hence the term "alexia without agraphia." *ICAD* Intracranial atherosclerosis.

HPI: 70-year-old woman with atrial fibrillation (adherent with apixaban), hypertension, hyperlipidemia, prediabetes, and a history of carotid endarterectomy presented with confusion and difficulty reading. Symptoms developed suddenly and persisted throughout the day. The patient's daughter was concerned when the patient was unable to read any text, despite having normal sounding speech. The patient was brought to the ED for evaluation. No numbness, tingling, weakness, dysarthria, dysphagia, or headache was reported.

Exam: Her blood pressure was 90/70 and glucose 106 (Hgb A1C 6.1%). She was alert and oriented, naming and repetition intact, as well as able to follow 2-step commands, but she had severe difficulty reading. She was able to write words without difficulty. The cranial nerve exam was normal, but the visual exam was notable for R homonymous hemianopsia. Strength and sensation were normal. Normal gait, no dysmetria.

Workup: CT head demonstrated no acute findings. (a, b) demonstrated severe atherosclerotic disease with a left P2 occlusion (white arrows). MRI-DWI (c) demonstrated diffusion restriction of the left splenium of the corpus callosum (orange arrow) and left occipital lobe consistent with acute infarct.

Management: Despite having multiple risk factors, the most likely etiology of her stroke was felt to be ICAD, given focal calcified atherosclerosis at the left P2 segment. She was outside the window for TNK as well as adherent with her apixaban, and she was not a candidate for thrombectomy. Her anticoagulation was initially held but restarted the day after the presentation, given the small size of the infarct on the MRI brain. There are no definitive guidelines on antithrombotic therapy for ICAD in patients already on anticoagulation. Since her stroke occurred despite taking apixaban, she was also started on aspirin 81 mg daily for secondary stroke prevention, with max dose statin. Her syndrome is classically referred to as "alexia without agraphia."

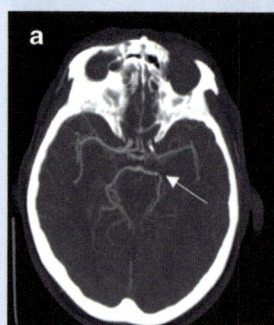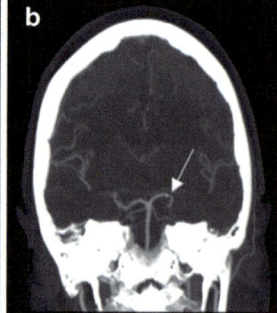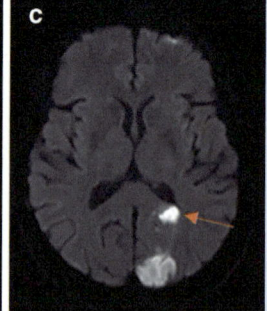

Case contributed by Dr. Barbara Gordon-Kundu

Thalamus: On imaging, the thalamus appears to be in the anterior circulation but is supplied mainly by branches of the PCA. While the most common symptom of a thalamic stroke is contralateral sensory loss, the thalamus is a complex structure. It acts as a highway for many other pathways affecting wakefulness, motor function, vision, and eye movements.

Clinical Pearls
- The initial presentation of lacunar infarcts can have a stuttering course where symptoms wax and wane.
- Visual symptoms attributed to the ipsilateral ICA, central retinal artery, ophthalmic artery, or posterior ciliary artery will be *monocular*.
- Left MCA syndromes will often involve language.
- Gaze deviation is ipsilateral to the stroke if it involves the frontal eye fields.
- Posterior circulation strokes will have varying presentations, most identifiable by associated cranial nerve and tract involvement in the brainstem.

Further Reading

Amin H, Schindler J. Vascular neurology board review: an essential study guide. 1st ed. Cham: Springer; 2020.

Chamorro A, Sacco RL, Mohr JP, et al. Clinical-computed tomographic correlations of lacunar infarction in the stroke data Bank. Stroke. 1991;22(2):175–81. https://doi.org/10.1161/01.str.22.2.175.

Gates P. The rule of 4 of the brainstem: a simplified method for understanding brainstem anatomy and brainstem vascular syndromes for the non-neurologist. Intern Med J. 2005;35(4):263–6. https://doi.org/10.1111/j.1445-5994.2004.00732.x.

Mendez MF, Clark DG. Neuropsychiatric aspects of aphasia and related disorders. In: Yudofsky SC, Hales RH, editors. The American Psychiatric Publishing Textbook of Neuropsychiatry and Behavioral Neurosciences. 5th ed. Washington, DC: American Psychiatric Publishing; 2007. p. 522.

Neuroradiology

4

Ajay Malhotra and Akash Patel

Identifying abnormal features on head and vessel imaging is essential in treating and managing acute stroke. But to identify the abnormal, one must first know what *normal* looks like. The confidence to say a scan is normal only comes after reviewing many hundreds of scans independently. Therefore, familiarizing oneself with various imaging techniques (CT, MRI, angiography, and ultrasound) will allow providers to rapidly review and interpret studies in real time to provide accurate and prompt patient care. Let's first review the basic views (or planes) before discussing the different types of imaging (Fig. 4.1).

- Sagittal: In this view, you look at the brain from the side.
- Coronal: In this "mirror" view, you look at the brain from the front to back (or vice versa).
- Axial: In this view, you look at the brain from the bottom to the top (or vice versa). Consider it a bird's eye view. This is often the default first view to review scans.
- Accurate interpretation of imaging allows clincans to answer the following questions regarding diagnosis, prognosis, and treatment:
- Diagnosis: Does the patient have an acute stroke? Is the stroke ischemic or hemorrhagic?
- Treatment selection: For ischemic strokes, would the patient benefit from thrombolysis, mechanical thrombectomy, or a combination thereof? What are the risks of bleeding with treatment? For hemorrhage, does the patient require blood pressure management, urgent surgery, or other treatments?
- Prognosis: What is the size of the stroke? Is the stroke large enough that the patient is likely to have a poor prognosis?

A. Malhotra (✉) · A. Patel
Yale School of Medicine, New Haven, CT, USA
e-mail: ajay.malhotra@yale.edu; akash.patel@yale.edu

© The Author(s), under exclusive license to Springer Nature Switzerland AG 2024
H. P. Amin (ed.), *Stroke for the Advanced Practice Clinician*,
https://doi.org/10.1007/978-3-031-66289-8_4

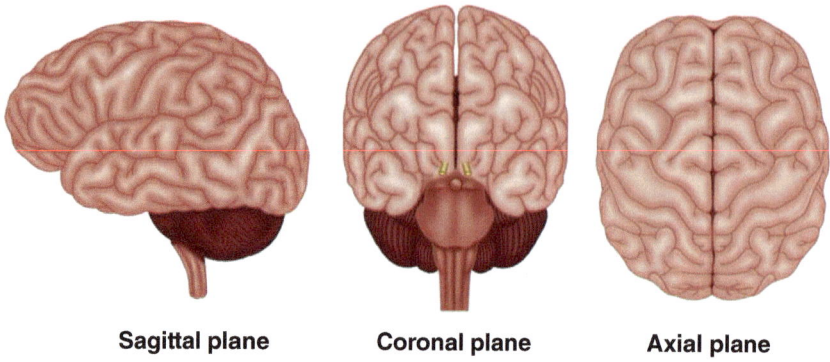

Sagittal plane   **Coronal plane**   **Axial plane**

Fig. 4.1 Standard viewing planes for imaging

The two main neuroimaging modalities used in acute stroke are CT and MRI. Although MRI is considered a more advanced technique, CT is the workhorse for acute stroke imaging. It is regarded as the first pass for stroke management due to its speed and ease of acquisition, 24/7 availability, lower cost, and the relative absence of contraindications compared to MRI. Options for CT studies used for stroke include noncontrast CT, CT angiography (CTA), and CT perfusion (CTP).

Noncontrast CT

The role of CT in an acute stroke situation is not to "rule in" acute ischemic stroke but to "rule out" hemorrhage. Therefore, excluding acute hemorrhage and understanding the typical imaging findings of acute ischemic stroke will assist providers in making decisions for intravenous thrombolytic therapy and endovascular thrombectomy (EVT). The CT scan of a patient with acute stroke symptoms should generally appear normal unless there is a large vessel occlusion, which may show a hyperdense vessel sign (Fig. 4.2). That is because ischemic changes will not appear on noncontrast CT until 3–6 h after symptom onset. Those changes include focal *hypo*dense (darker) areas, loss of gray-white differentiation, tissue swelling from edema, and effacement or blunting of the outer ridges (sulci) due to edema, and should correspond to the patient's clinical symptoms. How is this clinically relevant? Suppose you see hypodense areas in the brain that can be attributable to the patient's symptoms. In that case, chances are the symptoms have been going on for at least several hours, likely removing that patient from thrombolytic eligibility or increasing the risk of hemorrhage with thrombolysis. On CT scans, the grey matter is the outer area of the cortex with the gyri and sulci, and the white matter is the deeper territory. These two areas are normally separated by a clear border where the grey matter appears lighter and white matter appears darker on CT (yes, it does seem counter-intuitive). The loss of grey-white matter differentiation refers to the blurring between the grey and white matter due to the increased water content or edema.

Things that are hypodense or dark on CT include CSF, fat, and air. Acute blood, contrast, calcium, and bone are *hyper*dense or bright on CT (Fig. 4.3).

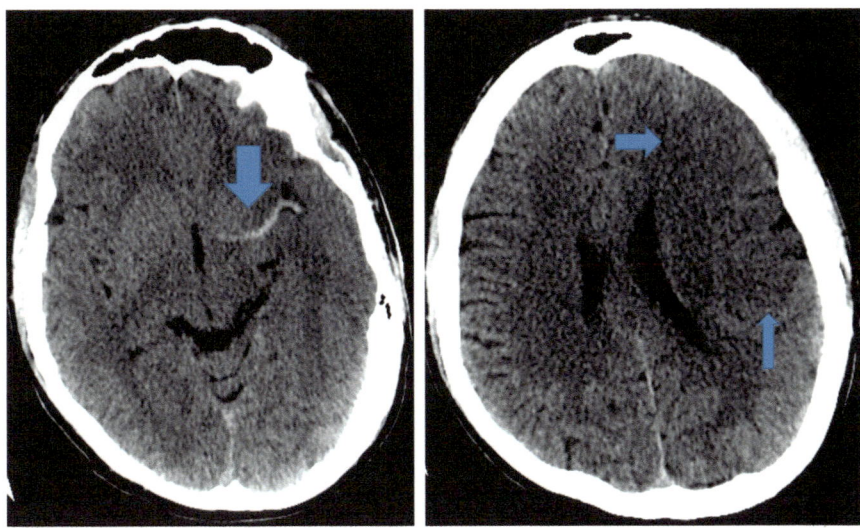

Fig. 4.2 Left: Axial noncontrast CT showed hyperdense (bright) left MCA, indicating acute thrombus (large blue arrow). Right: A wedge-shaped area of hypo (low) density in the left MCA territory, loss of grey-white differentiation and sulcal effacement (small blue arrows) is asymmetric compared to the right side. Note the clear sulci and gyri, and a distinct border between the grey and white matter, on the unaffected side

Fig. 4.3 Noncontrast head CT showing hyperdense hematoma and scattered hyperdense subarachnoid blood. Note the surrounding skull is also hyperdense (calcium/bone). The ventricles, filled with CSF, are hypodense (black)

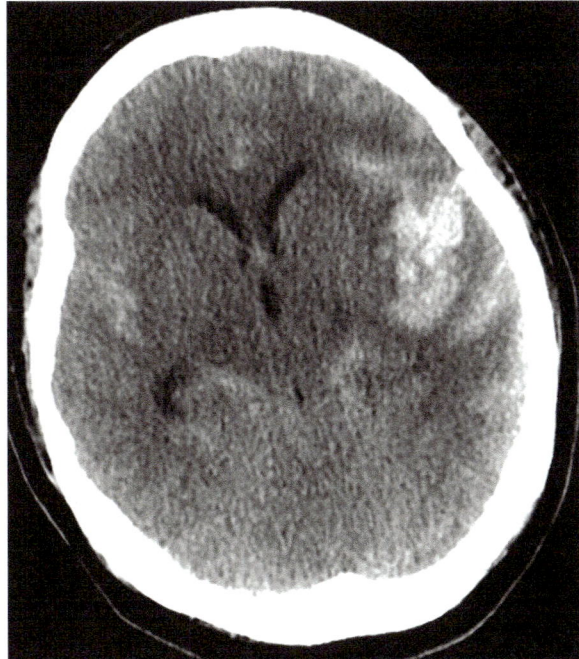

ASPECTS Score

One of the most widely used methods for quantifying the extent of ischemia on CT for the anterior circulation is the Alberta Stroke Program Early CT (ASPECTS) score. The ASPECTS score is a reproducible grading system to assess the presence and volume of ischemic changes (represented by darker or hypodense areas) on head CT and guide prognosis and treatment eligibility. The score can help guide decision-making regarding treatment with TPA/TNK and thrombectomy. Recall that one will not typically see hypodense areas in the brain in acute stroke situations. Such findings suggest a more prolonged duration of symptoms, or more rapid progression of ischemia, and require more caution before considering acute treatments. Opening up blood flow into an area of irreversible infarction can lead to hemorrhagic conversion (discussed below). Calculating the ASPECTS score requires looking at a total of ten regions of the MCA territory on two axial cuts on CT: one at the level of the basal ganglia and thalamus and another cut at the supragraganglionic level just above the level of the lateral ventricles.

Calculating an ASPECTS score consists of scoring ten areas supplied by the MCA (Fig. 4.4):

- Four subcortical structures: caudate, internal capsule, lentiform nucleus, and insula.
- Six cortical regions in the MCA territory.

Normal-appearing regions score one point each. If there are no hypodense areas, you have a max score of 10 points (normal scan). If you tell a colleague that a stroke

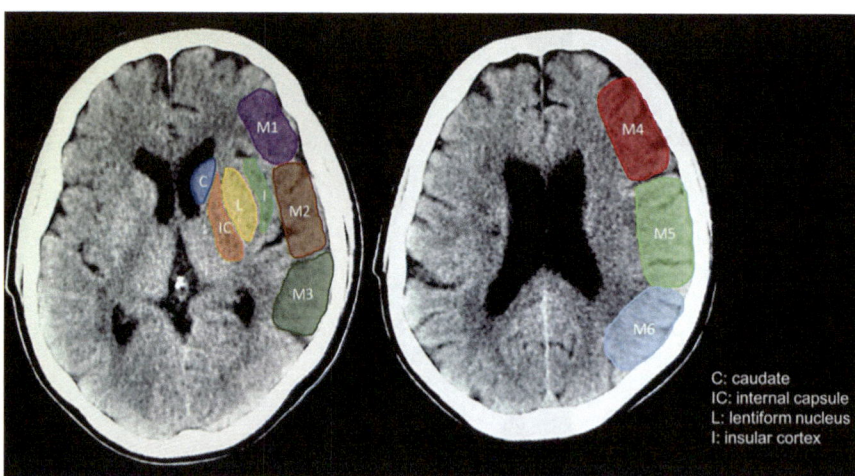

Fig. 4.4 Structures included in Aspects Score: C: caudate, IC: internal capsule, L: lentiform nucleus, I: insula, M1, M2, M3, and superior MCA territories (M4, M5, M6). Source: Bautista, M., Burger, R., Anderson, I.A. et al. ASPECT Score and Its Application to Vasospasm in Aneurysmal Subarachnoid Haemorrhage: a Case–Control Study. Transl. Stroke Res. 14, 94–99 (2023)

patient's CT has an ASPECTS score of 10, that colleague knows the CT scan looks normal; therefore, the patient has a low risk of hemorrhagic conversion, and all eligible treatment options are on the table. For each hypodense (presumably ischemic) area, you subtract one from 10. So, the more regions of ischemia seen on CT, the lower the ASPECTS score and the worse the overall prognosis. There is no established ASPECTS score "cutoff" when someone is no longer a candidate for thrombolytics or thrombectomy, but a score of <7 is generally associated with poorer outcomes despite recanalization. Note that the ASPECTS score is only for anterior circulation strokes. There is a version for the posterior circulation, but it is not widely used at this time.

Hemorrhagic Conversion

Hemorrhagic conversion (or transformation) is a complication of *ischemic* stroke that differs from a primary brain hemorrhage. Hemorrhagic conversion occurs when petechial (small amounts) or patchy bleeding occurs in an area of ischemia due to the breakdown of the blood-brain barrier in the arteries and leakage of blood. It can occur spontaneously or following thrombolysis or mechanical thrombectomy and appears as hyperdense material within a larger area of hypodense ischemia on CT. In other words, to suspect hemorrhagic transformation, you should see patchy blood within a larger area of ischemic tissue (Fig. 4.5).

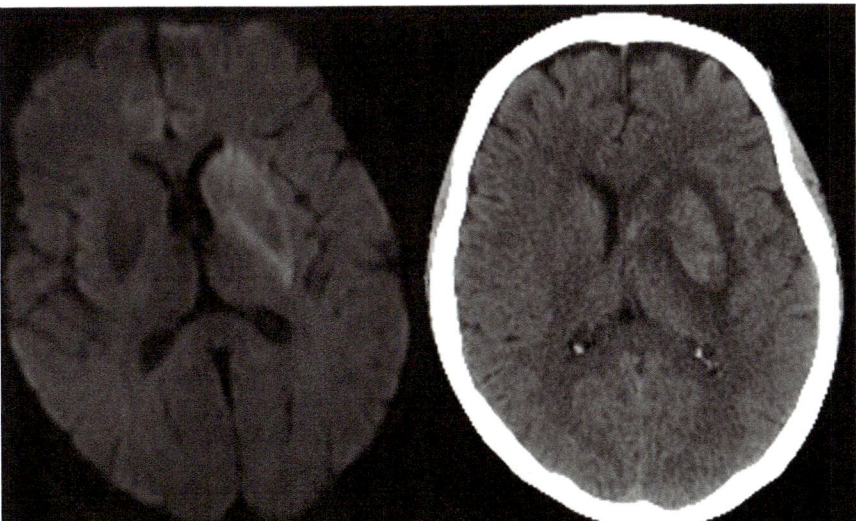

Fig. 4.5 Hemorrhagic conversion. MRI-DWI (left) demonstrates an ischemic infarct in the left basal ganglia. Head CT (right) 48 h later revealed hyperdense hemorrhage within the ischemic stroke bed. Note the rim of hypodensity around the hemorrhage, which is the larger ischemic infarct

CT Angiography (CTA)

CTA has become routine in suspected acute stroke to detect symptomatic stenosis or large-vessel-occlusion (LVO). CTA is fast and very sensitive in detecting carotid stenosis and LVO but requires the administration of iodinated contrast and exposes the patient to a small amount of radiation (as with all CT studies). Some patients may be allergic to iodine contrast and may need pretreatment with steroids and antihistamines if time permits. Some institutions will not allow contrast studies in patients with a history of impaired renal function. However, data show that true contrast-induced nephropathy is uncommon, and other issues like dehydration, diabetes, or medications are more likely culprits. Furthermore, getting an accurate view of the vasculature gives providers the best data to offer urgent treatments, which can be lifesaving or at least life-altering. Expert opinion is that routine kidney function testing before administering contrast in suspected acute stroke is unnecessary unless the patient has a history of chronic kidney disease (neurons over nephrons!).

CT Perfusion

For patients with large vessel occlusion (LVO) presenting more than a few hours after symptom onset or last known well, perfusion imaging helps identify permanently infarcted tissue, or core, versus the volume of salvageable brain tissue that is

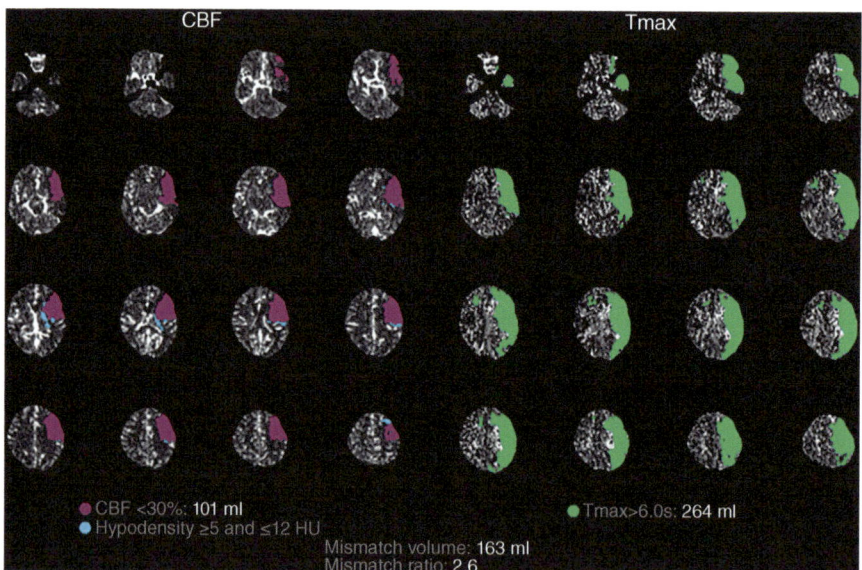

Fig. 4.6 CT perfusion demonstrates the core (magenta) and penumbra (green) tissue and mismatch volume in the left MCA territory

at risk of progressing to permanent infarct if not rescued, or penumbra (Fig. 4.6). The penumbra is made up of the tissue surrounding the infarct core. Thrombectomy is considered most beneficial in patients where the core is relatively small and the penumbra is large, also known as the mismatch volume or ratio. If the mismatch volume is small or zero (the core and penumbra are the same), those patients will not benefit from thrombectomy as no additional tissue is considered salvageable. We will not go into detailed perfusion measurements here, as many other sources are available.

Perfusion imaging can be done with both CT and MRI. The CTP is added to the CT and CTA in a stroke code. Again, perfusion imaging is most helpful when LVO patients arrive later in the treatment window (> 6 hours). Many centers will forego perfusion imaging for LVO patients if they present within a few hours of LKW or symptom onset, have a good ASPECTS score, and take the patient straight to thrombectomy.

Magnetic Resonance Imaging (MRI)

MRI utilizes a magnetic field and pulse radio waves to create images. Although MRI is a more time-consuming study compared to CT, it has a much higher sensitivity and specificity in diagnosing acute ischemic infarction, especially for posterior circulation infarcts, for which CT is relatively limited. Recall that CT is not very sensitive at identifying stroke in the hyperacute window (0–3 h). MRI, however, can detect an infarct minutes after stroke onset. MRI also clarifies the chronicity of the stroke. The key MRI sequences in stroke detection are diffusion-weighted imaging (DWI), apparent diffusion coefficient (ADC), fluid-attenuated inversion recovery (FLAIR), and susceptibility-weighted imaging (SWI).

DWI is considered the most sensitive sequence for acute stroke imaging. DWI measures the net movement of water in tissue due to Brownian molecular motion and shows a hyperintense/bright signal when the movement of water is restricted or trapped. This "restricted diffusion" is particularly true in ischemic stroke since there is cytotoxic edema, defined by intracellular entrapment of water molecules due to the dysfunction of sodium–potassium pumps in the blood-brain barrier. Occasionally, that hyperintense signal can be an artifact due to high T2 signal, referred to as the "shine-through" on DWI, and not actually a stroke. To rule this out, the bright signal on DWI must correlate with the *hypo*intense signal in the same area on ADC to determine whether the restricted diffusion is a true stroke (bright on DWI, dark on ADC). ADC measures the effect of diffusion without the T2 shine-through effect. When one sees a bright signal on DWI **and** a low signal on ADC in the same area, one can be confident that this represents restricted diffusion representing infarcted tissue (Fig. 4.7). Other conditions that cause restricted diffusion include bacterial abscesses or hypercellular tumors such as lymphoma, but the clinical presentation in those cases is different.

While the DWI sequence only picks up acute findings, the FLAIR sequence will demonstrate all subacute and chronic injuries in the brain over the patients' lifetime.

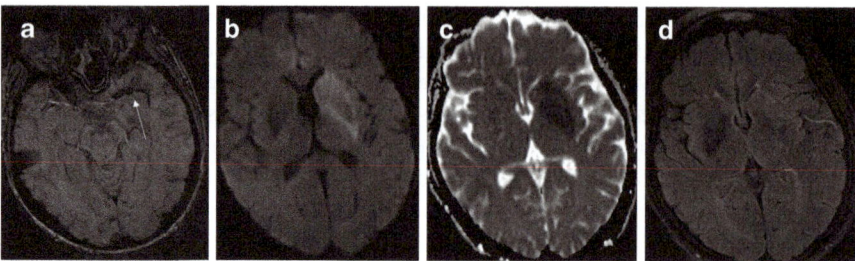

Fig. 4.7 Left MCA thrombus as seen on SWI (**a**) with restricted diffusion in left basal ganglia (**b**), corresponding hypointensity on ADC (**c**), and subtle increased signal on FLAIR (**d**). The clear infarct on DWI and ADC with only subtle FLAIR changes suggests the stroke is likely 4–6 h old (acute)

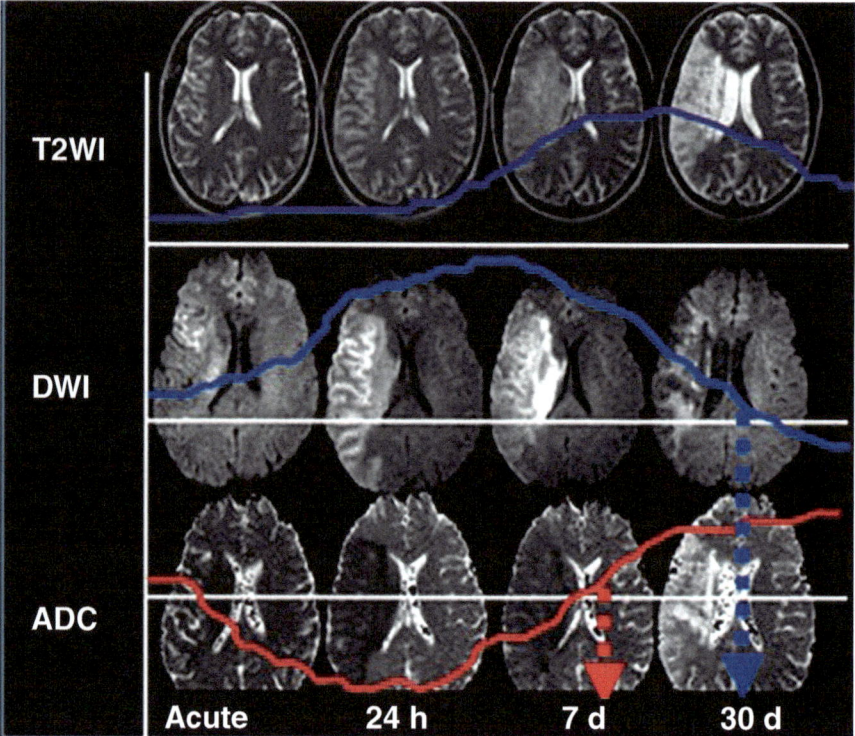

Fig. 4.8 Evolution of infarct on MRI over 30 days. Source: https://radiologyassistant.nl

FLAIR is also the sequence of choice to evaluate edema. Unlike DWI, FLAIR signal changes for acute stroke are only seen approximately 3–4.5 h after stroke onset. With the combination of DWI, ADC, and FLAIR imaging, one can distinguish acute, subacute, and chronic stroke (Fig. 4.7). ADC values are reduced in the first 7–10 days and then undergo pseudonormalization, in which the ADC signal progressively becomes brighter over time. Utilizing these principles, one can determine the age of the stroke, which is especially important in patients with an unclear "last known normal time" or those that present with wake-up strokes (Fig. 4.8). SWI is ideal for visualizing blood products, iron, and calcium. SWI is especially helpful in detecting microbleeds in the brain.

The size and pattern of the infarcted tissue are important to determine therapeutic and prognostic markers. Patients with smaller infarct cores have significantly better outcomes than patients with larger cores. The pattern of DWI lesions can help determine stroke etiology (Fig. 4.9). Multiple lesions in different vascular territories would suggest a cardioembolic etiology. Scattered lesions confined to one vascular territory could mean an unstable atheromatous plaque in the ipsilateral carotid artery or cardioembolic. Areas of ischemia in the border zone between different vascular territories would indicate watershed infarcts from significant vessel stenosis. A small, single infarct in the basal ganglia would be most compatible with a lacunar infarct due to hypertension, diabetes, etc.

Contrast is generally not required for acute stroke patients getting an MRI unless MR Perfusion imaging is being required. Acute infarcts do not show contrast enhancement, but subacute infarcts do. Other indications for contrast are outlined in Table 4.1.

MRI requires safety screening, which is critical but can be time-consuming. It involves screening patients for metallic foreign bodies, surgical clips, and pacemakers. MRI scan times can be long, and patients may experience claustrophobia or anxiety. The MRI scanner's magnetic field could reset or reprogram a cardiac implantable electronic device, causing loss of its preimaging settings (such as switching a pacemaker from a synchronous to an asynchronous mode or inhibiting pacing output), so it is essential to determine if the device is MRI safe.

Magnetic resonance angiography (MRA) of the *brain* is another option to evaluate intracranial blood vessels and routinely does not require contrast. However, evaluating the carotid and vertebral arteries in the *neck* with MRA is best

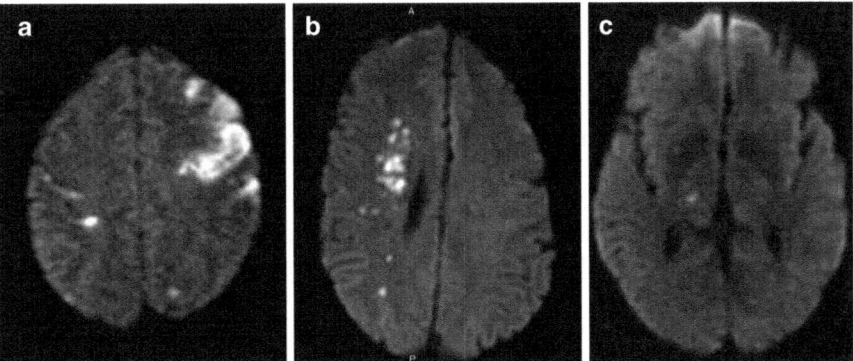

Fig. 4.9 Stroke patterns. (**a**) Bi-hemispheric multifocal infarcts concerning for cardioembolic source. (**b**) Right MCA/ACA watershed stroke due to ipsilateral carotid stenosis. (**c**) Small R thalamic lacunar stroke due to small vessel disease

Table 4.1 Indications for noncontrast and contrast-enhanced MRI

MRI without contrast	MRI with and without contrast
• Ischemic stroke	• Brain mass/metastatic disease
• Head trauma	• MR perfusion
• Syncope	• Infection (abscess, cerebritis, meningitis, encephalitis)
• MRA brain	
	• Inflammation (vasculitis)
	• Demyelinating disease (multiple sclerosis/optic neuritis)
	• MRA neck
	• Follow up after ICH
	• Seizure

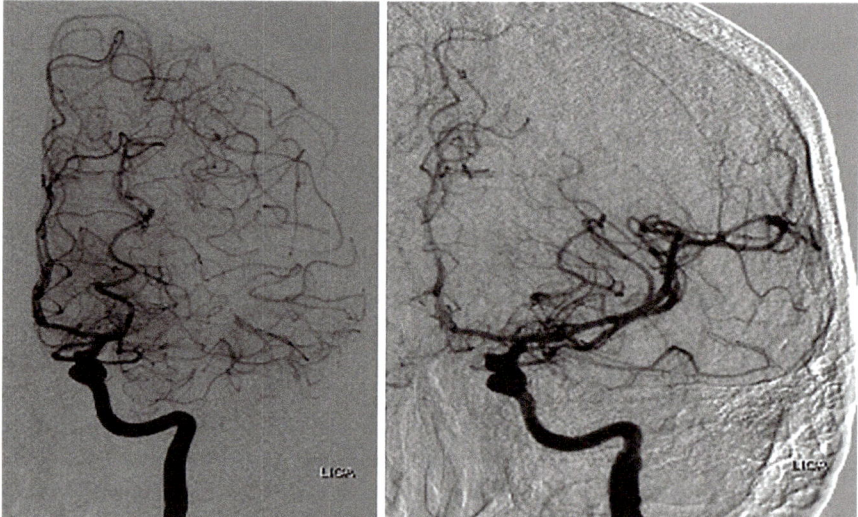

Fig. 4.10 Digital Subtraction Angiography (DSA). Coronal view, arterial phase, revealing left MCA occlusion (left), followed by normal flow after successful clot retrieval (right)

performed with contrast and can be helpful when assessing for carotid or vertebral dissections. MRA of the neck done without contrast is highly prone to motion artifact.

Digital subtraction angiography (DSA) or conventional angiography is the gold standard for brain vascular evaluation. It is an invasive procedure requiring vascular access and can result in complications, including access site hematomas. DSA is used during thrombectomy to map out the arteries before clot retrieval (Fig. 4.10), subarachnoid hemorrhage to evaluate for aneurysms, or intraparenchymal hemorrhages to look for underlying vascular malformations. It can be intimidating to scroll through the DSA images on your own. In a DSA, you follow the blood flow in real-time as it travels through the brain, instead of a single image like on CT or MRI. Blood flows first in arteries, then capillaries, then veins. There are three sequential phases for a DSA: arterial (you'll see all the arteries lit up), capillary (you'll see a blush of small vessels covering larger areas of the brain), and venous (the final draining vessels as blood is leaving the brain to return to the heart). Knowing which phase you are in is the first step, followed by the plane, right or left side, and finally, being able to identify an occluded vessel or aneurysm.

Carotid Ultrasound is a noninvasive, nonurgent, method to assess the carotid arteries without radiation or contrast and can be performed at the bedside. This test is often performed in outpatient or inpatient (not emergency room) settings. It is especially helpful to determine carotid stenosis, where flow velocities determine the degree of carotid stenosis. Think of a hose where your thumb partly covers the opening. The water flows out faster, right? So faster velocities in the carotids suggest carotid narrowing, and the speed can help stratify the degree of stenosis into mild (>50%), moderate (51–69%), or severe (>70%). However, critical stenosis (>95%) may have very low velocities, just like a kinked hose. Ultrasound can also detect the presence of intraplaque hemorrhage, which is a strong indicator of unstable carotid plaque and a risk of future stroke.

Clinical Pearls
- Noncontrast CT is highly sensitive to acute blood but not to hyperacute ischemic changes. CT is even less sensitive for posterior circulation infarcts.
- Vasogenic edema involves the subcortical white matter and spares the overlying cortex, while cytotoxic edema from acute ischemia involves gray matter early and to a greater extent than white matter.
- On MRI, hyperacute infarcts will be hyperintense on DWI and low signal on the ADC while not showing T2/FLAIR signal in the first 3 h since onset.
- Multiple foci of ischemia in different vascular territories suggest an embolic etiology.
- Areas of ischemia in the border zone between different vascular territories may indicate low perfusion from cardiac insufficiency or significant proximal vessel stenosis.

Stroke Codes

5

Emily Alston and Lee Chung

Introduction

The primary function of the stroke code (also known as code stroke, brain attack, or other names) is to rapidly determine if a patient suspected of experiencing a stroke is eligible for acute stroke reperfusion treatments. Treatment decisions are based on timing, exam findings, and imaging. The stroke code mantra is "time is brain," meaning the faster an eligible patient gets treatment, the better the outcome. To that end, it is necessary to obtain a concise history, perform an efficient examination, collect only essential clinical data, counsel and obtain informed consent from the patient and family, and prepare and administer initial therapy. An important concept to speed up care is to optimize the *parallel performance* of critical steps of the stroke code. Parallel performance, doing tasks simultaneously instead of one after the other, can dramatically speed up the process. Specific activities that may delay treatment even by a few minutes, and even if more broadly helpful to improve the patient's medical care, can wait until after reperfusion treatment. Each step of the stroke code process must be codified and scrutinized to minimize the time to initiate the optimal stroke treatment for each patient, and process metrics are invaluable to ensure continued care improvement (Table 5.1).

E. Alston · L. Chung (✉)
University of Utah, Salt Lake City, UT, USA
e-mail: Emily.Alston@hsc.utah.edu; lee.chung@hsc.utah.edu

Table 5.1 American Heart Association target: stroke initiative process metric goals (2010)

Process metric (time)	Goal (min)
Door-to-imaging	25
Door-to-imaging interpretation	45
Door-to-lab results	45
Door-to-needle	45
Door-to-device (LVO transfers in)	60
Door-to-device (LVO arriving direct)	90

LVO large vessel occlusion

Stroke Code Protocol

A typical stroke code protocol should be optimized to meet national guidelines for process metrics (Table 5.1).

Stages of the stroke code might proceed as mentioned in the following subsections:

Pre-arrival

A stroke code can be pre-activated in the field by EMS, at triage in the emergency room, or after a patient has been roomed in the emergency department. Once alerted, the unit clerk activates the stroke protocol notification sent to all relevant parties. Nursing will prepare patient labels and identification and bring the stroke code kit (which might contain basic equipment for alteplase administration, syringes, normal saline bag, blood pressure medications, checklists, and exam cards). The radiology tech will clear the scanner and hold the CT table for the stroke patient. The neurology code team leader will identify team members and roles, activate the stroke code and imaging order sets, and ensure the code runs smoothly and efficiently. Pre-made stroke code order sets are incredibly helpful in keeping all the correct and necessary orders in one checklist, avoiding mistakes and ensuring optimal adherence to core measures.

Code Activation at Triage or in the ED

Educating nurses at ED triage to identify stroke symptoms for walk-in patients will expedite evaluations. If an ED provider is concerned about potential stroke symptoms within a treatment window, activating a stroke code immediately will expedite imaging and neurological assessments. For hospitals that use telestroke or teleneurology, early communication with the telestroke provider *before* neuroimaging results in shorter times to stroke reperfusion therapy [1]. We will discuss telestroke in greater depth in another chapter. Many hospitals activate stroke codes for symptoms within 24 h, but check your hospital protocol for the window of symptoms for which to activate.

Initial Assessment

Nursing will place patient identification and verify or place peripheral IV access and can begin obtaining lab samples. The bedside provider will assess for hemodynamic stability, and the neurology consultant can begin some elements of the National Institutes of Health Stroke Scale (NIHSS) (Fig. 5.1) and obtain pertinent history.

Category	Score	Description
Level of Consciousness	0	Alert
	1	Drowsy
	2	Stuporous
	3	Coma
LOC Questions	0	Answers both correctly
	1	Answers one correctly
	2	Both incorrect
LOC Commands	0	Obeys both correctly
	1	Obeys one correctly
	2	Both incorrect
Best Gaze	0	Normal
	1	Partial gaze palsy
	2	Forced deviation
Visual Fields	0	No visual loss
	1	Partial Hemianopia (quadrantanopsia)
	2	Complete Hemianopia
	3	Bilateral hemianopia (blind)
Facial Paresis	0	Normal
	1	Minor (flat nasolabial fold)
	2	Partial (lower face)
	3	Complete (upper and lower face)
Motor Arm	0	No drift
*Score for each arm	1	Drift but does not hit bed
RIGHT:	2	Some antigravity but cannot sustain
LEFT:	3	No effort against gravity
	4	No movement
	X	Cannot assess due to orthopedic injury, amputation, etc.
Motor Leg	0	No drift
*Score for each leg	1	Drift but does not hit bed
RIGHT:	2	Some antigravity but cannot sustain
LEFT:	3	No effort against gravity
	4	No movement
	X	Cannot assess due to orthopedic injury, amputation, etc.
Limb Ataxia	0	No ataxia
	1	Present in one limb
	2	Present in two limbs
Sensory	0	Normal
	1	Partial loss (patient aware of touch but diminished)
	2	Dense (patient unaware of touch)
Best Language	0	Normal
	1	Mild to moderate aphasia
	2	Severe aphasia
	3	Mute
Dysarthria	0	Normal
	1	Mild to moderate slurring
	2	Near unintelligible speech
	X	cannot assess due to intubation or other physical barrier
Extinction and Inattention	0	No neglect
	1	Partial neglect (neglect or extinction to DSS in any modality)
	2	Profound or complete neglect
Total Score:		

Fig. 5.1 National Institutes of Health Stroke Scale (NIHSS)

The patient should be transported to the CT scanner the moment it is available. Many centers will continue the NIHSS on the way to the CT scanner.

The treatment clock begins at the symptom onset or last known well (LKW) time. Symptom *discovery* is not the same as symptom *onset*. For wake-up strokes (presumably, LKW when going to bed the night before), ask if the patient got up to use the bathroom overnight, or for hospitalized patients, talk to their nurse to determine LKW. If a patient is found in the morning at the breakfast table or dressed for the day, one might suspect they were ambulatory when waking up and could prepare breakfast or get dressed. Asking when the patient typically gets up might be helpful.

The NIHSS, though helpful in assessing stroke severity, has several limitations. It is biased toward anterior circulation symptoms and thus underrepresents the degree of disability caused by posterior circulation strokes [2, 3]. For example, visual field loss, ataxia, and dysphagia can all be disabling but score few or no points on the NIHSS. Remember that stroke mimics such as seizures, encephalopathy, or chronic symptoms from prior strokes will also score points on an NIHSS, so it is important to take the final score in context. Additionally, no precise number rules out the presence of stroke-related disability. A higher NIHSS score is felt to correlate with the size of the infarct, and an NIHSS ≥7 is more likely to have a large vessel occlusion.

Labs

If there is no history to suggest other labs will likely be abnormal, only a point-of-care glucose level is needed to rule out hypoglycemia as a stroke mimic before initiating thrombolysis. If there is a history of chronic kidney disease, thrombocytopenia, or other hematological disorder, warfarin use, or concern for a concurrent myocardial infarction, it would be necessary to ensure those laboratory results are available before thrombolysis [4].

Neuroimaging

A non-contrast CT scan of the brain is sufficient to determine eligibility for thrombolytics. Many centers perform CT and CTA together to ensure rapid large vessel occlusion (LVO) detection, and CT Perfusion for patients presenting > 6 hours from LKW with concern for LVO (Fig. 5.2). Adding CTA to the CT scan can increase total scan time by several minutes, especially if obtaining IV access is difficult. If there are barriers to getting a CTA in a patient who is otherwise a candidate for thrombolysis, get the non-contrast CT to rule out hemorrhage, then establish IV access, initiate thrombolysis, and get the CTA afterward.

While the patient is on the scanner, one can review the EMS report, obtain additional history from witnesses, and review the patient's chart. At larger centers, stroke team members may review the scans in real time while the patient is still in CT. With an experienced team, a formal radiology report is often unnecessary before making management decisions.

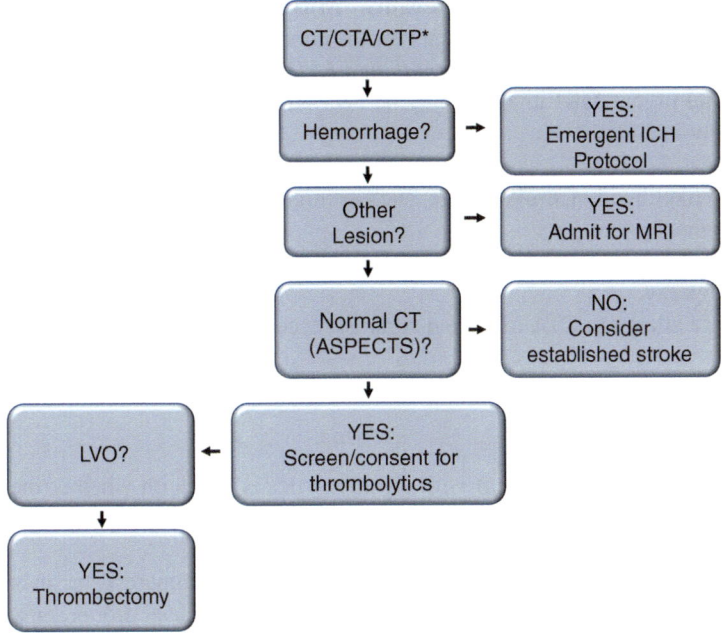

Fig. 5.2 Stroke code decision algorithm from imaging to treatment. *CTP ordering based on hospital protocol

If the patient is not eligible for thrombolysis due to bleeding risks (such as taking anticoagulation) or presenting between 4.5 and 24 h from LKW, placing an IV before neuroimaging is reasonable. For suspected LVO, most stroke imaging protocols will obtain a CT perfusion scan for patients within the 6–24 h window from LKW [5, 6]. However, there is emerging evidence that the ASPECTS score (see Chap. 4), calculated using the non-contrast head CT, can appropriately select patients likely to benefit from EVT without needing CT perfusion [7, 8].

Direct to MRI

Some centers have moved toward MRI as the first neuroimaging study. This approach, however, can introduce significant delays as it requires thorough MRI safety screening. Then there are 24/7 availability and feasibility issues, making MRI-based acute stroke protocols usually only successful in a handful of stroke centers. There are instances when obtaining additional urgent MRI after a CT scan and before treatment may be necessary. The Wake-Up trial included patients presenting >4.5 h from LKW but presenting to the hospital within 4.5 h of symptom discovery [9]. These patients received hyperacute MRI DWI and FLAIR imaging (taking less time than a full MRI). An acute stroke will show up almost instantly on the DWI sequence but takes 4–6 h to show up on FLAIR. The trial, therefore, looked for "DWI positive" but "FLAIR negative" MRI to infer that the stroke is less than 4.5 h old and consider those patients for thrombolysis. *Patients with stroke on DWI can still benefit from acute treatment if the FLAIR is negative.* Other instances where additional urgent MRI imaging may be necessary before determining reperfusion eligibility include:

- High likelihood of stroke mimic, such as migraine, encephalopathy, infection, or malignancy.
- High risk of bleeding with thrombolysis, such as with cerebral amyloid angiopathy.
- Severe allergy to CTA iodinated contrast, necessitating MRA to look for LVO.

Reperfusion Decision

The decision to treat a patient with thrombolytics is based on whether the patient perceives their symptoms as disabling and has no contraindications to thrombolytics (see Chap. 8 for more details).

Sometimes, the treatment decision is clear, such as hemiparesis or severe aphasia. Other times, the impairment can be more subtle, like facial droop, sensory deficits, or ataxia. If a patient can speak and comprehend, asking them if they feel their symptoms are disabling can be helpful. If the answer is yes, then thrombolytics should be considered. A low NIHSS score should not dissuade a provider from treating the patient. For example, mild aphasia or hand weakness may have a low NIHSS but still drastically affect day-to-day function.

After ruling out hemorrhage with neuroimaging, obtain the patient's weight. If the plan is to treat, order thrombolytics **immediately** after weighing and perform the remaining tasks in parallel. Including pharmacy in the stroke code process is vital to ensure proper ordering and reconstitution protocols to achieve target door-to-needle (DTN) times. Many centers use stretchers or boards equipped with scales (remember to zero the scale before weighing the patient). Do not visually estimate or rely on a weight in the medical chart.

After ordering and while awaiting drug delivery, nursing can transport the patient back to their room to perform an EKG and chest X-ray and draw any remaining labs. Document and monitor the patient's blood pressure (BP) during the code, and initiate blood pressure lowering treatment immediately if BP is above the threshold for thrombolytics (185/110 before administering, 180/105 after given). Note we have not mentioned blood pressure until now. Elevated blood pressure is a *relative* contraindication and can be treated *while waiting for drug delivery* so that thrombolytics can be given immediately when the BP is at goal. Elevated blood pressure should not delay the *ordering, mixing, or delivery* of thrombolytics. Typical agents for acute BP lowering include IV labetalol and nicardipine. Avoid oral medications as they will not work quickly enough. While thrombolytic dosing is confirmed and the drug is reconstituted, the stroke team can continue discussions to obtain informed consent for treatment. For patients with LVO, this is the time to activate the IR suite or start the transfer process. Additional advanced imaging like CTA or CTP, if necessary and not already performed with initial scans, should be performed after thrombolysis.

Thrombolysis: After reconstituting the thrombolytic agent, a quick time-out can help review all aspects of eligibility and risks before administering.

1. Symptom onset/Last known well.
2. Imaging results.
3. Bleeding risks.
4. Glucose and other lab values, if available (platelet count, PT, PTT, INR).
5. Informed consent or implied consent principles as applicable.
6. Thrombolytic dosage.
7. Current blood pressure (max <185/110 before bolus).

Change of Plan…

In cases where new information comes to light or the patient declines, drug manufacturers may replace unused medications like alteplase for free or provide reimbursement. To avoid concerns about ordering thrombolytics, confirm the reimbursement protocol with the hospital pharmacy.

After Lytics

After thrombolysis initiation, perform any subsequent neuroimaging or prepare for transport to EVT or another hospital. Patients receiving alteplase infusion following the bolus can be taken immediately to thrombectomy or placed in an ambulance for transfer to a thrombectomy-capable center with the infusion running. *Do not wait until the infusion is complete for the next stage of care!* Patients who receive tenecteplase do not require an infusion (more on that in Chap. 8).

Neuro Code Team Leader Checklist

- Introduces self and identifies each code team member (Table 5.2).
- Verifies use of the stroke code order set.
- Verifies with emergency/primary provider that patient is hemodynamically stable for neuroimaging transport.
- Coordinates team members to obtain a relevant patient history.
- Obtains NIHSS or assists telestroke consultant with NIHSS.
- Verifies correct imaging to be done based on history.
- Discusses neuroimaging findings with neuroradiology.
- Verifies thrombolytic dosing and order.
- Leads discussion for informed consent with patient/family.

Table 5.2 Stroke code roles

Stroke code team leader: The code team leader, who can be a physician or advanced practice clinician, is responsible for delegating code team roles and collecting information. They ensure that the code progresses to a stroke reperfusion decision safely and efficiently while coordinating team members and addressing potential delays. The code team leader leads time-outs, communicates with the attending physician, and ensures patient safety

Emergency provider or rapid response provider: A physician or advanced practice clinician must rapidly assess and stabilize the patient's hemodynamic and respiratory status

Nurses: Nurses experienced in stroke codes are essential for quick assessment and treatment of stroke patients. They have several responsibilities, including IV placement, vital sign monitoring, and patient preparation for neuroimaging. Nurses also gather additional history from the patient's family to identify bleeding risks. They administer thrombolytics and other medications and are critical in monitoring the patient's progress from presentation to post-thrombolytic care

Scribe: A designated scribe will be essential to mark essential time points during the stroke code, including arrival time, last known well (once determined from the history), start of neuroimaging, serial vital signs, and NIHSS, administration time of the thrombolytic, time of arrival to the EVT suite. This data is critical in identifying delays in the stroke code process

Laboratory/phlebotomy technicians: They will draw blood samples for rapid transport to the lab

Pharmacy: If available, the pharmacy can be instrumental in verifying the patient's medications and potential bleeding risks, reconstituting thrombolytics, or preparing antihypertensive medications. Pharmacy typically reconstitutes alteplase since it requires a bolus and infusion, but nurses can reconstitute tenecteplase since it is only a single bolus injection

EKG and X-ray tech: Techs or nurses should not perform EKGs or chest X-rays in the pre-treatment phase of stroke codes unless asked to. These studies should be done after the administration of lytics to minimize delays, as every minute wasted leads to an additional two million neurons lost

Radiology tech: The radiology technician will be responsible for clearing and holding the CT or MRI room to facilitate rapid neuroimaging

Neuroradiologist: A neuroradiologist and the stroke code team must be alerted to expect stat stroke imaging for immediate interpretation. Having specific names for stroke code imaging orders helps the neuroradiologist identify high-priority scans, such as "CT head STROKE TREATMENT CANDIDATE" or something similar

- Leads time-out before thrombolytic administration with emergency/primary provider, nurse, and pharmacist if available.
- Supervises rapid transfer to EVT if appropriate.
- Communicates end-of-stroke code to team members.

Parallel Processing

The stroke code protocol should be structured to optimize the fastest path to determining eligibility for stroke reperfusion therapies. Structuring as many tasks as possible to occur in parallel minimizes the effect of rate-limiting steps. Several steps may become rate-limiting, such as obtaining peripheral IV access, NIHSS, neuroimaging, laboratory results, reconstitution of thrombolytics, and obtaining consent for thrombolytics.

Fig. 5.3 Parallel processes
to save time and brain

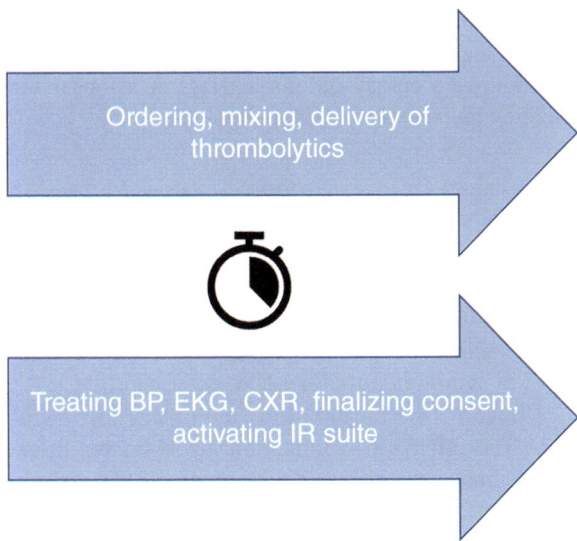

Stages of Parallel Processes

An efficient process can combine several key steps to occur in parallel, for example:

- PIV access, assessment of hemodynamic and respiratory status, initial history and initiation of NIHSS, obtaining dosing weight.
- Neuroimaging, obtaining collateral history from EMS and family members, continuing NIHSS between scan sequences, reviewing the chart, and discussing reperfusion eligibility with medical, neurology, and endovascular teams.
- Reconstitution of thrombolytic, discussion of diagnosis and obtaining informed consent for reperfusion therapy, management of hypertension, endovascular thrombectomy team preparation (Fig. 5.3).

Door In Door Out

Some patients will require transfer to a destination stroke center for admission or additional therapies. Patients with clinically suspected or imaging confirmed large vessel occlusion may require transfer to a thrombectomy capable center, or patients may require neurosurgical intervention or specialized neurocritical care. Door-in-door-out (DIDO) is a metric developed to assess and decrease the time a patient spends at the initial center before transfer. An accepted benchmark for an appropriate DIDO time is under 60 min. Some strategies for reducing DIDO time include establishing transfer agreements with receiving stroke centers for automated acceptance, initiating transfer discussion early in the stroke code process, such as exam findings suggesting large vessel occlusion (gaze deviation, aphasia, neglect), and

EMS agreements whereby the same crew may transport the patient on to the next facility, thereby reducing handoffs. Of course, educating EMS on LVO symptoms can improve accuracy and initial triage decisions to thrombectomy-capable centers, avoiding the need for transfer altogether.

Clinical Pearls
- A stroke code protocol should evaluate patients quickly and prioritize reperfusion therapies while avoiding unnecessary tasks.
- A stroke code team leader coordinates team members and resources, emphasizing parallel processing to minimize rate-limiting steps. The time of symptom onset or LKW is the most critical piece of history that often requires clarification from multiple family members or witnesses.
- The NIHSS has limitations in assessing stroke severity and disability, emphasizing the need for patient-specific assessment of current symptoms' impact on daily functioning to determine eligibility for thrombolysis.
- Non-contrast CT scan is sufficient to rule out intracranial hemorrhage before treatment.
- Urgent MRI may be necessary for some cases but comes with significant delays.
- Elevated BP should not delay thrombolytic ordering, reconstitution, and delivery. Treat the BP and administer thrombolytics when the BP is at goal if still within window.
- Established transfer agreements and early initiation of transfer protocols reduce the door-in-door-out time.

References

1. Jagolino-Cole AL, Bozorgui S, Ankrom CM, Vahidy F, Bambhroliya AB, Randhawa J, Trevino AD, Cossey TC, Savitz SI, Wu TC. Variability and delay in telestroke physician alert among spokes in a telestroke network: a need for metric benchmarks. J Stroke Cerebrovasc Dis. 2019;28(11):104332. https://doi.org/10.1016/j.jstrokecerebrovasdis.2019.104332. Epub 2019 Aug 19. PMID: 31439524
2. Hénon H, Godefroy O, Leys D, Mounier-Vehier F, Lucas C, Rondepierre P, Duhamel A, Pruvo JP. Early predictors of death and disability after acute cerebral ischemic event. Stroke. 1995;26(3):392–8. https://doi.org/10.1161/01.str.26.3.392. PMID: 7886712.
3. Inoa V, Aron AW, Staff I, Fortunato G, Sansing LH. Lower NIH stroke scale scores are required to accurately predict a good prognosis in posterior circulation stroke. Cerebrovasc Dis. 2014;37(4):251–5. https://doi.org/10.1159/000358869. Epub 2014 Mar 25. PMID: 24686370; PMCID: PMC4956480
4. Powers WJ, Rabinstein AA, Ackerson T, Adeoye OM, Bambakidis NC, Becker K, Biller J, Brown M, Demaerschalk BM, Hoh B, Jauch EC, Kidwell CS, Leslie-Mazwi TM, Ovbiagele B, Scott PA, Sheth KN, Southerland AM, Summers DV, Tirschwell DL. Guidelines for the early management of patients with acute ischemic stroke: 2019 update to the 2018 guidelines for the early management of acute ischemic stroke: a guideline for healthcare professionals from

the American Heart Association/American Stroke Association. Stroke. 2019;50(12):e344–418. https://doi.org/10.1161/STR.0000000000000211. Epub 2019 Oct 30. Erratum in: Stroke. 2019 Dec;50(12):e440-e441. PMID: 31662037

5. Albers GW, Marks MP, Kemp S, Christensen S, Tsai JP, Ortega-Gutierrez S, McTaggart RA, Torbey MT, Kim-Tenser M, Leslie-Mazwi T, Sarraj A, Kasner SE, Ansari SA, Yeatts SD, Hamilton S, Mlynash M, Heit JJ, Zaharchuk G, Kim S, Carrozzella J, Palesch YY, Demchuk AM, Bammer R, Lavori PW, Broderick JP, Lansberg MG, DEFUSE 3 Investigators. Thrombectomy for stroke at 6 to 16 hours with selection by perfusion imaging. N Engl J Med. 2018;378(8):708–18. https://doi.org/10.1056/NEJMoa1713973.

6. Nogueira RG, Jadhav AP, Haussen DC, Bonafe A, Budzik RF, Bhuva P, Yavagal DR, Ribo M, Cognard C, Hanel RA, Sila CA, Hassan AE, Millan M, Levy EI, Mitchell P, Chen M, English JD, Shah QA, Silver FL, Pereira VM, Mehta BP, Baxter BW, Abraham MG, Cardona P, Veznedaroglu E, Hellinger FR, Feng L, Kirmani JF, Lopes DK, Jankowitz BT, Frankel MR, Costalat V, Vora NA, Yoo AJ, Malik AM, Furlan AJ, Rubiera M, Aghaebrahim A, Olivot JM, Tekle WG, Shields R, Graves T, Lewis RJ, Smith WS, Liebeskind DS, Saver JL, Jovin TG, DAWN Trial Investigators. Thrombectomy 6 to 24 hours after stroke with a mismatch between deficit and infarct. N Engl J Med. 2018;378(1):11–21. https://doi.org/10.1056/NEJMoa1706442. Epub 2017 Nov 11. PMID: 29129157

7. Nguyen TN, Abdalkader M, Nagel S, et al. Noncontrast computed tomography vs computed tomography perfusion or magnetic resonance imaging selection in late presentation of stroke with large-vessel occlusion. JAMA Neurol. 2022;79(1):22–31. https://doi.org/10.1001/jamaneurol.2021.4082.

8. Porto GBF, Chen C, Al Kasab S, et al. Association of noncontrast computed tomography and perfusion modalities with outcomes in patients undergoing late-window stroke thrombectomy. JAMA Netw Open. 2022;5(11):e2241291. https://doi.org/10.1001/jamanetworkopen.2022.41291.

9. Thomalla G, Simonsen CZ, Boutitie F, Andersen G, Berthezene Y, Cheng B, Cheripelli B, Cho TH, Fazekas F, Fiehler J, Ford I, Galinovic I, Gellissen S, Golsari A, Gregori J, Günther M, Guibernau J, Häusler KG, Hennerici M, Kemmling A, Marstrand J, Modrau B, Neeb L, Perez de la Ossa N, Puig J, Ringleb P, Roy P, Scheel E, Schonewille W, Serena J, Sunaert S, Villringer K, Wouters A, Thijs V, Ebinger M, Endres M, Fiebach JB, Lemmens R, Muir KW, Nighoghossian N, Pedraza S, Gerloff C, WAKE-UP Investigators. MRI-guided thrombolysis for stroke with unknown time of onset. N Engl J Med. 2018;379(7):611–22. https://doi.org/10.1056/NEJMoa1804355. Epub 2018 May 16. PMID: 29766770

The Neuro Exam

6

Jennifer Bajek and William S. Musser

Introduction

A good history and physical exam are needed to diagnose most neurological disorders. A complete neurological exam takes considerable time to perform and to master, so much so that entire textbooks are written about it. For acute stroke patients, the acute onset of symptoms paired with an expedited exam is all that is needed to make a diagnosis, as CT imaging is often normal. The streamlined version of the neurological exam focusing on findings commonly associated with an acute stroke is the National Institutes of Health Stroke Scale (NIHSS) [1]. The NIHSS exam is an 11-item scale, scoring from 0 to 42 points, and takes about 5 min to perform. The NIHSS can be done by nurses, advanced practice clinicians, or physicians (in reality, all of these providers will perform the exam on the patient during their hospitalization). Web-based training on the NIHSS exam is readily available and has shown high inter-rater reliability for those who complete the training. The NIHSS exam is used during acute stroke evaluations, throughout the hospital course to monitor for clinical changes, and in outpatient follow-up.

Acute stroke exams are distilled and meant to be efficient, and they should be followed by more comprehensive neurological exams after the acute setting. In this chapter, we will review the main components of the acute stroke examination. They

J. Bajek · W. S. Musser (✉)
VA National Telestroke Program, Palo Alto VA Medical Center, California, CA, USA
e-mail: Jennifer.Bajek@va.gov; William.Musser@va.gov

include general appearance, mental status, speech, cranial nerves and visual fields, motor function (including reflexes), sensory function, cerebellar function, and gait evaluation.

The NIHSS

The NIHSS exam is a reliable tool used for initial stroke diagnosis and to monitor a patient's clinical condition over time. A change in exam may herald either clinical improvement or clinical deterioration. A sudden change in the NIHSS may signal either an extension of the original stroke or a recurrent event. An increase in NIHSS score may also suggest acute hemorrhage for patients treated with thrombolytic.

Inevitably, whether performing a complete neurological exam or the NIHSS, a patient may be unable or unwilling to perform a particular part of the exam. In these cases, one must document as best as possible what is observed and then move on to complete the remainder of the exam. It is helpful to know if the patient had any chronic deficits that could be included in the final score in order to separate new versus old findings.

Mental Status and Awareness

Simply observing the patient can yield a lot of helpful information. Is the patient alert and attentive, or are they inattentive, sleepy, or comatose? Do they look like they are in pain, or are they comfortable? You may notice that the patient is struggling to speak or not speaking at all, has forced eye deviation, or that an encephalopathic patient is not moving one side as much as the other. Most patients with acute ischemic strokes will be alert and attentive, except in cases of a large or malignant stroke with mass effect or strokes affecting the thalamus or brainstem. Patients with a hemorrhagic stroke causing mass effects are more likely to be sleepy.

Neglect is the lack of attention or awareness of one side of the body and world. Since neglect is most commonly seen with a right middle cerebral artery territory stroke, weakness tends to be left-sided. One can identify neglect by standing on the patient's left side, talking to them, or tapping their left shoulder. With true neglect, the patient will not acknowledge the examiner's presence if looking straight ahead. Having the patient interpret kitchen scene drawing in the NIHSS can uncover visual neglect. The patient may only describe the mother doing dishes (the right half of the picture) and completely ignore the children. A patient with neglect will squeeze all the numbers of a clock on the right half (Fig. 6.1).

Extinction is the inability to perceive multiple stimuli at the same time. To test for extinction, touch either the left or right side individually, followed by both sides (double simultaneous stimulation), and ask the patient to tell you where they feel you touching. Extinction occurs when the patient feels both sides when touched individually, but only the right side is felt when both are touched. The patient's eyes must be closed for this part of the exam to avoid giving away the answers!

Fig. 6.1 When asked to fill in the numbers on a clock, this patient with left-sided neglect filled in the numbers entirely on the right side of the clock

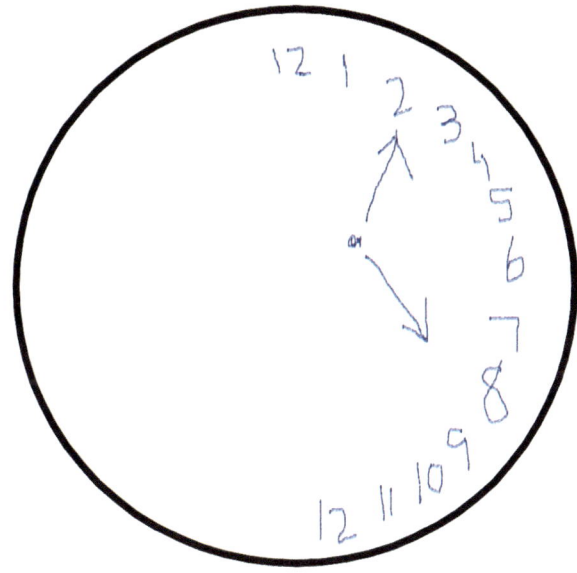

Speech

Aphasia, dysarthria, and neglect are three common findings on the exam of a patient experiencing a stroke. Aphasia, dysfunction in the production and processing of speech, may affect spontaneous speech, comprehension, reading, writing, and repeating and is often seen in occlusion of the dominant hemisphere's (usually left) middle cerebral artery. Broca's aphasia is due to a lesion in the inferior frontal lobe (Broca's area), and Wernicke's aphasia is due to a lesion in the superior temporal lobe (Wernicke's area).

To test aphasia, one often starts by just talking to the patient. Patients with Broca's (motor/expressive) aphasia will struggle to make or repeat any words and cannot string words together to create a sentence. To test comprehension, ask the patient to follow simple commands; just make sure you do not act out the command yourself. For repetition, start with short syllables (ma-ma, tip-top), followed by single words (thanks, huckleberry), and then sentences (the train arrived at the station 30 min late). Comprehension will be intact with Broca's, and these patients will often be frustrated by their impairment. On the other hand, patients with Wernicke's (sensory/receptive) aphasia will speak effortlessly, but their words will be nonsensical (word salad). They feel they are talking normally, are unaware of their deficit, and cannot follow commands or repeat words. Their frustration may be with the examiner, who cannot "understand" what they are saying. Transcortical aphasias are due to strokes adjacent to Broca's and Wernicke's areas and have preserved repetition that can be picked up with a careful speech exam. Figure 6.2 provides a roadmap for diagnosing specific aphasias.

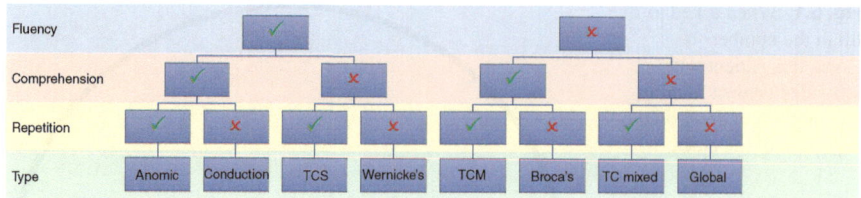

Fig. 6.2 Diagnosing aphasia type. Anomic: Difficulty naming objects. Conduction: Impaired repetition, paraphasic errors. *TCS* transcortical sensory, *TCM* transcortical motor, *TC mixed* transcortical mixed

Dysarthria, or slurred speech, is caused by the weakness of the bulbar muscles, which leads to impaired speech annunciation. Dysarthria often occurs with a facial droop and in both cortical and subcortical strokes. Words are thick and jumbled together but intelligible (except in severe cases), and patients have preserved comprehension and fluency. Patients with severe dysarthria often also have dysphagia (impaired swallowing).

Vision

Visual field defects are due to strokes in the occipital, inferior parietal, or superior temporal lobes. Visual field testing helps identify homonymous hemianopia (the same half of each visual field) or quadrantanopia (the same quarter of each visual field). First, have the patient cover either eye. Then, test visual fields by either using finger counting or visual threat (simply wiggling a finger) in all four quadrants to assess for blind spots while the patient stares directly at your nose (Fig. 6.1). The hemifields and quadrants are from the patient's perspective (Fig. 6.3). Know what quadrant you are testing for accurate documentation. If vision loss is detected, move that hand with fingers wiggling inward (toward the nose) until the patient sees the fingers. This method helps gauge how severe the field cut is and provides a reference point for future exams. In complete hemianopia, patients will only see wiggling fingers once they pass the midway point (nose) and not before, but this may improve somewhat over days or weeks. This method helps monitor for improvement in visual fields between exams. Moving fingers vertically and horizontally in a quadrantanopsia should delineate the point between the field cut and normal vision.

Complete vision loss in one eye is an orbital (as opposed to brain) problem, and acute painless vision loss is often a central retinal artery occlusion. The examination will have impaired reactivity to light in that pupil (afferent pupillary defect). An area of vision loss in *one eye only* may be due to a branch retinal artery occlusion. Both should have a stat ophthalmology consultation and consideration of thrombolytic therapy.

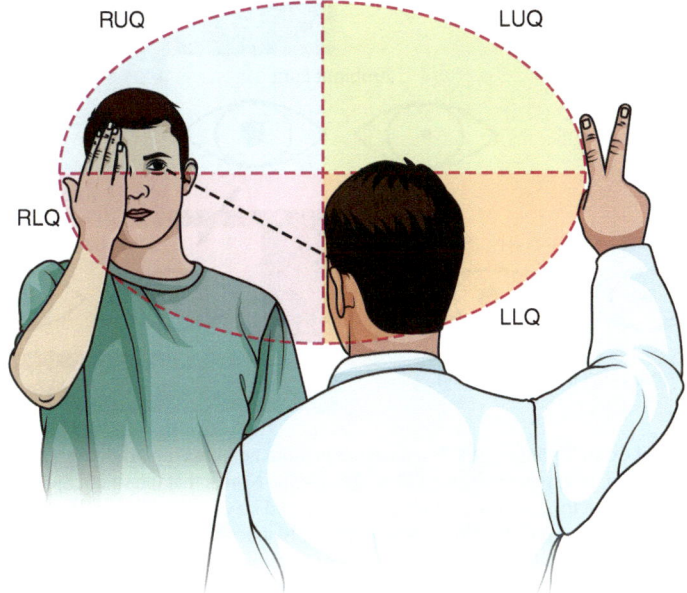

Fig. 6.3 Visual fields assessment. From the patient's viewpoint: *LUQ* left upper quadrant, *LLQ* left lower quadrant, *RUQ* right upper quadrant, *RLQ* right lower quadrant. Note the patient is looking straight at the examiner's nose

Pupils

Many stroke codes are called for isolated asymmetric pupils (anisocoria). However, isolated pupillary asymmetry without other deficits does not indicate an acute stroke. Pupils are usually normal in stroke unless the stroke is so large that it causes mass effect and herniation, in which case the patient will likely be lethargic or comatose.

That is not to say that anisocoria does not need an urgent evaluation. *With aniso-coria, the smaller pupil is not always the abnormal one.* To find out which pupil is abnormal, test them in bright light and in the dark (Fig. 6.4). Normal pupils should constrict in bright light. If the asymmetry is more apparent in bright light, then the dilated pupil is abnormal as it should constrict but cannot, which may be due to exposure to anti-cholinergic medications (scopolamine patch, pilocarpine, or aero-solized ipratropium contacting the sclera, common in hospitalized patients), or a compressive lesion on the oculomotor nerve, or Adie's (tonic) pupil. Normal pupils should dilate in the dark. If the anisocoria is more apparent in the dark, then the smaller pupil is abnormal as it cannot dilate. In that case, consider a Horner syndrome with sympathetic dysfunction from carotid dissection or brainstem stroke. A stroke, however, should have other deficits on the exam.

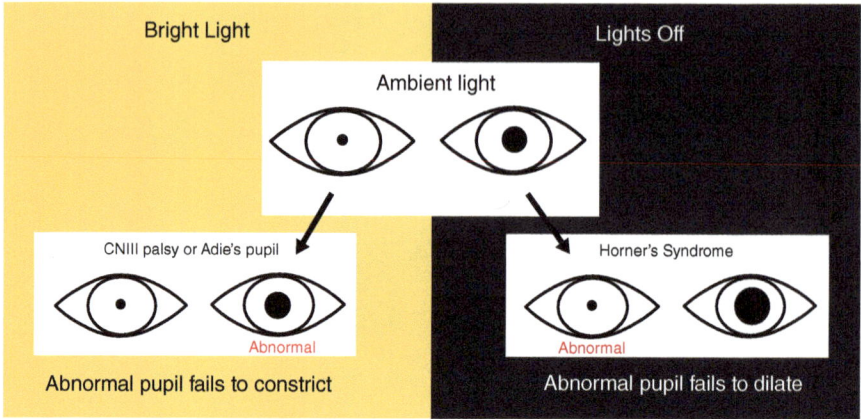

Fig. 6.4 Pupil exam for anisocoria. If anisocoria is more notable with bright light, consider CNIII palsy, Adie's pupil, or exposure to anticholinergic agents. Notice that the smaller pupil gets slightly smaller (normal), but the larger pupil fails to constrict and stays the same size. If anisocoria is more noticeable in the dark, consider Horner's Syndrome. Notice that the larger pupil gets larger (normal), but the smaller pupil fails to dilate and stays the same size

Eye Movements

Abnormalities in eye movement can occur with cortical, subcortical, or brainstem strokes. Typically, these will present with an ophthalmoparesis, a loss in the ability to move one or both eyes. Bilateral forced deviation to one side may suggest a lesion in the ipsilateral frontal eye field with stroke or contralateral eye field in a seizure. Strokes in the thalamus can lead to impaired vertical gaze. Strokes in the midbrain can lead to a third nerve palsy where the ipsilateral eye points downwards and out, possibly with a dilated pupil. Pontine strokes with a fourth nerve palsy where the *contralateral* eye points upwards and outwards, and patients may tilt their heads in the direction of the affected eye to fix their vertical diplopia. Pontine strokes with a sixth nerve palsy will lead to the inability of the ipsilateral eye to look outwards (abduct) on lateral gaze (e.g., with a "right sixth," the right eye cannot go past midline on rightward gaze).

Other Cranial Nerve Deficits

The most common cranial nerve abnormality seen with stroke is ipsilateral facial weakness due to cranial nerve seven palsy. The weakness may be apparent to the examiner when observing the patient's lower face just on general appearance. In most cases, facial weakness from a stroke will only affect the lower half of the face.

Medullary stroke causes tongue deviation from hypoglossal nerve palsy. Asking a patient with a medullary stroke to "stick out your tongue" may yield the finding of tongue deviation to the ipsilateral side. Because each half of the tongue is innervated by its respective hypoglossal nerve, a stroke may produce weakness in that half. So, instead of sticking straight out, the stronger side will push the tongue in the other direction (the same side as the stroke). While this finding is not always present, identifying it in an individual patient may help localize the stroke.

Motor

Hemiparesis is due to injury to the corticospinal tract in the cortex or brainstem and, except for spinal cord strokes, is contralateral to the stroke. It is weaker than the leg. This suggests a stroke involving the middle cerebral artery territory, while a pattern of leg greater than arm weakness suggests a stroke in the anterior cerebral artery territory. If both arm and leg are equally affected, this suggests either a large middle cerebral artery stroke or a subcortical lacunar infarct.

Sometimes, a stroke may present with a very subtle weakness that the patient notices but may not be identified through the NIHSS. Three exam techniques helpful in identifying subtle weakness are pronator drift testing, orbiting, and observing fine finger movements. Pronator drift is identified by having the patient fully extend and hold both arms out at 45 degrees for 10–20 s, hands fully supinated (palms pointed up as if holding a bowl of soup), next to but not touching each other, and with their eyes closed. With a pronator drift, one hand will turn and drift downward. If an arm drifts upwards and out, that suggests a cerebellar drift. For orbiting, ask the patient to rotate arms with elbows bent around each other as if they are hitting a punching bag. If one arm is weaker, the stronger arm will rotate more briskly, or orbit, around the weak arm. Fine finger movements are tested by having the patient tap the thumb and forefinger together and then tap the thumb to each of the remaining fingers sequentially. A positive finding is when the patient has difficulty with sequential tapping.

Note that scoring strength is very different when performing an NIHSS vs. a regular neurological exam (Table 6.1). In the NIHSS, the higher the number, the weaker the patient. The opposite is true in a formal neurological exam (to keep it interesting)!

Table 6.1 Motor testing scales

	NIHSS	Regular exam
0	Normal (no drift)	No muscle contractions
1	Drift but does not hit the bed	Minimal, muscle twitch
2	Drift and falls to the bed	Movement in the plane of the bed
3	No antigravity	Movement against gravity only (no resistance)
4	No movement (plegic)	Movement against gravity with resistance (with subjective gradation: 4−, 4, 4+)
5	N/A	Full/normal strength

Sensory

While the sensory exam includes several modalities (pinprick, light touch, vibration, and proprioception), generally, only light touch with fingertips or pinprick is used to examine acute stroke patients. The sensory exam, like the motor exam, helps to localize the stroke. An important caveat regarding sensory testing in stroke patients is that one should focus testing of sensation on the proximal part of each extremity (i.e., on the shoulders and thighs) rather than more distal areas as those may have sensory dysfunction for other reasons like diabetic or entrapment neuropathy. A good way to quantify sensory loss is to ask the patient, "If the normal side feels 100%, then how much does the affected side feel?" While this method is subjective, it can provide a reference point for future exams.

Cerebellar

Ataxia, a loss of coordination despite normal strength, is the most prominent abnormality seen in cerebellar stroke and is often seen in the ipsilateral arm or leg. Patients may describe this symptom as "weakness," which can be misleading. Finger-to-nose and heel-to-shin testing are standard tests for ataxia. Test finger-to-nose by having the patient *fully extend* their arm and reach to touch the examiner's index finger (Fig. 6.5). This allows the examiner to appreciate subtle dysmetria or a zig-zagging of the hand and arm on its way to the target. Not having the patient fully extend their arm risks missing this finding. Heel-to-shin testing requires the patient to take the heel of one foot, touch the knee of the other leg, and drag the heel up and down the shin, and vice versa. If the foot zig-zags along the shin, that is ataxia. Heel-to-shin might be difficult for patients with arthritis. Truncal ataxia (the patient cannot sit upright, and it looks like they are getting pulled to one side) is tested by having the patient sit upright in bed.

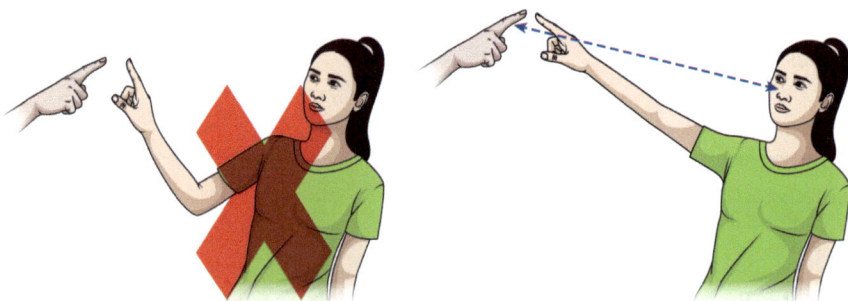

Fig. 6.5 Dysmetria testing. Note the incorrect method on the left, where the patient's arm is not fully extended. The correct method is on the right

Gait and Reflexes

While not a regular part of the NIHSS, asking the patient to walk (with staff assistance close by) is helpful if gait imbalance is a complaint. Gait testing can pick up mild leg weakness or ataxia, which may still be worthy of treatment with thrombolytics even if it does not score on the NIHSS. The muscle stretch reflex exam is part of the motor exam but is often of limited value in an acute stroke code. During an acute stroke, reflexes are diminished or absent in the affected limb, but they become hyperactive weeks later as tone increases.

Clinical Pearls
- The mental status provides the context for the rest of the exam.
- The components of an aphasia exam are fluency, comprehension, repetition, and naming.
- Ensure that all four visual fields are checked for each eye.
- Arm drift should be checked with eyes closed and both arms outstretched.
- Have the patient fully extend their arm and reach during the "finger-nose-finger" test.
- Sensation to soft touch should be checked in the proximal (upper) arms and legs during stroke exams to avoid confounding due to neuropathy.
- For anisocoria, use light and dark settings to determine which pupil is abnormal.

Reference

1. Lyden P. Using the national institutes of health stroke scale: A cautionary tale. Stroke. 2017;48(2):513–9. https://doi.org/10.1161/STROKEAHA.116.015434.

Telestroke

7

Jane Anderson and Hardik P. Amin

Introduction

In 1995, the National Institute of Neurological Disorders and Stroke (NINDS) rt-PA Stroke Trial demonstrated the effectiveness of the timely administration of alteplase (rt-PA) in reducing long-term disability for patients with acute ischemic stroke (AIS) [1]. At the time, however, less than 1.5% of stroke patients were treated with thrombolytics. Using telemedicine for AIS (Telestroke) was first described in 1999 to improve stroke care and expand the reach of stroke experts to rural communities to increase the utilization of rt-PA [2]. Initial questions focused on whether evaluating and treating patients via telemedicine was safe and effective. Several meta-analyses demonstrated that Telestroke was associated with reduced length of hospital stay, with similar rates of intracerebral hemorrhage and outcomes compared to patients receiving alteplase with in-person evaluations at stroke centers [3, 4]. A subsequent meta-analysis reviewing the efficacy of Telestroke, specifically in rural areas, demonstrated a two-fold increase in the utilization of alteplase, higher rates of functional outcomes, lower in-hospital mortality, and no differences in intracerebral hemorrhage rates [5]. Several trials have shown that utilizing Telestroke can lead to more accurate clinical diagnosis, improved process times, identification of stroke mimics, and interpretation of imaging with a high agreement between the Telestroke provider and radiologist [6–8]. Finally, the StrokeDOC trial demonstrated that video consultations provided higher accuracy than telephone consultations for determining alteplase eligibility.

J. Anderson
Baylor College of Medicine, Houston, TX, USA
e-mail: Jane.Anderson@va.gov

H. P. Amin (✉)
Hartford Hospital, Hartford, CT, USA
e-mail: hardik.amin@hhchealth.org

© The Author(s), under exclusive license to Springer Nature Switzerland AG 2024
H. P. Amin (ed.), *Stroke for the Advanced Practice Clinician*,
https://doi.org/10.1007/978-3-031-66289-8_7

Telestroke Models

The American Telemedicine Association released Telestroke Guidelines in 2017 to assist practitioners using Telestroke [9]. The guidelines detail the resources required to set up Telestroke at a site. Maintaining a Telestroke site requires financial and personnel support to implement and maintain video equipment, software, internet connectivity, managing patient records, licensing and credentialing fees, training, and physician call fees. Telestroke should be a service meant to complement (not replace) any existing services or providers. Most hospitals use Telestroke around the clock, but some use it for overnight or weekend coverage or when no in-house neurology providers are available. At a minimum, a Telestroke hospital should be able to perform head CT and administer thrombolytics around the clock.

Two models currently exist for Telestroke (Fig. 7.1). The more common "hub and spoke" model has a central institution (or hub), which is typically a high-volume academic center or comprehensive stroke center that provides acute Telestroke consultations to hospitals (spokes) *within a specified catchment or geographical area*. The Telestroke providers are typically affiliated with the hub hospital. It is customary for spoke hospitals to transfer patients requiring a higher level of care, such as endovascular intervention or admission to a stroke or intensive care unit, to the hub hospital. The second model is the "distributed" model. In this model, a decentralized telemedicine service (either an independent for-profit company or an organized group of providers) employs Telestroke providers at distant sites to provide hospital consultations through contracted services. In this case, the hospital utilizing Telestroke services would have an agreement with the closest comprehensive or thrombectomy-capable stroke center in its community for transfers. In both setups, acute stroke imaging (CT, CTA, CTP) should be immediately uploaded to a medical record or secure cloud-based imaging directory accessible by the Telestroke provider. Collaboration with teleradiology in a Telestroke network is effective in supporting rapid imaging interpretation for thrombolytic administration decision-making [10].

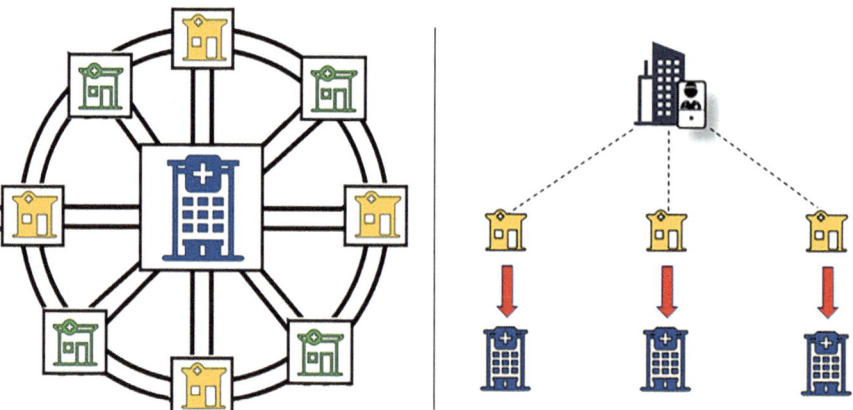

Fig. 7.1 Telestroke hub and spoke model (left) vs. distributed model (right)

The Telestroke Consult

Telestrokes can be activated in both the emergency department and inpatient settings. When does one activate Telestroke? When a patient presents with or is discovered to have new focal neurologic deficits, or the suspicion of acute stroke is high. Like a traditional stroke code, the primary purpose of a Telestroke consultation is to determine the likelihood that the patient is having a stroke and if the patient is a candidate for acute stroke treatment. A Telestroke consult should, therefore, be called within the stroke treatment "time window," which is up to 24 h from symptom onset. The traditional time window for alteplase or Tenecteplase is up to 4.5 h from the onset or "last known well (LKW)" time, and the treatment window for thrombectomy can be up to 24 h, depending on imaging findings. Therefore, most Telestroke protocols allow activation within 24 h of symptom onset or LKW time. When a patient presents with symptoms beyond 24 h, calling local neurology before activating Telestroke may be appropriate, but all parties should agree upon such a protocol.

For hospitals using Telestroke, activating a stroke code locally and calling Telestroke are two separate processes. Figure 7.2 has a common framework for Telestroke activations. When a patient presents with stroke symptoms, a hospital "stroke code" is activated by paging or calling the hospital operator, which will notify all necessary in-house medical staff, including specialized nurses and rapid response teams. These teams will assist with assessing, transporting, and administering lytic medication. CT scan technicians should also be notified so they can keep the scanner open for the patient. Notice that neurology has not been called yet to this point. Activating Telestroke requires a separate phone call to a response center, which then connects the caller to a vascular neurologist. Without this crucial second step, the in-house team will be left wondering where the neurologist is! The Telestroke specialist will then evaluate the patient via a Telestroke monitor connected to Wi-Fi. It is important to know where Telestroke monitors are kept in the hospital. Generally, there are two monitors—one in the emergency department and another one for inpatient codes, usually kept in an ICU. It is also crucial to know who is responsible for bringing the monitor to the patient's bedside in case of code activation.

After calling a stroke code, the patient should be quickly evaluated by bedside providers for medical stability, a brief neurological exam, and be taken to CT as soon as possible. Next, call Telestroke *as the patient is rolling to CT*. Calling Telestroke early is advantageous so the Telestroke provider can hear the history and review the chart while the patient is at scan. As the patient is rolling back from CT, the Telestroke provider can review the imaging so that when the patient returns, all that needs to be done is a focused neurological exam and a decision for treatment. Doing things in parallel can dramatically reduce treatment times!

Telestroke and teleneurology are two distinct services and should not be confused with each other. Teleneurology is a broader consultative service that can recommend studies and continue to follow a patient during their hospital stay. A Telestroke consultation is a one-time consultation, limited to the discrete episode of acute neurological symptoms, involving acute stroke imaging, exam, and

Fig. 7.2 Telestroke process

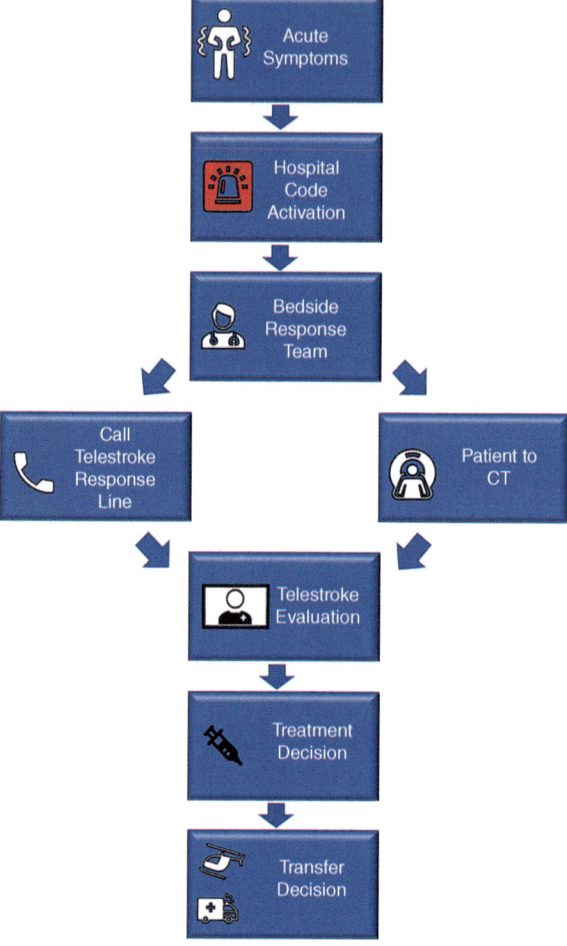

recommendations for acute stroke treatment. The consult begins with the bedside provider placing an initial telephone call to the Telestroke service/provider and ends when the final recommendations are made. The person making the initial phone call to the Telestroke physician must be a medical provider or nurse who has seen the patient and can provide first-hand information about the patient and the reason for activating a stroke code. *Administrative staff should not call Telestroke only to put the Telestroke provider on hold to wait for a bedside provider to come to the phone.* This wastes the Telestroke provider's time and delays patient care as Telestroke providers are often managing multiple cases simultaneously, especially in a hub and spoke model.

The following patient information should be known before calling Telestroke:

- Name, age.
- Presenting stroke symptoms.
- If the patient is an inpatient, what is the reason for admission?
- Time of symptom onset or Last Known Well (LKW) time.
- If a patient is "found" with new symptoms, the LKW time is critical.
- Vital signs.
- Blood glucose (obtained at the point of care via glucometer).
- If known, any pertinent cardiovascular or neurological history (prior stroke, brain tumor, epilepsy).
- Any pertinent medications (anticoagulation, anti-seizure medications).
- Any recent trauma or major surgery.

Timepoints are discussed in greater depth in the Chap. 5. For an actual "symptom onset" time, a patient must be able to verify when the change occurred or have it witnessed. If a patient is found with symptoms by family or a nurse, or wakes up with symptoms, the next question should be, "When was the patient last known well (at their baseline)?" The LKW time is when the treatment window would begin. For wake-up strokes, asking if a patient got up at any point in the night to use the bathroom might provide a more recent time point.

The Telestroke provider uses video-teleconference technology to connect virtually with the local care team at the patient's bedside. They will lead the bedside team in performing a focused exam, confirming history, reviewing imaging, and quickly ruling out treatment contraindications. The sooner the patient receives reperfusion therapy, the better the outcome.

The monitor should be placed at the foot of the patient's bed, and the head of the bed should be at 30° (Fig. 7.3). The exam should be efficient and focused on identifying any disabling symptoms. All bedside clinicians and nurses should undergo

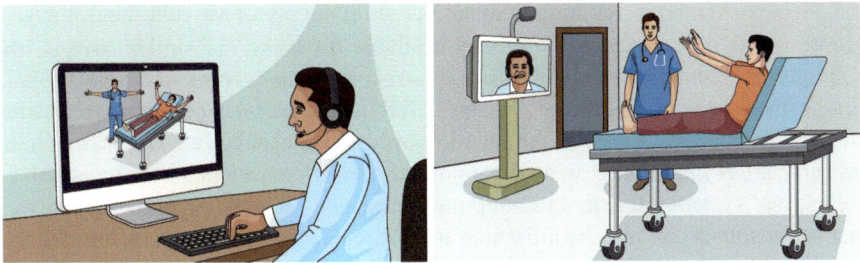

Fig. 7.3 Telestroke evaluation point of view for the Telestroke provider (left) and patient (right)

training in the NIHSS exam and be ready and willing to aid the Telestroke provider during the evaluation. Be prepared for the Telestroke provider to ask for assistance performing portions of the NIHSS like visual fields, sensation, dysmetria, extinction, and neglect. Refer to the Chap. 6 for guidance and tips on performing challenging parts of the exam.

Once a Telestroke consultation is complete, the local hospital team generally resumes care of the patient unless, of course, the patient is transferred.

Telestroke Triage

Telestroke services often have multiple consults simultaneously and may employ a triage process. Some Telestroke programs staff stroke-trained nurses to triage initial phone calls from consulting facilities for Telestroke consult eligibility based on symptom presentation and LKW time. Telestroke nurse triage is guided by an acute stroke consultation protocol. Cases within the treatment window are immediately forwarded to the on-call Telestroke provider. Cases outside the acute stroke treatment window might get referred to the consulting facility's neurology service. Suppose the consulting facility is rural and does not have a local neurology service. In that case, the Telestroke provider may agree to discuss nonacute consults by phone when able. When the Telestroke program does not have nurse triage, the Telestroke provider will triage consultations in a similar manner.

Telestroke in the United States

While Telestroke was initially developed to ensure access to stroke expertise in rural communities, recent data show a geographical disparity in the implementation of Telestroke systems. Interestingly, Telestroke is more available in metropolitan areas than rural areas, with 4 out of 5 rural counties in the United States without Telestroke systems [11]. The higher concentration of Telestroke units in metropolitan areas might be attributed to the high demand but short supply of vascular neurologists. There is only one vascular neurologist available for every 717 stroke cases in the United States, making it difficult to access stroke specialists across the country [12]. Large metropolitan healthcare systems establish Telestroke networks to ensure stroke expertise for their satellite locations in urban and suburban areas. Hospitals in rural areas unaffiliated with metropolitan networks are less likely to establish Telestroke systems. Barriers to adopting Telestroke services by rural and critical access hospitals can also be attributed to cost, capacity, technological limitations, and local, state, and federal policies and regulations [11]. However, research has demonstrated that hospitals with Telestroke capability are more likely to provide reperfusion treatment, highlighting its importance and growing need [13].

Clinical Pearls

- For Telestroke hospitals, calling Telestroke and activating a local stroke code are often two separate processes.
- Calling Telestroke prior to imaging helps expedite evaluation and treatment.
- Only providers or nurses who have seen the patient should call Telestroke.
- Proper positioning of the monitor and having a team member at the bedside to help with the exam are necessary.
- Ensure the monitor has adequate Wi-Fi connectivity and is plugged in when not in use to remain charged.

References

1. National Institute of Neurological Disorders and Stroke rt-PA Stroke Study Group. Tissue plasminogen activator for acute ischemic stroke. N Engl J Med. 1995;333(24):1581–7. https://doi.org/10.1056/NEJM199512143332401. PMID: 7477192
2. Levine SR, Gorman M. "Telestroke": the application of telemedicine for stroke. Stroke. 1999;30(2):464–9. https://doi.org/10.1161/01.str.30.2.464. PMID: 9933289
3. Baratloo A, Rahimpour L, Abushouk AI, Safari S, Lee CW, Abdalvand A. Effects of telestroke on thrombolysis times and outcomes: a meta-analysis. Prehosp Emerg Care. 2018;22(4):472–84. https://doi.org/10.1080/10903127.2017.1408728. Epub 2018 Jan 18. PMID: 29345529
4. Kepplinger J, Barlinn K, Deckert S, Scheibe M, Bodechtel U, Schmitt J. Safety and efficacy of thrombolysis in telestroke: a systematic review and meta-analysis. Neurology. 2016;87(13):1344–51. https://doi.org/10.1212/WNL.0000000000003148. Epub 2016 Aug 26. PMID: 27566746
5. Lazarus G, Permana AP, Nugroho SW, Audrey J, Wijaya DN, Widyahening IS. Telestroke strategies to enhance acute stroke management in rural settings: A systematic review and meta-analysis. Brain Behav. 2020;10(10):e01787. https://doi.org/10.1002/brb3.1787. Epub 2020 Aug 18. PMID: 32812380; PMCID: PMC7559631
6. Janícek M, Bruna J, Stěnhová H. Hodnocení změn denzity obratlového těla po nitrozilním podání kontrastní látky v průběhu rutinního CT vysetrení [evaluation of changes in the density of the vertebral body after intravenous administration of contrast medium during routine CT examination]. Cesk Radiol. 1984;38(4):243–7. PMID: 6488384
7. Meyer BC, Raman R, Hemmen T, Obler R, Zivin JA, Rao R, Thomas RG, Lyden PD. Efficacy of site-independent telemedicine in the STRokE DOC trial: a randomised, blinded, prospective study. Lancet Neurol. 2008;7(9):787–95. https://doi.org/10.1016/S1474-4422(08)70171-6. PMID: 18676180; PMCID: PMC2744128
8. Demaerschalk BM, Bobrow BJ, Raman R, Ernstrom K, Hoxworth JM, Patel AC, Kiernan TE, Aguilar MI, Ingall TJ, Dodick DW, Meyer BC. Stroke Team Remote Evaluation Using a Digital Observation Camera (STRokE DOC) in Arizona—The Initial Mayo Clinic Experience (AZ TIME) Investigators. CT interpretation in a telestroke network: agreement among a spoke radiologist, hub vascular neurologist, and hub neuroradiologist. Stroke. 2012;43(11):3095–7. https://doi.org/10.1161/STROKEAHA.112.666255. Epub 2012 Sep 13. PMID: 22984007; PMCID: PMC3502613
9. Demaerschalk BM, Berg J, Chong BW, Gross H, Nystrom K, Adeoye O, Schwamm L, Wechsler L, Whitchurch S. American telemedicine association: Telestroke guidelines. Telemed J E Health. 2017;23(5):376–89. https://doi.org/10.1089/tmj.2017.0006. Epub 2017 Apr 6. PMID: 28384077; PMCID: PMC5802246

10. Powers WJ, et al. Guidelines for the early management of patients with acute ischemic stroke: 2019 update to the 2018 guidelines for the early management of acute ischemic stroke: a guideline for healthcare professionals from the American Heart Association/American Stroke Association. Stroke. 2019;50(12):e344–418.
11. Machado S, et al. Abstract 14149: Access to neurology and telestroke services in rural America. Circulation. 2021;144(Suppl_1) https://doi.org/10.1161/circ.144.suppl_1.14149.
12. Leira EC, et al. The growing shortage of vascular neurologists in the era of health reform: planning is brain! Stroke. 2013;44(3):822–7.
13. Wilcock AD, Schwamm LH, Zubizarreta JR, et al. Reperfusion treatment and stroke outcomes in hospitals with telestroke capacity. JAMA Neurol. 2021;78(5):527–35. https://doi.org/10.1001/jamaneurol.2021.0023.

Acute Stroke Treatment: Thrombolytics

8

Samantha Salas, Razaz Mageid, and Hardik P. Amin

Introduction

Ischemic strokes occur when blood flow to the brain is interrupted. Often, this is due to an occlusion from a thrombus or embolism. A thrombus is a blood clot that develops at a site of injury in a blood vessel, over an ulcerated or unstable atherosclerotic plaque, from blood stasis or a hypercoagulable state. A thrombus leads to stenosis and can impair forward flow. On the other hand, an embolism occurs when a clump of red blood cells or platelets, or some other substance, travels through the bloodstream and blocks a vessel downstream. A thrombus in a deep leg vein can have a small piece break off. That small piece (the *thrombo*-embolism), then travels toward the heart and lungs, potentially causing a pulmonary embolism or travel through a PFO causing a stroke (more on that in the PFO chapter). Other examples of emboli include cardiac clots (cardioembolism), air, fat, amniotic fluid, or plaque (calcium) fragments.

Occluded arteries decrease cerebral blood flow, disrupting energy metabolism and causing neurological symptoms. The longer an artery remains occluded, the more brain tissue is irreversibly lost. The average human brain has about 100 billion neurons. The goal of acute thrombolytic therapy, therefore, is to dissolve the blood clot and reperfuse the brain before irreversible tissue death [1, 2]. Two million

S. Salas
Stanford Health, Stanford, CA, USA
e-mail: samantha.salas@yale.edu

R. Mageid (✉)
Beth Israel Lahey Health, Burlington, MA, USA
e-mail: razaz.h.mageid@lahey.org

H. P. Amin
Hartford Hospital, Hartford, CT, USA
e-mail: hardik.amin@yale.edu

neurons and 14 billion synapses (connections between neurons) are lost every minute an ischemic stroke goes untreated. Every hour an ischemic stroke goes untreated, the patient loses as many neurons as it does in almost 4 years of normal aging [3]!

Thrombolytics for Stroke

Researchers have been investigating clot-dissolving interventions since the 1950s. Alteplase, or tPA, approved by the FDA in 1996, was a significant advancement in treating acute ischemic stroke. tPA works by dissolving fibrin blood clots by converting plasminogen into plasmin, the enzyme that lyzes fibrin and breaks up clots [4]. The half-life of tPA is 5 min (meaning the drug itself leaves the body relatively quickly); however, since it also depletes the body's supply of fibrinogen, the risk of bleeding can last up to 24 h until the body replenishes its fibrinogen stores. Plasminogen activator inhibitor-1 (PAI-1) is the main inhibitory enzyme for tPA, limiting the drug's activity (provides checks and balances). The effect of PAI-1 is why the half-life of tPA is so short, and the hour-long infusion is needed to keep enough drugs in the system to be effective [5].

Tenecteplase (TNK), like tPA, is a plasminogen activator. It is a variant of tPA with three engineered mutations. Tenecteplase is the preferred thrombolytic therapy for ST-elevation myocardial infarctions but is not currently FDA-approved for use in ischemic stroke. However, many studies have demonstrated several advantages of TNK over alteplase. It is more resistant to PAI-1 than tPA, giving it a longer half-life than tPA (i.e., TNK hangs around longer in the body) so administration is more straightforward than alteplase, only requiring a single bolus and no infusion. It also has higher fibrin specificity (more selective clot dissolution), is cheaper, and has less depletion of systemic fibrinogen (so there is less systemic bleeding risk). Data have found TNK to be just as effective for stroke as tPA. As a result, many stroke centers around the country have transitioned to TNK as the main thrombolytic for acute ischemic stroke. Table 8.1 provides a side-by-side comparison of the two agents.

Table 8.1 A comparison of alteplase and tenecteplase

	Alteplase	Tenecteplase
FDA approved	Stroke, MI, high-risk PE	MI
Half-life	5 min	20 min
Administration	• 0.09 mg/kg total dose • 10% given as an IV bolus over 1 min • 90% given as a continuous infusion over 1 h • Maximum dose 90 mg	• 0.25 mg/kg • Administered IV push over 5 min • Maximum dose 25 mg
Fibrin specificity	Intermediate	High
Resistance to PAI-1	Low	High
Fibrinogen depletion	Intermediate	Low
Access and administration	2× peripheral IV IV bolus +60-min infusion	Single peripheral IV Single 5–10 s IV bolus

Evaluation and Administration

The priority during an acute stroke code is identifying the patient's focal neurological deficits with the NIHSS score and getting them to the CT scanner. The goal of obtaining a CT head is to rule out a hemorrhage, a major contraindication to intravenous thrombolysis. For acute stroke patients, the history and exam are crucial to making time-sensitive treatment decisions. The administration of thrombolytics, either tPA or TNK, is time-based depending on symptom onset or last known well (LKW) time. The treatment window is 3 h from symptom onset or LKW. That window can be extended to 4.5 h for a selected group of patients.

A meta-analysis showed that tPA administration by 3 h had the most favorable outcomes for stroke patients in terms of minimal disability at 3–6 months and the lowest risk of tPA-associated hemorrhage. Patients given tPA within 90 min of symptom onset are three times more likely to have favorable outcomes compared to patients given tPA toward the end of the 4.5-h window [6]. This critical point is often overlooked, leading to less urgency from medical providers for patients arriving early in the window because "there is time." Administration of lytics after 4.5 h has no benefit and increases the risk of hemorrhage [7].

Understanding the distinctions between the different time points is essential to determine eligibility. The clock does not start when a patient's symptoms are *discovered* by family or medical staff, but rather when the patient was last known well (LKW). For wake-up strokes, the LKW was when the patient went to bed unless they mentioned getting up in the middle of the night to use the bathroom. For inpatients, this may mean calling overnight nurses to determine when the patient was truly confirmed at baseline. Asking pointed questions like, "Was the patient truly speaking fluently when you saw them at 3 am," or "Were they truly moving their right side without any problems during your last nursing check," avoids the pitfall of assuming patients were at baseline without a specific function being evaluated. Again, symptom discovery does not equal symptom onset.

How Effective Are tPA and TNK?

In the late 1980s and early 1990s, multiple clinical trials established the efficacy and safety of tPA. In 1995, the NINDS tPA stroke trial was the first randomized, double-blind, placebo-controlled trial of IV-tPA in acute ischemic stroke within 3 h of the last known well [8]. This study showed a significant difference in 3-month outcome measures (Barthel Index, mRS NIHSS, and Glasgow outcome score). They found that patients treated with tPA were at least 30% more likely to have minimal or no disability at 3 months. Regarding safety outcomes, the NINDS tPA trial found a 6.4% symptomatic intracerberal hemorrhage (ICH) rate at 36 h compared to 0.6% in the placebo group. When discussing the risks and benefits of tPA with patients, some providers will quote a "1 in 3" chance of improving outcomes over 3 months and a 6% chance of ICH.

tPA is only FDA-approved for 0–3 h from the last known well, but in practice, it is administered up to 4.5 h from LKW. The ECASS III trial (2008) demonstrated the safety and efficacy of tPA 3–4.5 h from the last known well. This European study randomized patients administered tPA vs. placebo at 3–4.5 h from symptom onset. The primary outcome was a 90-day favorable outcome (mRS 0–1) vs. unfavorable (mRS 2–6), with the primary outcome favoring the tPA arm (52.4% favorable outcome in the tPA group vs. 45.2% in the placebo group). ICH was also more common in the tPA arm [9]. They excluded patients > 80 years old, with NIHSS > 25, history of stroke and diabetes, and are on any anti-coagulant regardless of INR. So, these patients currently would not qualify for thrombolytics in the extended window.

It is also notable that tPA does not work well for larger clots (>8 mm), which tend to lodge in the larger arteries like the distal ICA and proximal MCA. tPA is least effective when clots occlude the distal ICA with about a 4–10% recanalization rate, followed by the M1 and M2 segments of the MCA with 20–30% recanalization (Fig. 8.1). Clots in the vertebrobasilar arteries have a 31% recanalization rate [10]. The more proximal vessels have larger diameters than more distal vessels; therefore, the more proximal the occluded artery, the larger the clot and the less responsive it is to tPA. Fortunately, today, thrombectomy is an option, but for patients in the pre-thrombectomy era, no other treatment was available for persistent clots.

TNK is not FDA-approved, but many institutions are starting to transition following multiple trials demonstrating noninferiority of TNK compared to tPA (NOR-TEST, ATTEST, TRACE-2 trials). This means that TNK is thought to be just as good as tPA for treating acute stroke, same risk of ICH, with some added

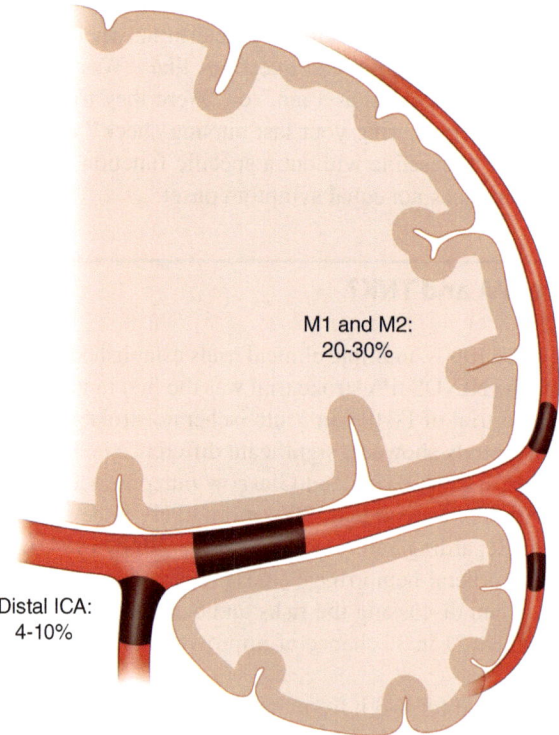

Fig. 8.1 Efficacy of alteplase based on clot location

advantages. Evidence also suggests that TNK has a better recanalization rate in the setting of large vessel occlusion (EXTEND-IA TNK) than tPA. See Table 8.1 for other advantages of TNK.

A small, randomized trial of tenecteplase vs. alteplase for acute ischemic stroke (TAAIS 2012) was the first trial to show the superiority of tenecteplase with LVO. The tenecteplase group had a 79.3% reperfusion rate at 2 h on CT angiography compared to 55.4% in the alteplase group, but the study was very small. There was no statistically significant difference in ICH rates between the two groups [11]. EXTEND-IA TNK found that patients with LVO who were given TNK within 4.5 h of stroke had significantly higher rates of spontaneous reperfusion without needing thrombectomy compared to tPA (22% vs. 10%, respectively). A large retrospective study of 54 academic medical centers found that patients treated with TNK had lower mortality rates, lower risk of systemic bleeding requiring transfusions, and no difference in ICH at 30 days post-stroke than patients treated with tPA [12]. And to drive it home, after switching to TNK, a 10-hospital regional network in Texas demonstrated shorter door-to-needle times, shorter transfer times, a higher percentage of patients able to be discharged home, and overall reduced cost per stay compared to patients who received tPA [13].

Who Should Not Get Thrombolytics?

The 2019 American Heart Association/American Stroke Association Guidelines state tPA is indicated for anyone >18 with suspected ischemic stroke with last known well $\leq$4.5 h (recall tPA is not FDA approved for the 3–4.5-h window). Before administration, patients must have CT without evidence of brain hemorrhage and no known contraindications suggesting increased systemic bleeding risk (Table 8.2). Many contraindications are based on patient exclusion from tPA trials, not proven high risk of bleeding. So things like history of ICH, surgery, head trauma, known aneurysms or tumors, and recent GI bleeding should warrant further risk/benefit discussions with relevant teams before the final decision. Note the additional contraindications for the extended 3–4.5-h window.

Table 8.2 Contraindications to thrombolytic therapy (per 2019 AHA/ASA guidelines) [14]

0–3 h	3–4.5 h (per ECASS (III criteria)
ICH/SAH/SDH on CT	Criteria in 0–3 h plus below:
History of ICH	Age >80
Surgery/head trauma or major stroke in the last 3 months	History of DM and prior stroke
BP >185/110	Any anticoagulant use
Platelet count <100,000	NIHSS >25
INR > 1.7	CT involving $\frac{1}{3}$ MCA territory
DOAC use within the last 48 h	
Major surgery in the last 14 days	
Known AVM, brain tumor, or aneurysm	
Heparin within the last 48 h with elevated PTT	
Recent/active internal bleeding	
Serum glucose <50 or >400	
Seizure (relative exclusion)	

What About Beyond 4.5 H?

The onset time of stroke symptoms is unknown in many cases. In some instances, symptoms are identified upon waking. Approximately 20% of strokes are classified as wake up strokes [15]. This would remove many patients from thrombolytic eligibility because giving thrombolytics to a stroke more than 4.5 h old is not only unhelpful but can cause hemorrhage. But what if the stroke occurred 30 min before someone woke up? How can we determine if someone might still be in the treatment window if we do not have time points? Recall that a stroke will show up almost immediately on DWI-MRI but only after about 4–6 h on FLAIR-MRI sequences. Therefore, if a patient with new stroke symptoms shows changes in DWI but not normal FLAIR sequence (called DWI-FLAIR mismatch), stroke onset was likely within the past few hours. It is believed that thrombolytics carry a lower risk of bleeding when no FLAIR changes are present.

Recent trials sought to identify patients outside the traditional treatment window who might still benefit from thrombolytic therapy. The MR WITNESS trial evaluated the safety of administering tPA to patients with stroke of LKW 4.5–24 h prior. These patients must have presented to the hospital within 4.5 h of symptom discovery and MRI with DWI-FLAIR mismatch. The trial demonstrated that giving tPA was safe in patients who met these criteria, with symptomatic hemorrhage occurring in 1.3% and asymptomatic hemorrhage in 26.3% (similar to the ECASS III trial results) [16]. The WAKE-UP trial evaluated the efficacy and outcomes after administering tPA in the same group of patients. It demonstrated significantly better functional outcomes at 90 days (mRS of 0–1 in 53% of the tPA group and 41% of the placebo group) [17]. The challenge, however, is that most hospitals cannot get such rapid MRIs on patients to identify potential patients. Even if hospitals can get rapid MRIs, imaging every stroke patient in an extended window would significantly strain resources. Finally, there may be variability in interpreting FLAIR sequences between readers.

Despite these barriers, the lessons learned from these trials improve our understanding of "tissue-based" rather than "time-based" treatment decisions. As a result, some comprehensive stroke centers have started implementing MRI protocols to allow for the safe administration of tPA outside of the 4.5 LKW time.

Post-tPA Care

Monitoring patients after tPA administration is essential for detecting neurologic exam changes that could indicate hemorrhagic transformation or anaphylaxis. Post-TNK care is the same as for post-tPA. Standard practice is to monitor post-tPA patients in an intensive care unit or intermediate care unit for at least 24 h due to frequent vital signs and neurological monitoring. Per the alteplase manufacturer guidelines, recommendations for post-thrombolytic care are as follows [18]:

- Vital signs and NIHSS every 15 min for 2 h, then every 30 min for 6 h, then every 1 h for 16 h, then provider discretion.
- Continue to check for major and/or minor bleeding.
- Obtain a follow-up CT scan or magnetic resonance imaging (MRI) 24 h before starting anticoagulants or antiplatelet agents.
- Continue to monitor for signs of hypersensitivity.

The recommended blood pressure goal following thrombolytic administration is <180/105 mmHg for the following 24 h, and antiplatelet therapy with aspirin is started within 24–48 h [19].

How Do You Manage Complications?

The NINDS study estimated a 6.4% risk of intracerebral hemorrhage [8]. Suspect hemorrhage in patients with an abrupt decrease in consciousness, severe headache, nausea/vomiting, seizure, sudden BP rise, or worsening NIHSS/Glasgow Coma Scale. Swift action must be taken if hemorrhage is suspected (Table 8.3).

Allergic reactions with IV tPA infusion, while rare, are seen more often in patients taking ACE inhibitors like lisinopril. tPA induces the production of bradykinin, a potent vasodilator that promotes inflammation and the release of histamines. ACE inhibitors inhibit bradykinin breakdown. Increased bradykinin levels can cause mild to severe reactions like rash, urticaria, angioedema, hypotension, bronchospasm, and shock. Rapid treatment is required for moderate to severe reactions (Table 8.4). Angioedema is a type of swelling that occurs under the skin. It can happen several hours after tPA infusion is completed and often affects the tongue and lips on the opposite side of the infarct, as well as the cheeks and pharynx.

Table 8.3 Protocol for suspected hemorrhage following thrombolytics (per AHA/ASA 2019 guidelines)

STOP infusion
Check CBC, PT (INR), aPTT, fibrinogen level, and type and cross-match
Obtain STAT head CT
If hemorrhage detected, administer cryoprecipitate: 10 U infused over 10–30 min; if fibrinogen level <150, administer an additional dose of cryoprecipitate. Every ten units of cryoprecipitate should increase fibrinogen by almost 50 mg/dL
If blood products are declined (cryo has FFP) or cryoprecipitate is not available, alternatives include tranexamic acid 1000 mg over 10 min or ε-aminocaproic acid 4–5 g over 1 h, followed by 1 g IV until bleeding is controlled
Hematology and neurosurgery consultations
Supportive therapy: Blood pressure management, ICP, CPP, MAP, temperature, and glucose control

Table 8.4 Protocol for angioedema following thrombolytics (per 2019 AHA/ASA guidelines)

Stop tPA infusion

Assess and secure airway, breathing, and circulation

High flow oxygen; nebulizer for bronchospasm; consider intubation if edema involves the larynx, palate, floor of mouth, or oropharynx

Administer IV methylprednisolone 125 mg, IV diphenhydramine 50 mg, and IV ranitidine 50 mg or famotidine 20 mg

If an increase in angioedema is seen, administer epinephrine (0.1%) 0.3 mL subcutaneously or 0.5 mL via nebulizer

Supportive care

Challenging Situations

1. *"Too good to treat."* A common reason not to treat a patient is unimpressive exam findings or low NIHSS. For example, a 70-year-old right-handed musician with a sudden onset of right-sided numbness that started 1-h prior to presentation. CTH negative for hemorrhage, no contraindications to tPA. NIHSS 1. Given his low NIHSS, one may think the risk outweighs the benefit of tPA administration. After further discussion, the patient revealed that he plays the guitar. He expressed concern that if his symptoms continued, he would be unable to play the guitar during performances. Since this would be considered a disabling symptom, a discussion was held with the patient, and it was decided that tPA should be administered. For milder symptoms, ask *the patient* if they would consider their symptoms disabling should they remain. If yes, treatment remains an option. Likewise, someone with isolated aphasia may only have an NIHSS of 2, but it is fair to say most people would consider that disabling. A low NIHSS does *not* exclude a patient from eligibility.

2. *Direct Acting Oral Anticoagulants such as Apixaban, Rivaroxaban or Dabigatran (DOACs).* Since there is no rapid, universally accepted test to test for DOAC use, the current guidelines recommend not giving thrombolytics to patients who have taken a dose within the last 48 h. For aphasic patients without anyone else at the bedside, this would be hard to confirm. Calling the patient's family or a care facility may be helpful. While there is emerging safety data for thrombolytics in patients taking DOACs, most centers will not treat them unless someone can confirm when the last dose was taken. Reversal agents should not be given in order to then administer thrombolytic therapy.

3. *Hypotension.* Hypotension in a stroke patient is an independent poor prognostic factor as it can expand the infarct size. Low blood pressure should prompt investigation into the possibility of cardiogenic hypotension, such as from concurrent myocardial infarction or aortic dissection. Hypotension may also be due to vasodilatory hypotension, such as from sepsis. If signs of sepsis are present, this should prompt consideration of concurrent infective endocarditis and associated septic emboli as the possible stroke etiology, which is also a contraindication due to an association with high rates of intracerebral hemorrhage after thrombolysis.

4. *Recent surgery.* Any recent procedure should, at a minimum, warrant a call to the surgeon to discuss the risks of thrombolytic therapy. If the benefit of treatment outweighs the risks of bleeding into a surgical site and given the go-ahead by surgery, patients can be treated with clear documentation and close monitoring.

5. *Lecanemab.* Lecanemab is a monoclonal antibody recently approved by the FDA for the treatment of Alzheimer's disease. A case report was published in 2023 of a 65-year-old patient treated with lecanemab who died of intracerebral hemorrhage after being treated with tPA [20]. The patient did not have any other contraindications to tPA. This case has led to concerns over lecanemab as a potential risk factor for hemorrhage for patients treated with tPA.

Stroke Transfers

If a tPA patient requires a transfer to another hospital, patients can be transported while the infusion is running. Waiting until after the infusion is complete leads to unnecessary delays in care, especially if the patient requires a thrombectomy.

Notable Trials

NINDS (1995): Double-blinded, randomized controlled trial of 624 patients with acute ischemic stroke to determine if administration of tPA within 3 h of stroke onset reduces morbidity and mortality. The trial was divided into two parts. Part 1 tested whether tPA led to neurologic improvement within 24 h. Part 2 assessed outcomes at 3 months. No significant difference in outcomes was seen in Part 1 (24 h), but a benefit was seen for tPA patients in Part 2 compared to placebo. The trial found that administration of tPA within 3 h of stroke onset improved clinical outcomes at 3 months in all four measures (Barthel Index, Modified Rankin Scale, Glasgow Outcome Scale, NIHSS), but had no effect on mortality. Symptomatic intracerebral hemorrhage occurred in 6.4% of patients who received tPA [8].

ECASS III (2008): Double-blinded, randomized controlled trial of 821 patients with acute ischemic stroke to determine the efficacy and safety of tPA 3–4.5 h after stroke onset. Stricter exclusion criteria: previous stroke *and* concomitant diabetes, National Institutes of Health Stroke Scale (NIHSS) >25, age >80, and warfarin use (irrespective of INR). The study found that patients in the tPA group were more likely to have favorable outcomes compared to the placebo group. The incidence of symptomatic intracerebral hemorrhage occurred in 2.4% of patients who received tPA [9].

NOR-TEST (2017): Randomized trial of TNK vs. alteplase for acute ischemic stroke. Tenecteplase was given at 0.4 mg/kg. A total of 1100 patients total found that TNK was noninferior to alteplase in terms of favorable outcomes, safety, and mortality [21].

Extend-IA TNK (2018): A randomized controlled trial comparing 0.25 mg/kg TNK to standard dose alteplase for patients with confirmed LVO enrolled

202 patients. TNK or alteplase was given, and the patient was then taken to thrombectomy. The primary outcome was >50% spontaneous reperfusion of clot in the symptomatic vessel. The study found that 22% of patients who received TNK had spontaneous reperfusion of the vessel, compared to 10% of alteplase patients, leading to higher overall reperfusion rates in the TNK arm when including thrombectomy. Overall, 64% of patients in the TNK group went on to independent recovery compared to 51% of the alteplase group [22].

Clinical Pearls
- IV thrombolytics should be considered for acute stroke patients who present within 4.5 of LKW with no contraindications, regardless of NIHSS score.
- Patients treated within 90 min of symptom onset are 3× more likely to have better outcomes than those treated at the end of the treatment window.
- TNK has a lower risk of systemic bleeding, a longer half-life, is easier to administer, and is less expensive than tPA.
- For thrombolytic-associated hemorrhage, immediately stop the infusion, check fibrinogen, and administer cryoprecipitate.

References

1. Hui C, et al. National Library of Medicine, StatPearls Publishing. In: Ischemic stroke; 2022. www.ncbi.nlm.nih.gov/books/NBK499997/. Accessed 16 Dec 2023.
2. Kuriakose D, Xiao Z. Pathophysiology and treatment of stroke: present status and future perspectives. Int J Mol Sci. 2020;21(20):7609. https://doi.org/10.3390/ijms21207609. Accessed 16 Dec 2023
3. Saver JL. Time is brain-qualified. Stroke. 2006;37(1):263–6. https://doi.org/10.1161/01.STR.0000196957.55928.ab. Epub 2005 Dec 8
4. Barreto AD. Intravenous thrombolytics for ischemic stroke. Neurotherapeutics. 2011;8(3):388–99.
5. Jilani TN, Siddiqui AH. Tissue plasminogen activator. StatPearls Publishing; 2020. www.ncbi.nlm.nih.gov/books/NBK507917/#:~:text=Mechanism%20of%20Action. Accessed 16 Dec 2023
6. Hacke W, Donnan G, Fieschi C, Kaste M, von Kummer R, Broderick JP, Brott T, Frankel M, Grotta JC, Haley EC Jr, Kwiatkowski T, Levine SR, Lewandowski C, Lu M, Lyden P, Marler JR, Patel S, Tilley BC, Albers G, Bluhmki E, Wilhelm M, Hamilton S, ATLANTIS Trials Investigators; ECASS Trials Investigators; NINDS rt-PA Study Group Investigators. Association of outcome with early stroke treatment: pooled analysis of ATLANTIS, ECASS, and NINDS rt-PA stroke trials. Lancet. 2004;363(9411):768–74. https://doi.org/10.1016/S0140-6736(04)15692-4. PMID: 15016487
7. Emberson J, Lees KR, Lyden P, Blackwell L, Albers G, Bluhmki E, Brott T, Cohen G, Davis S, Donnan G, Grotta J, Howard G, Kaste M, Koga M, von Kummer R, Lansberg M, Lindley RI, Murray G, Olivot JM, Parsons M, Tilley B, Toni D, Toyoda K, Wahlgren N, Wardlaw J, Whiteley W, del Zoppo GJ, Baigent C, Sandercock P, Hacke W, Stroke Thrombolysis Trialists'

Collaborative Group. Effect of treatment delay, age, and stroke severity on the effects of intravenous thrombolysis with alteplase for acute ischaemic stroke: a meta-analysis of individual patient data from randomised trials. Lancet. 2014;384(9958):1929–35.

8. National Institute of Neurological Disorders and Stroke rt-PA Stroke Study Group. Tissue plasminogen activator for acute ischemic stroke. N Engl J Med. 1995;333(24):1581–7.

9. Hacke W, Kaste M, Bluhmki E, Brozman M, Dávalos A, Guidetti D, Larrue V, Lees KR, Medeghri Z, Machnig T, Schneider D, von Kummer R, Wahlgren N, Toni D, Investigators ECASS. Thrombolysis with alteplase 3 to 4.5 hours after acute ischemic stroke. N Engl J Med. 2008;359(13):1317–29.

10. Bhatia R, Hill MD, Shobha N, Menon B, Bal S, Kochar P, Watson T, Goyal M, Demchuk AM. Low rates of acute recanalization with intravenous recombinant tissue plasminogen activator in ischemic stroke: real-world experience and a call for action. Stroke. 2010;41(10):2254–8.

11. Warach SJ, Dula AN, Milling TJ Jr. Tenecteplase thrombolysis for acute ischemic stroke. Stroke. 2020;51(11):3440–51.

12. Murphy LR, Hill TP, Paul K, Talbott M, Golovko G, Shaltoni H, Jehle D. Tenecteplase versus alteplase for acute stroke: mortality and bleeding complications. Ann Emerg Med. 2023;82(6):720–8. https://doi.org/10.1016/j.annemergmed.2023.03.022. Epub 2023 May 12

13. Warach SJ, Dula AN, Milling TJ, Miller S, Allen L, Zuck ND, Miller C, Jesser CA, Misra LR, Miley JT, Mawla M, Ding MC, Bertelson JA, Tsui AY, Jefferson JR, Davison HM, Shah DN, Ellington KT, Padrick MM, Nova AS, Krishna VR, Davis LA, Paydarfar D. Prospective observational cohort study of tenecteplase versus alteplase in routine clinical practice. Stroke. 2022;53(12):3583–93. https://doi.org/10.1161/STROKEAHA.122.038950. Epub 2022 Sep 23

14. Powers WJ, Rabinstein AA, Ackerson T, Adeoye OM, Bambakidis NC, Becker K, Biller J, Brown M, Demaerschalk BM, Hoh B, Jauch EC, Kidwell CS, Leslie-Mazwi TM, Ovbiagele B, Scott PA, Sheth KN, Southerland AM, Summers DV, Tirschwell DL. Guidelines for the early management of patients with acute ischemic stroke: 2019 update to the 2018 guidelines for the early management of acute ischemic stroke: a guideline for healthcare professionals from the American Heart Association/American Stroke Association. Stroke. 2019;50(12):e344–418.

15. Rehani B, Ammanuel SG, Zhang Y, Smith W, Cooke DL, Hetts SW, Josephson SA, Kim A, Hemphill JC 3rd, Dillon W. A new era of extended time window acute stroke interventions guided by imaging. Neurohospitalist. 2020;10(1):29–37.

16. Schwamm LH, Wu O, Song SS, Latour LL, Ford AL, Hsia AW, Muzikansky A, Betensky RA, Yoo AJ, Lev MH, Boulouis G, Lauer A, Cougo P, Copen WA, Harris GJ, Warach S, MR WITNESS Investigators. Intravenous thrombolysis in unwitnessed stroke onset: MR WITNESS trial results. Ann Neurol. 2018;83(5):980–93.

17. Thomalla G, Simonsen CZ, Boutitie F, Andersen G, Berthezene Y, Cheng B, Cheripelli B, Cho TH, Fazekas F, Fiehler J, Ford I, Galinovic I, Gellissen S, Golsari A, Gregori J, Günther M, Guibernau J, Häusler KG, Hennerici M, Kemmling A, Marstrand J, Modrau B, Neeb L, Perez de la Ossa N, Puig J, Ringleb P, Roy P, Scheel E, Schonewille W, Serena J, Sunaert S, Villringer K, Wouters A, Thijs V, Ebinger M, Endres M, Fiebach JB, Lemmens R, Muir KW, Nighoghossian N, Pedraza S, Gerloff C, WAKE-UP Investigators. MRI-guided thrombolysis for stroke with unknown time of onset. N Engl J Med. 2018;379(7):611–22.

18. Hughes RE, et al. TPA therapy. Nih.gov, StatPearls Publishing, 22 Mar. 2019, www.ncbi.nlm. nih.gov/books/NBK482376/. Accessed 16 Dec 2023.

19. Monitoring Patients in the First 24 Hours | Activase® (Alteplase). Www.activase.com. www. activase.com/ais/dosing-and-administration/patient-monitoring.html. Accessed 17 Dec 2023.

20. Reish NJ, Jamshidi P, Stamm B, Flanagan ME, Sugg E, Tang M, Donohue KL, McCord M, Krumpelman C, Mesulam MM, Castellani R, Chou SH. Multiple cerebral hemorrhages in a patient receiving lecanemab and treated with t-PA for stroke. N Engl J Med. 2023;388(5):478–9. https://doi.org/10.1056/NEJMc2215148. Epub 2023 Jan 4. PMID: 36599061; PMCID: PMC10228637

21. Nicola L, et al. Tenecteplase versus alteplase for management of acute ischaemic stroke (NOR-TEST): a phase 3, randomised, open-label, blinded endpoint trial. Lancet Neurol. 16(10):781–88
22. Bruce CVC, et al. "Tenecteplase versus Alteplase before Thrombectomy for Ischemic Stroke." NEJM. 2018;378(17):1573–82. https://doi.org/10.1056/nejmoa1716405.

Acute Stroke Treatment: Thrombectomy

9

Nicole Veltri, Safa Hakim Elnazer, and Adam De Havenon

What Is a Large Vessel Occlusion?

A large vessel occlusion (LVO) typically refers to the occlusion of a larger intracranial vessel, such as the middle cerebral artery (MCA) or distal internal carotid artery (ICA), typically due to a larger clot (Fig. 9.1). LVO occurs in about one-third of all acute ischemic stroke patients, and is the indication for thrombectomy. The remaining two-thirds of ischemic stroke patients will have occlusions in smaller, more distal branches that are more responsive to thrombolytic therapy and typically beyond the reach of currently used catheter devices.

N. Veltri
Yale New Haven Hospital, New Haven, CT, USA
e-mail: Nicole.veltri@yale.edu

S. H. Elnazer · A. De Havenon (✉)
Yale School of Medicine, New Haven, CT, USA
e-mail: safa.abdelhakim@yale.edu; adam.dehavenon@yale.edu

© The Author(s), under exclusive license to Springer Nature Switzerland AG 2024
H. P. Amin (ed.), *Stroke for the Advanced Practice Clinician*,
https://doi.org/10.1007/978-3-031-66289-8_9

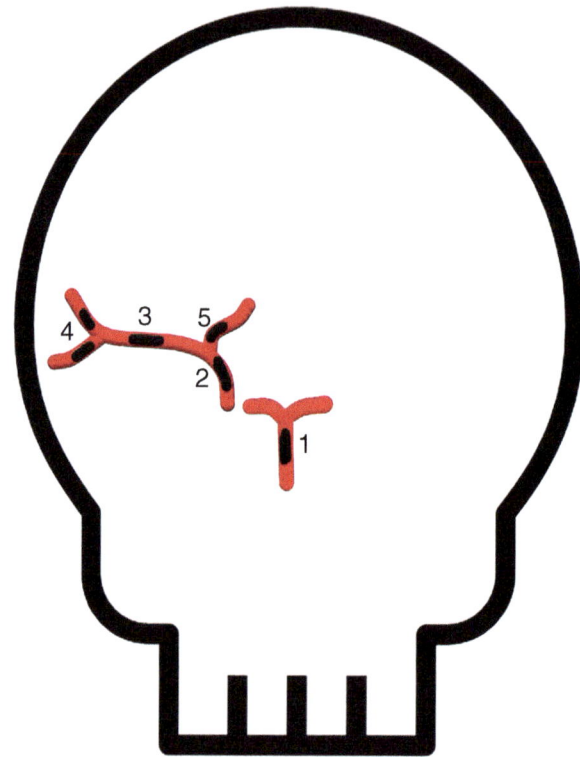

Fig. 9.1 LVO locations. (1) Basilar artery, (2) Distal internal carotid artery, (3) Middle cerebral artery M1 segment, (4) Middle cerebral artery M2 segments, (5) Anterior cerebral artery A1 segment

What Is a Thrombectomy?

An endovascular thrombectomy (EVT) is an invasive catheter-based procedure that retrieves the clot and opens the occluded vessel. Once a large vessel occlusion is identified clinically and via CTA, a neurologist and a neuro-interventionalist collaborate to determine if the procedure is appropriate.

Who Is Eligible for Thrombectomy?

Thrombectomy has a wide therapeutic time window (up to 24 h from symptom onset or LKW) and can be performed concurrently with thrombolytic therapy. Patients who are candidates for thrombolytic therapy should receive it even if there is an LVO and a thrombectomy is planned. Thrombectomy should not be delayed to assess for response to thrombolysis. In other words, eligible LVO patients should get thrombolytic therapy and go immediately for EVT; for alteplase, that means going to the endovascular suite while the infusion is running. Data have shown that concomitant use of IV alteplase and thrombectomy can improve outcomes [1]. Another reason to administer thrombolytics for eligible patients is that while thrombectomy success rates are very good, procedural success is not guaranteed.

Per the 2018 AHA Guidelines for Management of Acute Ischemic Stroke, patients should receive thrombectomy if they meet the following eligibility criteria: pre-stroke mRS score 0–1 (although clinical practice can vary and patients with higher mRS are sometimes included), causative occlusion of the ICA or MCA segment, ≥ 18 years of age, NIHSS ≥6, ASPECTS of ≥6 (which is discussed in the Chap. 4), and ideally initiation of treatment within 6 h of symptoms onset (Table 9.1) [2]. Patients who do not strictly meet the AHA recommendations for EVT may still be eligible but would require further consideration of risk versus benefit. For example, a patient who uses a wheelchair with new onset aphasia and arm weakness from LVO would still benefit from a thrombectomy. In addition to these guidelines, thrombectomy can be considered in patients within the 6-h window of symptom onset found to have an occlusion of the M2 or M3 segments of the MCA, the anterior cerebral artery (ACA) or within the posterior circulation due to occlusion of the vertebral artery, basilar artery, or posterior cerebral artery. However, the benefits of EVT in these vessels are less certain [2].

There are logistical aspects to keep in mind regarding the thrombectomy procedure. The first is availability. If thrombectomy is not available, the patient must be transferred emergently to the nearest thrombectomy-capable or comprehensive

Table 9.1 Thrombectomy eligibility criteria

Indications for EVT 0–6 h from onset	• Pre-stroke mRS score of 0–1[a]
	• Occlusion of internal carotid or MCA segment 1 (M1)
	• Age more ≥18 years
	• NIHSS score ≥6
	• ASPECTS ≥6
	• Treatment initiation within 6 h
	• The benefits of EVT should be discussed if
	  – Occlusion of MCA segment 2 (M2) or MCA segment 3 (M3)
	  – Occlusion of the anterior cerebral artery, vertebral arteries, basilar artery, or posterior cerebral arteries

Indications for EVT 6–24 h from onset	• Age ≥18 years
	• Failed or contraindicated for IV tPA
	• NIHSS ≥10
	• Pre-stroke -mRS 0–1
	• Time last seen well: 6–24 h
	  – Infarct size <1/3 MCA territory by CT or MRI
	• ICA-T or MCA-M1 occlusion
	  – Clinical imaging mismatch:
	    Age ≥80 years, NIHSS ≥10 + core <21 mL on CTP
	    Age <80 years, NIHSS ≥10 + core <31 mL on CTP
	    Age <80 years, NIHSS ≥20 + core <51 mL on CTP

[a] mRS alone should not be the sole determinant, as much as a proper understanding of the disability and whether the procedure might still salvage a vital function

stroke center. The next factor is time. If a patient presents 6 h or more from symptom onset or last known well (LKW) time, further imaging with CT Perfusion (CTP) can be beneficial to detect the presence of an ischemic core and penumbra. CTP is discussed in greater detail in the Chap. 4, but in brief, a patient with a small core infarct and large penumbra is usually a good candidate for the procedure.

Who Is Not Eligible for Thrombectomy?

At this time, patients with clear ischemia on CT (downstream to the occluded vessel, and that explains the patient's symptoms) and unfavorable CTP profiles typically would not benefit from thrombectomy. Not only is there limited benefit, but opening up a vessel for an established stroke can risk hemorrhagic conversion. Newer data are emerging, however, showing that carefully selected patients with "unfavorable" imaging may still benefit. Patients with severe disability at baseline are unlikely to gain benefit. Clots in distal portions of vessels (i.e., the M3 segment of the MCA or A1 segment of the ACA) are often felt to be too distal for current devices to reach.

How Does the Procedure Work?

A thrombectomy is a catheter-based procedure that requires transporting the patient to a sterile interventional suite. Catheter access for the thrombectomy procedure is often through the femoral artery in the groin. In this approach, a catheter is threaded through the aortic arch, up the carotid or vertebral artery, and passed through the occluded segment. The most recent version of catheters is the stent retriever, or "stentriever," where a mesh "stent" is deployed into the clot, which expands to stretch the artery's walls and captures the clot. The stent is then pulled back and retrieved, bringing the clot with it into a larger catheter that is then completely removed from the artery. The interventionalist, after the clot is retrieved, injects contrast through the artery to ensure it is fully recanalized. Several attempts, or "passes," to remove the clot may be necessary. Another approach is direct suctioning or aspiration of the clot instead of using stent retrievers, whereby a catheter is brought directly up to the location of the clot and suctioned back [3]. The interventionalist will often discuss the most appropriate approach with a stroke neurologist.

What Is the Data?

Historically, the strict time window of up to 4.5 h from symptom onset has determined eligibility for acute stroke treatment. There has been a paradigm shift with an extension of the time window from symptom onset up to 24 h for thrombectomy, using advanced perfusion imaging in determining thrombectomy eligibility in the extended window. MR CLEAN is one of the earlier thrombectomy trials that enrolled patients within 6 h of stroke symptoms. However, later trials, like DEFUSE 3 and DAWN, expanded the window from symptom onset for selected patients and still demonstrated significant functional benefit (Table 9.1) [4–6]. The 2018 AHA guidelines had new EVT recommendations based on the DAWN and DEFUSE 3 trials, which expanded the LKW window to 24 h in patients with an LVO in the anterior circulation (distal ICA or MCA) [2]. Although patients who are treated as quickly as possible from symptom onset time tend to have better clinical outcomes, these trials had neuroimaging inclusion criteria that allowed for the identification of a large group of LVO patients who still derive benefit from thrombectomy in the 6–24-h window where brain tissue had not yet completely infarcted [2].

How Do You Interpret the ASPECTS Score and Perfusion Imaging?

Various aspects of the patient presentation determine if a patient would benefit from thrombectomy, including the NIH Stroke Scale (NIHSS), Alberta Stroke Program Early CT Score (ASPECTS) score, clinical-imaging mismatch, and perfusion-imaging mismatch. ASPECTS is a 10-point scoring system with anatomic regions distributed over the MCA territory (exact locations are reviewed in Chap. 4). One point is subtracted for early ischemic changes in any of the ten anatomic areas to calculate the ASPECTS score, with lower numbers indicating more infarcted tissue and 10 being a completely normal CT scan [7]. The thinking that more early infarcted tissue is less likely to benefit from treatment led to the exclusion of LVO patients with ASPECTS of 5 or lower from most EVT trials. New data, however, suggest that patients with lower ASPECTS may still benefit from thrombectomy [8].

An additional important factor to consider is the collateral supply of blood flow for the compromised tissue. When a patient has an LVO, the downstream tissue could still get blood flow through additional blood vessels, known as "collateral supply." The degree of collateral flow is probably based on individual genetics, not lifestyle or health conditions. Think of collaterals as bypass routes or detours on a highway with a section closed down. Robust collaterals (more roads) allow blood flow (traffic) to keep moving, whereas fewer collateral vessels will lead to less blood flow and traffic jams. The presence of robust collaterals, therefore, can help keep at-risk brain tissue downstream to an LVO salvageable for more extended periods, and lack of collaterals probably leads to faster progression to irreversible stroke. Patients with robust collaterals, not surprisingly, tend to have better outcomes after reperfusion treatments, including alteplase and thrombectomy [9].

On perfusion imaging, one can identify the ischemic core, which is a tissue that is irreversibly injured and would not benefit from revascularization, and ischemic penumbra, which is ischemic (symptomatic) tissue that is receiving less blood flow compared to normal brain tissue but is still viable. The penumbra is the target of EVT to prevent a smaller core from growing to the size of the penumbra. Perfusion imaging using MRI or CT can evaluate the ischemic core versus penumbra, with the

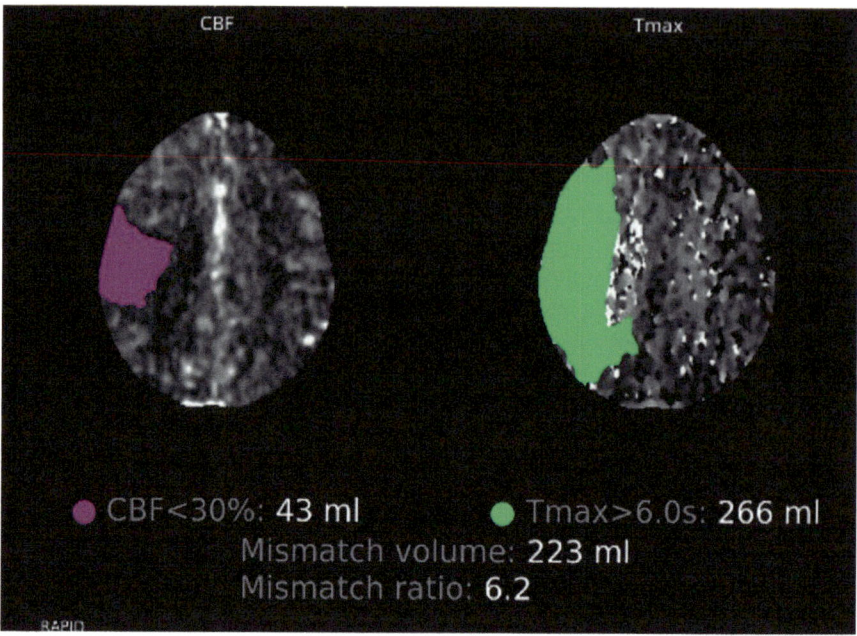

Fig. 9.2 CTP demonstrates a small core (magenta) and large penumbra (green) with a large mismatch volume (potentially salvageable tissue)

latter being more readily available. The cerebral blood flow (CBF) is less than 30% of normal levels in the ischemic core [10]. A large difference (or mismatch) between the core and penumbra indicates salvageable tissue that would benefit from thrombectomy (Fig. 9.2).

How Do You Describe the Results of a Thrombectomy?

Thrombectomy aims to re-establish blood flow through the previously occluded vessel. Following the procedure, a reperfusion score is determined based on the resulting flow through the previously blocked artery, called the Thrombolysis in Cerebral Infarction (TICI) Scale (Table 9.2), with a goal score of TICI3 indicating complete revascularization [11]. Reperfusion success correlates with patient outcomes, although the established "core" stroke before thrombectomy and patient factors such as age and medical comorbidities also impact outcomes [12]. It is essential to document the TICI score and communicate it to other providers taking care of the patient following a thrombectomy.

Table 9.2   Thrombolysis in cerebral infarction (TICI) scoring system

Treatment in cerebral ischemic (TICI) scale	
0	No reperfusion
1	Flow beyond occlusion without distal branch reperfusion
2a	Reperfusion of less than half of the downstream target arterial territory
2b	Reperfusion of more than half, yet incomplete, in the downstream target arterial territory
2c	Near complete perfusion without clearly visible thrombus but with delay in contrast run-off
3	Complete reperfusion of the downstream target arterial territory, including distal branches with slow flow

What Are the Post-Procedure Considerations?

Following EVT, providers may target specific blood pressure goals based on the TICI score or additional patient factors, including the patient's initial blood pressure. Evidence suggests that patients with lower blood pressure post-treatment may have better outcomes than those with higher ones. However, a universal approach to an exact target blood pressure goal is challenging to determine. For example, a patient with a large core infarct is at higher risk for reperfusion injury (additional damage to the already infarcted tissue due to the abrupt return of blood supply to the area) and may benefit from lower target blood pressure. On the other hand, it is essential to avoid rapid, aggressive lowering of blood pressure as it may lead to worse outcomes [13]. Aiming for systolic blood pressure of <180 for patients with successful recanalization with high TICI scores is reasonable, especially for patients who received thrombolytics.

As with any invasive procedure, there are peri-procedural and post-procedural risks and complications associated with thrombectomy. Patients may have allergies to iodinated contrast (1–12%), although severe reactions are rare. Contrast-induced nephropathy is a possible complication, although relatively uncommon [14]. Intra-procedural complications may occur, including re-occlusion of the target artery, vasospasm of the vessel, vessel perforation from the catheter wire, intracranial hemorrhage, cerebral edema, or death. Clots might also embolize after catheter manipulation, lodging in smaller downstream vessels and increasing stroke burden. Complications may also occur at the catheter access site, including bleeding and hematoma formation, pseudoaneurysm, or retroperitoneal hemorrhage [14]. Bleeding may be controlled with local pressure, but more complex complications may require surgical treatment.

Early detection with neurological and vascular monitoring should detect complications following thrombectomy. Neurovascular checks include evaluating distal pulses, hematoma, bleeding, or ecchymosis at the access site. They should be completed every 15 min for 2 h, every 30 min for 6 h, and then every hour for 16 h. In addition, NIHSS and pupil checks should be completed and documented using the same timeline [14].

Clinical Pearls
- Thrombectomy increases the likelihood of functional recovery for patients with a large vessel occlusion.
- Patients are candidates for EVT if pre-stroke mRS score is 0–1, causative occlusion of the ICA or MCA segment 1, >/= 18 years of age, NIHSS >/= 6, ASPECTS of >/= 6, and initiation of treatment is ideally within 6 h of symptoms onset.
- Thrombectomy can be considered in patients beyond 6 h with a favorable perfusion profile, other vessel occlusions (ACA, PCA, and Basilar artery), and lower ASPECTS scores.
- Factors to consider while making thrombectomy decisions include the clinical exam, mismatch between core infarct and penumbra on CTP, baseline functional status, and goals of care.
- Treatment in Cerebral Ischemic Scale (TICI) scores assess reperfusion success to intracranial vessels, with TICI 0 being the lowest and TICI 3 being the highest.
- There are various complications to be aware of after thrombectomy, including vasospasm of the vessel, vessel perforation, intracranial hemorrhage, and cerebral edema.
- Post-thrombectomy patients need clear blood pressure parameters and frequent neurological monitoring in an ICU setting to detect and manage any complications.

Notable Trials Summary

- Hermes meta-analysis: A meta-analysis pooled data from five thrombectomy trials: MR CLEAN, ESCAPE, REVASCAT, SWIFT PRIME, and EXTEND IA. Patients who presented with proximal large vessel occlusion were assigned to receive thrombectomy versus medical therapy within 12 h of symptom onset. Forty-six percent of patients achieved functional independence at 90 days in the thrombectomy group compared to 27% in the medical management group [15].
- DEFUSE 3: Multicenter, randomized, open-label trial that compared outcomes in patients managed 6–16 h from last known well with a proximal MCA or ICA occlusion, who had an NIHSS ≥6 and a radiologic mismatch between the penumbra and core infarct, who received thrombectomy versus medical management. Perfusion imaging helped to assess the eligibility of patients who would undergo thrombectomy. Patients had to have an infarct size of less than 70 ml and a ratio of the volume of the brain tissue at risk (penumbra) to the volume of

infarcted tissue of 1.8 or more. Forty-five percent of patients in the thrombectomy group achieved functional independence at 90 days, compared to only 17% in the medical therapy group. Ninety-day mortality was also less in the thrombectomy group [5].

- DAWN: A multicenter, prospective randomized open-label trial comparing outcomes in patients with an intracranial ICA occlusion or a proximal middle cerebral artery occlusion 6–12 h from last known well who had a mismatch between their clinical deficits and imaging treated with thrombectomy versus medical management. Patients had to have NIHSS ≥ 10, and a maximum infarct volume of 51 ml. Forty-nine percent of patients in the thrombectomy group achieved functional independence at 90 days compared to 13% in the medical therapy group. The selective criteria are difficult to generalize [6].

References

1. Masoud HE, Dehavenon A, et al. 2022 Brief practice update on intravenous thrombolysis before thrombectomy in patients with large vessel occlusion acute ischemic stroke: a statement from society of vascular and interventional neurology guidelines and practice standards (GAPS) committee. Stroke Vasc Interv Neurol. 2022;2:e000276. https://doi.org/10.1161/SVIN.121.000276.
2. Powers WJ, Rabinstein AA, Ackerson T, et al. Guidelines for the early management of patients with acute ischemic stroke: 2019 update to the 2018 guidelines for the early management of acute ischemic stroke: a guideline for healthcare professionals from the American Heart Association/American Stroke Association [published correction appears in stroke. 2019;50(12):e440-e441]. Stroke. 2019;50(12):e344–418. https://doi.org/10.1161/STR.0000000000000211.
3. Turk AS 3rd, Siddiqui A, Fifi JT, et al. Aspiration thrombectomy versus stent retriever thrombectomy as first-line approach for large vessel occlusion (COMPASS): a multicentre, randomised, open label, blinded outcome, non-inferiority trial. Lancet. 2019;393(10175):998–1008. https://doi.org/10.1016/S0140-6736(19)30297-1.
4. Fransen PS, Beumer D, Berkhemer OA, et al. MR CLEAN, a multicenter randomized clinical trial of endovascular treatment for acute ischemic stroke in The Netherlands: study protocol for a randomized controlled trial. Trials. 2014;15:343. Published 2014. https://doi.org/10.1186/1745-6215-15-343.
5. Albers GW, Marks MP, Kemp S, et al. Thrombectomy for stroke at 6 to 16 hours with selection by perfusion imaging. N Engl J Med. 2018;378(8):708–18. https://doi.org/10.1056/NEJMoa1713973.
6. Nogueira RG, Jadhav AP, Haussen DC, et al. Thrombectomy 6 to 24 hours after stroke with a mismatch between deficit and infarct. N Engl J Med. 2018;378(1):11–21. https://doi.org/10.1056/NEJMoa1706442.
7. Pexman JH, Barber PA, Hill MD, et al. Use of the alberta stroke program early CT score (ASPECTS) for assessing CT scans in patients with acute stroke. AJNR Am J Neuroradiol. 2001;22(8):1534–42.
8. Goyal M, Menon BK, van Zwam WH, et al. Endovascular thrombectomy after large-vessel ischaemic stroke: a meta-analysis of individual patient data from five randomised trials. Lancet. 2016;387(10029):1723–31. https://doi.org/10.1016/S0140-6736(16)00163-X.
9. Lima FO, Furie KL, Silva GS, et al. The pattern of leptomeningeal collaterals on CT angiography is a strong predictor of long-term functional outcome in stroke patients with

large vessel intracranial occlusion. Stroke. 2010;41(10):2316–22. https://doi.org/10.1161/STROKEAHA.110.592303.

10. González RG. Imaging-guided acute ischemic stroke therapy: from "time is brain" to "physiology is brain". AJNR Am J Neuroradiol. 2006;27(4):728–35.

11. Wintermark M, Albers GW, Alexandrov AV, et al. Acute stroke imaging research roadmap. AJNR Am J Neuroradiol. 2008;29(5):e23–30. https://doi.org/10.1161/STROKEAHA.107.512319.

12. Goyal M, Fargen KM, Turk AS, et al. 2C or not 2C: defining an improved revascularization grading scale and the need for standardization of angiography outcomes in stroke trials. J Neurointerv Surg. 2014;6(2):83–6. https://doi.org/10.1136/neurintsurg-2013-010665.

13. Peng TJ, Ortega-Gutiérrez S, de Havenon A, Petersen NH. Blood pressure management after endovascular thrombectomy. Front Neurol. 2021;12:723461. Published 2021 Sep 3. https://doi.org/10.3389/fneur.2021.723461.

14. Jadhav AP, Molyneaux BJ, Hill MD, Jovin TG. Care of the post-thrombectomy patient. Stroke. 2018;49(11):2801–7. https://doi.org/10.1161/STROKEAHA.118.021640.

15. Goyal M, Menon BK, van Zwam WH, Dippel DW, Mitchell PJ, Demchuk AM, Dávalos A, Majoie CB, van der Lugt A, de Miquel MA, Donnan GA, Roos YB, Bonafe A, Jahan R, Diener HC, van den Berg LA, Levy EI, Berkhemer OA, Pereira VM, Rempel J, Millán M, Davis SM, Roy D, Thornton J, Román LS, Ribó M, Beumer D, Stouch B, Brown S, Campbell BC, van Oostenbrugge RJ, Saver JL, Hill MD, Jovin TG, HERMES Collaborators. Endovascular thrombectomy after large-vessel ischaemic stroke: a meta-analysis of individual patient data from five randomised trials. Lancet. 2016;387(10029):1723–31. https://doi.org/10.1016/S0140-6736(16)00163-X. Epub 2016 Feb 18

Transient Ischemic Attack

10

Mary Ann Harmon, Neeharika Thottempudi, and Hardik P. Amin

Definition

The traditional definition of transient ischemic attack (TIA) is "focal neurological dysfunction confined to an area of the brain or eye, presumed to be of vascular origin perfused by a specific cerebral artery and symptoms lasting for less than 24 h" [1]. This time-based definition of < 24 h has been debated since the 1980s. Several studies showed that diffusion-weighted imaging (DWI) changes on brain MRI can still occur in about one-third of patients with transient neurologic symptoms, which changes the diagnosis from TIA to stroke. The tissue-based definition is now widely accepted, which describes TIA as a transient episode of neurological dysfunction caused by focal brain, spinal cord, or retinal ischemia without evidence of acute infarction on DWI [1]. If the MRI is positive, the diagnosis changes from TIA to stroke with resolved symptoms.

A transient ischemic attack (TIA) should be considered a warning of an imminent stroke, with subsequent stroke risk estimates ranging from 7.5% to 17.3% in the first 3 months and at least half of those events occurring in the first 2 days [1].

M. A. Harmon
Yale New Haven Hospital, New Haven, CT, USA
e-mail: maryann.harmon@yale.edu

N. Thottempudi
Carson Tahoe Health, Carson City, NV, USA
e-mail: neeharika.thottempudi@yale.edu

H. P. Amin (✉)
Hartford Hospital, Hartford, CT, USA
e-mail: hardik.amin@hhchealth.org

© The Author(s), under exclusive license to Springer Nature Switzerland AG 2024
H. P. Amin (ed.), *Stroke for the Advanced Practice Clinician*,
https://doi.org/10.1007/978-3-031-66289-8_10

Furthermore, MRI positivity can suggest a sixfold increase in recurrent stroke risk in 1 year, which is why the tissue-based definition can help identify higher risk patients [2]. The challenge in accurately diagnosing a TIA is that symptoms may have resolved when a patient gets medical attention. Despite symptoms being transient or even mild, one should not take that to mean that the underlying problem is benign. When discussing the implications of a TIA with a patient, point out what a TIA *represents*: that some medical condition (either sub-optimally treated or even undiagnosed at the time) is putting them at risk of a future disabling or fatal stroke, and that is an emergency. TIA and stroke have the same risk factors: hypertension, diabetes, smoking, carotid disease, cardiac arrhythmia, and older age, to name a few. Some risk factors (carotid stenosis, arrhythmia) can lead to a full-blown stroke fairly quickly after an initial TIA. Therefore, both deserve an expedited evaluation with the rapid implementation of a secondary stroke prevention plan. Deferring a TIA workup to the routine outpatient setting can delay the detection and treatment of important risk factors, placing that patient at higher risk of a preventable stroke.

Epidemiology and Risk Factors

The true incidence of TIA is difficult to determine given the lack of a standardized monitoring system and the transitory nature of symptoms, which makes accurate diagnosis challenging. A large 2002 population-based study conservatively estimated a yearly incidence of 240,000 TIAs in the United States [3]. The study also found that the incidence of TIA appears to increase with age, regardless of race or gender. Additionally, there are well-documented racial and ethnic disparities in stroke and TIA, which will be discussed in greater depth in the Chap. 38. Black patients have approximately twice the risk of stroke incidence and higher mortality than Caucasians. Other cohort studies have demonstrated higher stroke risk in Hispanic/Latino Americans than Caucasians [4, 5].

Like stroke, TIA risk factors are categorized into modifiable (medical and behavioral) and nonmodifiable groups (Table 10.1) [4]. The nonmodifiable (untreatable) risk factors include age, sex, race, ethnicity, and certain hereditary conditions. Since any of these risk factors can contribute to a TIA or stroke, it is incumbent on the provider to perform a comprehensive risk factor evaluation.

Table 10.1 Modifiable risk factors for TIA

Medical	Behavioral
Hypertension	Smoking
Diabetes mellitus	Substance abuse (including alcohol)
Carotid stenosis	Sedentary lifestyle
Atrial fibrillation	Diet/nutrition
Hyperlipidema	
Hematological disorders	
Obstructive sleep apnea	

How Do You Differentiate a TIA from Other Diagnoses?

The main criteria for diagnosing TIA require a history with symptoms attributable to a brain vascular territory and normal brain imaging. It can be challenging to differentiate stroke or TIA from mimics such as migraine, vertigo, seizures followed by Todd's paralysis, multiple sclerosis, hypoglycemia, or peripheral nerve injury. Cerebrovascular events are typically painless and acute in onset. Symptoms are often maximal at onset or might "stutter" after onset and resolve quickly. Factors that *might* point to a TIA mimic are a young patient with no vascular risk factors, dizziness only triggered by movement that resolves with rest, a history of seizures followed by weakness, pain or migraine headache with neurological symptoms, brain tumor, or symptoms spreading from one site to another (Jacksonian march suggesting seizure) (Table 10.2). Stroke mimics are discussed in greater detail in their own chapter. With nonspecific symptoms, the key is to dig for any focal symptoms like double vision with both eyes open (binocular diplopia), dysequilibrium at rest, ataxia, aphasia, dysmetria, or hemiparesis that might raise suspicion for a vascular process. In cases with diagnostic uncertainty or a lack of neurovascular expertise, it would be appropriate to still perform a complete neurovascular workup for a suspected TIA [6].

Table 10.2 Symptoms suggestive of stroke vs stroke mimics. This table should be used as a guide only and should not supersede clinical judgment

Stroke	Stroke mimics
Sudden onset and maximal symptoms on presentation	Symptoms spreading from one site to another (suggestive of seizure)
Vertigo with ataxia/dysmetria and cranial nerve deficits	Isolated vertigo with positional component
Sudden onset loss of consciousness with pupillary changes, hemodynamic instability	Loss of consciousness with triggering factors and prodromal symptoms, quick return to baseline
Facial droop with associated hemiparesis/other cranial nerve deficits	Isolated upper and lower facial weakness – peripheral seventh nerve palsy
Sudden onset severe thunderclap headache	Gradual onset headache preceded by visual or sensory aura
Headache, neck pain with ptosis, miosis might suggest dissection	

Table 10.3 ABCD^2 score for TIA risk stratification, with a max score of 7

Age ≥ 60 years	1 point
BP ≥ $\frac{140}{90}$ mmHg	1 point
Clinical features of TIA	Unilateral weakness: +2 points
	Speech disturbance without weakness: +1 point
	Other symptoms: 0 points
Duration of symptoms	<10 min: 0 points
	10–59 min: +1 point
	≥60 min: +2 points
History of diabetes	1 point

Determining Risk of Stroke Following a TIA

Clinical risk stratification tools such as the ABCD^2 score help stratify patients into low, moderate, and high risk of an early recurrent stroke [7]. The ABCD^2 score gives a numerical value based on the clinical and medical history and provides an aggregate score that places the patient into a low (0–3), moderate (4–5), or high-risk (6–7) group (Table 10.3). High and moderate-risk patients have an 8.1% and 4.1% risk of stroke in the following 2 days, respectively [6, 7]. Therefore, patients in the moderate or high-risk groups warrant hospitalization for closer monitoring and expedited workup. However, the ABCD^2 score has its limitations. It does not include brain or vascular imaging results, history of recurrent events (sometimes called "dual TIA"), or atrial fibrillation. These are all considered strong risk factors (and treatable in the case of AF or carotid stenosis) that can be missed if the decision to discharge a patient from the ED is based on the ABCD^2 score alone. Even a patient with a low ABCD^2 score can be at high risk without a thorough evaluation with proper imaging and a detailed history.

Performing an Expedited Work-up for a TIA Patient

All patients with suspected TIA should get imaging, laboratory, and cardiac testing. Initial lab studies should include point-of-care glucose testing, complete blood count, chemistry panel, hemoglobin A1c, and lipid profile. Patients over the age of 50 years who report visual symptoms need erythrocyte sedimentation rate (ESR) and C-reactive protein (CRP) to assess for temporal arteritis [3].

After basic laboratory testing, a noncontrast head CT rules out hemorrhage or any structural causes that could explain the patient's symptoms. Based on the current tissue-based definition of TIA, all patients should undergo an MRI of the brain imaging to look for acute stroke on the DWI sequence (which would not be seen on CT). If an MRI is available quickly, skipping a CT is reasonable for a patient *with completely resolved symptoms* who would otherwise not be a candidate for thrombolytics. An MRI should be done while the patient is in the ED to guide disposition

(MRI positivity means stroke and typically warrants full admission). If an MRI is unavailable from the ED within a reasonable timeframe (a few hours), admitting the patient for an expedited MRI within 24 h is reasonable.

Vessel imaging with a CT angiogram of the head and neck is a rapid way to rule out symptomatic intracranial and cervical carotid disease, and requires iodinated contrast. If a patient cannot receive iodinated contrast due to allergy or severe kidney disease, an MRA head without contrast can be obtained, but this only views the intracranial vessels. MRA neck to view the carotid arteries requires gadolinium contrast for a quality study. An alternative for neck vessels is a carotid duplex ultrasound, which is only available for inpatients but may be available through a dedicated TIA observation unit.

A cardiac examination should also be completed. ECG can help rule out acute myocardial infarction and evaluate for atrial fibrillation, although the sensitivity of a single 10-s ECG to detect atrial fibrillation is only 1.5% [8]. A transthoracic echocardiogram (TTE) is required to rule out structural heart disease, but for a low-risk patient without acute cardiac concerns, this could be arranged as an outpatient if done promptly. If an arrhythmia is suspected, 30-day cardiac monitoring will evaluate for atrial fibrillation [6]. For TIA patients with negative MRI, suspect a cardioembolic process like atrial fibrillation for older patients (typically >60) with normal vasculature, especially if the episode includes aphasia, monocular vision loss, or homonymous hemianopia. Aphasia, vision loss, neglect, and gaze deviation are symptoms often caused by an embolic process. A 30-day cardiac monitor will increase the sensitivity of detecting AF to 55% and can be arranged through a stroke/TIA clinic or cardiologist [8].

Admit Vs. Discharge?

Deciding to admit or discharge a TIA patient from the ED is challenging. *Most institutions will admit patients with MRI-positive findings or ipsilateral carotid stenosis of >50%.* Refer to Fig. 10.1 for a potential pathway. Disposition for the TIA patient depends on factors such as $ABCD^2$ score representing low versus high-risk TIA, imaging results, available resources to obtain a timely TTE, and availability of rapid stroke/TIA clinic follow-up. A patient with a low $ABCD^2$ score (0-3), normal vessel imaging, and negative MRI could be appropriate for ED discharge as long as timely outpatient TTE and follow-up are arranged. Studies have shown that managing selected low-risk patients in outpatient TIA clinics (if available) can be safe and cost-effective, avoiding the need for hospitalization [10]. The decision to admit or discharge a patient will ultimately depend on the resources available to a particular center and its risk tolerance.

Patients discharged from the ED should ideally be scheduled to follow up in stroke prevention or TIA clinic within 2 weeks of ED discharge. For admitted patients seen by neurologists in the hospital, the neurologist will recommend the timing of follow-up. Many areas do not have rapid access to an in-person neurology

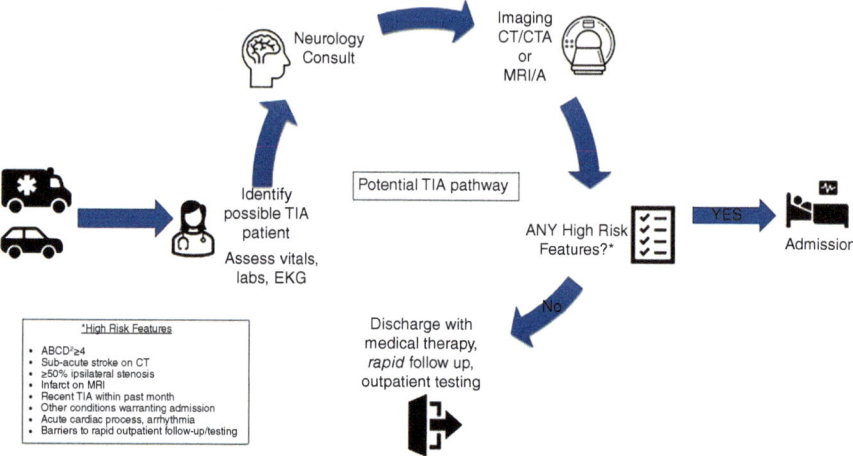

Fig. 10.1 A potential TIA pathway that incorporates clinical evaluation, imaging, and risk stratification to guide disposition decisions. Modifications are expected when rapid neurology consult or MRI is not available [9]

clinic, if at all. If possible, consider a telemedicine referral with a stroke specialist at the closest stroke center or academic hospital in these situations.

Secondary Stroke Prevention

Understanding why the patient had a TIA will guide the secondary stroke prevention strategy. Secondary stroke prevention strategies include antithrombotic agents, statins, anti-hypertensives, and diabetes treatment [6]. Patients with presumed symptomatic carotid artery stenosis should be evaluated for revascularization. Consider anticoagulation for patients with a history of atrial fibrillation; otherwise, antiplatelet is usually reasonable. A comprehensive secondary stroke prevention strategy can lead to an 80% reduction in stroke risk after a TIA [6]. We will briefly review the main points here, but a subsequent chapter covers secondary stroke prevention for ischemic stroke in greater depth.

1. **Antithrombotics:** Antiplatelet therapy is the standard of care for most TIA patients who do not have AF and should start within 24 h of presentation. Monotherapy with aspirin is appropriate for low-risk TIA, determined by an $ABCD^2$ score <4 [6, 11]. Dual antiplatelet therapy using aspirin plus clopidogrel can be considered for the first 21 days (followed by aspirin monotherapy) in those with high-risk TIA, defined as an $ABCD^2$ score ≥ 4 [12, 13]. For patients with known or newly diagnosed atrial fibrillation, immediate initiation of anticoagulation from the ED is safe, assuming the patient has a negative MRI.

2. **Hyperlipidemia:** The SPARCL trial demonstrated the role of statins in primary and secondary stroke prevention [14]. The target LDL for TIA and stroke patients

should be <70 mg/dL. The Treat Stroke to Target trial showed that an LDL goal of <70 mg/dL had a 28% lower relative risk of stroke compared to <100 mg/dL [15]. Patients may report side effects when starting statins, such as myopathy (muscle aches and weakness) or GI symptoms. While all statins might cause myopathy, rosuvastatin (Crestor) tends to have lower rates than others [16]; therefore, simply switching statins might resolve the symptoms. Interestingly, a recent meta-analysis demonstrated that most reports of muscle symptoms by patients taking statins were not due to their use; therefore, it is essential to rule out other causes as well [17]. For patients who are intolerant to all statins (and after ruling out any other reversible causes), consider ezetimibe or PCSK-9 inhibitors. The utility of statins is uncertain for patients already at goal LDL without any atherosclerosis on imaging.

3. **Hypertension:** Many patients with TIA and stroke will present with elevated blood pressure. It is important, however, not to reduce blood pressure acutely until carotid stenosis is ruled out. Aggressively lowering BP for someone with severe stenosis might lead to a recurrence of stroke symptoms. Long-term blood pressure goals in the outpatient setting, with a target of less than 130/80, are achieved over weeks by working closely with the patient's primary care provider. Achievement of this goal has shown a reduction in recurrent stroke risk by 22% [6].

4. **Diabetes:** A screening hemoglobin A1c is recommended for all patients with suspected TIA, with a goal A1c of <6 [3]. Those who require medications may start on metformin along with a recommendation for lifestyle optimization, including a referral to nutrition [6].

5. **Referrals:** All patients who have experienced a TIA should be seen by a neurologist, ideally trained in stroke. Some patients may require cardiology referrals for extended cardiac monitoring, uncontrolled hypertension, or newly diagnosed arrhythmia or heart disease. Consider referrals to nutrition and endocrinology clinics for poorly controlled diabetics. Patients with reliance on tobacco, alcohol, and other substances should be referred to outpatient counseling services [6]. Consider a sleep study for those suspected of having sleep apnea, an often-overlooked risk factor for stroke and TIA.

Role of the Advanced Practice Clinician (APC)

The demand for high-quality care for all TIA patients continues to challenge healthcare providers. The APC can be an excellent resource for the TIA patient since the demand for physicians far exceeds the current supply. A well-prepared APC can provide rapid follow-up and quality, evidence-based care for TIA patients in outpatient transitional care clinics [18].

Research has shown that APC stroke clinics can influence hospital readmissions in several ways. The APC can spend more patient-centered time completing detailed physical examinations and medication reconciliation, assuring the patient has filled prescriptions. APCs can explain prescribed medications, ensure the patient is compliant with directions, and follow up on referrals. In addition, the APC can spend more time reviewing test results and imaging with the patient and family [18].

> **Clinical Pearls**
> - A TIA represents a higher risk of future stroke.
> - Counseling patients on the importance of a TIA workup to reduce stroke risk helps facilitate rapid completion of the workup.
> - TIA symptoms should be referred to the emergency room.
> - Risk scores have limitations and should not be used in isolation to identify a low-risk patient.
> - Resolved symptoms with positive MRI findings is no longer a TIA, but a stroke with resolved symptoms.
> - Discharging a TIA patient from the ED requires negative imaging results, no significant risk factors, and availability of close outpatient follow-up.

References

1. Degan D, Ornello R, Tiseo C, De Santis F, Pistoia F, Carolei A, Sacco S. Epidemiology of transient ischemic attacks using time- or tissue-based definitions: a population-based study. Stroke. 2017;48(3):530–6. https://doi.org/10.1161/STROKEAHA.116.015417. Epub 2017 Jan 31. PMID: 28143922
2. Cucchiara BL, Messe SR, Taylor RA, Pacelli J, Maus D, Shah Q, Kasner SE. Is the ABCD score useful for risk stratification of patients with acute transient ischemic attack? Stroke. 2006;37(7):1710–4. https://doi.org/10.1161/01.STR.0000227195.46336.93. Epub 2006 Jun 8. PMID: 16763186
3. Kleindorfer DO, Towfighi A, Chaturvedi S, Cockroft KM, Gutierrez J, Lombardi-Hill D, Kamel H, Kernan WN, Kittner SJ, Leira EC, Lennon O, Meschia JF, Nguyen TN, Pollak PM, Santangeli P, Sharrief AZ, Smith SC Jr, Turan TN, Williams LS. 2021 guideline for the prevention of stroke in patients with stroke and transient ischemic attack: a guideline from the American Heart Association/American Stroke Association. Stroke. 2021;52(7):e364–467.
4. Boehme AK, Esenwa C, Elkind MS. Stroke risk factors, genetics, and prevention. Circ Res. 2017;120(3):472–95. https://doi.org/10.1161/CIRCRESAHA.116.308398. PMID: 28154098; PMCID: PMC5321635
5. Cruz-Flores S, Rabinstein A, Biller J, Elkind MS, Griffith P, Gorelick PB, Howard G, Leira EC, Morgenstern LB, Ovbiagele B, Peterson E, Rosamond W, Trimble B, Valderrama AL, American Heart Association Stroke Council; Council on Cardiovascular Nursing; Council on Epidemiology and Prevention; Council on Quality of Care and Outcomes Research. Racial-ethnic disparities in stroke care: the American experience: a statement for healthcare professionals from the American Heart Association/American Stroke Association. Stroke. 2011;42(7):2091–116. https://doi.org/10.1161/STR.0b013e3182213e24. Epub 2011 May 26. PMID: 21617147
6. Coutts SB. Diagnosis and management of transient ischemic attack. Continuum (Minneap Minn). 2017;23(1, Cerebrovascular Disease):82–92. https://doi.org/10.1212/CON.0000000000000424. PMID: 28157745; PMCID: PMC5898963
7. Johnston SC, Rothwell PM, Nguyen-Huynh MN, Giles MF, Elkins JS, Bernstein AL, Sidney S. Validation and refinement of scores to predict very early stroke risk after transient ischaemic attack. Lancet. 2007;369(9558):283–92. https://doi.org/10.1016/S0140-6736(07)60150-0. PMID: 17258668

8. Diederichsen SZ, Haugan KJ, Kronborg C, Graff C, Højberg S, Køber L, Krieger D, Holst AG, Nielsen JB, Brandes A, Svendsen JH. Comprehensive evaluation of rhythm monitoring strategies in screening for atrial fibrillation: insights from patients at risk monitored long term with an implantable loop recorder. Circulation. 2020;141(19):1510–22. https://doi.org/10.1161/CIRCULATIONAHA.119.044407. Epub 2020 Mar 2. PMID: 32114796

9. Amin HP, Madsen TE, Bravata DM, Wira CR, Johnston SC, Ashcraft S, Burrus TM, Panagos PD, Wintermark M, Esenwa C, American Heart Association Emergency Neurovascular Care Committee of the Stroke Council and Council on Peripheral Vascular Disease. Diagnosis, workup, risk reduction of transient ischemic attack in the emergency department setting: a scientific statement from the American Heart Association. Stroke. 2023;54(3):e109–21.

10. Lavallée P, Amarenco P. TIA clinic: a major advance in management of transient ischemic attacks. Front Neurol Neurosci. 2014;33:30–40. https://doi.org/10.1159/000351890. Epub 2013 Oct 11. PMID: 24157555

11. Kargiotis O, Tsivgoulis G. The 2020 breakthroughs in early secondary prevention: dual antiplatelet therapy versus single antiplatelet therapy. Curr Opin Neurol. 2021;34(1):45–54.

12. Wang Y, Wang Y, Zhao X, Liu L, Wang D, Wang C, Wang C, Li H, Meng X, Cui L, Jia J, Dong Q, Xu A, Zeng J, Li Y, Wang Z, Xia H, Johnston SC, CHANCE Investigators. Clopidogrel with aspirin in acute minor stroke or transient ischemic attack. N Engl J Med. 2013;369(1):11–9. https://doi.org/10.1056/NEJMoa1215340. Epub 2013 Jun 26. PMID: 23803136

13. Johnston SC, Easton JD, Farrant M, Barsan W, Conwit RA, Elm JJ, Kim AS, Lindblad AS, Palesch YY, Clinical Research Collaboration, Neurological Emergencies Treatment Trials Network, and the POINT Investigators. Clopidogrel and aspirin in acute ischemic stroke and high-risk TIA. N Engl J Med. 2018;379(3):215–25. https://doi.org/10.1056/NEJMoa1800410. Epub 2018 May 16. PMID: 29766750; PMCID: PMC6193486

14. Bhattacharya P, Chaturvedi S. Dyslipidemia management. Continuum. 2011;17(6, Secondary Stroke Prevention):1242–54. https://doi.org/10.1212/01.CON.0000410033.42100.db.

15. Amarenco P, Kim JS, Labreuche J, Charles H, Abtan J, Béjot Y, Cabrejo L, Cha JK, Ducrocq G, Giroud M, Guidoux C, Hobeanu C, Kim YJ, Lapergue B, Lavallée PC, Lee BC, Lee KB, Leys D, Mahagne MH, Meseguer E, Nighoghossian N, Pico F, Samson Y, Sibon I, Steg PG, Sung SM, Touboul PJ, Touzé E, Varenne O, Vicaut É, Yelles N, Bruckert E, Treat Stroke to Target Investigators. A comparison of two LDL cholesterol targets after ischemic stroke. N Engl J Med. 2020;382(1):9. https://doi.org/10.1056/NEJMoa1910355. Epub 2019 Nov 18. PMID: 31738483

16. Abed W, Abujbara M, Batieha A, Ajlouni K. Statin induced myopathy among patients attending the National Center for diabetes, endocrinology, and genetics. Ann Med Surg (Lond). 2022;74:103304. https://doi.org/10.1016/j.amsu.2022.103304. PMID: 35145672; PMCID: PMC8818528

17. Cholesterol Treatment Trialists' Collaboration. Effect of statin therapy on muscle symptoms: an individual participant data meta-analysis of large-scale, randomized, double-blind trials. Lancet. 2022;400(10355):832–45. https://doi.org/10.1016/S0140-6736(22)01545-8. Epub 2022 Aug 29. Erratum in: Lancet. 2022 Oct 8;400(10359):1194. PMID: 36049498; PMCID: PMC7613583

18. McClain JV 4th, Chance EA. The advanced practice nurse will see you now: impact of a transitional care clinic on hospital readmissions in stroke survivors. J Nurs Care Qual. 2020;35(2):147–52.

Blood on CT

11

Carrie Crowder and William S. Musser

Introduction

Patients presenting to the emergency room with acute neurological symptoms require an emergent computerized tomography (CT) scan of the head before considering options for acute stroke treatment. When reviewing a scan during an acute stroke evaluation, one often expects to see normal brain tissue, perhaps some early ischemic changes, or a hyperdense vessel. But what happens when the CT reveals a hemorrhage? Blood on CT requires an immediate shift in management from an ischemic stroke to a hemorrhagic stroke protocol. Knowing how to "shift gears" into managing an acute hemorrhage is essential and can significantly impact the patient's course and outcome.

Overview of ICH

Common types of intracranial hemorrhage include intracerebral (or intraparenchymal) hemorrhage (ICH), subdural and epidural hematoma (SDH and EDH), and subarachnoid hemorrhage (SAH). Cerebral amyloid angiopathy (CAA) is an example of a less common cause. The location and the mechanism of hemorrhage will guide further workup and monitoring, and treatment options vary accordingly (Fig. 11.1). This chapter will focus on the management of ICH, the most common, and we will also review SDH. We will discuss the management of SAH in another chapter.

C. Crowder
VA National Telestroke Program, Palo Alto VA Medical Center, Palo Alto, CA, USA
e-mail: Carrie.Crowder@va.gov

W. S. Musser (✉)
VA National Telestroke Program, Palo Alto VA Medical Center, California, CA, USA
e-mail: William.Musser@va.gov

© The Author(s), under exclusive license to Springer Nature Switzerland AG 2024
H. P. Amin (ed.), *Stroke for the Advanced Practice Clinician*,
https://doi.org/10.1007/978-3-031-66289-8_11

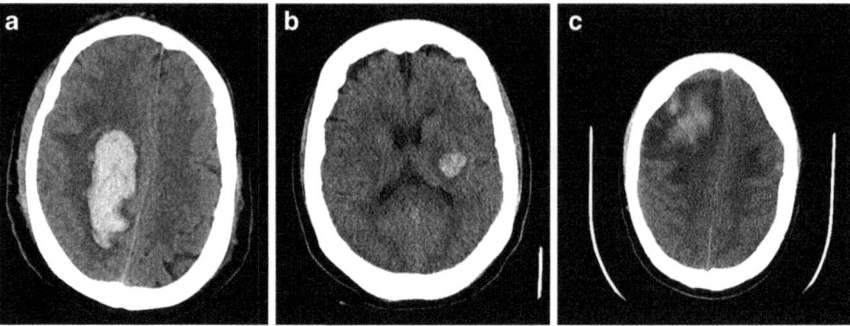

Fig. 11.1 Three examples of intracerebral hemorrhage on non-contrast head CT. (**a**) 84-year-old man with dementia with sudden left-sided weakness. CT demonstrates a right hemispheric lobar hemorrhage, likely from CAA. (**b**) A 56-year-old man with severe HTN, sudden right-sided numbness, dizziness, and headache. His systolic blood pressure is greater than 200 mmHg. CT demonstrates a right thalamic hemorrhage, likely hypertensive hemorrhage. (**c**) A 77-year-old man with atrial fibrillation, not on anticoagulation, with sudden left-sided weakness and right gaze deviation. CT demonstrates a patchy right frontal hyperdensity superimposed on a larger hypodense area, which is concerning for hemorrhagic conversion of an ischemic stroke, as well as a resulting midline shift due to mass effect

In ICH, the bleeding is *within* the brain tissue. ICH is associated with both higher morbidity and higher mortality than acute ischemic stroke (AIS). Symptoms may overlap, but onset varies slightly. AIS symptoms present instantaneously, while the symptoms of ICH may develop over several minutes [1]. ICH is the second most common type of stroke after AIS, making up about 20% of all strokes [2, 3]. The extravasated (escaped) blood damages the brain tissue, and the resulting edema and mass effect can further compound the injury. Every additional millimeter of edema volume can double the odds of a poor functional outcome [1]. Outcomes vary based on the size and location of the hemorrhage, the degree of surrounding edema, and the resulting compression of any adjacent structures. Unlike the secondary hemorrhages seen after an acute stroke where the hemorrhage most often confines itself to the area of the original stroke, hematomas from primary ICH may expand rapidly, most often within the first 24 hours, and are associated with poor outcomes [4]. Therefore, acute interventions for ICH are directed at decreasing the risk of continued expansion.

How Does ICH Present?

The clinical presentation of ICH often involves an acute focal deficit, a change in mental status, or both. Figure 11.2 is an MRI of a patient who presented with a seizure and left gaze deviation, found to have right frontal lobe hemorrhage due to a metastatic lesion. Recall that traditionally the gaze deviation is towards the stroke. But in this case the right frontal eye field was experiencing a seizure and overpowered the contralateral eye field, pushing the eyes to the left (so gaze deviation is towards a stroke, away from a seizure). Many ICHs are associated with severe hypertension (HTN), headache, nausea and vomiting, vertigo, depressed level of consciousness, or even a seizure (Table 11.1). Neurological history and examination cannot reliably distinguish ICH from AIS, so rapid imaging is needed.

Fig. 11.2 Brain MRI demonstrating a right frontal lobe hemorrhage with surrounding edema. This ICH was due to metastatic disease from testicular cancer. Note the significant edema surrounding the hemorrhage

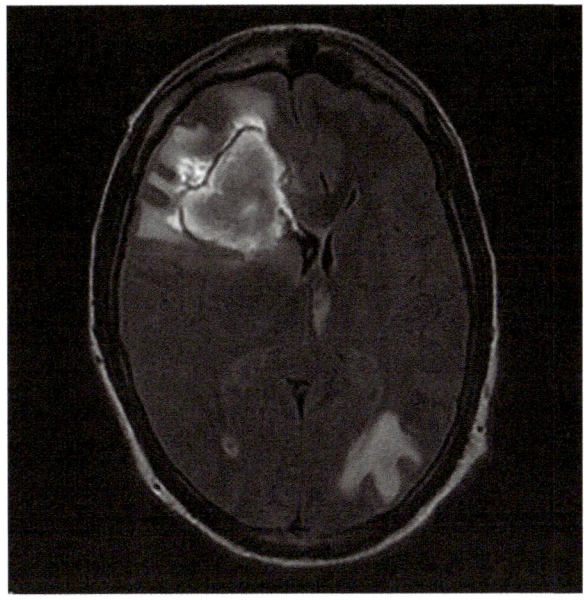

Table 11.1 Clinical signs of hemorrhagic stroke

- Severe headache/nausea/vomiting
- Profound hypertension
- Lethargy/unconsciousness
- Nuchal rigidity
- Seizure

How Do You Characterize an ICH?

A noncontrast CT head is the fastest and most widely available method to diagnose ICH. First, determine in which compartment(s) the bleeding is occurring: intraparenchymal, subarachnoid, subdural, epidural, or intraventricular (IVH). Is the blood cortical (sometimes called lobar, because the hematoma involves most or all of an entire lobe or lobes), or in the deeper structures like the basal ganglia, cerebellum, or brainstem? The shape also matters. Is it circular or ovoid shape, irregularly shaped, or does it have varying shades of brightness to suggest acute and subacute bleeding? Unusual shapes or locations may indicate vascular lesions warranting further imaging, such as angiography, to rule out an underlying lesion or suggest an underlying coagulopathy like anticoagulation-related hemorrhage. Each of these details helps determine underlying mechanism and treatment plan. For example, intraparenchymal blood is often due to HTN or CAA, whereas subarachnoid hemorrhage is often due to aneurysm, and subdural/epidural hematomas are often due to trauma.

Next, determine if the hemorrhage is pushing or compressing adjacent brain tissue, also known as mass effect which is due to edema or a large hematoma. All hemorrhages will be surrounded by some degree of edema, but significant edema may indicate an underlying mass lesion (Fig. 11.2). Compression of the ventricles can lead to hydrocephalus, a feared complication of large hemorrhage or ischemic stroke, which is both a neurological and neurosurgical emergency.

Hemorrhage size can be described as small, moderate, or large. For an exact measurement, use the formula ABC/2, where A = maximum length (in cm), B = width perpendicular to A on the same head CT slice (in cm), and C = the number of slices in which the hematoma is visible multiplied by the slice thickness in cm [5]. Start by answering: Is the ICH larger or smaller than 30 cc? Less than 30 cc would signify a smaller quantity if supratentorial, but 15–30 cc could be devastating in the posterior fossa since there is less room to accommodate the hemorrhage. Size matters! Severity and risks increase with size and location, and volumes >50 cc are associated with poor prognosis.

Vessel Imaging in Acute ICH

CT angiography (CTA) of the head and neck is a standard component in the evaluation of patients with acute stroke symptoms and is also helpful in identifying secondary causes of ICH like aneurysms or vascular malformations, unless the amount of blood obscures the underlying lesion. CTA can identify extravasation of contrast into the hemorrhage, demonstrated by the "spot sign," which raises the risk of hematoma expansion (Fig. 11.3). CTA can also change medical management if it identifies rare findings for example, the finding of mycotic aneurysms underlying a hemorrhage would suggest a diagnosis of endocarditis. CTA can be done rapidly with CT during a stroke code, but MRA is another option for those with iodine contrast allergies.

Fig. 11.3 Spot sign. A hyperdense focus (spot) within an area of hemorrhage (yellow arrow) is thought to imply a higher risk of further hematoma expansion. (Image credit to Dr. Ashu Jadhav)

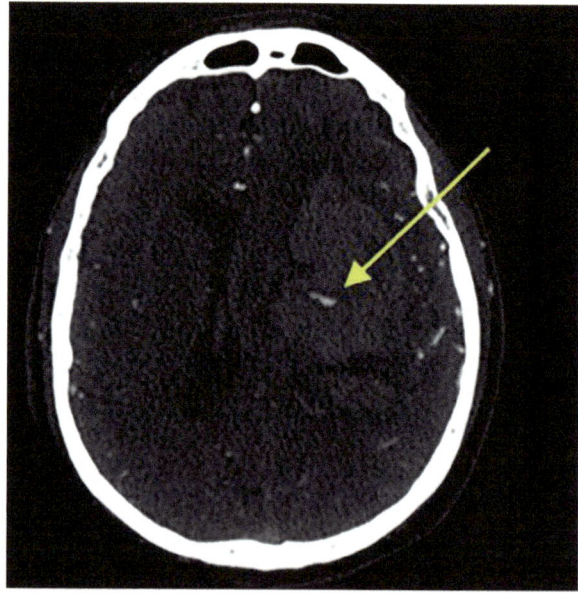

If a hemorrhage appears outside a traditional arterial vascular territory or has a lot of surrounding edema, a CT venogram can rule out cerebral venous sinus thrombosis (CVST). Consider CVST in patients with a history of clotting or cancer (discussed in more depth in the venous sinus thrombosis chapter). Recall that veins drain blood away from the brain. Hemorrhage and edema from venous thrombosis occur due to outflow obstruction, which causes smaller draining veins to burst from increased pressure. Ruling out CVST acutely for an atypical hemorrhage is important because, despite the presence of blood, the underlying problem is a thrombosis that typically requires urgent anticoagulation.

Utility of MRI

Most patients will require an MRI when stable to further evaluate the cause of the hemorrhage. MRI is typically not done acutely, but it can reliably identify hemorrhage and better determine the age of the hemorrhage [6]. MRI frequently surpasses a CT's ability to rule out underlying causes for ICH, and this topic is discussed in more depth in a later chapter. MRIs are also more sensitive for identifying cortical microhemorrhages due to cerebral amyloid angiopathy, underlying infectious lesions like abscesses, vascular syndromes such as posterior reversible leukoencephalopathy syndrome (PRES), and acute infarcts with hemorrhagic transformation.

Initial Management

The acute management of ICH should focus on preventing hematoma expansion. Expansion is most common within the first few hours and is associated with a higher risk of mortality and poor outcomes. ICH protocols are helpful to ensure all necessary parties (neurosurgery, neurology, and ICU) are alerted and necessary steps are taken (Table 11.2). Upon arrival for a stroke code, start with ABCs, confirm IV access, and monitor blood pressure and central line needs. Ensure that the airway is

Table 11.2 Initial actions when hemorrhage is detected

- Ensure airway and hemodynamic stability
- Activate ICH protocol (notifies all necessary teams like neurosurgery, neurology, and ICU)
- Ensure coagulation labs are sent
- Immediate and consistent management of systolic blood pressure (SBP)
- Discontinuation of AC, AP, and NSAIDs
- Reversal of AC effects
- Clinical screenings for signs/symptoms of ICP and initiating ICP monitoring when indicated
- Screening and addressing coagulopathies or other hematologic disorders

AC anticoagulants, *AP* antiplatelet, *NSAIDs* nonsteroidal anti-inflammatory drugs, *ICP* intracranial pressure

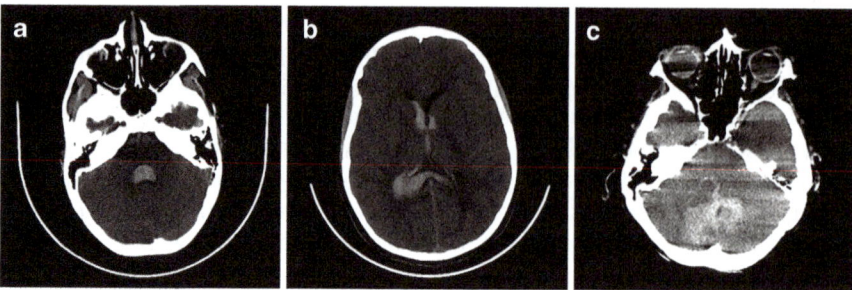

Fig. 11.4 Posterior fossa hemorrhage extending into the fourth ventricle (**a**) with edema, mass effect, IVH in third and lateral ventricles with obstructive hydrocephalus (**b**), and brainstem herniation (**c**). (Photo credit to Dr. Ashu Jadhav)

safe. Initiate blood pressure monitoring every 10–15 min. With an altered level of consciousness (LOC), consider sending an arterial blood gas (ABG), performing a sepsis workup, and using a bedside or continuous electroencephalogram (EEG) to rule out subclinical seizure activity. Necessary labs include a comprehensive metabolic profile with liver function tests, complete blood count with differential, coagulation panel, toxicology/drug screen, ESR, CRP, cardiac enzymes, pregnancy test for women of childbearing age, and a type and screen [7]. Place the patient's head of bed between 30 and 45° to help mitigate elevations in the intracranial pressure (laying flat may raise intracranial pressure), and gravity will help support cerebral venous drainage and reduce the risk of edema formation [8].

Every ICH requires a neurosurgical consult to determine the need for emergent surgery. Indications for urgent surgery include significant edema with mass effect, herniation, or ventricular extension of the hemorrhage leading to hydrocephalus. Posterior fossa hemorrhage in the cerebellum or brainstem requires special surgical attention since brainstem compression carries higher morbidity and mortality (Fig. 11.4) [1]. However, the risk may outweigh the benefit of neurosurgical intervention like in clinical situations where the hemorrhage is due to CAA, as there is a high risk of rebleeding [9].

Disposition

If the neurosurgery team determines that no surgical intervention is necessary, then it is recommended that the patient be admitted to an intensive care unit, ideally a neurological ICU. This is important for proper neurologic and critical care surveillance and management, which can provide a full range of high-acuity care and expertise to achieve better outcomes [7]. Most patients will require surveillance imaging within 4–6 h of presentation. Frequent neurologic checks, hourly to start, should include an NIHSS or Glasgow coma score (GCS) for those with altered levels of consciousness. Ongoing clinical screenings for signs/symptoms of increased ICP can determine the need for ICP monitoring and drainage. Serial examinations can help staff to recognize any suggestion of an acute demise. ICH patients should not remain at hospitals without ICU or neurosurgical capabilities.

Next, we will review some patient-specific factors that increase risk and may require more urgent management in the ED.

The Hypertensive Patient

Acute management of hypertension in patients with ICH is of singular importance and should begin immediately after diagnosis of ICH. Patients who present with SBP between 150 and 220 mmHg should have a target of 140 mmHg within the first hour of presentation to maintain BP in a range of 130–150 mmHg [7]. If the presenting SBP is >220 mmHg, get the BP < 220 mmHg immediately and between 140 and 160 mmHg over the next few hours (Fig. 11.5). It is essential to communicate with nursing and to be notified if the SBP falls below or exceeds the specified parameters. After meeting the established BP goal, continue clinically monitoring the patient with serial NIHSS or GCS examinations.

The INTERACT-2 trial demonstrated that patients in the more intensive BP-lowering group did have improved functional outcomes and quality of life [10]. The ATACH-2 trial, however, did not find benefit in outcomes with aggressive BP reduction to <140 mmHg and noted higher rates of kidney injury in the intensive BP reduction group with SBPs <130. The difference in outcomes and adverse effects may be due to a more rapid and aggressive decrease in blood pressure early on in patients from the ATACH-2 trial [11]. The takeaway is that SBP < 130 may not be helpful acutely, and overaggressive BP reduction can raise the risk of kidney injury. Persistently elevated blood pressure risks hematoma expansion. The challenge for the treating team, therefore, is to keep the blood pressure within the target range.

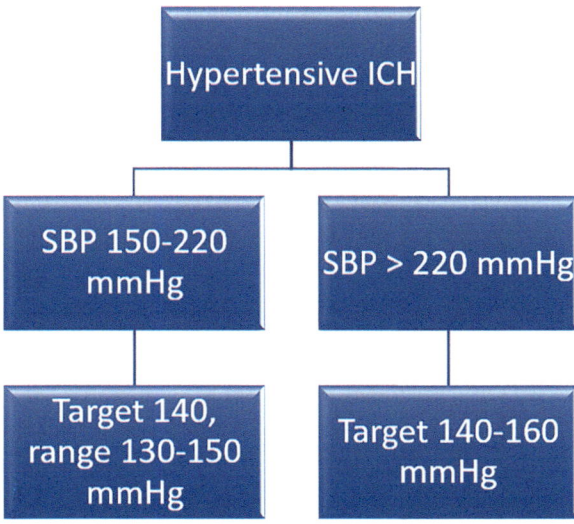

Fig. 11.5 BP targets for hypertensive ICH

Vacillating blood pressure can lead to neurologic deterioration, so keeping BP stable within a target range is vital. Steady blood pressure control may be the most effective interventional tool for giving the patient the best chance at a functional recovery. IV blood pressure meds like labetalol, nicardipine, clevidipine, and esmolol have advantages over oral agents, including rapid onset, quick titration, and usefulness for patients with swallowing difficulty. Avoid nitroglycerin and nitroprusside as they are more centrally acting and cause vasodilation, increasing the risk of raised intracranial pressure [12].

The Patient on Anticoagulation and Antiplatelets

ICH can occur in patients treated with anticoagulants, such as vitamin K antagonists (warfarin), heparin, direct factor Xa inhibitors (apixaban and rivaroxaban), and direct thrombin inhibitors (dabigatran). To treat bleeding caused by anticoagulants, providers must decide on acute reversal agents based on the type of anticoagulant. The anticoagulant must be discontinued immediately. The pharmacology chapter provides more information on dosage and administration of reversal agents.

For warfarin reversal (a vitamin K antagonist), four-factor prothrombin complex concentrate (4F-PCC) administration is the agent of choice, or fresh frozen plasma if 4F-PCC is unavailable, plus intravenous vitamin K. 4F-PCC has been shown to normalize INR rapidly. Administering vitamin K does little in the acute setting but helps lower bleeding risk over 24 h as the body makes more vitamin K-dependent factors (so administer it with an acute reversal agent, but not alone).

For factor Xa inhibitors (Eliquis and Xarelto) or direct thrombin inhibitors (dabigatran), initial management depends on the timing of the last dose. Activated charcoal is helpful if the last dose of anticoagulation is within 2 h. If the last dose was taken more than 2 h before the presentation, consider using andexanet alfa for the factor Xa inhibitors and idarucizumab for dabigatran. Many protocols may go directly to the reversal agent regardless of the time from last dose. Andexanet alfa reverses the effects of the factor Xa inhibitors. It has been shown to decrease hematoma size by approximately one-third in approximately 8% of patients treated with the drug [13]. Idarucizumab is a monoclonal antibody that binds to the dabigatran molecule, quickly rendering it inactive. Idarucizumab is considered beneficial for ICH; however, it has yet to be specifically studied in this population. Since they are new, these reversal agents may not be on the formulary at many smaller hospitals. In that case, consider 4F-PCC or fresh frozen plasma. Protamine sulfate is the recommended agent for heparin-associated ICH.

For ICH patients on aspirin, one might assume that a platelet transfusion should help decrease the risk of hematoma expansion; however, this does not appear to be the case. The PATCH trial randomized patients on antiplatelet therapy within 6 h of ICH onset to either standard care or standard care with platelet transfusion [14]. The authors found that administering platelets to all patients may be harmful, with death and dependency higher in the platelet transfusion group. However, platelet transfusion may be appropriate in patients with thrombocytopenia or who need emergent neurosurgical procedures.

The Seizing Patient

Acute hemorrhage increases the risk of seizures. An EEG is required for all ICH patients with witnessed seizure activity and initiating intravenous antiseizure medication (ASM). The Post-Stroke Epilepsy chapter covers this in detail, including options for ASM. Acute seizures require treatment for one week, followed by weaning off if stable without further seizure activity. Empiric treatment with ASM for ICH patients without seizures is not indicated and may be harmful [7].

ICH Prognosis

For devastating hemorrhages, goals of care conversations should still be started early, especially for older patients. The ICH score can be used as a communication tool with family but should not be used as a formal prognostic scale (Table 11.3). Early rapport with the patient and family is essential, especially when risks are high from large volume hemorrhages, expanding hematomas, and factors leading to high ICH scores. Navigating this topic will be detailed further in a subsequent chapter.

Table 11.3 ICH score [15]

Component	Score	Points
GCS score	3–4	2
	5–12	1
	13–15	0
ICH volume (mL)	>30	1
	<30	0
IVH	Present	1
	Absent	0
Infratentorial ICH	Yes	1
	No	0
Age (years)	>80	1
	<80	0
Total Points	**30-day mortality (%)**	
5+	100	
4	97	
3	72	
2	26	
1	13	
0	0	

Fig. 11.6 (right)
Left-sided SDH causing
mass effect, with lethargy
and right-sided weakness.
The blood is outside the
brain but can still cause
mass effect if large enough

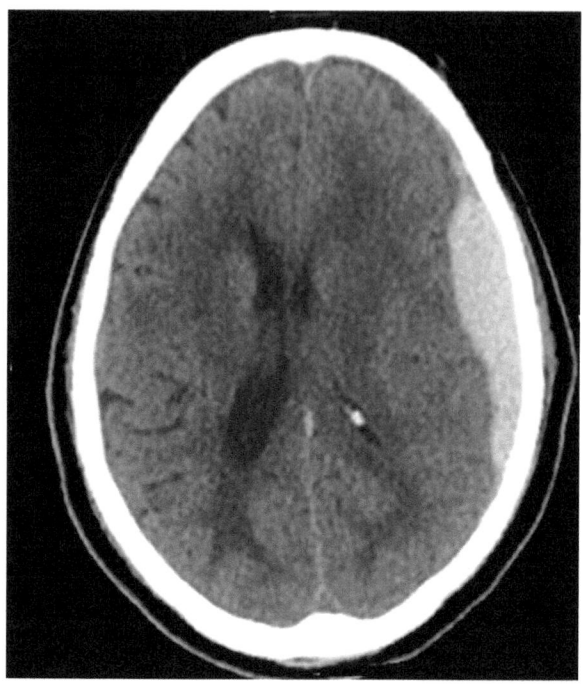

SDH Overview

In contrast to ICH, where there is bleeding within the brain parenchyma, a subdural hemorrhage (SDH), or hematoma, occurs *outside* the brain between the dura and arachnoid meningeal layers. The brain has three protective meningeal layers. The pia mater directly overlies the brain, the arachnoid mater is the middle layer, and dura mater is the outermost layer that attaches to the skull. The spaces between the pia and arachnoid, and between the arachnoid and dura mater provide added cushioning, but have blood vessels that can rupture with trauma. Depending on size, the SDH can lead to mass effect and cause focal neurological symptoms (Fig. 11.6). The meningeal arteries supply the dura mater, and their structure makes them susceptible to acceleration-deceleration injuries like falls or motor vehicle accidents. Bridging veins in the subdural compartment bridge the superior sagittal sinus to the brain surface for venous brain drainage. Brain atrophy can cause these bridging veins to be under more tension, which increases the risk of rupture or tear.

SDH Presentation

SDH usually occurs after a clear head injury or significant shifts in momentum. Due to the low arterial pressure, it may take days to weeks before hemorrhage grows to the point that the patient becomes symptomatic. SDHs often present with headaches, lethargy, malaise, and possibly focal findings like weakness, speech disturbance, or neglect. Regardless of location, the main concern about SDHs is the risk of further bleeding, mass effect/compression, and neurological decline.

SDH Management

Neurosurgery must be notified once an SDH is detected. Expansion may occur with any significant fluid shifts, as potentially seen with dehydration or congested heart/renal failure patients. Therefore, fluid balance should be thoughtfully restored and maintained [16]. Abrupt and significant shifts in the body's fluid balance should be avoided. Hematoma expansion can lead to worsening symptoms and even progress to a herniation syndrome. Rapid clinical decline, increased midline shift, or compression of vital structures can all be indications for neurosurgical intervention. In the past, neurosurgical management consisted mainly of placing a burr hole and a drain. However, some less invasive options, like ligation of the middle meningeal artery, are now available.

Relevant ICH Study Summaries

ATACH-2 Trial: The ATACH-2 trial evaluated the role of SBP lowering in patients after an ICH. The study showed that acute lowering of SBP in patients with ICH to the range of 110–139 mmHg was not beneficial in decreasing rates of death or less disability than a target of 140–179 mmHg. In addition, acute renal injuries were reported to be higher frequency in patients randomized to the intensive treatment (110–139 mmHg) group. Therefore, a cautionary note for close medical monitoring during crisis management is needed [11].

INTERACT-2 Trial: The INTERACT-2 trial further evaluated the role of SBP control after ICH by randomizing patients to SBP <140 versus SBP <180 mmHg. It showed that intentionally lowering SBP to <140 mm Hg does not improve clinical outcomes of death or severe disability [10].

PATCH Trial: The PATCH trial was designed to evaluate the role of platelet transfusions in patients with ICH. Patients on antiplatelet therapy were randomized within 6 h of ICH onset to either standard care or standard care with platelet transfusion. The authors found that death and degree of dependency were higher in the group receiving platelet transfusions, so empiric use of platelet transfusions is not recommended [14].

Conclusion

Blood on CT during a stroke code requires a rapid shifting of gears to an ICH protocol, with a focus on patient stability, surgical evaluation, and minimizing the risk of hematoma expansion (Fig. 11.7). Management reflects the underlying mechanism, which may not always be apparent early on but should be standardized into well-established protocols.

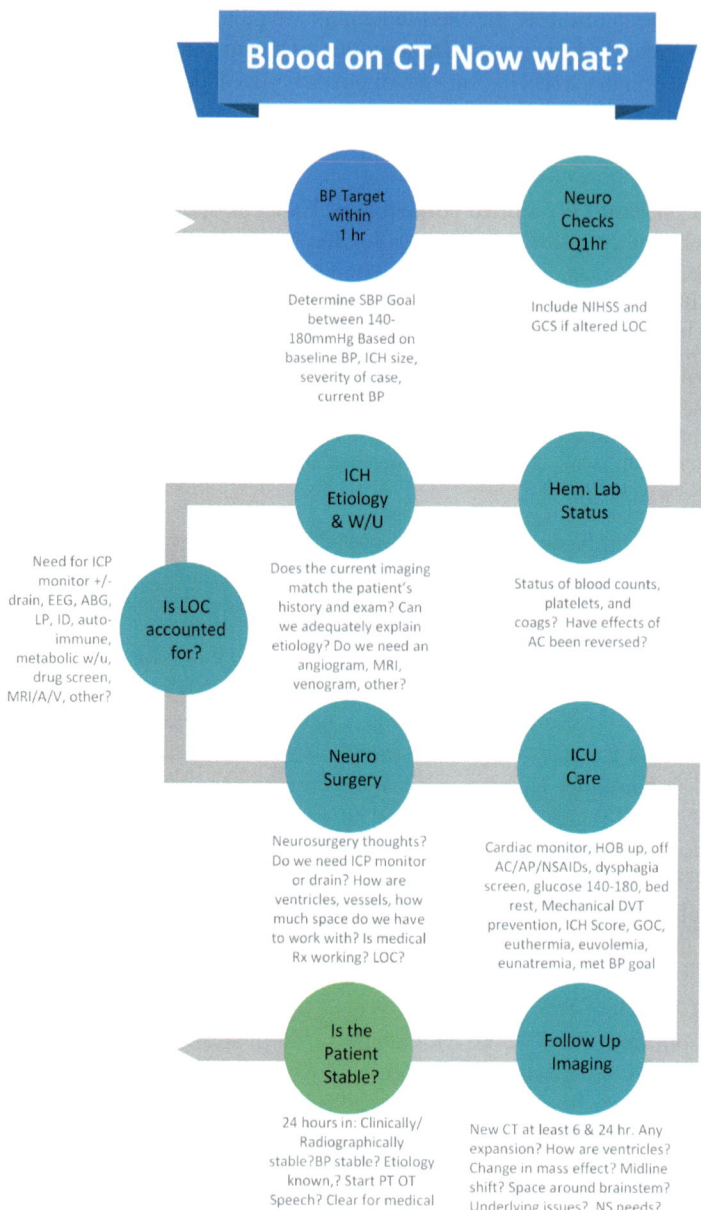

Fig. 11.7 Blood on CT algorithm

Clinical Pearls
- Ischemic and hemorrhagic strokes can have similar presentations, but severely elevated blood pressure, headache, and depressed mental status are more common with ICH
- Blood pressure management is critical with acute ICH, as are reversal agents for patients on anticoagulation
- ICH protocols help streamline rapid management and notify all pertinent parties
- ICH patients should be at a hospital that has 24–7 neurosurgical capabilities

References

1. Sheth KN, Ropper AH. Review article: spontaneous intracerebral hemorrhage. N Engl J Med. 2022;387(17):1589–96. https://doi.org/10.1056/NEJMra2201449.
2. Virani SS, Alonso A, Benjamin EJ, Bittencourt MS, Callaway CW, Carson AP, Chamberlain AM, et al. Heart disease and stroke statistics—2020 update: a report from the American Heart Association. Circulation. 2020;141(9):e139. https://doi.org/10.1161/CIR.0000000000000757.
3. Feigin VL, Lawes CMM, Bennett DA, Barker-Collo SL, Parag V. Worldwide stroke incidence and early case fatality reported in 56 population-based studies: a systematic review. Lancet Neurol. 2009;8(4):355–69. https://doi.org/10.1016/S1474-4422(09)70025-0.
4. Davis SM, Broderick J, Hennerici M, Brun NC, Diringer MN, Mayer SA, Begtrup K, Steiner T, for the Recombinant Activated Factor VII Intracerebral Hemorrhage Trial Investigators. Hematoma growth is a determinant of mortality and poor outcome after intracerebral hemorrhage. Neurology. 2006;66(8):1175–81. https://doi.org/10.1212/01.wnl.0000208408.98482.99.
5. Kothari RU, Brott T, Broderick JP, Barsan WG, Sauerbeck LR, Zuccarello M, Khoury J. The ABCs of measuring intracerebral hemorrhage volumes. Stroke. 1996;27(8):1304–5. https://doi.org/10.1161/01.STR.27.8.1304.
6. Fiebach JB, Schellinger PD, Gass A, Kucinski T, Siebler M, Villringer A, Ölkers P, et al. Stroke magnetic resonance imaging is accurate in hyperacute intracerebral hemorrhage: a multicenter study on the validity of stroke imaging. Stroke. 2004;35(2):502–6. https://doi.org/10.1161/01.STR.0000114203.75678.88.
7. Greenberg SM, Ziai WC, Cordonnier C, Dowlatshahi D, Francis B, Goldstein JN, Claude Hemphill J, et al. 2022 guideline for the management of patients with spontaneous intracerebral hemorrhage: a guideline from the American Heart Association/American Stroke Association. Stroke. 2022;53(7):e282. https://doi.org/10.1161/STR.0000000000000407.
8. Cook AM, Morgan Jones G, Hawryluk GWJ, Mailoux P, McLaughlin D, Papangelou A, et al. Guidelines for the acute treatment of cerebral edema in neurocritical care patients. Neurocrit Care. 2020;32(3):647–66. https://doi.org/10.1007/s12028-020-00959-7.
9. Arishima H, Neishi H, Kodera T, Kitai R, Kikuta K-i. Cerebral amyloid angiopathy causing large contralateral hemorrhage during surgery for lobar hemorrhage: a case report. J Stroke Cerebrovasc Dis. 2015;24(3):e83–5. https://doi.org/10.1016/j.jstrokecerebrovasdis.2014.11.015.
10. Anderson CS, Heeley E, Huang Y, Wang J, Stapf C, Delcourt C, Lindley R, et al. Rapid blood-pressure lowering in patients with acute intracerebral hemorrhage. N Engl J Med. 2013;368(25):2355–65. https://doi.org/10.1056/NEJMoa1214609.
11. Qureshi AI, Palesch YY, Barsan WG, Hanley DF, Hsu CY, Martin RL, Moy CS, et al. Intensive blood-pressure lowering in patients with acute cerebral hemorrhage. N Engl J Med. 2016;375(11):1033–43. https://doi.org/10.1056/NEJMoa1603460.

12. Vitt JR, Trillanes M, Claude Hemphill J III. Management of blood pressure during and after recanalization therapy for acute ischemic stroke. Front Neurol. 2019;10:138. https://doi.org/10.3389/fneur.2019.00138.
13. Demchuk AM, Yue P, Zotova E, Nakamya J, Lizhen X, Milling TJ, Ohara T, et al. Hemostatic efficacy and anti-FXa (factor Xa) reversal with Andexanet alfa in intracranial hemorrhage: ANNEXA-4 substudy. Stroke. 2021;52(6):2096–105. https://doi.org/10.1161/STROKEAHA.120.030565.
14. Baharoglu MI, Cordonnier C, Salman RA-S, de Gans K, Koopman MM, Brand A, Majoie CB, et al. Platelet transfusion versus standard care after acute stroke due to spontaneous cerebral haemorrhage associated with antiplatelet therapy (PATCH): a randomised, open-label, phase 3 trial. Lancet. 2016;387(10038):2605–13. https://doi.org/10.1016/S0140-6736(16)30392-0.
15. Hemphill JC III, Bonovich DC, Besmertis L, Manley GT, Johnston SC. The ICH score: a simple, reliable grading scale for intracerebral hemorrhage. Stroke. 2001;32:891–7.
16. Alshora W, Alfageeh M, Alshahrani S, Alqahtani S, Dajam A, et al. Diagnosis and management of subdural hematoma: a review of recent literature. Int J Commun Med Public Health. 2018;5(9):3709–14.

Stroke Mimics

12

Trista Pennington and Daniel C. Brooks

Introduction

A stroke mimic is a condition that resembles a stroke but is ultimately determined to be due to a nonvascular cause [1]. To be considered a stroke mimic, the condition needs to cause focal neurological deficits, meaning symptoms or signs that could localize to specific parts of the brain, such as aphasia, vertigo, eye movement disorders, and (usually unilateral) weakness, sensory change, and visual field loss [1]. Isolated encephalopathy and decreased level of consciousness are much less likely to be due to ischemia, as these are often caused by global cerebral dysfunction (rather than focal), such as in most cases of metabolic or infectious encephalopathy [1].

Stroke mimics are extremely common. As many as 30% of all presentations of presumed acute stroke are eventually determined to be due to an alternative diagnosis [1]. Prompt recognition of stroke mimics can ideally reduce the risk of patient harm and decrease healthcare expenditures by (a) treating and hopefully reversing the symptoms of the mimic and (b) avoiding unnecessary tests, hospitalizations, and treatments.

Diagnosing stroke mimics can be challenging. First, caution should be taken to not rule out a vascular event too early in the setting of brief or resolved symptoms, given that a transient ischemic attack (TIA), by its very nature, both clinically resolves and leaves no evidence of injury on imaging [2]. Second, brain imaging, particularly magnetic resonance imaging (MRI), often plays a central role in differentiating stroke from a stroke mimic, but brain imaging does have limitations. Computed tomography (CT) of the head is ideal for ruling out acute

T. Pennington
Bridgeport Hospital, Bridgeport, CT, USA
e-mail: Trista.Pennington@YNHH.ORG

D. C. Brooks (✉)
Providence Specialty Medical Group, Santa Monica, CA, USA

© The Author(s), under exclusive license to Springer Nature Switzerland AG 2024   127
H. P. Amin (ed.), *Stroke for the Advanced Practice Clinician*,
https://doi.org/10.1007/978-3-031-66289-8_12

intracranial hemorrhage, with a sensitivity close to 100% in the hyperacute phase, but not for acute ischemic stroke (AIS), with a detection rate near 67% when performed within 3 h of symptom onset [3, 4]. The CT is likely to be normal for most acute stroke and stroke mimic patients alike. Brain MRI is much more helpful in ruling out AIS, with a sensitivity of approximately 90–94%. However, the clinician must know that MRI carries a false-negative rate for AIS of approximately 6–10% [5, 6]. MRI may miss tiny strokes (10 mm or less), hyperacute (with MRI less than 48 hours after symptom onset), or located in the posterior circulation [6, 7]. Therefore, if no stroke mimic is identified in a patient with acute neurological deficits, it is reasonable that TIA or AIS stroke remains on the differential even if the initial MRI brain is negative.

Evaluation and treatment of AIS and stroke mimics are time-sensitive—frequently an emergency—and necessitate prompt consideration of intravenous thrombolysis (IVT). Therefore, it is reassuring that IVT appears safe in patients with stroke mimics, with a low risk of symptomatic intracranial hemorrhage [8]. According to current guidelines, prompt treatment with IVT is reasonable if a patient presents with stroke-like symptoms within the time window eligible for IVT, has a measurable neurological deficit deemed disabling, and does not meet any exclusionary criteria for IVT [9].

In this chapter, we will discuss common stroke mimics. Where appropriate, we will address epidemiology and pathophysiology (how the condition causes stroke-like/focal neurological symptoms), what to look for in the history and examination, how they may differ from stroke, and testing, diagnosis, and possible treatment options.

Migraine with Aura

Migraine is a common condition that affects females and younger adults more frequently than males and older adults [10]. Up to one-third of patients with migraines experience an aura, a neurological symptom that may occur before or during the headache part of the migraine [11]. The pathophysiology of aura is a phenomenon known as cortical spreading depression, the depolarization of cells within the brain with a subsequent period of neuronal suppression leading to focal neurological symptoms [11, 12]. Aura symptoms may be "positive" or "negative" and can affect vision, sensation, motor function, and speech and may also localize to the brainstem and cause vertigo [13]. Positive symptoms occur with preserved normal functioning, like flashing lights or colors in the visual field with otherwise intact vision or headaches. Examples of positive symptoms include photopsia (flashes of light) or fortification (straight, jagged lines). Negative symptoms involve loss of function, like vision loss, aphasia, and weakness. Patients may also experience multiple different aura symptoms (e.g., visual, sensory, and speech symptoms). Unlike symptoms due to stroke, multiple aura symptoms typically occur sequentially rather than simultaneously [13]. Each aura symptom normally lasts 5–60 min, although motor symptoms may last longer [13].

Features that may help distinguish migraine aura from AIS include an established history of aura with similar symptoms as well as the presence of a headache, especially a headache with classic migrainous features (pulsatile, unilateral, and associated with phonophobia, photophobia, nausea, or vomiting) occurring after the onset of aura-related symptoms. Additionally, multiple aura symptoms, as mentioned above, typically occur in a slow, successive pattern, whereas AIS typically presents with acute development of symptoms occurring nearly simultaneously [13]. The characteristics of visual symptoms are also helpful. Visual aura is the most common type of aura, and it frequently presents as gradual, positive symptoms such as a fortification spectrum (a zig-zag pattern at the point of fixation that can expand in either direction) followed by a scotoma [13]. Isolated, acute-onset visual loss (negative symptom) should raise suspicion for ischemia rather than visual aura [2]. Vision loss with headache, especially in an older patient, should raise concern for giant cell arteritis. Finally, brain MRI helps distinguish migraine with aura from AIS with high sensitivity, as migraine is not typically associated with diffusion restriction [14].

While a migraine headache should be treated, avoid specific migraine therapies if cerebral ischemia is still in the differential diagnosis. Trying migraine therapy to see if the symptoms improve is not the best way to diagnose a migraine. Triptans, commonly used to treat migraine attacks, can potentially worsen ischemia through vasospasm [15]. Use conservative pain control measures, such as acetaminophen, magnesium, and antinausea agents, until the team has definitively ruled out stroke.

Seizure

Seizures are common in the general population and responsible for approximately 14–22% of presentations identified to be stroke mimics [16, 17]. About 8–10% of the population will suffer at least one seizure [18]. Seizures can cause focal neurological dysfunction (and thus mimic stroke) by two mechanisms: the active ictal (seizing) period, characterized by neuronal hyperactivity or impaired neuronal inhibition that leads to pathologic firing leading to forced gaze deviation, abnormal speech, and motor symptoms, followed by the postictal period, which can cause focal neurological dysfunction through a cerebral "burnout" phenomenon in which the electrical hyperactivity of the seizure leads to neuronal exhaustion which can be focal and last minutes to hours [19]. History is critical for distinguishing seizure (both the ictal and postictal periods) from stroke. A history of epilepsy or seizures, witnessed convulsive activity, urinary incontinence, and tongue or lip bite should all raise suspicion for seizure but are not 100% predictive.

The examination, specifically the relationship between the direction of horizontal gaze deviation or gaze preference and other neurological symptoms (such as vision loss, sensory change, and especially weakness), can differentiate between seizure and stroke. Gaze deviation occurs from injury in the cerebral hemispheres or brainstem, and the underlying mechanism may be ischemia (such as in acute stroke), metabolic hyperactivity (such as in an active seizure), or metabolic depletion (the postictal period) [20, 21]. To understand gaze, we must discuss the frontal eye fields (FEFs) located in the frontal lobes of both hemispheres. The job of each FEF is to direct gaze to the contralateral side (so the right FEF directs both eyes to the left, and vice versa). Now imagine a stroke in the right frontal lobe that (in addition to other symptoms) deactivates the right FEF. This leads to unopposed action by the left FEF, forcing the eyes to the right. So, a right-sided stroke leads to right-gaze deviation (and left-sided weakness). Conversely, a frontal lobe seizure leads to hyperactivation of the ipsilateral FEF, overcoming the opposing FEF and forcing gaze deviation to the contralateral side. An active seizure from the left cerebral hemisphere may cause forced gaze deviation to the patient's right side and convulsions or weakness of the patient's right side as well. So, you look "towards a stroke and away from a seizure." If the eyes point to the same side as the motor symptoms, the patient is likely having a seizure. Finally, a patient actively seizing is unlikely to follow commands. If the patient is alert, follows commands, and has these deficits, stroke is a consideration.

Severe metabolic derangements like hyponatremia, hypoglycemia, or hyperammonemia may favor a provoked seizure. Arterial and brain imaging can be helpful. The absence of a large vessel occlusion and the presence of hyperperfusion (due to higher metabolic activity on the seizure side) on CT perfusion are suggestive of seizure rather than ischemia [22]. While seizures can cause diffusion-weighted hyperintensity on MRI, similar to AIS, the pattern typically presents as gyriform cortical hyperintensity that does not respect typical vascular distributions [23].

Active seizures often require treatment with abortive agents like benzodiazepines. If a patient presents acutely with binocular horizontal gaze deviation to the same side as weakness, it would not be unreasonable to consider empiric treatment with a benzodiazepine as active seizure would be high on the differential. However, arterial imaging, brain imaging, and possibly rapid application of electroencephalography should all be considered.

Dizziness and Vertigo

The terms dizziness and vertigo are often used interchangeably, so we will try to differentiate them. Patients often describe dizziness as lightheadedness or a sense of instability, but, by definition, it is merely a catch-all term for a feeling of disequilibrium [24]. Vertigo, on the other hand, is typically defined as a false sense of motion, frequently with a sense of spinning or rotation [24]. Dizziness and vertigo are extremely common and responsible for at least 3.3% of emergency department visits in the United States annually [25].

Dizziness has numerous causes, many of which are systemic rather than neurologic, such as orthostasis, cardiac disorders, medication toxicity, and metabolic disturbance [25, 26] (see Table 12.1). Vertigo can either be peripheral or central in origin. "Peripheral vertigo" arises from a pathology of the peripheral vestibular system (primarily the semicircular canals, structures adjoining the semicircular canals, and the vestibular nerves) [27]. Conditions causing peripheral vestibulopathy

Table 12.1 Common causes of dizziness. Dizziness can be broadly categorized into central, peripheral, and systemic causes

Central	Peripheral	Systemic
• Posterior circulation infarct • Tumor • Multiple sclerosis • Migraine aura	• Vestibular neuritis/ labyrinthitis • Meniere's disease • BPPV • Acoustic neuroma	• Orthostatic hypotension • Medication toxicity • Arrhythmia

include vestibular neuritis and benign paroxysmal positional vertigo (BPPV). "Central vertigo" arises from a central lesion in the brain, such as stroke/TIA, demyelinating disease, migraine, and toxic-metabolic encephalopathies.

Differentiating true vertigo (vestibular dysfunction) from dizziness can be challenging. However, a thorough history, including triggers and alleviating factors, presence of other focal symptoms, prior similar episodes, medication review, and review of orthostatic vital signs, can be very helpful. It is important to note that patients' descriptions or interpretations of their dizziness vary widely and do not reliably distinguish vertigo from dizziness [28]. Symptoms of dizziness that arise purely when standing up suggest orthostasis, warranting a review of medications (beta blockers) and fluid volume status [26]. Vision loss, diplopia, sensory change, weakness, hearing loss, dysarthria, dysphagia, or ataxia should increase suspicion of a central cause of vertigo, such as stroke [29, 30].

Distinguishing a peripheral from a central cause of AVS can be challenging, as many signs and symptoms overlap between the two [29, 30]. Brief episodes of vertigo triggered specifically with head movement and resolved with rest (typically after seconds to minutes) suggest BPPV, which is responsible for 10% of all cases presenting to the ED with dizziness [31, 32]. The Dix-Hallpike maneuver has good sensitivity in diagnosing BPPV, specifically for patients with short, motion-triggered episodes of vertigo. The Dix-Hallpike maneuver is only appropriate for patients with no other neurological findings and who are asymptomatic if sitting still. There are excellent online videos on how to perform this test.

New-onset isolated vertigo that is continuous, prolonged, and associated with nausea and vomiting, exacerbated by head turning but still present at rest, should raise a concern for stroke, especially with vomiting that is out of proportion to the vertigo [33, 34]. Also concerning for stroke is bidirectional (the fast phase goes in the direction of gaze in both directions), vertical, or torsional nystagmus, as is the presence of skew deviation (vertical misalignment of the eyes) [33]. Unidirectional nystagmus (fast phase in one direction no matter the direction of gaze) is not specific for either peripheral or central vertigo [33].

When evaluating a patient with hours or days of continuous vertigo, nausea, and vomiting, the examination technique is the HINTS + hearing loss (head impulse, nystagmus, and test of skew) test. The first step is to look for nystagmus. To test for nystagmus, have the patient look to the right and then to the left. The direction of the nystagmus is based on which way the "fast phase" is pointing. Unidirectional nystagmus, suggestive of a peripheral process, means the fast phase goes in the same direction no matter which way the patient is looking. Bidirectional nystagmus occurs when the fast phase is in the same direction as the gaze. Bidirectional and vertical nystagmus should raise concern for stroke. HINTS (along with hearing evaluation) can reliably distinguish peripheral vestibulopathy from stroke [26].

The HINTS examination should only be performed on a patient with continuous vertigo and spontaneous nystagmus (nystagmus at resting forward gaze). Like Dix-Hallpike, there are excellent videos online for this examination as well.

1. The head impulse test (HIT) evaluates the vestibulocochlear nerve and the vestibulo-ocular reflex (VOR), which keeps an object in the line of sight despite head movement. Perform the HIT by holding the vertiginous patient's head in your hands while facing them and asking the patient to look at the tip of your nose. Then, quickly move the head 20–30° first to the same side as the direction of the nystagmus. Then, bring the head back to midline and quickly turn it in the opposite direction.

   Suppose the patient has peripheral vertigo (i.e., a viral inflammation of CN VIII or vestibular neuritis). In that case, the VOR will likely be impaired; the eyes will move with the head as it turns, requiring corrective saccades (a quick jump) back toward the tip of your nose. In vestibular neuritis, the direction of the nystagmus is almost always away from the affected ear, and the corrective saccade will occur when the head is turned toward the affected ear, with the corrective saccade in the same direction as the nystagmus. So, in a patient with vestibular neuritis of the left ear, the direction of the nystagmus will be to the right, and corrective saccades will be seen when turning the head quickly to the left. If the VOR is preserved in a patient with ongoing vertigo, the eyes will remain fixed on your nose, meaning the cause of the patient's vertigo is not inflammation of CN VIII but likely a stroke. *In other words, the abnormal finding is more reassuring for a benign process!* HIT should not be performed in patients with significant neck issues or concerns about cervical artery dissection.
2. Determine the direction of the nystagmus by having the patient look to the left and right. The direction of the fast phase is the direction of the nystagmus. In a patient with peripheral vertigo, nystagmus is either only in one direction, or the fast phase is in the same direction regardless of the gaze direction.
3. To test for skew, have the patient look at your nose. With your hand, cover one eye and then the other. If there is any vertical movement of either eye when you move your hand away, that is worrisome for a stroke.
4. Recently, the addition of acute hearing loss by finger rub to the HINTS examination (HINTS plus) has been shown to be more accurate than MRI in ruling out stroke [33, 34].

A reassuring HINTS examination requires a positive or abnormal head impulse test AND unidirectional nystagmus AND no skew deviation AND no acute hearing loss and has been shown to reliably rule out central etiologies of AVS with a sensitivity of 99% [33, 34]. Any abnormal findings should get stroke imaging. In many cases, however, it is very difficult to differentiate a peripheral from a central process. In those situations, an MRI can be helpful. However, as discussed in the introduction section, MRI has limitations: The false-negative rate for AIS is approximately 6–10%, and the strokes most likely to be missed by MRI are exactly the strokes most likely to cause AVS—acute, small, and located in the posterior circulation [5–7, 34]. Therefore, AIS should remain on the differential if a patient with AVS has a negative MRI if HINTS plus hearing loss testing suggests a central process [35].

Metabolic Mimics

Metabolic disarray can produce focal neurological deficits, especially hypoglycemia and, to a lesser extent, hyperglycemia [36, 37]. Hypoglycemia can lead to sedation, difficulty speaking, weakness, and seizures. The mechanism by which these conditions mimic stroke still needs to be fully understood, with one theory being decreased global cerebral perfusion paired with multiple mechanisms of cellular metabolic dysfunction [37]. Patients with stroke-like symptoms should have a point-of-care blood glucose test and require prompt correction of any significant abnormality. You do not want to give the patient thrombolytics if they only need some glucose! The American Heart Association suggests (class of recommendation IIa) intravenous thrombolysis for eligible patients with acute stroke-like symptoms when there is diagnostic uncertainty regarding stroke versus stroke mimic; the exception to this recommendation is when the patient's initial blood glucose is less than 50 or greater than 400. Still, the patient can simultaneously have an acute ischemic stroke and be hypoglycemic. In that situation, thrombolysis can be considered if the patient continues to have disabling neurological deficits despite correction of the hypoglycemia or hyperglycemia [9].

Other metabolic abnormalities linked with focal neurological deficits include hyponatremia, hypernatremia, and hepatic encephalopathy [38]. Hyponatremia and hypernatremia result in neurological dysfunction through cellular swelling and shrinkage, respectively [39]. In cases of low or elevated electrolyte levels, particularly disorders of sodium, care should be taken to correct these derangements slowly, as rapid correction in either direction can worsen neurological dysfunction and, in extreme cases, cause permanent neurological damage [39]. Hepatic encephalopathy is also associated with focal neurological deficits resulting from elevated levels of toxic metabolites within the CNS, leading to neuronal dysfunction [40].

Demyelinating Disease

An acute and focal central nervous system (CNS) demyelinating lesion can often present with signs and symptoms that mimic stroke, such as visual disturbance, ophthalmoplegia, vertigo, dysarthria, and motor and sensory symptoms [41]. However, this disease process is unlikely to produce the classic cortical signs associated with a large vessel occlusion (such as aphasia) or cognitive dysfunction [42].

CNS demyelinating diseases (DDs) are common, particularly multiple sclerosis (MS), which affects approximately 2.5 million people worldwide [43]. Historical features that may raise suspicion for CNS DD, such as MS rather than AIS, include relatively young age, a known history of MS, a family history of MS, symptoms suggestive of optic neuritis, bilateral motor or sensory symptoms, or bladder or bowel dysfunction (which may indicate spinal cord involvement) [41, 44–47]. Paroxysmal symptoms of MS are typically shorter than those of a TIA (seconds to minutes vs. minutes to hours) and can occur between 10 and 20 times per day [47].

MRI of the brain with and without contrast and MRI of the spine are the studies of choice when the diagnosis of DD is uncertain. MRI findings suggesting acute DD rather than AIS are lesion(s) that typically do not restrict diffusion, enhance with gadolinium contrast, and do not respect an identifiable vascular territory. The T2/FLAIR sequence may show multifocal white matter lesions (juxtacortical, periventricular, infratentorial, and in the spinal cord) that do not appear consistent with small vessel ischemic disease [41, 48]. Early demyelinating lesions, abscesses, and tumors can all demonstrate restricted diffusion and postcontrast enhancement on MRI [49].

Tumors

Approximately 25 people per 100,000 are newly diagnosed with an intracranial tumor yearly; fortunately, most are benign [50]. Intracranial tumors can cause focal neurological deficits mimicking stroke via multiple mechanisms, including direct disruption of normal brain parenchyma, tumor-associated edema, local mass effect on adjacent intracranial structures, increased intracranial pressure (which can cause "focal" symptoms near to or distant from the mass), and inducing seizures [51]. Tumor-associated neurological deficits often start with subtle symptoms days to weeks before presentation, except for seizures, which are more acute in onset. In addition to focal deficits, tumors may show signs of increased intracranial pressure due to edema and hydrocephalus, like headache (tumor-associated headaches are worse when the patient lays flat), lethargy, vomiting, or blurred vision [51, 52].

Imaging, particularly contrast-enhanced MRI, is critical for differentiating tumors from AIS. Tumors, both primary and metastatic, have significant contrast enhancement with surrounding vasogenic edema ("finger-like projections" of swelling) and have variable DWI/ADC values depending on tumor type [53]. Highly cellular tumors like high-grade gliomas and primary CNS lymphoma can demonstrate restricted diffusion like AIS [54]. Acute AIS may have minimal enhancement (but typically not as intense as a tumor), cytotoxic edema (more confluent), and fit a vascular distribution [53]. Thus, while specific imaging characteristics strongly suggest a tumor, sometimes it is unclear, and obtaining tissue via biopsy/resection to confirm diagnosis may be necessary. Neurosurgery and neuro-oncology consultations are warranted in this setting.

Abscess

An abscess is a walled-off collection of pus and immune cells. MRI demonstrates a large round or ovoid structure outside of a typical vascular territory, with surrounding edema and mass effect, a ring of contrast enhancement, and restricted diffusion on DWI, with the potential backdrop of infection with fever, meningismus (neck stiffness), and leukocytosis [55]. An abscess can occur in the context of fever, bacterial meningitis, endocarditis with septic embolism, immunocompromised state, or drug use. Prompt diagnosis of an abscess is essential, as this condition can be lethal if intervention (antibiotics ± surgical drainage) is not implemented expeditiously [55]. Neurosurgery and infectious disease consults are required here. These patients often belong in an ICU setting during their initial course.

Hypertensive Encephalopathy

Hypertensive encephalopathy (HE) refers to neurological symptoms and signs that arise due to a profound elevation in blood pressure [56]. Every patient has a baseline blood pressure (BP) range within which cerebral perfusion pressure (CPP) is maintained relatively constantly via brain autoregulatory mechanisms [56, 57]. However, a sustained BP increase above that baseline range may result in cerebral autoregulatory failure, vascular damage, and vasogenic edema within the brain [56, 57]. Notice we use the term "baseline," which focuses on the individual patient's physiology, and not "normal," which implies the same range for everyone. HE frequently leads to nonlocalizing symptoms of increased intracranial pressure, such as headache, nausea, vomiting, blurriness of vision, and fluctuating levels of confusion [57]. The confusion in HE is often misinterpreted as aphasia because both have abnormal speech. To differentiate encephalopathy from aphasia, a clinical pearl is to determine the patient's attentiveness. Patients with aphasia are alert and attentive to the examiner but have a clear speech deficit. On the other hand, encephalopathic patients may ignore the examiner, have a depressed level of alertness, and often ramble incoherently without appearing to struggle to speak.

Both HE and AIS frequently present with very elevated BP [58]. Prompt lowering of BP by up to 25% is the appropriate treatment for HE—and this intervention often leads to improvement of neurological symptoms in HE—but rapid BP lowering in the setting of AIS can lead to worsened symptoms and enlargement of the stroke [56, 58]. Therefore, when uncertain about the diagnosis, it is reasonable to gather more history, monitor the patient carefully, and pursue imaging of the arteries and brain MRI to rule out stroke if the patient is still eligible for acute thrombolytics.

Recrudescence Syndrome

Patients with prior stroke may experience reemergence of previously resolved (or nearly resolved) focal neurological deficits termed recrudescence [59]. While the exact mechanism is unclear, recrudescence may result from impairment of compensatory neurological pathways developed following stroke by some physiological stress [60]. Symptoms should not differ from or exceed the severity of the patient's prior stroke presentation [61]. Recrudescence should no longer be considered if the symptoms are different or worse than the patient has experienced before and no identifiable exacerbating trigger is identified, such as infection, fatigue, hypotension/dehydration, medication (sedatives, narcotics), and metabolic disturbance (hypoglycemia, hyponatremia) [62]. Without a clear trigger, recrudescence is unlikely and should prompt consideration of a new ischemic event.

Milder forms of recrudescence are common and many times are expected. Patients with aphasia will often notice more difficulty with speech production if they are fatigued or try to speak faster in a heightened emotional state. Patients may notice worsening weakness or balance towards the end of the day or if they have been ambulating or standing for extended periods of time. Counsel the patient that symptoms should resolve with rest, to speak slower, and to remove oneself from the emotional situations if possible.

Functional Mimics/Conversion Disorder

Functional (psychogenic) neurological syndromes can present with a variety of neurological symptoms and are reported to account for up to 10% of all stroke mimics [60]. Various focal deficits can be observed, with a prevalence of motor and sensory deficits, which in a functional patient can be inconsistent between repeated examinations [60]. However, these deficits have no identifiable underlying neurological cause after appropriate workup. Each presentation of functional symptoms should be handled carefully. Providers should validate the patient's symptoms and understand that they are frequently quite disabling [63]. However, the deficit results from abnormal functioning rather than permanent damage to the brain, which may be reassuring to the patient [63]. Consultation with a mental health provider is indicated for functional disorders, and physical or speech therapy may also be helpful [63] (Table 12.2).

Table 12.2 Key points summarizing stroke mimics

Mimic	Pearls
General principles	• A condition causing focal neurological deficits not caused by stroke is termed a stroke mimic • In the setting of transient symptoms, TIA should remain on the differential • MRI is very useful to rule out AIS but does have a false-negative rate of 6–10%. Small AISs in the posterior circulation are particularly associated with false-negative MRI • Patients presenting with an acute focal neurological deficit suspicious for stroke mimic but with disabling symptoms should be considered candidates for thrombolytic therapy, as the rate of symptomatic hemorrhage in stroke mimics is low
Migraine with aura	• Occurs via cortical spreading depression • Aura can occur before, during, or after a migrainous headache or may occur without a headache • Aura symptoms may be positive or negative, with positive visual symptoms being the most common • Negative visual symptoms are more suggestive of AIS than migraine • Aura symptoms occur slowly and progressively, with different symptoms occurring in a sequential fashion • Symptoms of AIS are typically rapid onset with multiple focal symptoms occurring nearly simultaneously rather than sequentially • Migraine does not typically cause restricted diffusion on MRI, except in rare cases of migrainous infarction • Care should be taken in ruling out TIA, as both TIA and migraine aura cause transient neurological deficits without restricted diffusion on MRI, but TIA typically does not cause headache • Genetic testing (mutations in *CACNA1A*, *ATP1A2*, and *SCN1A* have been associated with familial hemiplegic migraine
Seizures	• Seizures result from neuronal hyperactivity followed by hypoactivity in the postictal period • Assessment of gaze deviation can help differentiate stroke from seizure • An active seizure in one hemisphere may result in contralateral limb shaking or weakness and contralateral gaze deviation, whereas hemispheric stroke can cause contralateral weakness and ipsilateral gaze deviation • The postictal phase may mimic hemispheric stroke due to residual hypoactivity in the postictal hemisphere, resulting in contralateral weakness and ipsilateral gaze deviation • A brainstem infarction may result in both contralateral weakness and contralateral gaze deviation, thereby mimicking an active seizure • Seizures may cause cortical hyperintensity on MRI, often in a gyriform pattern that does not respect a vascular territory, sometimes associated with ipsilateral thalamic hyperintensity, features which are not characteristic of stroke

(continued)

Table 12.2 (continued)

Mimic	Pearls
Dizziness and vertigo	• History is critical and should include "timing and triggers" • Association with additional focal neurologic deficits suggests central rather than peripheral etiology • Symptoms such as intensity of the spinning sensation, worsening or lessening of the vertigo with head position or movement, presence of nausea/vomiting, and imbalance with ambulation do not reliably differentiate peripheral from central vertigo • Acute vestibular syndrome (AVS) is defined as new onset, prolonged, and continuous vertigo that may be central (as in AIS) or peripheral (as in vestibular neuritis) • The HINTS + hearing examination has 99% sensitivity for central etiology of vertigo and should be performed on all patients presenting with AVS • The HINTS + hearing examination is significantly more sensitive than MRI for posterior circulation AIS when MRI is performed within the first 48 h of symptom onset
Metabolic mimics	• Both hypoglycemia and hyperglycemia can produce focal neurological deficits • All patients presenting with stroke-like symptoms should have point-of-care glucose testing performed • Patients with acute focal neurological deficits and blood glucose less than 50 or greater than 400 should have blood glucose corrected first and symptoms reassessed before consideration of IV thrombolysis • Hyponatremia and hypernatremia may also produce focal neurological deficits
Demyelinating disease (DD)	• Historical features suggestive of DD include young age, family history, symptoms of optic neuritis, and bilateral motor or sensory symptoms • MS can rarely present with transient focal deficits similar to TIA, but episodes are typically shorter (seconds to minutes) and much more frequent (10–20 times per day) than with TIA • MRI findings suggesting DD include T2/FLAIR white matter hyperintensities in the juxtacortical, periventricular, and infratentorial regions and in the spinal cord that do not appear consistent with leukoaraiosis • Acute demyelinating lesions usually do not restrict diffusion on MRI and typically enhance with contrast, whereas AIS does restrict diffusion and typically does not enhance with contrast until several days after symptom onset
Mass lesions	• Focal symptoms can be caused by direct disruption of brain tissue, edema, local mass effect, increased intracranial pressure, and seizures • If intracranial pressure is sufficiently increased, focal symptoms may be accompanied by headache (particularly when supine), blurry vision, vomiting, or lethargy • On MRI, tumors frequently enhance with contrast, are associated with vasogenic edema, and usually do not restrict diffusion (but there are exceptions). AIS typically does not enhance with contrast in the hyperacute/early acute phase, respects vascular/arterial territories, may have surrounding cytotoxic edema, and restricts diffusion • Abscesses present in a similar fashion to tumors but are often accompanied by an infectious picture and, on MRI, typically appear as ring-enhancing lesions with diffusion restriction and vasogenic edema

Table 12.2 (continued)

Mimic	Pearls
Hypertensive encephalopathy (HE)	• HE occurs when the brain's autoregulatory mechanisms are overwhelmed and lead to vascular damage and edema within the brain • This does not typically cause focal neurological symptoms, but the extreme elevation of BP in HE combined with neurological dysfunction may suggest both HE and AIS • When the diagnosis is uncertain, caution with BP lowering is advised, as this may improve symptoms due to HE but may worsen stroke symptoms
Recrudescence	• Prior neurological deficits associated with encephalomalacia may reemerge in the setting of metabolic, infectious, or toxic disturbance • These deficits should not exceed the degree of the prior deficit • Imaging is often required to assess for new ischemic stroke
Functional mimics	• Account for up to 10% of all stroke mimics • Can present with ANY focal neurological deficit with a prevalence of motor and sensory symptoms • Examination findings may be inconsistent between exams • Imaging may be needed for diagnosis • Arm drift without pronation • Giveaway weakness • Inverse pyramidal pattern: Limb weakness with upper extremity extensor > flexor weakness and lower extremity flexor > extensor weakness • Nonreproducible speech pattern disturbances/inconsistencies • Facial lip pulling • Hoover's sign

References

1. Vilela P. Acute stroke differential diagnosis: stroke mimics. Eur J Radiol. 2017;96:133–44.
2. Edlow JA. Managing patients with transient ischemic attack. Ann Emerg Med. 2018;71(3):409–15.
3. Dubosh NM, et al. Sensitivity of early brain computed tomography to exclude aneurysmal subarachnoid hemorrhage. Stroke. 2016;47(3):750–5.
4. Latchaw RE, et al. Recommendations for imaging of acute ischemic stroke: a scientific statement from the American Heart Association. Stroke. 2009;40(11):3646–78.
5. Brunser AM, et al. Accuracy of diffusion-weighted imaging in the diagnosis of stroke in patients with suspected cerebral infarct. Stroke. 2013;44(4):1169–71.
6. Edlow BL, Hurwitz S, Edlow JA. Diagnosis of DWI-negative acute ischemic stroke: a meta-analysis. Neurology. 2017;89(3):256–62.
7. Choi J-H, et al. Early MRI-negative posterior circulation stroke presenting as acute dizziness. J Neurol. 2018;265(12):2993–3000.
8. Tsivgoulis G, et al. Safety of intravenous thrombolysis in stroke mimics: prospective 5-year study and comprehensive meta-analysis. Stroke. 2015;46(5):1281–7.
9. Powers WJ, et al. Guidelines for the early management of patients with acute ischemic stroke: 2019 update to the 2018 guidelines for the early management of acute ischemic stroke: a guideline for healthcare professionals from the American Heart Association/American Stroke Association. Stroke. 2019;50(12):e344–418.
10. Ashina M, et al. Migraine: epidemiology and systems of care. Lancet. 2021;397(10283):1485–95.

11. Kissoon NR, Cutrer FM. Aura and other neurologic dysfunction in or with migraine. Headache. 2017;57(7):1179–94.
12. Hadjikhani N, et al. Mechanisms of migraine aura revealed by functional MRI in human visual cortex. Proc Natl Acad Sci U S A. 2001;98(8):4687–92.
13. Headache Classification Committee of the International Headache Society (IHS). The international classification of headache disorders, 3rd edition. Cephalalgia. 2018;38(1):1–211.
14. Wolf ME, et al. Clinical and MRI characteristics of acute migrainous infarction. Neurology. 2011;76(22):1911–7.
15. Diener H-C. The risks or lack thereof of migraine treatments in vascular disease. Headache. 2020;60(3):649–53.
16. Kim T, Jeong HY, Suh GJ. Clinical differences between stroke and stroke mimics in code stroke patients. J Korean Med Sci. 2022;37(7):e54.
17. Keselman B, et al. Intravenous thrombolysis in stroke mimics: results from the SITS International Stroke Thrombolysis Register. Eur J Neurol. 2019;26(8):1091–7.
18. Gavvala JR, Schuele SU. New-onset seizure in adults and adolescents: a review. JAMA. 2016;316(24):2657–68.
19. Tarabar AF, ASU, D'Onofrio G. Seizure. In: Emergency medicine: clinical essentials. Saunders; 2013. p. 857–869.
20. Singer OC, et al. Conjugate eye deviation in acute stroke: incidence, hemispheric asymmetry, and lesion pattern. Stroke. 2006;37(11):2726–32.
21. Olaciregui Dague K, et al. Gaze palsy as a manifestation of Todd's phenomenon: case report and review of the literature. Brain Sci. 2020;10(5):298.
22. Kataoka S, et al. Paramedian pontine infarction. Neurological/topographical correlation. Stroke. 1997;28(4):809–15.
23. Lansberg MG, et al. MRI abnormalities associated with partial status epileptics. Neurology. 1999;52(5):1021–7.
24. Karatas M. Central vertigo and dizziness: epidemiology, differential diagnosis, and common causes. Neurologist. 2008;14(6):355–64.
25. Newman-Toker DE, et al. Spectrum of dizziness visits to US emergency departments: cross-sectional analysis from a nationally representative sample. Mayo Clin Proc. 2008;83(7):765–75.
26. Steenerson KK. Acute vestibular syndrome. Continuum (Minneap Minn). 2021;27(2):402–19.
27. Thompson TL, Amedee R. Vertigo: a review of common peripheral and central vestibular disorders. Ochsner J. 2009;9(1):20–6.
28. Newman-Toker DE, et al. Imprecision in patient reports of dizziness symptom quality: a cross-sectional study conducted in an acute care setting. Mayo Clin Proc. 2007;82(11):1329–40.
29. Searls DE, et al. Symptoms and signs of posterior circulation ischemia in the New England Medical Center posterior circulation registry. Arch Neurol. 2012;69(3):346–51.
30. Kerber KA. Acute vestibular syndrome. Semin Neurol. 2020;40(1):59–66.
31. Saber Tehrani AS, et al. Diagnosing stroke in acute dizziness and vertigo: pitfalls and pearls. Stroke. 2018;49(3):788–95.
32. Voetsch B, Sehgal S. Acute dizziness, vertigo, and unsteadiness. Neurol Clin. 2021;39(2):373–89.
33. Kattah JC. Use of HINTS in the acute vestibular syndrome. An overview. Stroke Vasc Neurol. 2018;3(4):190–6.
34. Newman-Toker DE, et al. HINTS outperforms ABCD2 to screen for stroke in acute continuous vertigo and dizziness. Acad Emerg Med. 2013;20(10):986–96.
35. Kattah JC, et al. HINTS to diagnose stroke in the acute vestibular syndrome. Stroke. 2009;40(11):3504–10.
36. Lee H. Isolated vascular vertigo. J Stroke. 2014;16(3):124–30.
37. Rossi S, et al. Acute stroke-like deficits associated with nonketotic hyperglycemic hyperosmolar state: an illustrative case and systematic review of literature. Neurol Sci. 2022;43(8):4671–83.
38. Singh R-J, Doshi D, Barber PA. Hypoglycemia causing focal cerebral hypoperfusion and acute stroke symptoms. Can J Neurol Sci. 2021;48(4):550–2.
39. Magauran BG Jr, Nitka M. Stroke mimics. Emerg Med Clin North Am. 2012;30(3):795–804.

40. Adrogué HJ, Tucker BM, Madias NE. Diagnosis and management of hyponatremia: a review. JAMA. 2022;328(3):280–91.
41. Ford H. Clinical presentation and diagnosis of multiple sclerosis. Clin Med. 2020;20(4):380–3.
42. Toledano M, Weinshenker BG, Solomon AJ. A clinical approach to the differential diagnosis of multiple sclerosis. Curr Neurol Neurosci Rep. 2015;15(8):57.
43. Dendrou CA, Fugger L, Friese MA. Immunopathology of multiple sclerosis. Nat Rev Immunol. 2015;15(9):545–58.
44. Filippi M, et al. Multiple sclerosis. Nat Rev Dis Primers. 2018;4(1):43.
45. Cotsapas C, Mitrovic M, Hafler D. Chapter 46—Multiple sclerosis. In: Geschwind DH, Paulson HL, Klein C, editors. Handbook of clinical neurology. Elsevier; 2018. p. 723–730.
46. Katz Sand I. Classification, diagnosis, and differential diagnosis of multiple sclerosis. Curr Opin Neurol. 2015;28(3):193–205.
47. Zhang Y, et al. Paroxysmal symptoms as the first manifestation of multiple sclerosis mimicking a transient ischemic attack: a report of two cases. Front Neurol. 2017;8:585.
48. Balashov KE, Lindzen E. Acute demyelinating lesions with restricted diffusion in multiple sclerosis. Mult Scler. 2012;18(12):1745–53.
49. Karonen JO, et al. Evolution of MR contrast enhancement patterns during the first week after acute ischemic stroke. AJNR Am J Neuroradiol. 2001;22(1):103–11.
50. Ostrom QT, et al. CBTRUS statistical report: primary brain and other central nervous system tumors diagnosed in the United States in 2015-2019. Neuro Oncol. 2022;24(Suppl 5):v1–v95.
51. Rees JH. Diagnosis, and treatment in neuro-oncology: an oncological perspective. Br J Radiol. 2011;84 Spec No 2(Spec Iss 2):S82–9.
52. Dostovic Z, et al. Brain edema after ischaemic stroke. Med Arch. 2016;70(5):339–41.
53. Adam G, et al. Magnetic resonance imaging of arterial stroke mimics: a pictorial review. Insights Imaging. 2018;9(5):815–31.
54. Gaddamanugu S, et al. Clinical applications of diffusion-weighted sequence in brain imaging: beyond stroke. Neuroradiology. 2022;64(1):15–30.
55. Muzumdar D, Jhawar S, Goel A. Brain abscess: an overview. Int J Surg. 2011;9(2):136–44.
56. Solar P, et al. Blood-brain barrier alterations and edema formation in different brain mass lesions. Front Cell Neurosci. 2022;16:922181.
57. Miller JB, et al. New developments in hypertensive encephalopathy. Curr Hypertens Rep. 2018;20(2):13.
58. Suneja M, Sanders ML. Hypertensive emergency. Med Clin North Am. 2017;101(3):465–78.
59. Dupre CM, et al. Stroke chameleons. J Stroke Cerebrovasc Dis. 2014;23(2):374–8.
60. Pohl M, et al. Ischemic stroke mimics: a comprehensive review. J Clin Neurosci. 2021;93:174–82.
61. Topcuoglu MA, et al. Recrudescence of deficits after stroke: clinical and imaging phenotype, triggers, and risk factors. JAMA Neurol. 2017;74(9):1048–55.
62. Tanaka T, Ihara M. Post-stroke epilepsy. Neurochem Int. 2017;107:219–28.
63. Popkirov S, Stone J, Buchan AM. Functional neurological disorder. Stroke. 2020;51(5):1629–35.

Disposition Decisions

13

Darshna Patel and Michael Lyerly

Following initial stabilization and provision of acute interventions in the Emergency Department, the next critical decision is determining the optimal setting where the patient can receive safe and effective care. Whenever possible, admission to a primary or comprehensive stroke center is the goal for stroke patients. Primary stroke centers (PSCs) can care for all stroke patients who receive thrombolytic therapy or are not eligible for acute reperfusion therapies. In contrast, comprehensive stroke centers (CSCs) provide a higher level of care for those requiring endovascular interventions and more complex neurocritical care. Standardized patient care protocols, organized stroke units, and well-educated staff knowledgeable in acute stroke care management and neurologic monitoring lead to optimal care regardless of the center's certification level.

Stroke Centers

Stroke Centers were first developed in the early 2000s to enhance the delivery of guideline-concordant stroke care. Stroke centers are required to demonstrate cohesive, interdisciplinary stroke teams, the use of standardized stroke protocols, and the formation of a dedicated care area called a stroke unit [1]. With the advent of endovascular therapy, protocols now also focus on early vessel imaging, cloud-based image sharing, and early mobilization of transport resources to rapidly identify and triage patients with large vessel occlusions requiring endovascular therapies. Primary Stroke Centers (PSCs) are suited to care for most stroke patients, including those with transient ischemic attack and cerebral infarcts not requiring neurointensive care services. Many stroke units in these hospitals are equipped to monitor those who have received intravenous thrombolytics (i.e., alteplase or tenecteplase)

D. Patel · M. Lyerly (✉)
University of Alabama, Birmingham, AL, USA
e-mail: dhpatel@uabmc.edu; mlyerly@uabmc.edu

© The Author(s), under exclusive license to Springer Nature Switzerland AG 2024   143
H. P. Amin (ed.), *Stroke for the Advanced Practice Clinician*,
https://doi.org/10.1007/978-3-031-66289-8_13

in a medical ICU. Although over 1000 PSCs have been designated nationwide, most are clustered in more urban areas, leading to geographic disparities in access.

The expansion of endovascular therapies has led to the rise of more Comprehensive Stroke Centers (CSCs) nationwide. These hospitals provide endovascular therapies, post-procedural care, and can manage associated complications in a dedicated neurological ICU [2]. These hospitals have access to neurosurgical and neurocritical care expertise and can manage complex ischemic strokes (e.g., those with cerebral edema or high risk of deterioration) and intracerebral hemorrhages. Thrombectomy Capable Centers (TSC) have recently emerged as facilities that can provide endovascular interventions (although frequently not 24/7) but without the full scope of resources as a CSC. Understanding the patient's needs and surrounding stroke centers' resources should help triage and transfer patients to the appropriate locations.

Interhospital Transfer

Many hospitals are neither PSCs nor CSCs but are acute stroke-capable (or acute stroke-ready), meaning they can evaluate, image, and treat stroke patients with thrombolytics in the ED. However, patients will then require transfer to a higher level of care for ongoing management. Acute stroke telemedicine has enabled many hospitals to become acute stroke-capable by expanding access to vascular neurology expertise. Telestroke is discussed in depth in another chapter. Guidelines for non-stroke-ready hospitals or satellite urgent care centers recommend transporting suspected stroke patients to the nearest stroke-capable hospital. For patients with clinically suspected large vessel occlusions (aphasia, gaze deviation, or neglect in addition to weakness or numbness; LVO), bypassing a PSC in favor of a CSC is reasonable as long as the additional transport time does not exceed 15 min [3]. Patients with LVO who present to PSCs will still require a second transport to a CSC. Door-in-door-out (DIDO) time is a metric measuring how much time a patient spends in an ED from when they arrive to when they leave to go to another hospital. All non-CSCs use DIDO as a performance measure to monitor quality and efficiency not just for stroke but for other conditions as well. Shorter DIDO times with a streamlined evaluation, imaging, treatment, and communication process are associated with higher reperfusion rates and lower mortality rates [4].

Levels of Care Within Hospitals

Designating the most appropriate level of care for the patient based on stroke severity and treatments administered helps prevent complications and maximizes outcomes. Each level of care has criteria for patient needs and nursing ratios (Table 13.1). A severity-based level of care determined by a certified stroke neurologist may include the following:

Table 13.1 Levels of care based on patient severity and needs

Capacity	NICU	Step-down	General ward
Nurse patient ratio	1:2	1:3	1:5
Hemodynamic monitoring	Every 1 h	Every 1–4 h	Every 4 h
Neurological monitoring	Every 1 h	Every 1–4 h	Every 4 h
Arterial line for BP monitoring	Yes	No	No
External ventricular drain	Yes	No	No
IV medications	Sedation, Pressors, Heparin, or Insulin drips	Some Pressors, Heparin, or Insulin drips	No drips
Expertise	Neuro critical care team, Stroke team, and Neurosurgery	Stroke team and Neurosurgery	Stroke team

1. Neuro intensive care unit
2. Stroke Stepdown unit (intermediate care unit)
3. Acute care stroke unit (general ward)

Neuro-intensive care units offer access to critical care intensivists or neuro-intensivists, as well as more dedicated nursing care and monitoring. They are best suited for those requiring mechanical ventilation, invasive monitoring (e.g., intracranial pressure monitors, arterial blood pressure monitors), medication drips (e.g., antihypertensives, pressors, or insulin), and patients with evidence of multiorgan dysfunction. Ischemic stroke patients with (or at risk for) significant cerebral edema belong in a neuro-intensive care unit, as do most patients with cerebral hemorrhage. The ICU is often the only setting where hourly neuro checks can be performed because of a lower nurse-to-patient ratio (typically 1:1 or 2:1). Therefore, patients at risk for neurologic worsening (see below) who need more frequent neuro checks should be considered for ICU level of care. Most hospitals will admit patients who received thrombolytics to the ICU for 24 h or more for frequent neuro-checks, while others may have step-down units equipped to handle straightforward thrombolytic patients. Finally, patients who have undergone endovascular thrombectomy require ICU for adequate post-procedure management and monitoring for complications such as vessel re-occlusion or hemorrhagic transformation. Situations where neuro checks change management include emergent thrombectomy for vessel occlusion or stat craniectomy for expansion of hemorrhage or edema.

A neuro-intensive care unit can provide continuous hemodynamic monitoring and critical care expertise to manage patients at high risk for worsening. These units are also best suited to implement acute interventions such as hyperosmolar therapies for cerebral edema, correction of metabolic abnormalities, or hemodynamic augmentation.

Many hospitals have implemented intermediate care (sometimes called step-down) units to manage stroke patients. These came about as a more cost-effective means to manage patients who have received intravenous thrombolytics but do not otherwise have critical care needs. These units also have a low nurse-to-patient ratio (typically 3:1 or 4:1). They can offer more frequent neurologic monitoring than a "floor" bed (usually every 2 h). Most non-critically ill stroke patients are appropriate for this level of care for the initial portion of their hospitalization. In hospitals without intermediate care units, the provider must evaluate which unit, the general ward or ICU, more closely meets the patient's needs.

The final option for stroke admission is a general medical or neurological ward (sometimes called a "floor" bed). These units have standard nursing care (nurse-to-patient ratio typically ≥4:1); therefore, frequent neurological assessments beyond once or twice a shift are not possible. Regular floor beds should provide continuous telemetry monitoring, which all stroke patients need to monitor for arrhythmias.

Most stroke centers have a designated stroke unit staffed by a multidisciplinary team of specialists in the care of stroke patients [5]. Patients admitted to a dedicated stroke unit have reduced morbidity and mortality compared to those admitted to non-stroke units. A multidisciplinary team improves communication, a crucial factor in exceptional patient care, and reduces adverse patient outcomes. Nurses in stroke units are better trained to educate patients on stroke-specific risk factors. By having stroke patients in one centralized area, the multidisciplinary team of providers, nurses, social workers, case managers, and therapists can frequently interact to determine the best possible next steps in a patient's stroke care and disposition.

Neurological Worsening

Neurological worsening occurs in up to 25% of patients during the first 24–48 h after stroke, regardless of the unit setting [6]. The challenge is anticipating which patients are more likely to worsen and placing them in a higher level of care to catch worsening quickly. Predictors of early deterioration include higher initial stroke severity, multiple medical comorbidities, seizures, large vessel occlusions or stenosis, and hemorrhage. Patients with critical stenosis in the cervical or intracranial vasculature are also at risk of worsening during hemodynamic fluctuations and hypoperfusion.

Clinical Pearls
- Certified primary or comprehensive stroke centers, with dedicated stroke units, specialized nursing, stroke expertise, and multidisciplinary management teams, are associated with better patient outcomes.
- For patients who require inter-hospital transfer for a higher level of care, quality efforts should focus on DIDO times to minimize delays in care.
- Providers should be familiar with the resources for patient management in different hospital areas to match the appropriate level of care to the patient's needs and risk for neurological deterioration.

References

1. Alberts MJ, Hademenos G, Latchaw RE, Jagoda A, Marler JR, Mayberg MR, et al. Recommendations for the establishment of primary stroke centers. Brain attack coalition. JAMA. 2000;283:3102–9.
2. Alberts MJ, Latchaw RE, Selman WR, Shephard T, Hadley MN, Brass LM, et al. Recommendations for comprehensive stroke centers: a consensus statement from the brain attack coalition. Stroke. 2005;36:1597–616.
3. Powers WJ, Rabinstein AA, Ackerson T, Adeoye OM, Bambakidis NC, Becker K, et al. Guidelines for the early management of patients with acute ischemic stroke: 2019 update to the 2018 guidelines for the early management of acute ischemic stroke: a guideline for health-care professionals from the American Heart Association/American Stroke Association. Stroke. 2019;50:e344–418.
4. McTaggart RA, Moldovan K, Oliver LA, Dibiasio EL, Baird GL, Hemendinger ML, et al. Door-in-door-out time at primary stroke centers may predict outcomes for emergent large vessel occlusion patients. Stroke. 2018;49:2969–74.
5. Langhorne P. The stroke unit story: where have we been and where are we going? Cerebrovasc Dis. 2021;50:636–43.
6. Seners P, Turc G, Oppenheim C, Baron JC. Incidence, causes, and predictors of neurological deterioration occurring within 24 h following acute ischaemic stroke: a systematic review with pathophysiological implications. J Neurol Neurosurg Psychiatry. 2015;86:87–94.

Stroke Centers and Certification

14

Susan Ashcraft and Kiffon Keigher

Introduction

Obtaining stroke center certification has become the hallmark of demonstrating that a healthcare facility provides organized, evidence-based care, regardless of size or location. Certification of stroke centers has been linked to better functional outcomes [1]. Various organizations like The Joint Commission (TJC), Net Norske Veritas (DNV), Healthcare Facilities Accreditation Program (HFAP), and some state-run organizations offer certifications or designations for a stroke program. The requirements for certification vary between agencies, including differences in survey frequency, patient and treatment volumes, availability of specific resources, and clinicians' experience. As an advanced practice clinician (APC), it is essential to understand the stroke program's certification status and the APC's role in providing stroke care.

Four different levels of stroke center certification exist, including Acute Stroke-Ready Hospitals (ASRH), Primary Stroke Centers (PSCs), Thrombectomy-Capable Stroke Centers (TSC), and Comprehensive Stroke Centers (CSCs). An ASRH provides an organized system of care that expedites diagnostic workup for treatment decisions and can administer thrombolytic therapy to eligible ischemic stroke patients. They may or may not be able to admit patients after thrombolysis. These centers can transfer patients to other stroke centers for ongoing care or advanced treatments like thrombectomy. Facilities designated ASRH are commonly located in rural, less densely populated areas or where there is a significant distance from centers with advanced stroke care. The next level of stroke certification is the PSC,

S. Ashcraft (✉)
Novant Health, Charlotte, NC, USA
e-mail: sjashcraft@novanthealth.org

K. Keigher
Downers Grove, IL, USA
e-mail: Kiffon.Keigher@aah.org

© The Author(s), under exclusive license to Springer Nature Switzerland AG 2024
H. P. Amin (ed.), *Stroke for the Advanced Practice Clinician*,
https://doi.org/10.1007/978-3-031-66289-8_14

which has a dedicated team for emergent stroke diagnostic workup and treatment, plus a dedicated stroke unit to provide ongoing inpatient care. TSC meet all requirements for a PSC but also have an on-call interventionalist team to provide mechanical thrombectomy care with a dedicated critical care unit to monitor and care for ischemic stroke patients post-procedure. CSCs are considered the most advanced and provide care to both ischemic and hemorrhagic stroke patients, with practitioners with extensive expertise in vascular neurology, neurocritical care, and neurosurgery. In addition, CSCs have a skilled, comprehensive team of bedside clinicians who provide care to these complex patients.

A stroke program's capabilities for delivering evidence-based care will determine the level of certification. Certification requirements by level are outlined in Table 14.1. As stroke care continues to evolve rapidly, the requirements are often modified. Keeping up with the most up-to-date benchmarks will ensure adherence to level-specific standards.

Table 14.1 Stroke program-level requirements

Requirements	ASRH	PSC	TSC	CSC
Stroke volumes	No requirements	No requirements	Thrombectomy procedures and post-intervention care volume requirements	Thrombectomy procedures, post-intervention care, aneurysmal SAH treatment, and securement volume requirements
Specialty resources	No requirements	Designated Stroke Beds/Unit	Designated Stroke Beds/Unit Designated Neuro Intensive Care Beds/ Unit	Designated Stroke Beds/Unit Designated Neuro Intensive Care Beds/ Unit
Imaging/ Diagnostics	CT MRI, if required by protocol 24/7 lab results Electrocardiogram	CT/CTA/MRI/ MRA Transthoracic echocardiogram 24/7 lab results Electrocardiogram	Catheter angiography Carotid duplex Trans-thoracic and esophageal echocardiogram CT/CTA/MRI/MRA Transcranial doppler	Catheter angiography Carotid duplex Trans-thoracic and esophageal echocardiogram CT/CTA/MRI/MRA Transcranial doppler
Treatment availability	Thrombolytic administration	Thrombolytic administration time frame requirements	Thrombolytic administration Cerebral angiography Thrombectomy	Thrombolytic administration Cerebral angiography Thrombectomy Endovascular and surgical aneurysm repair Carotid endarterectomy and stenting

Table 14.1   Continued

Requirements	ASRH	PSC	TSC	CSC
Expertise availability	ED providers Access to cerebrovascular expertise via Telemedicine	If it provides neurosurgery services—a written plan and call schedule	24/7 access to: ED providers Neurointerventionalist Neurocritical care providers If it provides neurosurgery services—a written plan and call schedule	24/7 access to: ED providers Neurosurgeons Neuroradiologists Neurointerventionalist Neurovascular Physicians Neurocritical Care Providers Physiatrist or equivalent Pharmacist Nurse CM, SW OT/PT/ST APC that supports the program
Quality metrics	Standardized measures Focus on the implementation of EBP care and processes	Standardized measures Focus on implementation of EBP care, processes, and complications post-thrombolytics	Standardized measures Focus on implementing EBP care, processes, and outcomes post-thrombolytics and endovascular therapy	Standardized measures Focus on implementing EBP care, processes, and outcomes post-thrombolytics, thrombectomy, CEA/ CAS, ventriculostomy, and aneurysm treatment
Clinical stroke research	No	No	No	Yes
Educational offerings	Pre-hospital personnel education	Pre-hospital personnel education Public educational activities/year	Pre-hospital personnel education Public educational activities/year	Public educational activities/year Professional educational activities for internal or external participants

APC Advanced Practice Clinician, *ASRH* Acute Stroke Ready Hospital, *CAS* Carotid Artery Stent, *CEA* Carotid Endarterectomy, *CM* Case Manager, *CT* Computerized Tomography, *CTA* Computed Tomography Angiography, *CSC* Comprehensive Stroke Center, *ED* Emergency Department, *EBP* Evidence-based practice, *MRA* Magnetic Resonance Angiography, *MRI* Magnetic Resonance Imaging, *OT* Occupational Therapy, *PT* Physical Therapy, *PSC* Primary Stroke Center, *TSC* Thrombectomy Capable Stroke, *SW* Social Work, *ST* Speech Therapy, *SAH* Subarachnoid Hemorrhage

National Agency and State-Level Certifications

In the United States, all 50 states and Washington D.C. have hospitals certified as stroke centers. Most states require certification by a national agency such as TJC, DNV, or HFAP. APPs in clinical and leadership positions within a stroke program are vital for adherence to standards and certification requirements, which ensures the implementation of evidence-based care for patients.

Certification Considerations for the Hospital APP Leader

The success of stroke certification requires hospital leaders' engagement, vision, and support. Different types of leaders will evaluate and strategize the program's design based on their unique leadership roles. The lens by which executive leadership and clinical operations leaders will approach certification is helpful to recognize, as APCs may occupy many of these positions within organizations. As a service line leader, designing a strategy encompassing resource allocation, clinical operations, capital needs, and financial success is critical. A review and understanding of market share, growth opportunities, and impact of the stroke program is necessary for service line and executive c-suite leaders alike.

For APCs that may serve in operations, the primary focus will be a review of staffing, partnerships, technologies, education and training, data capture, and compliance. Multi-disciplinary collaborative work is the hallmark of stroke programs. The operations leader must be able to design teams and workflows that support collaboration, safety, and evidence-based practice for the best patient outcomes and to maintain regulatory compliance. Special attention to the needs of clinical operations, including nursing management, is critical.

The stroke coordinator leader has ultimate oversight of the program. Coordinators must have a broad lens over the program to help keep all key stakeholders engaged and aware of outcomes. The focus of the coordinator role varies based on other hospital resources allocated to the stroke program. In general, stroke coordinators spend much of their time on program management, data collection, analytics and reporting, patient education, and competencies of staff and providers (Table 14.2) [2].

Table 14.2 Roles of the stroke coordinator

- Entering/abstraction of Data
- Education: Patients, community, staff, MD, EMS
- Quality Improvement
- Development of policies and procedures based on EBP
- Research
- Re-certification
- Clinical: Stroke codes, inpatient, outpatient
- Face of stroke programs

Training for a Stroke Program Reviewer

The training and onboarding of stroke program reviewers for the different regulatory agencies is not standardized. While there is a great deal of literature on the education and training of hospital staff to provide stroke care, there are virtually no reports from regulatory bodies on how they prepare reviewers to serve in these governing roles. Each agency is assumed to have a robust onboarding and orientation process with ongoing annual training and seminars to ensure expertise and compliance.

Disease-specific stroke reviewers must be experts in the field. Most reviewers are APCs, nurses, or physicians who served in clinical roles in the field they are reviewing. It is a core requirement that all program reviewers have a robust understanding of current guidelines that drive the delivery of care. Additionally, and equally important, reviewers must understand best practices and current research in the field and master the required resources for each type of stroke certification. Ultimately, the goal of the review is to determine compliance, the safety of care, and adherence to established guidelines, leading to good outcomes. To ensure best practices, ongoing training for stroke program reviewers focuses on comprehension and interpretation of the data.

Keen observation, thoughtful listening, and sharing constructive direction, knowledge, and feedback are defining traits of stroke reviewers. The goal is to ensure compliance and provide a collaborative discussion with direction for programs on methods that may help with continued growth and sound strategy. The APC will need to be an active participant with excellent communication skills.

Summary

The role of the APC has far-reaching capabilities in the healthcare environment. The approach to stroke program design and development as an APC hospital leader requires a unique skillset compared to that of the APC stroke program regulatory agency reviewer. However, each requires a robust understanding of clinical guidelines and the resources needed for these complex and multi-disciplinary teams.

Clinical Pearls
- Stroke center certification has been shown to improve outcomes and ensures adherence to evidence-based practice
- Understanding the resources required for each level of certification is critical for a reviewer
- Thrombectomy Capable Stroke Centers can perform thrombectomies and care for uncomplicated patients, whereas CSCs can care for the entire spectrum of stroke patients, including hemorrhages
- Advancing in leadership roles allows an APP to make a larger impact on stroke care in their hospital

References

1. Raychev R, Sun JL, Schwamm L, Smith EE, Fonarow GC, Messé SR, Xian Y, Chiswell K, Blanco R, Mac Grory B, Saver JL. Performance of thrombectomy-capable, comprehensive, and primary stroke centers in reperfusion therapies for acute ischemic stroke: report from the get with the guidelines-stroke registry. Circulation. 2023;148(25):2019–28.
2. Purvis T, Middleton S, Alexandrov AW, et al. Understanding coordinator roles in acute stroke care: a national survey. J Stroke Cerebrovasc Dis. 2021;12:106111. https://doi.org/10.1016/j.jstrokecerebrovasdis.2021.106111.

Core Measures and Data Collection

15

Karin V. Nyström and Adam S. Jasne

Introduction

Over the past several decades, examining the quality of clinical care has become an important initiative for practitioners and healthcare organizations. The significance for optimal outcomes in quality clinical practice and excellence in care include public recognition (Hospital-of-Choice), desired patient outcomes (CMS mortality and morbidity statistics), public reporting opportunities ("Best Clinician," U.S. News and World Report), and financial incentives (Pay for Performance) [1]. Research initiatives and publications have evaluated variability in stroke care, in order to standardize stroke practice to improve patient-related and process-related outcomes [2].

The organization of stroke programs and stroke systems of care has revolutionized the approach to stroke care, leading to the use of disease-specific order sets, care pathways, electronic medical record (EMR)-generated databases/repositories, and a plethora of performance improvement platforms. This has significantly strengthened the quality of stroke care across the U.S. and worldwide [3]. Looking ahead, this chapter will explore the inpatient hospital environment as the domain that has driven much of this work. It is anticipated that over the next 10 years, there will be an increased focus towards primary and secondary prevention metrics driven by ambulatory clinicians and outpatient-specific healthcare programs.

K. V. Nyström
Yale New Haven Hospital, New Haven, CT, USA
e-mail: Karin.nystrom@yale.edu

A. S. Jasne (✉)
Yale School of Medicine, New Haven, CT, USA
e-mail: adam.jasne@yale.edu

Table 15.1 Source: Institute of Medicine (IOM): Crossing the quality chasm, 2001 [4]

Six domains of healthcare quality
- *Safe*: Avoiding harm to patients from the care intended to help them
- *Effective*: Providing services based on scientific knowledge to all who could benefit and refraining from providing services to those not likely to benefit (avoiding underuse and misuse, respectively)
- *Patient-centered*: Proving care that is respectful of and responsive to individual patient preferences, needs, and values and ensuring that patient values guide all clinical decisions
- *Timely*: Reducing wait times and sometimes harmful delays for those who receive and give care
- *Efficient*: Avoiding waste, including waste of equipment, supplies, ideas, and energy
- *Equitable*: Providing care that does not vary in quality because of personal characteristics such as gender, ethnicity, geographic location, and socioeconomic status

Setting the Stage for Healthcare Quality

At the turn of the twenty-first century, a series of publications and novel treatment paradigms significantly impacted the healthcare field and stroke care. The Institute of Medicine (IOM) published *Crossing the Quality Chasm* in 2000, introducing six healthcare quality domains with recommendations to address the gaps in healthcare practices (Table 15.1) [4]. These domains set the stage for healthcare organizations to formalize their mission, strategic vision, and patient-centered values for delivering quality care.

Alongside this framework, the Brain Attack Coalition (BAC) published the first stroke "guideline" in 2000, supporting the establishment of Primary Stroke Centers and the components necessary for delivering evidence-based care [5]. A key element included in the recommendations was using a database or registry to track selected aspects of performance that could be measured, trended over time, and benchmarked with external sources. An accompanying quality improvement program was also recommended to measure selected patient-related and system-related outcomes.

This publication followed two landmark efforts: the 1996 FDA approval of alteplase for suspected acute ischemic stroke patients and the 1998 establishment of the American Stroke Association as a part of the American Heart Association [6, 7]. In line with the work in the cardiology field to develop performance measures and quality metrics from the published clinical practice guidelines, stroke experts and several other organizations developed performance metrics that aligned with the evidence-based clinical practice guidelines [8, 9]. Over the years, stroke performance measures became standardized in that they have precisely defined specifications, meet established evaluation criteria, can be uniformly adopted for use, and are selected to be part of the larger set of requirements for recognition by Centers for Medicare and Medicaid Services (CMS), the National Quality Forum (NQF), the Veterans Administration Stroke Quality Enhancement Research Initiative, as well as certification organizations such as The Joint Commission (TJC), Det Norske Veritas (DNV) and Healthcare Facilities Accreditation Program (HFAP).

Types of Performance Measures

- *Standardized Measures*: Standardized performance measures are expert-driven and endorsed by agencies like the Joint Commission. They have precisely defined specifications, have standardized data collection protocols, meet established evaluation criteria, and can be uniformly adopted. Where applicable, standardized measures replace non-standardized measures and must be uniform.
- *Clinical Measures*: For hospitalists not using standardized measures, selected clinical measures evaluate processes and outcomes of care associated with the delivery of clinical services. They allow for intra- and inter-organizational comparisons that can be used to continuously improve patient health outcomes and focus on the appropriateness of clinical decision-making and implementation of those decisions. These measures must be condition—or procedure-specific or address essential functions of patient care, such as medication use, infection control, patient assessment, and patient safety.

History and Development of Stroke Centers

The call to formalize the delivery of acute and recovery stroke care outlined in the 2000 BAC publication paved the way for the "tiered" stroke center recognition programs across the U.S. today. While there was a common goal to deliver rapid, efficient, and quality care to acute stroke patients, it was evident that healthcare facilities across the country had varying resources and capacities and could only provide some of the acute and recovery stroke care elements. As with other medical conditions, patients needing complex stroke care often benefit from initial acute care treatment and transfer to a higher level of care for further management. Following the original 2000 BAC publication for the recommendations for Primary Stroke Centers, additional levels of stroke center certification have been established, which will be discussed in greater depth in another chapter. Figure 15.1 maps out the locations of all stroke centers in the U.S. as of 2018. Note the relatively high concentrations along the coasts [11]. Figure 15.1 represents the stroke center certification tiers ranging from the Acute Stroke Ready Hospital to the Comprehensive Stroke Center. It broadly describes the criteria and resources needed to meet the standards for certification [10].

Databases/Registries

Whether local, regional, or national, databases and registries are critical tools for improving our understanding of disease states and the quality of stroke care. They are used to evaluate selected data to report incidence, track interventions, and describe outcomes. Databases can highlight the demographics of stroke patients, what risk factors offer opportunities for better control, and where clinicians can best target education, particularly in the context of disparities in access to care. Databases

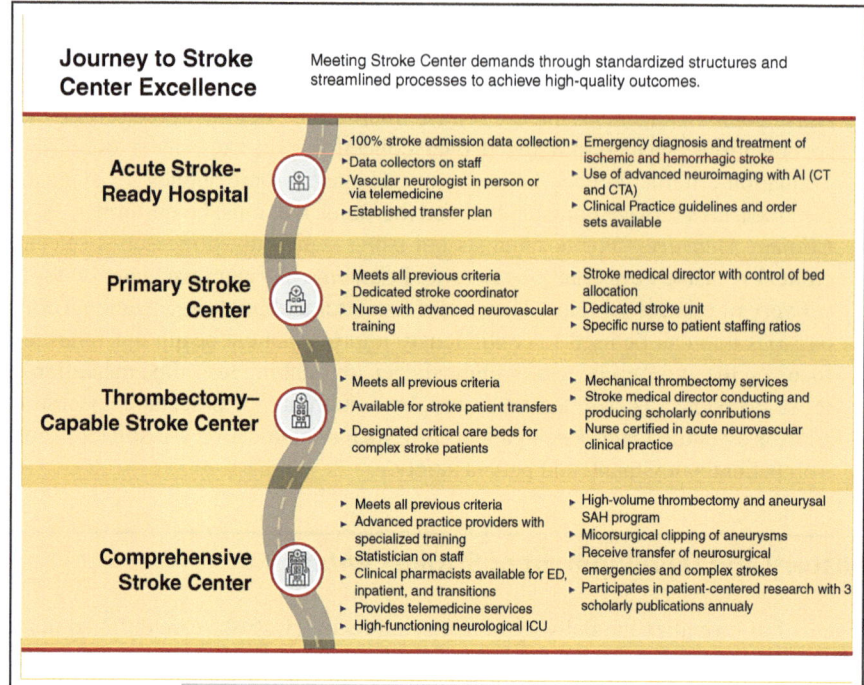

Figure 1. Journey to stroke center excellence.
Creating standard criteria for the structure of stroke centers enhances system efficiency and patient outcomes. AI indicated artificial intelligence; CT, computed tomography; CTA, computed tomographic angiography; ED, emergency department; ICU, intensive care unit; and SAH subarachnoid hemorrhage.

Fig. 15.1 The Journey to Stroke Center Excellence (reprinted with permission) [10]

and registries can also track the best interventions to improve patient outcomes. While research trials can offer insight into these subjects, databases, and registries provide real-world and more location-specific data.

Following the BAC's publication of stroke center recommendations, two registries were launched in the U.S. to support the work on stroke care quality. The Centers for Disease Control and Prevention's Paul Coverdell National Acute Stroke Registry rolled out in 2001, targeting states that could collect pre-hospital and acute stroke care data and develop quality improvement initiatives to enhance stroke care. Get-With-the-Guidelines-Stroke (GWTG) is a popular registry for hospitals to compile data-specific standardized stroke performance measures. It has since expanded to include practice parameters supported by stroke clinical guidelines and evidence-based practice [12]. While not feasible for all hospitals, voluntary participation in certification programs increases guideline adherence [13, 14].

Measuring Performance

Why measure health care performance? In part, practice measurements help inform internal stakeholders, such as clinicians and stroke program leadership, about how effectively selected practices are delivered. Performance measures also inform external stakeholders, such as patients, payors, and government agencies, about the health system and have clinical and financial support implications. Implementing these performance guidelines and selected measures has been associated with improved outcomes, such as length of stay and risk-adjusted hospital mortality [15]. Components for improvement in healthcare models have been summarized by Donabedian's model, which outlines three components: *structure*, *process*, and *outcome* [16]. *Structure* refers to a healthcare system's physical environment, equipment, and personnel resources. *Process* refers to the interactions between providers and patients or the direct delivery of care. *Outcome* refers to the impact or result of the interactions or services provided to patients by healthcare providers (see Table 15.2).

The American Heart Association Task Force on Performance Measures defined *quality metrics* as measures that "promote self-assessment and subsequent

Table 15.2 Components for improvement in healthcare models [16]

Structural Measures

Structural measures give consumers a sense of a health care provider's capacity, systems, and processes to provide high-quality care. For example:
- Whether the health care organization uses electronic medical records or medication order entry systems
- The number or proportion of board-certified physicians
- The ratio of providers to patients

Process Measures

Process measures indicate what a provider does to maintain or improve health, either for healthy people or for those diagnosed with a health care condition. These measures typically reflect generally accepted recommendations for clinical practice. For example:
- The percentage of people receiving preventive services (such as mammograms or immunizations)
- The percentage of people with diabetes who had their blood sugar tested and controlled

Process measures can inform consumers about medical care they may expect to receive for a given condition or disease, and can contribute toward improving health outcomes. The majority of health care quality measures used for public reporting are process measures

Outcome Measures

Outcome measures reflect the impact of the health care service or intervention on the health status of patients. For example:
- The percentage of patients who died as a result of surgery (surgical mortality rates)
- The rate of surgical complications or hospital-acquired infections

Outcome measures may seem to represent the "gold standard" in measuring quality, but an outcome is the result of numerous factors, many beyond providers' control. Risk-adjustment methods—mathematical models that correct for differing characteristics within a population, such as patient health status—can help account for these factors. However, the science of risk adjustment is still evolving. Experts acknowledge that better risk-adjustment methods are needed to minimize the reporting of misleading or even inaccurate information about health care quality improvement among healthcare providers and their respective healthcare systems" [17]. The Task Force further defined *performance measures* as "practice measures vetted by a formal review process and designed to be benchmarked with other similar healthcare facilities as well as reportable for public awareness" [9].

While recognizing the importance of quality throughout the stroke care continuum, from hyper-acute and acute/recovery care to rehabilitation and long-term recovery, early work to standardize performance measures has focused on the care of patients recovering from ischemic stroke. Standardized stroke metrics related to short-term and long-term outcomes have been part of stroke centers' overall quality and performance improvement programs for over two decades. Stroke programs have multiple standardized performance measures with mapped algorithms for determining the denominator and numerator and specific inclusion and exclusion criteria for each metric incorporated into the performance plans and improvement initiatives [2].

Metrics are "built" using a definition and rationale for the measure (derived from evidence-based practice guidelines), describing the metric type (structure, process, or outcome), whether the improvement direction should be positive (more patients receiving DVT prophylaxis) or negative (fewer patients with hemorrhagic transformation), and what elements would include or exclude the patient. A ratio or fraction is then created based on the patient population that meets the metric and the larger patient population that is eligible for the metric. A detailed description of a standard metric, "Venous Thromboembolism" VTE Prophylaxis is outlined in Fig. 15.2), and includes the rationale (clinical evidence) for the measure as well as the measure type and the desired direction (i.e., an increase in the rate). Process metrics are typically included as items in an order-set or pathway so that clinicians include them in the overall care plan. Tracking metrics compliance from an electronic medical record allows for the abstraction of this data from "queryable" fields and supports both the abstraction and the reporting process. The data extraction algorithm described in Fig. 15.3 provides a sequential approach to considering possible exclusion criteria so that the final numerator accurately includes patients for whom the metric would be clinically relevant. In this example, patients who might be deemed

---

Performance Measure Name: Venous Thromboembolism (VTE Prophylaxis)

Description: Ischemic or hemorrhagic stroke patients who received VTE prophylaxis or have documentation why no VTE prophylaxis was given the day of or the day after hospital admission

Rationale: Stroke patients are at increased risk of developing venous thromboembolism (VTE). One study noted proximal deep vein thrombosis in more than a third of patients with moderately severe stroke. Reported rates of occurrence vary depending on the type of screening used. Prevention of VTE, through the use of prophylactic therapies, in at risk patients is a noted recommendation in numerous clinical practice guidelines. For acutely ill stroke patients who are confined to bed, thromboprophylaxis with low-molecular-weight heparin (LMWH), low-dose unfractionated heparin (LDUH), or fondaparinux is recommended if there are no contraindications. Aspirin alone is not recommended as an agent to prevent VTE.

Type Of Measure: Process

Improvement Noted As: Increase in the rate

Numerator Statement: Ischemic or hemorrhagic stroke patients who received VTE prophylaxis or have documentation why no VTE prophylaxis was given on the day of or the day after hospital admission.

Included Populations: Not applicable

Excluded Populations: None

Fig. 15.2 Venous thromboembolism metric. (Source: Specifications Manual for Joint Commission National Quality Measures (v2023A))

STK-1: Venous Thromboembolism Prophylaxis

Numerator: Ischemic or hemorrhagic stroke patients who received VTE prophylaxis or have documentation why no VTE prophylaxis was given on the day of day after hospital admission.

Denominator: Ischemic or hemorrhagic stroke patients

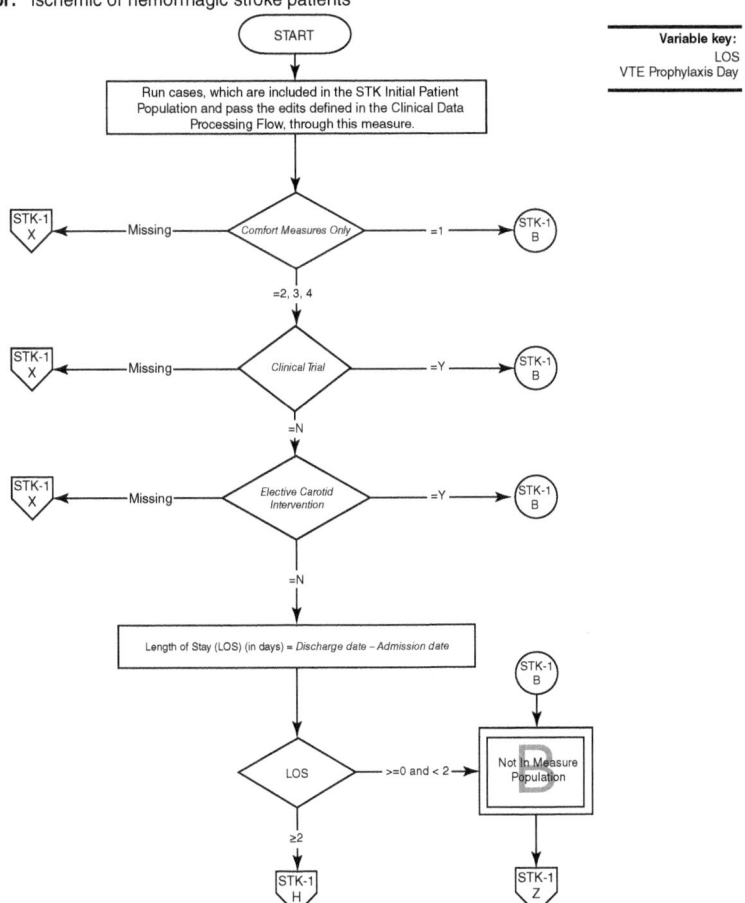

Fig. 15.3 VTE algorithm mapping the metric used to abstract data from the electronic medical record. (Source: *Specifications Manual for Joint Commission National Quality Measures (v2023A)*)

CMO (or "comfort measures only") would be excluded since this metric would not be clinically meaningful as a treatment option.

Stroke Measures

Standardized metrics for stroke care for Primary Stroke Centers, Thrombectomy-Capable Stroke Centers, and Comprehensive Stroke Centers are typically highlighted in protocols or clinical pathways and built into stroke sub-type-specific order sets to ensure compliance. These measures align with elements of clinical practice guidelines and are standard features of quality improvement activities. Process metrics can be evaluated over time with improvement in compliance and are designed to affect outcome metrics. Table 15.3 outlines each measure, describing the practice metric (the numerator) within the stroke subtype (the denominator). Measures are reported as a percentage of patients that "meet the measure," with organizations or certification requirements setting target benchmark data.

Advanced practice clinicians (APCs) with expertise in stroke care should know the specific stroke performance measures and how they impact daily practice and documentation. As described earlier in this chapter, the GWTG-Stroke is a commonly used stroke registry. Since its inception, more than five million patient records have been entered into this platform by stroke coordinators, data abstractors, and selected members of a hospital's quality team. This has resulted in a robust databank that can highlight broad practices among healthcare programs throughout

Table 15.3 Joint Commission stroke measures

Stroke measure	Stroke type	Metric class
STK-1.DVT prophylaxis administered by the end of Hospital Day #2	Ischemic Hemorrhagic	Process measure
STK-2. Antithrombotics prescribed at discharge	Ischemic	Process measure
STK-3. Anticoagulant prescribed for Afib-flutter or hx of Afib-flutter at discharge	Ischemic	Process measure
STK-4. Thrombolytic therapy is administered within 3 h of arrival to patients within 2 h of symptom onset	Ischemic	Process measure
STK-5. Anti-thrombotic therapy administered by the end of H.D. #2	Ischemic Hemorrhagic	Process measure
STK-6. Statin therapy is prescribed at discharge for patients with LDL > 70 or not documented	Ischemic	Process measure
STK-8. Stroke education before discharge, addressing personal risk factors, warning signs, emergency medical services activation, follow-up appointments, and medications	Ischemic Hemorrhagic	Process measure
STK-10. Assessment for rehabilitation before discharge	Ischemic Hemorrhagic	Process measure
CSTK-01. NIHSS is performed within 12 h of arrival or before an acute intervention	Ischemic	Process measure

Source: Specifications Manual for Joint Commission National Quality Measures (v2023A)
STK Stroke Core Measures, *CSTK* Comprehensive Stroke Measures

the country. Benchmarking against other "same" facilities, trending metric compliance over time, and answering important research questions are just a few advantages of utilizing this platform. Historically, abstractors were assigned to review the medical records of stroke patients (as determined by principal discharge diagnosis of stroke) and to record demographics in addition to whether or not there was evidence of compliance with defined metrics. The prior reference to determining compliance with VTE prophylaxis is a specific example abstractors would record by validating the use of either sequential compression devices or chemical prophylaxis (such as subcutaneous heparin) and then entering the (compliance with) this metric into the database. Many of these selected metrics are now electronically queried for efficiency and as an option by CMS. Beyond tracking hospital performance metrics, the registry can also help evaluate individual or provider group performance and provide patient education tools.

Order sets and daily care plans should reflect an accounting of the metrics relevant to their patient panel. Selected metrics may be contraindicated or felt unsafe in certain situations. For example, one crucial metric applicable to all certified stroke centers is identifying the percentage of patients with atrial fibrillation/flutter who are prescribed anticoagulation at the time of hospital discharge (as a secondary stroke prevention strategy). However, it may not be clinically appropriate to discharge a patient in atrial fibrillation on an anticoagulant (AC) in the setting of a recent large ischemic stroke, and the clinician may wish to wait some period of time before starting AC. Guidelines and embedded metrics are meant to guide care, not dictate it; if an intervention is inappropriate or unnecessary for a patient, one should use clinical judgment supported by appropriate documentation. It is strongly recommended that APCs are generally familiar with the abstraction process and are provided with feedback related to their compliance with the organization's metric targets as it may be an option for driving ongoing provider performance evaluations.

Given the expanded use of electronic medical records, the dynamics of clinical decision-making, disease-specific order sets, and tabulation and analysis of metric compliance as a Quality Improvement initiative for public reporting have become streamlined [18]. In stroke centers, there is a constant rotation of doctors and trainees. This is where the Advanced Practice Clinicians (APCs) come in, who provide a consistent presence on stroke teams, hospitalist teams, and Emergency Departments. APCs familiar with order sets and quality metrics can educate trainees on a stroke or medicine service who may not appreciate the importance of standardized metrics.

Standardizing Care with Order Sets

Order sets will naturally vary by country, region, and institution. In general, they serve to streamline routine processes, such as guideline-driven neurologic and vital signs assessments after thrombolytic therapy or admission order sets for stroke patients, including standard evaluations (such as diabetes or cholesterol screens), precautions (such as NPO pending swallow evaluation), or interventions (therapy evaluations, antithrombotic medications). Clinical pathways may provide similar benefits. Standardized documentation provides evidence that the center uses guideline-based care (or provides the rationale for variation). These tools are not meant to replace clinical judgment or intuition but should improve patient care while streamlining the clinician's workflow. Clinical leadership should ensure that order sets reflect the most up-to-date nationally endorsed clinical practice guidelines, with revisions made within 6 months of publication or annually as needed.

Clinical Pearls
- Stroke quality metrics and disease-specific order sets help standardize care and measure patient-related and system-related outcomes.
- Using metrics and order sets results in a significant increase in the utilization of acute stroke treatments, increased patient survival, and a greater number of patients prescribed secondary stroke prevention care.
- Tracking and reporting such outcomes is challenging and requires significant resources and commitment from all stakeholders.

References

1. Poisson SN, Josephson SA. Quality measures in stroke. Neurohospitalist. 2011;9(2):71–7.
2. Yu AXY, Bravata DM, Norrving B. Measuring stroke quality: methodological considerations in selecting, defining and analyzing quality measures. Stroke. 2022;53:3214–21.
3. Chatterjee P, Joynt KE. Do cardiology quality metrics improve patient outcomes? J Am Heart Assoc. 2014;3:1–9.
4. Institute of Medicine (U.S.) Committee on Quality of Health Care in America. Crossing the quality chasm: a new health system for the 21st century. Washington, DC: National Academies Press (U.S.); 2001.
5. Alberts MJ, Hademenos G, Latchaw RE, et al. Recommendations for the establishment of primary stroke centers. Brain Attack Coalition. JAMA. 2000;283(23):3102–9.
6. The National Institutes of Neurological Disorders and Stroke rtPA Study Group. Tissue plasminogen activator for acute ischemic stroke. N Engl J Med. 1995;333:1581–8.
7. Lesparre MA. Century of the AHA. Hosp Health Netw. 1998;72(2):36–48.
8. Krumholz HM, Keenan PS, Brush JE, et al. Standards for measures used for public reporting of efficiency in health care. J Am Coll Cardiol. 2008;52(18):1518–28.
9. Reeves MJ, Parker C, Fonarow GC, et al. Development of stroke performance measures; definitions, methods, and current measures. Stroke. 2010;41:1573–8.
10. Dusenbury W, Mathiesen C, Whaley M, et al. Ideal foundational requirements for stroke program development and growth; a scientific statement from the American Heart Association. Stroke. 2023;54:e175–87.
11. Boggs KM, Vogel BT, Zachrison KS, Espinola JA, Faridi MK, Cash RE, Sullivan AF, Camargo CA Jr. An inventory of stroke centers in the United States. J Am Coll Emerg Physicians Open. 2022;3(2):e12673. https://doi.org/10.1002/emp2.12673. PMID: 35252972; PMCID: PMC8886184.
12. Moore KD, Summers D, Wilson S. Improving stroke measures compliance and outcomes through hospital collaboration. Stroke. 2023;54:1160–70.
13. Jasne AS, Sucharew H, Alwell K, et al. Stroke center certification is associated with improved guideline concordance. Am J Med Qual. 2019;34(6):585–9.

14. Howard G, Schwamm LH, Donnelly JP, et al. Participation in get with the guidelines-stroke and its association with quality of care for stroke. J Am Med Assoc Neurol. 2018;75(11):1331–7.
15. Fonarow GC, Reeves MJ, Smith EE, et al.; The GWTG-Stroke Steering Committee and Investigators. Characteristics, performance measures, and in-hospital outcomes of the first one million stroke and transient ischemic attack admissions in get with the guidelines-stroke. Circ Cardiovasc Qual Outcomes. 2010;3(3):291–302.
16. Donabedian A. The quality of care: how can it be assessed? JAMA. 1988;260(12):1743–8.
17. Heidenriech PA, Fonarow GC, Breathett K. 2020 ACC/AHA clinical performance and quality measures for adults with heart failure. Circ Cardiovasc Qual Outcomes. 2020;13(11):919–56.
18. Bravata DM, Purvis T, Kilkenny M. Advances in stroke; quality improvement. Stroke. 2022;53:1767–171.

Stroke Care in the Intensive Care Unit

16

Amber Robinson, Mohammed W. Al-Dulaimi, and Rachel Beekman

Introduction

Neurocritical care is a subspecialty focusing on the optimal management of life-threatening diseases of the nervous system [1]. Advanced Practice Clinicians (APCs) are vital members of the modern Neuro Intensive Care Unit (NICU). APPs in the NICU must understand acute stroke pathophysiology, treatment decisions, expected complications and comorbid diseases, and criteria for transition out of the NICU. This chapter reviews the early management of acute ischemic stroke (AIS) and intracerebral hemorrhage (ICH), indications for NICU admission, and transfer criteria.

Indications for Admission to the ICU

The NICU plays a critical role in the management of acute cerebrovascular disease. Patients at risk for neurologic deterioration, requiring frequent neurologic assessments, and patients with a systemic critical illness (respiratory failure, sepsis, arrhythmia with hemodynamic compromise) require admission to the ICU. Acute stroke patients are at higher risk for systemic critical illness, which can either be the cause or a consequence of the stroke.

A. Robinson
Yale New Haven Hospital, New Haven, CT, USA
e-mail: Amber.ROBINSON@YNHH.ORG

M. W. Al-Dulaimi
Inova Fairfax Hospital, Falls Church, VA, USA

R. Beekman (✉)
Yale School of Medicine, New Haven, CT, USA
e-mail: Rachel.beekman@yale.edu

Neurological Indications for ICU Admission
- Treatment with intravenous (IV) thrombolytics or endovascular thrombectomy (EVT)
- Cerebral edema in "Malignant" large cerebral hemisphere strokes involving >2/3 of a cerebral hemisphere or >50% of MCA territory
- Symptomatic hemorrhagic transformation of AIS
- Large posterior fossa stroke at risk for development of hydrocephalus
- Herniation
- Failure to protect the airway
- Symptomatic large vessel occlusion or stenosis
- Rapidly progressive or dynamic vasculopathy (cerebral vasculitis, reversible cerebrovascular constriction syndrome, infectious vasculopathy, blood pressure dependency with severe stenosis)
- Hemorrhagic stroke with high-risk features: large hemispheric intraparenchymal hemorrhage (IPH), intraventricular hemorrhage with risk for hydrocephalus, infratentorial IPH, radiographic or clinical deterioration, and coagulopathy
- Aneurysmal subarachnoid hemorrhage
- High-risk anticoagulation (i.e., with large ischemic stroke)

Cardiopulmonary Indications for ICU Admission
- Hemodynamic monitoring ± need for blood pressure augmentation
- High risk for cardiopulmonary collapse (pulmonary embolism, myocardial infarction)
- Symptomatic cardiomyopathy or cardiac arrhythmia
- Respiratory failure

Other Systemic ICU Needs
- Neurovascular assessment (compartment syndrome, pseudoaneurysm)
- Glycemic management (diabetic ketoacidosis, hyperosmolar hyperglycemic syndrome)
- Need for renal replacement therapy

Post-thrombolytic or Endovascular Thrombectomy Care

Up to 11.8% of all AIS patients in the United States receive IV thrombolysis [2]. Admission to an ICU following IV thrombolysis or endovascular thrombectomy (EVT) varies depending on local health practices and the availability of resources. Stroke patients who receive inpatient care in an organized stroke unit have better outcomes with a shorter hospital stay [3].

Table 16.1 Blood pressure management after thrombolysis

Blood pressure is close to the goal of <180/105 mmHg	Labetalol 10–20 mg IV over 1–2 min (may repeat dose) In patients with bradycardia, consider Hydralazine 10 mg IV
Inadequate response to IV push or blood pressure significantly above goal	Nicardipine 5 mg/h IV; may increase by 2.5 mg/h every 5–15 min (maximum dose: 15 mg/h) Clevidipine 1–2 mg/h IV; may double rate every 90 s until close to BP goal, then increase by smaller increments every 5–10 min (maximum dose: 32 mg/h)

Post-thrombolytic Monitoring

- Measure blood pressure (BP) and perform neurological assessments every 15 min during and after IV thrombolysis bolus and infusion for 2 h, then every 30 min for 6 h, then hourly until 24 h after IV thrombolysis therapy [4].
- Maintain BP at <180/105 mmHg during the first 24 h. Increase the frequency of BP measurements if SBP > 180 mmHg or DBP > 105 mmHg. Administer anti-hypertensive medications to maintain BP at or below these levels (Table 16.1).
- Perform a follow-up CT scan at 24 h to rule out interval hemorrhagic conversion (unless an MRI can be done instead around the same timeframe). Avoid antico-agulant and antithrombotic agents, such as heparin, warfarin, direct oral antico-agulants, antiplatelet drugs, and
- Subcutaneous DVT prophylaxis until the 24-h follow-up scan.

Post-EVT Monitoring

- Immediate post-EVT blood pressure goals are usually determined case by case. There are two thresholds for systolic blood pressure: the upper and lower limits. Exceeding the upper limit risks hemorrhage, and falling below the lower limit risks stroke expansion and worse outcomes. Lower limits are particularly impor-tant for patients with symptomatic large vessel stenosis or unsuccessful EVT. No clear fixed thresholds can apply to all post-EVT patients. BP goals for each case should be based on a thorough case assessment and discussion between the stroke neurologist, neuro intensivist, and interventionalist.
- One general concept is that if a vessel remains occluded or severely stenotic after EVT, the upper and lower SBP limits will likely remain higher than if a vessel is completely recanalized (open) after EVT [5–8].
- Factors that influence BP goal include EVT include the Thrombolysis in Cerebral Infarction (TICI) score, presence of penumbral tissue, baseline BP, infarct size, the status of collaterals (assessed by CT, DSA, CTP, TCDs), cerebral pressure autoregulation, and procedural compilations.
- Regardless of EVT outcome, IV thrombolysis patients must achieve a BP < 180/105. In patients with successful revascularization (TICI of 2b or higher), a BP upper limit of ≤140 to 160 mmHg can be considered.

- If a patient with a blood pressure-dependent exam becomes symptomatic at a specific SBP, their lower limit should be raised with BP support with IV fluids or pressors.
- Blood pressures at either extreme (hypertension /hypotension) and wide fluctuations are associated with worse functional outcomes. Intensive control of systolic blood pressure to <120 mmHg is associated with neurologic deterioration and major disability at 90 days; therefore, a common lower limit threshold is often >120 mmHg.

Nursing Assessments
- Nursing should perform neurologic examinations hourly, including a full National Institute Health Stroke Scale (NIHSS) every 15 min for 2 h, every 30 min for 6 h, and hourly for 16 h [4, 9].
- The femoral artery in the groin is the most common site of access for mechanical thrombectomy. Risks of arterial puncture include bleeding, ecchymosis, hematoma, and thrombosis. Therefore, the arterial puncture site must be monitored for signs of bleeding, ecchymosis, and hematoma.
- Additionally, distal pulse checks to identify thrombosis should be performed every 15 min for 2 h, every 30 min for 6 h, and hourly for 16 h.
- For femoral access, interventionalists often recommend keeping the patient supine (flat on their back) for 2–6 h, depending on the risk of access-site hemorrhage. A leg immobilizer prevents limb manipulation that could result in bleeding. If a hematoma develops at the access site, pressure should be applied proximal (higher) to the vessel access point.

Common Complications of Acute Stroke Treatments

Intracranial hemorrhage (ICH): Symptomatic ICH is reported in 2.4–6.4% after IV thrombolysis. ICH can present as an acute neurological deterioration (increase in NIHSS, decline in the level of consciousness, headache, nausea, emesis, and sudden increase in BP). ICH most commonly occurs within 24 h of receiving IV thrombolysis therapy [4, 10–14]. When suspected, obtain head CT urgently and stop thrombolytic infusion if still going. The protocol for reversing alteplase-associated ICH is outlined in the Thrombolytics chapter.

Angioedema: Typically mild, involving the face and the mouth; rarely severe orolingual angioedema can occur, leading to airway compromise [4, 15, 16]. The risk of angioedema is higher in patients taking Angiotensin-Converting Enzyme inhibitors (ACEi) like lisinopril. Assess severity, involvement of the mouth and tongue, airway, breathing, and circulation, secure airway (when applicable), discontinue IV thrombolysis and ACE-inhibitor, and consider IV methylprednisolone 125 mg, diphenhydramine 50 mg, and ranitidine 50 mg or famotidine 20 mg.

Malignant Stroke (Cerebral Edema)

Cerebral edema is an increase in the brain tissue water content that results in brain swelling. Cerebral edema can be classified *as cytotoxic* and *vasogenic* (Fig. 16.1). *Cytotoxic edema* is cell swelling. Stroke causes dysfunction of cell membrane transporters (specifically the sodium–potassium pump), responsible for keeping sodium and water out of the cells; uncontrolled entry of sodium and, subsequently, water results in cell swelling. *Vasogenic edema* occurs due to vascular leakage and interstitial swelling [17, 18]. Stroke results in the breakdown of the blood-brain barrier, causing extravasation of water into the interstitial space. Both processes will eventually result in brain parenchymal swelling (cerebral edema). AIS and ICH have mixed edema with both cytotoxic and vasogenic components. Cytotoxic edema can occur within hours, whereas vasogenic edema forms within 2–3 days and peaks in 3–5 days [19].

The contents of the cranium include the brain, blood, and cerebrospinal fluid, all contained within a fixed skull. The Monro-Kellie doctrine states that the sum of volumes of these components should remain constant. In a neurologically healthy individual, an increase in the volume of one of these components can be compensated for by decreased production of CSF or increased venous drainage of blood to keep the "total volume" constant. This ability to compensate for a volume change is called compliance and is ultimately limited by the skull. Once the compliance threshold is met, the rise in volume leads to increased intracranial pressure (ICP). The most common situation for raised ICP is cerebral edema. Cerebral edema can have life-threatening consequences due to limited space within the cranium, potentially leading to midline shift, herniation, and brainstem compression (referred to as malignant edema).

Predicting which patient with a large stroke will develop a malignant course is challenging. Table 16.2 summarizes risk factors.

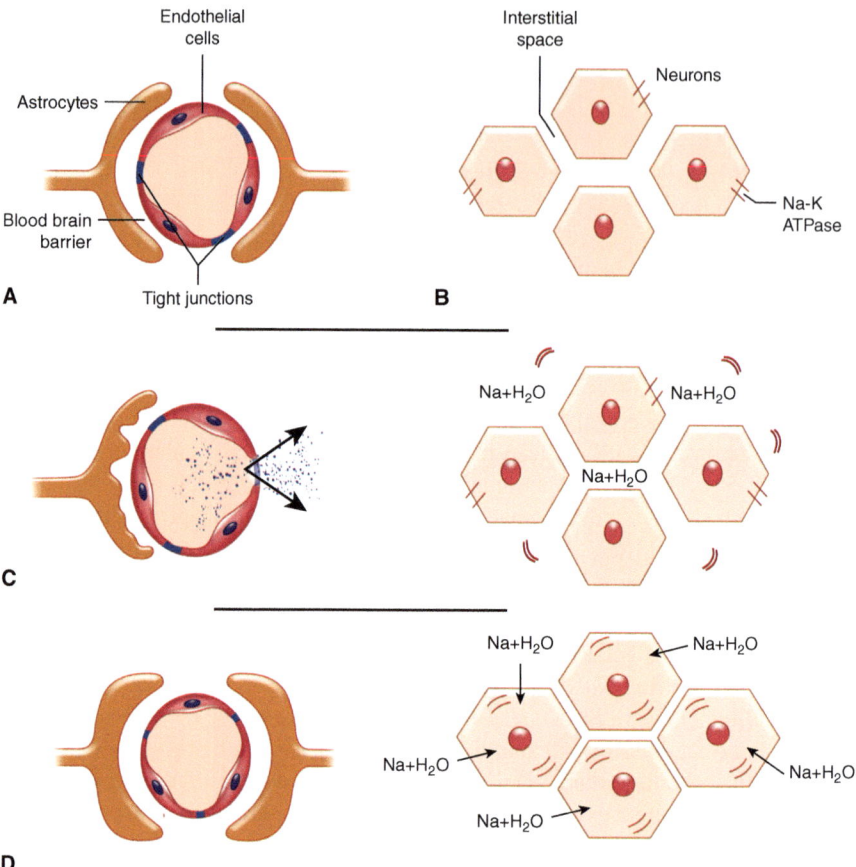

Fig. 16.1 Cytotoxic and vasogenic edema. (**a**) A drawing of the blood-brain barrier. (**b**) Neurons with functioning sodium–potassium pump. (**c**) Vasogenic edema due to dysfunction of the blood-brain barrier, resulting in interstitial swelling. (**d**) Cytotoxic edema due to dysfunction of the sodium potassium pump, resulting in cellular swelling

Table 16.2 Risk factors for malignant cerebral edema [20, 21]

Age < 60 years
NIHSS >11–20
Stroke with internal carotid artery occlusion
Poor collateral score (poor collaterals mean less backup blood flow, causing more rapid tissue ischemia)
Inability to revascularize large vessel occlusion
Radiologic parameters:
– Infarct size on diffusion weighted imaging (DWI) on MRI of >80 mL within 6 h or >145 mL within 14 h of stroke onset
– >2/3 of the middle cerebral artery (MCA) distribution or >50% of the cerebral hemisphere with compression of the ventricles or midline shift

Table 16.3 Description of mental status examination terms

Term	Description
Lethargy	Difficulty maintaining a state of wakefulness but arouses to vocal stimuli
Obtundation	Blunted state of alertness when responding to stimuli other than pain
Stupor	Responsive only to painful stimuli that are forceful and continuous
Coma	Unresponsive to painful stimuli

The most concerning sign of clinically significant cerebral edema and midline shift is depression in the level of consciousness [22]. Hyperosmolar therapy should be considered when patients become sleepy or lethargic. Obtundation or worse (see degrees of mental status in Table 16.3) should raise concern for herniation and prompt consideration for decompressive hemicraniectomy (DHC), which is the removal of a bone flap of the skull to alleviate the raised pressure. While DHC has been shown to reduce mortality, it does not reduce morbidity or severe disability, meaning patients may live longer but more likely in a severely disabled state.

Therefore, patients appropriate for decompressive craniectomy should have a reasonable pre-stroke functional status, no active medical comorbidities, low surgical risk, and acceptable quality of life. Patients with high mRS before the stroke or who are medically ill are less suitable for DHC. It is best to identify patients at high risk of developing malignant edema early and assess the suitability of DHC with neurosurgery before decompensation occurs.

Medical management of cerebral edema includes attention to airway, breathing, circulation, medical management of raised ICP (head of bed elevation, avoiding hyper- and hypocapnia, minimizing compression of the internal jugular veins to promote venous drainage, and use of hyperosmolar therapy).

The posterior fossa area represents a smaller intracranial sub-compartment occupied mainly by the brainstem and cerebellum. Cerebellar vascular injuries (AIS and ICH) can carry a relatively good prognosis if they spare the brainstem. However, the posterior fossa has very little compliance, and even a modest degree of cerebral edema carries the risk of life-threatening brainstem compression and obstructive hydrocephalus by compressing the fourth ventricle [23]. Due to the timeline of cerebral edema after AIS, the highest risk for obstructive hydrocephalus and brainstem compression after large cerebellar AIS is within 2–7 days. Lethargy, confusion, and dysphagia are early symptoms of lower brainstem compression and development of hydrocephalus [24].

Clinical Vignette

HPI: 85-year-old male with a history of atrial fibrillation not on anticoagulation who was brought to the ED after being found down at home by his son. He was last seen well the prior day.

Exam: BP: 137/75, HR 88. He was lethargic but oriented to self, month, and location. He had severe dysarthria with a left facial droop. He had mild weakness in the left arm and leg. Severe dysmetria in L arm and difficulty with heel to shin with the left leg.

Workup: CT head revealed a large established left cerebellar infarct with hemorrhagic conversion (**a**, red arrow) and mass effect on the fourth ventricle (white arrow) with hydrocephalus (**b**, white arrows).

Management: The etiology of his stroke was likely cardioembolic from AF. During goals of care discussions, the family stated they did not wish to pursue surgical interventions. He was started on hyperosmolar therapy and repeat head CT (**c**) revealed increasing mass effect in the posterior fossa and evolving hydrocephalus. After further discussion, the patient was transitioned to comfort measures and passed away shortly thereafter.

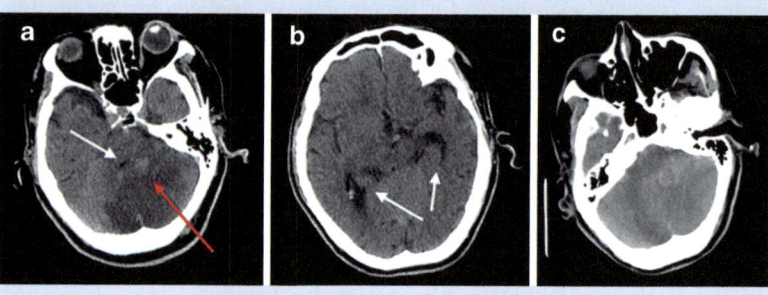

Hyperosmolar therapy (fluids with higher concentration of solutes than plasma) is indicated when a neurologic deterioration is attributed to cerebral edema. Hyperosmolar therapy draws water out of the brain parenchyma and into the vasculature (from lower concentration to higher concentration), where it gets drained, decreasing overall intracranial volume [19, 23, 25]. The neurological exam is crucial to determine the effectiveness of hyperosmolar therapy and its impact on cerebral edema through clinical findings. Options for hyperosmolar therapy include hypertonic saline and Mannitol (Table 16.4).

Neurosurgical intervention for malignant anterior circulation stroke is a *Decompressive Hemicraniectomy* [4, 26–30]. Decompressive craniectomy is a life-saving neurosurgical procedure that removes a portion of the skull and expands the dura to allow room for cerebral edema. While guidelines suggest that

Table 16.4 Options and considerations for hyperosmolar therapy

Hypertonic saline: 1.5%, 3%, 23.4%	Mannitol
• Duration of effect: 90 min–4 h • Continuous drip, bolus (23.4% given as 30 mL IV push over 10–20 min) • Requires monitoring of sodium every 4–6 h • Prolonged sodium >160 mEq/L should be avoided • Concentrations of 3% or above require central access • Adverse reactions: pulmonary edema, acute kidney injury, metabolic acidosis, osmotic demyelination	• Duration of effect: 90 min–6 h • Dosing:1 g/kg, IV piggyback over 15–30 min • Requires monitoring of osmolality (goal <320) and osmolar gap (goal <15–20 mOsm/L) • Prolonged use can result in rebound edema on discontinuation • It can be administered through peripheral access, but central access is preferred • Adverse reactions: acute kidney injury, dehydration, hypotension, pseudohyponatremia

decompressive craniectomy should be performed within 48 hours of AIS, data suggests that the outcome of patients with decompressive craniectomy after 48 hours in malignant MCA stroke is not worse. Numerous observational studies investigated the role of decompressive craniectomy in AIS patients with cerebral edema. Table 16.5 includes a summary of 5 trials showing the survival benefit of decompressive craniectomy in patients with malignant edema secondary to AIS.

Neurosurgical intervention for malignant posterior fossa stroke is a *Suboccipital Craniectomy* [4, 19]. For acute hydrocephalus, an external ventricular drain (EVD) is placed for CSF diversion. This neurosurgical intervention is usually done at the same time or shortly prior to suboccipital decompressive craniectomy. In such circumstances, suboccipital decompression is a lifesaving procedure that improves neurologic outcomes.

An EVD is a temporary catheter inserted into the ventricular system through a burr hole in the skull and removes CSF that cannot otherwise circulate or get reabsorbed normally. CSF diversion, the use of an EVD to remove CSF, is a treatment for hydrocephalus as the catheter bypasses the obstruction. In patients with cerebellar edema and obstruction of the fourth ventricle, CSF diversion can cause upward herniation when surgical management (suboccipital decompression) is not also performed. Post-operative imaging to assess the adequacy of surgical decompression is essential, as some patients will require hyperosmolar therapy post-operatively.

Treatment with corticosteroids does not improve functional outcomes and may result in adverse effects, such as gastrointestinal bleeding, infection, and hyperglycemia. There is no evidence to suggest using steroids to improve brain edema related to AIS [31].

Table 16.5 Decompressive craniectomy trials [28, 29, 32, 33]

Trial	Type of management	Population	Outcomes measures	Findings
HeADDFIRST trial	Surgical decompression (n = 15) Medical treatment only (n = 10)	Aged 18–75 years (median age 55), NIHSS item 1a <2, unilateral MCA, hypodensity involves ≥50% of MCA territory on CT, ≥4 mm of pineal shift and deterioration in level of arousal or ≥7.5 mm of anteroseptal shift within 96 h of stroke onset	Mortality at 21 days Mortality at 6 months mRS at 6 months	Mortality at 21 days was lower in the surgical arm (21% vs. 40%). This difference is less evident at 90 days (36% vs. 40%) and did not meet statistical significance due to the small sample size
HAMLET trial	Surgical decompression (n = 32) Medical management only (n = 32)	Adults aged 18– 60 years (mean = 48.7 years, SD = 9.05 years), R-MCA NIHSS ≥16/ L-MCA NIHSS ≥21, CTH ≥ 2/3 of MCA	Primary mRS at one year Mortality at one year Quality of life at one year	Craniectomy reduced the risk of death at one year (ARR 38%) but did not affect the likelihood of good functional outcomes
DESTINY trial	Surgical decompression (n = 17) Medical management only (n = 15)	Adults aged 18–60 years, NIHSS non-dominant >18/ dominant >20, NIHSS 1a ≥1, Prestroke mRS score <2	Mortality at 30 days and one year mRS at 6 months and one year	Craniectomy reduced mortality at 30 days (12% vs 53%). There was an improved functional outcome (mRS 0–3) at 60 days in the surgical group (47% vs. 27%). The study was terminated after a joint analysis of the 3 European craniectomy trials
DECIMAL trial	Surgical decompression (n = 20) Medical management only (n = 18)	Adults aged 18 to 55 years (mean = 43.4), clinical and CT evidence of full MCA infarct, DWI infarct volume > 145 mL	Mortality at 6 months and one year mRS at 6 months and one year	Craniectomy was associated with reduced mortality (ARR 52.8%) and improved functional outcome at 6 months and one year (surgical vs. medical groups mRS 0–3 at 6 months 25% vs. 5.6%; at 1-year 50% vs. 22.2%)

Table 16.5 (continued)

Trial	Type of management	Population	Outcomes measures	Findings
DESTINY II trial	Surgical decompression (*n* = 49) Medical management only (*n* = 63)	Age 61 and above (median 70), unilateral MCA, NIHSS non-dominant >14, dominant >19, radiological infarct >2/3 of MCA, Prestroke mRS score <2	Mortality at one year mRS at 6 months and one year Quality of life at one year	Craniectomy increased survival (33% vs. 70%). Craniectomy improved survival with functional outcomes, defined by mRS 0–4 (38% vs. 18%). Survivors in the craniectomy group were more likely to have a mRS of 4

Post-stroke Seizure

Ischemic stroke patients have a 3–6% risk of developing acute seizures and up to 12% risk of delayed seizures [34, 35]. Post-stroke epilepsy is discussed in greater depth in another chapter. Acute symptomatic seizures occur within the first week of stroke and are more frequent after ICH than AIS because blood is a strong irritant to brain tissue. Seizure development is associated with mortality and poor neurologic outcomes and requires immediate anti-seizure medication (ASM) treatment. Electroencephalography (EEG) can detect subclinical seizures in patients with an unexplained neurologic decline, fluctuation in the clinical neurologic examination, or neurologic exam out of proportion to imaging findings.

ICH Management in the NICU

We will review high-yield points in the ICU management of ICH. Please refer to the ICH chapter for more details regarding the workup of ICH. Here, we will only discuss spontaneous (non-traumatic) ICH. Spontaneous ICH accounts for 10% of all strokes in the US [36], with up to 50% mortality rate at 30 days [37].

CT has 97–100% sensitivity in diagnosing acute ICH [38, 39]. ICH score (see Blood on CT chapter for table) is helpful for early prediction of outcomes based on aggregate score, with scores >4 carrying >97% mortality risk [40, 41]. The ICH score must be used with caution, however, given the risk of self-fulfilling prophecy bias. Self-fulfilling prophecy bias is when a prediction becomes true because a scoring system influences the provider's judgment on prognosis and treatment plans; for example, a high ICH score may predict a high likelihood of death, resulting in withdrawal of life-sustaining therapy. A retrospective study evaluated the actual predictive value of the ICH score in patients who had delayed goals of care conversations (all patients received full ICU interventions for 5 days) and found that observed mortality was significantly lower than predicted (60% relative mortality risk reduction compared to predicted [42].

Factors Associated with ICH Expansion

ICH expansion is common in the first 24 h, and early expansion is associated with worse outcomes. Clinical changes warrant urgent repeat CT imaging; otherwise, a follow-up CT scan at 4–6 h and 24 h is recommended for patients with a stable examination [14]. If the follow-up scan shows interval expansion, evaluate the need for surgery. Otherwise, CT should be repeated at 4–6 h intervals until radiological stability is achieved. Early or more frequent follow-up scans are indicated with clinical or radiological signs suggesting a high risk for hematoma expansion.

A high-risk finding on CT is the spot sign, defined as contrast extravasation into the hematoma on a CT angiogram, which predicts hematoma expansion [43]. See the Blood on CT chapter for an example. Coagulopathy is associated with hematoma expansion and worse outcomes; early reversal of coagulopathy is critical for improving outcomes (Table 16.6). Of note, DVT prophylaxis effectively protects from thromboembolic complications without significantly increasing the risk of volume expansion in patients with ICH [44, 45]. If no other contraindications exist (such as active gastrointestinal bleeding), practitioners should consider starting thromboembolism prophylaxis within 24–48 h of radiographic stability of the ICH.

Hypertension is the common cause of ICH, and persistently elevated blood pressures increase the risk of ICH expansion. Most ICH patients will present with elevated blood pressure from pre-existing uncontrolled hypertension, reflex hypertension due to the hemorrhage, or both. Current AHA recommendations for blood pressure management are based on two trials: Intensive Blood Pressure

Table 16.6 Reversal of coagulopathy

Agent	Reversal
Vitamin K antagonist (Coumadin)	Prothrombin complex concentrate (PCC): 1500–2000 units based on weight and INR; can give additional 500 units if repeat INR is >1.4 and bleeding persists Vit K 10 mg IV (can repeat for 3 daily doses) Repeat INR 2 h after PCC and on daily basis for 3 days If PCC is not available, give FFP 2 units IV by rapid infusion. Check INR 15 min after completion of infusion
Dabigatran	If <2 h from ingestion: activated charcoal (25–100 g) Idarucizumab 5 g IV (2.5 g × 2 doses)
Factor Xa inhibitors (apixaban, rivaroxaban, edoxaban)	If <2 h from ingestion: activated charcoal (25–100 g) Andexanet alfa 400–800 mg bolus followed by 4–8 mg/min infusion depending on patient dosing If Andexanet is unavailable, treat with PCC 25–50 units/kg IV
Heparin (Unfractionated heparin and low molecular weight heparin LMWH)	Protamine 1 mg IV for every 100 units of heparin administered in the pat 2–2.5 h (max dose 50 mg)
Aspirin	For those requiring emergent neurosurgery, platelet transfusion might be considered to reduce post-operative mortality If no emergent surgery is required, platelet transfusions should be avoided as they may cause harm [48]

Reduction in Acute Cerebral Hemorrhage Trial INTERACT2 and Antihypertensive Treatment of Acute Cerebral Hemorrhage II ATACH-2 [46, 47]. In the hyperacute phase, dropping systolic blood pressure to 130–140 mmHg is safe and improves outcome. However, dropping blood pressure < 130 mmHg in patients presenting with ICH and elevated blood pressure is potentially harmful and should be avoided [14].

Patients with ICH with associated intraventricular hemorrhage, hydrocephalus, or infratentorial hemorrhage are better cared for in a facility with neurosurgical and NICU capabilities. For patients with supratentorial ICH volume >20–30 mL and Glasgow coma scale score of 5–12, minimally invasive approaches for evacuation have demonstrated reductions in mortality, but improvement in functional outcome is uncertain [14, 49]. In patients with supratentorial ICH who are in a coma, have large hematomas with significant midline shift or have elevated intracranial pressure refractory to medical management, decompressive craniectomy with or without hematoma evacuation can reduce mortality, but improvement in functional outcomes is uncertain [50]. In patients with cerebellar hemorrhage, indications for immediate surgical evacuation with or without an external ventricular drain to reduce mortality include ICH volume >15 mL and neurological deterioration, brainstem compression, and hydrocephalus. Surgical decompression with hematoma evacuation is considered in patients with clinical deterioration, brain stem compression, hydrocephalus, or ICH volume ≥15 mL [51].

Clinical Pearls
- Initial imaging is essential for determining the etiology of ICH based on radiologic characteristics and assessing complications and prognostic markers.
- Hematoma expansion is most common in the first 6 h after ICH and is associated with increased mortality.
- Reversal of coagulopathy, blood pressure control, and close monitoring for neurologic deterioration is critical to improve outcomes.
- In ICH patients presenting blood pressure >180, a reasonable target for blood pressure reduction is SBP 130–150. Over-aggressive blood pressure reduction (below 130 mmHg systolic) can increase the risk of acute kidney injury.

Hyponatremia

Hyponatremia can worsen cerebral edema and increase the risk of seizures in patients with AIS and ICH. Hyponatremia requires prompt identification, evaluation of etiology, and treatment. The most common causes of hyponatremia in patients with stroke are hypovolemia, syndrome of inappropriate antidiuretic hormone secretion (SIADH), cerebral salt wasting, or complications of medical comorbidities such as kidney injury or congestive heart failure. The workup for hyponatremia

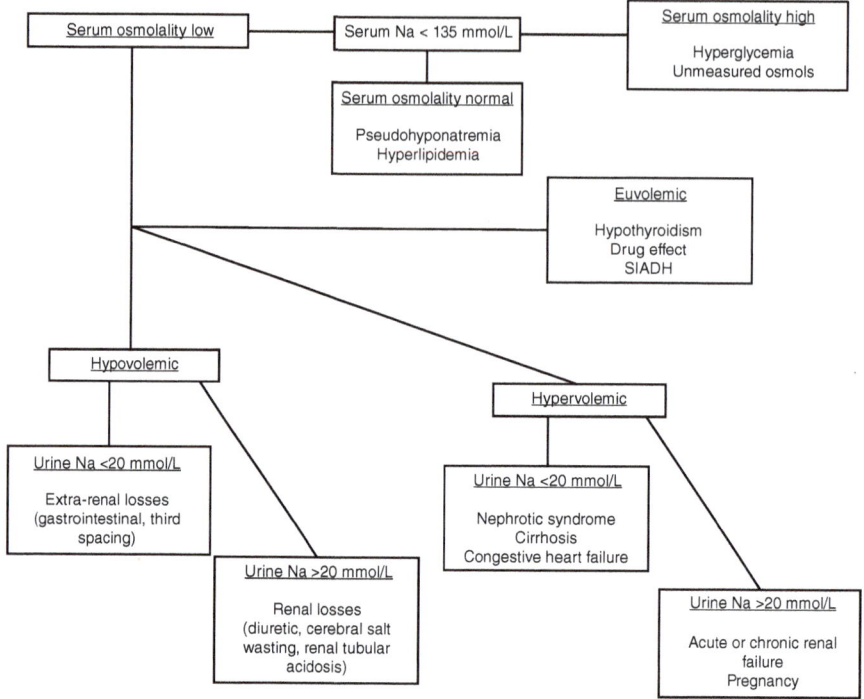

Fig. 16.2 Hyponatremia assessment of serum osmolality, urine sodium, and volume status

includes an assessment of serum osmolality, urine sodium, and volume status (Fig. 16.2). Treatment of hypovolemic hyponatremia includes fluid resuscitation, treatment of SIADH includes fluid restriction, free water restriction ± salt tabs and urea to assist with removal of free water, and the treatment of cerebral salt wasting includes fluid resuscitation, sodium replacement ± fludrocortisone.

Indications for Transfer to Step-Down Unit or Floor

The optimal time window for patients to leave the intensive care unit is unknown, and clinical judgment, individualized to the patient, is essential. There are "hard" criteria (not requiring mechanical ventilation or non-invasive ventilatory support, hemodynamic support) and "soft" criteria (clinical stability, lower risk for neurologic or respiratory decline without needing the frequency of monitoring offered by the ICU). In patients who are no longer requiring ICU-level care but in whom transfer to the floor may pose a higher risk, disposition to the step-down unit may be appropriate, where patients get more frequent monitoring and often a smaller nurse-to-patient ratio. A high-level sign-out (Table 16.7), upon transfer, is critical to ensure a continuation of care in these medically and neurologically complex patients.

Table 16.7 Key components of sign-out

A brief synopsis of HPI and ICU course

Details of work up to date (including results), current understanding of etiology, and pending work up

Current neurologic exam (including best and worst if fluctuating)

Medications and recent changes (if applicable, the rationale for choices and next steps if a change is needed)

Key parameters (hemodynamic, sodium goals)

Family communications, goals of care, decision maker (if not the patient)

References

1. Moheet AM, Livesay SL, Abdelhak T, Bleck TP, Human T, Karanjia N, Lamer-Rosen A, Medow J, Nyquist PA, Rosengart A, Smith W, Torbey MT, Chang CWJ. Standards for neurologic critical care units: a statement for healthcare professionals from the Neurocritical Care Society. Neurocrit Care. 2018;29(2):145–60. https://doi.org/10.1007/s12028-018-0601-1. Erratum in: Neurocrit Care 2019 May 22. PMID: 30251072.

2. Anand SK, Benjamin WJ, Adapa AR, Park JV, Wilkinson DA, Daou BJ, Burke JF, Pandey AS. Trends in acute ischemic stroke treatments and mortality in the United States from 2012 to 2018. Neurosurg Focus. 2021;51(1):E2. https://doi.org/10.3171/2021.4.FOCUS21117. PMID: 34198248.

3. Langhorne P, Ramachandra S, Stroke Unit Trialists' Collaboration. Organised inpatient (stroke unit) care for stroke: network meta-analysis. Cochrane Database Syst Rev. 2020;4(4):CD000197. https://doi.org/10.1002/14651858.CD000197.pub4. PMID: 32324916; PMCID: PMC7197653.

4. Powers WJ, Rabinstein AA, Ackerson T, Adeoye OM, Bambakidis NC, Becker K, Biller J, Brown M, Demaerschalk BM, Hoh B, Jauch EC, Kidwell CS, Leslie-Mazwi TM, Ovbiagele B, Scott PA, Sheth KN, Southerland AM, Summers DV, Tirschwell DL. Guidelines for the early management of patients with acute ischemic stroke: 2019 update to the 2018 guidelines for the early management of acute ischemic stroke: a guideline for healthcare professionals from the American Heart Association/American Stroke Association. Stroke. 2019;50(12):e344–418. https://doi.org/10.1161/STR.0000000000000211. Epub 2019 Oct 30. Erratum in: Stroke. 2019 Dec;50(12):e440-e441. PMID: 31662037.

5. Cernik D, Sanak D, Divisova P, Kocher M, Cihlar F, Zapletalova J, Veverka T, Prcuchova A, Ospalik D, Cerna M, Janousova P, Kral M, Dornak T, Prasil V, Franc D, Kanovsky P. Impact of blood pressure levels within first 24 hours after mechanical thrombectomy on clinical outcome in acute ischemic stroke patients. J Neurointerv Surg. 2019;11(8):735–9. https://doi.org/10.1136/neurintsurg-2018-014548. Epub 2019 Feb 6. PMID: 30728203.

6. Yang P, Song L, Zhang Y, Zhang X, Chen X, Li Y, Sun L, Wan Y, Billot L, Li Q, Ren X, Shen H, Zhang L, Li Z, Xing P, Zhang Y, Zhang P, Hua W, Shen F, Zhou Y, Tian B, Chen W, Han H, Zhang L, Xu C, Li T, Peng Y, Yue X, Chen S, Wen C, Wan S, Yin C, Wei M, Shu H, Nan G, Liu S, Liu W, Cai Y, Sui Y, Chen M, Zhou Y, Zuo Q, Dai D, Zhao R, Li Q, Huang Q, Xu Y, Deng B, Wu T, Lu J, Wang X, Parsons MW, Butcher K, Campbell B, Robinson TG, Goyal M, Dippel D, Roos Y, Majoie C, Wang L, Wang Y, Liu J, Anderson CS, ENCHANTED2/MT Investigators. Intensive blood pressure control after endovascular thrombectomy for acute ischaemic stroke (ENCHANTED2/MT): a multicentre, open-label, blinded-endpoint, randomised controlled trial. Lancet. 2022;400(10363):1585–96. https://doi.org/10.1016/S0140-6736(22)01882-7. Epub 2022 Oct 28. Erratum in: Lancet. 2022 Dec 3;400(10367):1926. PMID: 36341753.

7. Maïer B, Dargazanli C, Bourcier R, Kyheng M, Labreuche J, Mosimann PJ, Puccinelli F, Taylor G, Le Guen M, Riem R, Desilles JP, Boisseau W, Fahed R, Redjem H, Smajda S, Ciccio G, Escalard S, Blanc R, Piotin M, Lapergue B, Mazighi M, ASTER Trial. Effect of steady

and dynamic blood pressure parameters during thrombectomy according to the collateral status. Stroke. 2020;51(4):1199–206. https://doi.org/10.1161/STROKEAHA.119.026769. Epub 2020 Mar 11. PMID: 32156204.

8. Peng TJ, Ortega-Gutiérrez S, de Havenon A, Petersen NH. Blood pressure management after endovascular thrombectomy. Front Neurol. 2021;12:723461. https://doi.org/10.3389/fneur.2021.723461. PMID: 34539562; PMCID: PMC8446280.

9. Jadhav AP, Molyneaux BJ, Hill MD, Jovin TG. Care of the post-thrombectomy patient. Stroke. 2018;49(11):2801–7. https://doi.org/10.1161/STROKEAHA.118.021640. PMID: 30355218.

10. National Institute of Neurological Disorders and Stroke rt-PA Stroke Study Group. Tissue plasminogen activator for acute ischemic stroke. N Engl J Med. 1995;333(24):1581–7. https://doi.org/10.1056/NEJM199512143332401. PMID: 7477192.

11. Hacke W, Kaste M, Bluhmki E, Brozman M, Dávalos A, Guidetti D, Larrue V, Lees KR, Medeghri Z, Machnig T, Schneider D, von Kummer R, Wahlgren N, Toni D, ECASS Investigators. Thrombolysis with alteplase 3 to 4.5 hours after acute ischemic stroke. N Engl J Med. 2008;359(13):1317–29. https://doi.org/10.1056/NEJMoa0804656. PMID: 18815396.

12. Yaghi S, Boehme AK, Dibu J, Leon Guerrero CR, Ali S, Martin-Schild S, Sands KA, Noorian AR, Blum CA, Chaudhary S, Schwamm LH, Liebeskind DS, Marshall RS, Willey JZ. Treatment and outcome of thrombolysis-related hemorrhage: a multicenter retrospective study. JAMA Neurol. 2015;72(12):1451–7. https://doi.org/10.1001/jamaneurol.2015.2371. PMID: 26501741; PMCID: PMC4845894.

13. Yaghi S, Eisenberger A, Willey JZ. Symptomatic intracerebral hemorrhage in acute ischemic stroke after thrombolysis with intravenous recombinant tissue plasminogen activator: a review of natural history and treatment. JAMA Neurol. 2014;71(9):1181–5. https://doi.org/10.1001/jamaneurol.2014.1210. PMID: 25069522; PMCID: PMC4592535.

14. Greenberg SM, Ziai WC, Cordonnier C, Dowlatshahi D, Francis B, Goldstein JN, Hemphill JC 3rd, Johnson R, Keigher KM, Mack WJ, Mocco J, Newton EJ, Ruff IM, Sansing LH, Schulman S, Selim MH, Sheth KN, Sprigg N, Sunnerhagen KS, American Heart Association/American Stroke Association. 2022 guideline for the management of patients with spontaneous intracerebral hemorrhage: a guideline from the American Heart Association/American Stroke Association. Stroke. 2022;53(7):e282–361. https://doi.org/10.1161/STR.0000000000000407. Epub 2022 May 17. PMID: 35579034.

15. Hurford R, Rezvani S, Kreimei M, Herbert A, Vail A, Parry-Jones AR, Douglass C, Molloy J, Alachkar H, Tyrrell PJ, Smith CJ. Incidence, predictors and clinical characteristics of orolingual angio-oedema complicating thrombolysis with tissue plasminogen activator for ischaemic stroke. J Neurol Neurosurg Psychiatry. 2015;86(5):520–3. https://doi.org/10.1136/jnnp-2014-308097. Epub 2014 Jul 12. PMID: 25016564.

16. Engelter ST, Fluri F, Buitrago-Téllez C, Marsch S, Steck AJ, Rüegg S, Lyrer PA. Life-threatening orolingual angioedema during thrombolysis in acute ischemic stroke. J Neurol. 2005;252(10):1167–70. https://doi.org/10.1007/s00415-005-0789-9. Epub 2005 Sep 27. PMID: 16184341.

17. Qureshi AI, Suarez JI, Yahia AM, Mohammad Y, Uzun G, Suri MF, Zaidat OO, Ayata C, Ali Z, Wityk RJ. Timing of neurologic deterioration in massive middle cerebral artery infarction: a multicenter review. Crit Care Med. 2003;31(1):272–7. https://doi.org/10.1097/00003246-200301000-00043. PMID: 12545028.

18. Hacke W, Schwab S, Horn M, Spranger M, De Georgia M, von Kummer R. 'Malignant' middle cerebral artery territory infarction: clinical course and prognostic signs. Arch Neurol. 1996;53(4):309–15. https://doi.org/10.1001/archneur.1996.00550040037012. PMID: 8929152.

19. Torbey MT, Bösel J, Rhoney DH, Rincon F, Staykov D, Amar AP, Varelas PN, Jüttler E, Olson D, Huttner HB, Zweckberger K, Sheth KN, Dohmen C, Brambrink AM, Mayer SA, Zaidat OO, Hacke W, Schwab S. Evidence-based guidelines for the management of large hemispheric infarction: a statement for health care professionals from the Neurocritical Care Society and the German Society for Neuro-intensive Care and Emergency Medicine. Neurocrit Care. 2015;22(1):146–64. https://doi.org/10.1007/s12028-014-0085-6. PMID: 25605626.

20. Huang X, Yang Q, Shi X, Xu X, Ge L, Ding X, Zhou Z. Predictors of malignant brain edema after mechanical thrombectomy for acute ischemic stroke. J Neurointerv Surg. 2019;11(10):994–8. https://doi.org/10.1136/neurintsurg-2018-014650. Epub 2019 Feb 23. PMID: 30798266.
21. Wu S, Yuan R, Wang Y, Wei C, Zhang S, Yang X, Wu B, Liu M. Early prediction of malignant brain edema after ischemic stroke. Stroke. 2018;49(12):2918–27. https://doi.org/10.1161/STROKEAHA.118.022001. PMID: 30571414.
22. Plum F, Posner JB. The diagnosis of stupor and coma. Contemp Neurol Ser. 1972;10:1–286. PMID: 4664014.
23. Wijdicks EF, Sheth KN, Carter BS, Greer DM, Kasner SE, Kimberly WT, Schwab S, Smith EE, Tamargo RJ, Wintermark M, American Heart Association Stroke Council. Recommendations for the management of cerebral and cerebellar infarction with swelling: a statement for healthcare professionals from the American Heart Association/American Stroke Association. Stroke. 2014;45(4):1222–38. https://doi.org/10.1161/01.str.0000441965.15164.d6. Epub 2014 Jan 30. PMID: 24481970.
24. Arch AE, Weisman DC, Coca S, Nystrom KV, Wira CR 3rd, Schindler JL. Missed ischemic stroke diagnosis in the emergency department by Emergency Medicine and Neurology Services. Stroke. 2016;47(3):668–73. https://doi.org/10.1161/STROKEAHA.115.010613. Epub 2016 Feb 4. Erratum in: Stroke 2016 Mar;47(3):e59. PMID: 26846858.
25. Cook AM, Morgan Jones G, Hawryluk GWJ, Mailloux P, McLaughlin D, Papangelou A, Samuel S, Tokumaru S, Venkatasubramanian C, Zacko C, Zimmermann LL, Hirsch K, Shutter L. Guidelines for the acute treatment of cerebral edema in neurocritical care patients. Neurocrit Care. 2020;32(3):647–66. https://doi.org/10.1007/s12028-020-00959-7. PMID: 32227294; PMCID: PMC7272487.
26. Ayling OGS, Alotaibi NM, Wang JZ, Fatehi M, Ibrahim GM, Benavente O, Field TS, Gooderham PA, Macdonald RL. Suboccipital decompressive craniectomy for cerebellar infarction: a systematic review and meta-analysis. World Neurosurg. 2018;110:450–459.e5. https://doi.org/10.1016/j.wneu.2017.10.144. Epub 2017 Dec 2. PMID: 29104155.
27. Goedemans T, Verbaan D, Coert BA, Kerklaan B, van den Berg R, Coutinho JM, van Middelaar T, Nederkoorn PJ, Vandertop WP, van den Munckhof P. Outcome after decompressive craniectomy for middle cerebral artery infarction: timing of the intervention. Neurosurgery. 2020;86(3):E318–25. https://doi.org/10.1093/neuros/nyz522. PMID: 31943069; PMCID: PMC7061200.
28. Jüttler E, Schwab S, Schmiedek P, Unterberg A, Hennerici M, Woitzik J, Witte S, Jenetzky E, Hacke W, DESTINY Study Group. Decompressive surgery for the treatment of malignant infarction of the middle cerebral artery (DESTINY): a randomized, controlled trial. Stroke. 2007;38(9):2518–25. https://doi.org/10.1161/STROKEAHA.107.485649. Epub 2007 Aug 9. PMID: 17690310.
29. Vahedi K, Vicaut E, Mateo J, Kurtz A, Orabi M, Guichard JP, Boutron C, Couvreur G, Rouanet F, Touzé E, Guillon B, Carpentier A, Yelnik A, George B, Payen D, Bousser MG, DECIMAL Investigators. Sequential-design, multicenter, randomized, controlled trial of early decompressive craniectomy in malignant middle cerebral artery infarction (DECIMAL trial). Stroke. 2007;38(9):2506–17. https://doi.org/10.1161/STROKEAHA.107.485235. Epub 2007 Aug 9. PMID: 17690311.
30. Hofmeijer J, Kappelle LJ, Algra A, Amelink GJ, van Gijn J, van der Worp HB, HAMLET investigators. Surgical decompression for space-occupying cerebral infarction (the Hemicraniectomy after middle cerebral artery infarction with life-threatening edema trial [HAMLET]): a multicentre, open, randomised trial. Lancet Neurol. 2009;8(4):326–33. https://doi.org/10.1016/S1474-4422(09)70047-X. Epub 2009 Mar 5. PMID: 19269254.
31. Sandercock PA, Soane T. Corticosteroids for acute ischaemic stroke. Cochrane Database Syst Rev. 2011;2011(9):CD000064. https://doi.org/10.1002/14651858.CD000064.pub2. PMID: 21901674; PMCID: PMC7032681.
32. Frank JI, Schumm LP, Wroblewski K, Chyatte D, Rosengart AJ, Kordeck C, Thisted RA, HeADDFIRST Trialists. Hemicraniectomy and durotomy upon deterioration from infarction-related swelling trial: randomized pilot clinical trial. Stroke. 2014;45(3):781–7. https://doi.

org/10.1161/STROKEAHA.113.003200. Epub 2014 Jan 14. PMID: 24425122; PMCID: PMC4033520.

33. Jüttler E, Unterberg A, Woitzik J, Bösel J, Amiri H, Sakowitz OW, Gondan M, Schiller P, Limprecht R, Luntz S, Schneider H, Pinzer T, Hobohm C, Meixensberger J, Hacke W, DESTINY II Investigators. Hemicraniectomy in older patients with extensive middle-cerebral-artery stroke. N Engl J Med. 2014;370(12):1091–100. https://doi.org/10.1056/NEJMoa1311367. PMID: 24645942.

34. Holtkamp M, Beghi E, Benninger F, Kälviäinen R, Rocamora R, Christensen H, European Stroke Organisation. European Stroke Organisation guidelines for the management of post-stroke seizures and epilepsy. Eur Stroke J. 2017;2(2):103–15. https://doi.org/10.1177/2396987317705536. Epub 2017 Apr 19. PMID: 31008306; PMCID: PMC6453212.

35. Zöllner JP, Schmitt FC, Rosenow F, Kohlhase K, Seiler A, Strzelczyk A, Stefan H. Seizures and epilepsy in patients with ischaemic stroke. Neurol Res Pract. 2021;3(1):63. https://doi.org/10.1186/s42466-021-00161-w. PMID: 34865660; PMCID: PMC8647498.

36. Virani SS, Alonso A, Benjamin EJ, Bittencourt MS, Callaway CW, Carson AP, Chamberlain AM, Chang AR, Cheng S, Delling FN, Djousse L, Elkind MSV, Ferguson JF, Fornage M, Khan SS, Kissela BM, Knutson KL, Kwan TW, Lackland DT, Lewis TT, Lichtman JH, Longenecker CT, Loop MS, Lutsey PL, Martin SS, Matsushita K, Moran AE, Mussolino ME, Perak AM, Rosamond WD, Roth GA, Sampson UKA, Satou GM, Schroeder EB, Shah SH, Shay CM, Spartano NL, Stokes A, Tirschwell DL, VanWagner LB, Tsao CW, American Heart Association Council on Epidemiology and Prevention Statistics Committee and Stroke Statistics Subcommittee. Heart disease and stroke statistics—2020 update: a report from the American Heart Association. Circulation. 2020;141(9):e139–596. https://doi.org/10.1161/CIR.0000000000000757. Epub 2020 Jan 29. PMID: 31992061.

37. Fogelholm R, Murros K, Rissanen A, Avikainen S. Long term survival after primary intracerebral haemorrhage: a retrospective population based study. J Neurol Neurosurg Psychiatry. 2005;76(11):1534–8. https://doi.org/10.1136/jnnp.2004.055145. PMID: 16227546; PMCID: PMC1739413.

38. Romanova AL, Nemeth AJ, Berman MD, Guth JC, Liotta EM, Naidech AM, Maas MB. Magnetic resonance imaging versus computed tomography for identification and quantification of intraventricular hemorrhage. J Stroke Cerebrovasc Dis. 2014;23(8):2036–40. https://doi.org/10.1016/j.jstrokecerebrovasdis.2014.03.005. Epub 2014 Jul 30. PMID: 25085346; PMCID: PMC4214254.

39. Kidwell CS, Chalela JA, Saver JL, Starkman S, Hill MD, Demchuk AM, Butman JA, Patronas N, Alger JR, Latour LL, Luby ML, Baird AE, Leary MC, Tremwel M, Ovbiagele B, Fredieu A, Suzuki S, Villablanca JP, Davis S, Dunn B, Todd JW, Ezzeddine MA, Haymore J, Lynch JK, Davis L, Warach S. Comparison of MRI and CT for detection of acute intracerebral hemorrhage. JAMA. 2004;292(15):1823–30. https://doi.org/10.1001/jama.292.15.1823. PMID: 15494579.

40. Hemphill JC 3rd, Bonovich DC, Besmertis L, Manley GT, Johnston SC. The ICH score: a simple, reliable grading scale for intracerebral hemorrhage. Stroke. 2001;32(4):891–7. https://doi.org/10.1161/01.str.32.4.891. PMID: 11283388.

41. McCracken DJ, Lovasik BP, McCracken CE, Frerich JM, McDougal ME, Ratcliff JJ, Barrow DL, Pradilla G. The intracerebral hemorrhage score: a self-fulfilling prophecy? Neurosurgery. 2019;84(3):741–8. https://doi.org/10.1093/neuros/nyy193. PMID: 29762777.

42. Morgenstern LB, Zahuranec DB, Sánchez BN, Becker KJ, Geraghty M, Hughes R, Norris G, Hemphill JC 3rd. Full medical support for intracerebral hemorrhage. Neurology. 2015;84(17):1739–44. https://doi.org/10.1212/WNL.0000000000001525. Epub 2015 Mar 27. PMID: 25817842; PMCID: PMC4424123.

43. Phan TG, Krishnadas N, Lai VWY, Batt M, Slater LA, Chandra RV, Srikanth V, Ma H. Meta-analysis of accuracy of the spot sign for predicting hematoma growth and clinical outcomes. Stroke. 2019;50(8):2030–6. https://doi.org/10.1161/STROKEAHA.118.024347. Epub 2019 Jul 5. PMID: 31272327.

44. Paciaroni M, Agnelli G, Venti M, Alberti A, Acciarresi M, Caso V. Efficacy and safety of anticoagulants in the prevention of venous thromboembolism in patients with acute cerebral

hemorrhage: a meta-analysis of controlled studies. J Thromb Haemost. 2011;9(5):893–8. https://doi.org/10.1111/j.1538-7836.2011.04241.x. PMID: 21324058.

45. Chi G, Lee JJ, Sheng S, Marszalek J, Chuang ML. Systematic review and meta-analysis of thromboprophylaxis with heparins following intracerebral hemorrhage. Thromb Haemost. 2022;122(7):1159–68. https://doi.org/10.1055/s-0042-1744541. Epub 2022 Jun 19. PMID: 35717948.

46. Qureshi AI, Palesch YY. Antihypertensive treatment of acute cerebral hemorrhage (ATACH) II: design, methods, and rationale. Neurocrit Care. 2011;15(3):559–76. https://doi.org/10.1007/s12028-011-9538-3. PMID: 21626077; PMCID: PMC3340125.

47. Qureshi AI, Palesch YY, Barsan WG, Hanley DF, Hsu CY, Martin RL, Moy CS, Silbergleit R, Steiner T, Suarez JI, Toyoda K, Wang Y, Yamamoto H, Yoon BW, ATACH-2 Trial Investigators and the Neurological Emergency Treatment Trials Network. Intensive blood-pressure lowering in patients with acute cerebral hemorrhage. N Engl J Med. 2016;375(11):1033–43. https://doi.org/10.1056/NEJMoa1603460. Epub 2016 Jun 8. PMID: 27276234; PMCID: PMC5345109.

48. Baharoglu MI, Cordonnier C, Al-Shahi Salman R, de Gans K, Koopman MM, Brand A, Majoie CB, Beenen LF, Marquering HA, Vermeulen M, Nederkoorn PJ, de Haan RJ, Roos YB, PATCH Investigators. Platelet transfusion versus standard care after acute stroke due to spontaneous cerebral haemorrhage associated with antiplatelet therapy (PATCH): a randomised, open-label, phase 3 trial. Lancet. 2016;387(10038):2605–13. https://doi.org/10.1016/S0140-6736(16)30392-0. Epub 2016 May 10. PMID: 27178479.

49. Hanley DF, Thompson RE, Rosenblum M, Yenokyan G, Lane K, McBee N, Mayo SW, Bistran-Hall AJ, Gandhi D, Mould WA, Ullman N, Ali H, Carhuapoma JR, Kase CS, Lees KR, Dawson J, Wilson A, Betz JF, Sugar EA, Hao Y, Avadhani R, Caron JL, Harrigan MR, Carlson AP, Bulters D, LeDoux D, Huang J, Cobb C, Gupta G, Kitagawa R, Chicoine MR, Patel H, Dodd R, Camarata PJ, Wolfe S, Stadnik A, Money PL, Mitchell P, Sarabia R, Harnof S, Barzo P, Unterberg A, Teitelbaum JS, Wang W, Anderson CS, Mendelow AD, Gregson B, Janis S, Vespa P, Ziai W, Zuccarello M, Awad IA, MISTIE III Investigators. Efficacy and safety of minimally invasive surgery with thrombolysis in intracerebral haemorrhage evacuation (MISTIE III): a randomised, controlled, open-label, blinded endpoint phase 3 trial. Lancet. 2019;393(10175):1021–32. https://doi.org/10.1016/S0140-6736(19)30195-3. Epub 2019 Feb 7. Erratum in: Lancet. 2019 Apr 20;393(10181):1596. PMID: 30739747; PMCID: PMC6894906.

50. Yao Z, Ma L, You C, He M. Decompressive craniectomy for spontaneous intracerebral hemorrhage: a systematic review and meta-analysis. World Neurosurg. 2018;110:121–8. https://doi.org/10.1016/j.wneu.2017.10.167. Epub 2017 Nov 10. PMID: 29129764.

51. Kuramatsu JB, Biffi A, Gerner ST, Sembill JA, Sprügel MI, Leasure A, Sansing L, Matouk C, Falcone GJ, Endres M, Haeusler KG, Sobesky J, Schurig J, Zweynert S, Bauer M, Vajkoczy P, Ringleb PA, Purrucker J, Rizos T, Volkmann J, Müllges W, Kraft P, Schubert AL, Erbguth F, Nueckel M, Schellinger PD, Glahn J, Knappe UJ, Fink GR, Dohmen C, Stetefeld H, Fisse AL, Minnerup J, Hagemann G, Rakers F, Reichmann H, Schneider H, Rahmig J, Ludolph AC, Stösser S, Neugebauer H, Röther J, Michels P, Schwarz M, Reimann G, Bäzner H, Schwert H, Claßen J, Michalski D, Grau A, Palm F, Urbanek C, Wöhrle JC, Alshammari F, Horn M, Bahner D, Witte OW, Günther A, Hamann GF, Hagen M, Roeder SS, Lücking H, Dörfler A, Testai FD, Woo D, Schwab S, Sheth KN, Huttner HB. Association of surgical hematoma evacuation vs conservative treatment with functional outcome in patients with cerebellar intracerebral hemorrhage. JAMA. 2019;322(14):1392–403. https://doi.org/10.1001/jama.2019.13014. PMID: 31593272; PMCID: PMC6784768.

Inpatient Stroke Workup

17

Jeremy Bingham and Deborah Kerrigan

The TOAST Criteria

Following the acute treatment phase, the workup to discover the mechanism (or source) of the stroke begins. Identifying the mechanism of a stroke is necessary to initiate appropriate secondary prevention and prevent a future stroke. The TOAST Criteria, a systematic method to classify the mechanism of ischemic stroke, was developed for the study "Trial of Org10172 in Acute Stroke Treatment (TOAST)". The TOAST criteria divide ischemic strokes into mechanisms: those caused by large-artery atherosclerosis, cardioembolism, lacunar small vessel disease, a stroke of other determined etiology (meaning the source of the stroke is something other than the aforementioned), or a stroke of undetermined etiology. Undetermined etiology (also known as cryptogenic stroke) includes strokes with no identified cause, more than one potential cause, or those with an incomplete evaluation [1] (Table 17.1). Stroke specialists will agree that this classification is not perfect since a stroke could be due to multiple mechanisms, so each patient still requires a thoughtful, comprehensive approach to their workup.

Brain Imaging

In most cases of acute stroke, the initial non-contrast computed tomography (NCCT) will be normal because it takes several hours for signs of ischemia to show up in this study. In some cases, with a keen eye on the correct location based on symptoms, one can identify loss of gray versus white matter differentiation, and sulcal effacement might be seen in the acute setting. Stroke is clearly visible on CT by around 6 h of symptom onset in around 80% of cases [2].

J. Bingham · D. Kerrigan (✉)
Vanderbilt University Medical Center, Nashville, TN, USA
e-mail: Jeremy.Bingham@va.gov; Deborah.L.Kerrigan@vumc.org

© The Author(s), under exclusive license to Springer Nature Switzerland AG 2024   187
H. P. Amin (ed.), *Stroke for the Advanced Practice Clinician*,
https://doi.org/10.1007/978-3-031-66289-8_17

Table 17.1 Toast classification of subtypes of acute ischemic stroke

Large-artery atherosclerosis (includes carotid and intracranial)
Cardioembolism (high-risk/medium-risk)
Small-vessel occlusion (lacune)
Stroke of other determined etiology
Stroke of undetermined etiology
    (a)   Two or more causes identified
    (b)   Negative evaluation
    (c)   Incomplete evaluation

In contrast, stroke can usually be seen on MRI within minutes of symptom onset [3]. The appearance of infarcted tissue on the different MRI sequences can help determine the stroke's mechanism and chronicity. Within minutes of cerebral ischemia, the apparent diffusion coefficient (ADC) sequence becomes dark (hypointense), followed quickly by diffusion-weighted imaging (DWI) hyperintensity correlating well with the core infarct size. After about 6 h, the infarct becomes visible on T2 imaging (easier seen of T2 fluid-attenuated inversion recovery [FLAIR] sequences). Beyond the acute phase, refer to Table 17.2 to predict how a stroke evolves on MRI. It is important to note that in a tiny stroke (especially in the brainstem), the infarcted tissue may be located between the slices of the MRI, leading to an "MRI negative" stroke [4, 5]. MRI can still miss small strokes, especially in the brainstem, so if the history and symptoms fit an acute stroke, it could very well still be the diagnosis.

MRI helps potentially indicate the stroke's source. Flow-limiting stenosis of a large artery (internal carotid artery [ICA], vertebral artery, or basilar artery) can lead to "watershed" or "border-zone" appearing strokes. A ruptured plaque in an ICA can lead to multifocal strokes, but all in the ipsilateral hemisphere. In contrast, single infarcts less than 20 mm in the basal ganglia, thalamus, cerebellum, or brainstem are indicative of a lacunar infarction due to poorly controlled vascular risk factors such as hypertension, hyperlipidemia, diabetes, obesity, tobacco use, or sleep apnea [6]. Strokes due to a cardioembolic source often present as multiple foci involving different vascular territories (either bilateral or in both the anterior and posterior distributions). It is prudent to consider further cardiac or hypercoagulability workup in these cases.

For patients with cardiac implantable electronic devices such as an implantable cardiac defibrillator or pacemaker, a "pacer-protocol" MRI can be arranged (if available), but it takes extra time and may extend the length of stay. It is more expensive and should only be considered if it will truly guide management and workup despite the risks, and at centers that have the proper experience and personnel [7]. Alternatively, a "poor man's" MRI is a delayed CT scan 24–48 h after symptom onset where the infarct volume is more clearly visible. When might a pacer protocol MRI be needed? If a patient has multiple risk factors, an MRI might point to a cardiac source vs. a symptomatic carotid, or a concern for an alternative process (tumor, infection, demyelination) requiring more detailed brain imaging. Avoid extending hospital stays or inter-hospital transfers for pacer protocol MRIs if they will not ultimately change management.

Table 17.2 Evolution of infarct on MRI

MRI sequence	Minutes	6 h	1 Week	3 Weeks	1 Week to 4 Months	4 Months+
ADC	Dark (Hypointense)	Dark (Hypointense)	Resolves (Isointense)	Resolved (Isointense)	Resolved (Isointense)	Resolved (Isointense)
DWI	Bright (Hyperintense)	Bright (Hyperintense)	Bright (Hyperintense)	Resolves (Isointense)	Resolved (Isointense)	Resolved (Isointense)
T2 or FLAIR	No Change (Isointense)	Bright (Hyperintense)	Bright (Hyperintense)	Bright (Hyperintense)	Bright (Hyperintense)	Bright (Hyperintense) or dark (Hypointense) in the setting of encephalomalacia
T1 with Contrast	No Change (Isointense)	No Change (Isointense)	No Change (Isointense)	No Change (Isointense)	Bright (Hyperintense)	Resolved (Isointense)

Vascular Imaging

Vascular imaging is imperative for stroke patients to rule out symptomatic carotid or intracranial disease and assess collateral blood flow. Detecting a large vessel occlusion acutely is critical for determining candidacy for endovascular thrombectomy. Identification of hemodynamically significant carotid or intracranial arterial stenosis helps establish blood pressure parameters to prevent aggressive over-reduction in BP (which can lead to worsening ischemia), guide antithrombotic therapy, and consider revascularization procedures. Assessment of collateral vessels (separate blood vessels that form over time and co-supply brain tissue along with the native cerebral vessels) is important to recognize, as patients with poor collateral blood flow tend to have larger infarcts than those with more established collaterals [8].

Currently, there are four imaging modalities available to assess the vasculature in stroke: computed tomography angiography (CTA), magnetic angiogram angiography (MRA), ultrasonography (carotid ultrasound [CUS], transcranial doppler [TCD]), and cerebral angiography also known as digital subtraction angiography (DSA). CTA is often done in the emergency department (ED) simultaneously with NCCT and requires iodinated contrast. MRA (performed with MRI) is an option for patients with iodine contrast allergy but can take longer to arrange and might not be possible for some patients. With a good-quality CTA from the ED, MRA is not necessary. MRA neck requires gadolinium contrast, but MRA brain does not. Compared to MRA, CTA has a higher sensitivity for detecting intravascular occlusion and vascular stenosis [8, 9]. For patients who are neither able to get CTA nor MRA, CUS and TCD use ultrasonography to measure blood velocities both extracranially and intracranially respectively to determine degree of stenosis.

A DSA is an invasive catheter-based procedure for dynamic visualization of blood flow and should not be a first-line option to screen for vascular disease. The procedure for a DSA is the same as for a thrombectomy; only in the latter, we are removing a clot. DSA can be helpful in conditions like suspected vasculitis, Moya Moya vasculopathy, reversible cerebrovascular syndrome, and intracranial atherosclerosis. It can help determine the actual degree of stenosis for a suspected symptomatic vessel (cervical or intracranial) and its suitability for an intervention like stenting. DSA is routinely performed in most patients with spontaneous subarachnoid hemorrhage to exclude an aneurysm or an arteriovenous malformation [10]. Table 17.3 compares the non-invasive modalities of vascular imaging.

Table 17.3 Options for vascular imaging [8]

	CTA	MRA	CUS and/or TCD
Time requirement for acquisition and interpretation	3–5 min	~30 min (screening, preparing, imaging time)	10–30 min
Accessibility	Most hospitals, 24×7 availability, mostly near EDs	Not typically available 24×7	Dependent on operator availability and experience, TCD is only able to be performed if the patient has reliable acoustic windows
Safety	Low radiation risk, contrast induced nephropathy occurring in 3% of patients, and iodine contrast allergy in 1/10,000 patients	No risk (assuming proper screening)	No risk
Use in ICH management	Rules out secondary causes (aneurysm, AVM), CTA "spot sign" indicative of active contrast extravasation into the hemorrhagic demonstrating active bleeding		
Occlusion detection	High accuracy proximally	Less accuracy distally than CTA	Proximal occlusion only

Echocardiography

Echocardiography evaluates for structural causes of cardioembolic stroke, systolic heart failure, left ventricular thrombus, and intra-cardiac tumors such as atrial myxomas, papillary fibroelastomas, and rhabdomyosarcomas [11]. Transthoracic echocardiogram (TTE) is also the imaging technique used to screen for patent foramen ovale, which is present in about 25% of the population and, in *some* cases, might be associated with stroke. Detection of left atrial dilation is correlated with an increased incidence of atrial fibrillation and left ventricular wall thickening is seen with chronic hypertension [12].

A transesophageal echocardiogram (TEE) is indicated when there is a concern for valvular pathology, recurrent embolic strokes, or a high-risk structural lesion. TEE has a sensitivity of 99% to detect a left atrial appendage thrombus, which is where most cardioembolic clots develop in atrial fibrillation. TEE is superior to TTE in detecting vegetations or thrombus in either infective or marantic endocarditis. TEE is also the gold standard for evaluating patent foramen ovale due to its higher diagnostic accuracy, but this indication should be reserved for younger patients with embolic strokes and no other risk factors [11]. Patients getting a TEE must be Nil Per Os (NPO, no food or liquid) for at least 6 hours prior to the procedure. Refer to the Cardioembolic stroke chapter for a more detailed comparison of TTE and TEE.

Arrhythmia Monitoring

All admitted stroke patients require telemetry monitoring to detect arrhythmias like atrial fibrillation or atrial flutter. However, in-hospital telemetry monitoring has variable utility because it depends on non-cardiology providers regularly reviewing the rhythms, patient movement, and removal of leads either inadvertently or when patients go for tests. Any concerning runs on telemetry monitoring should be accompanied by a bedside EKG and consideration of a formal cardiology evaluation.

For suspected embolic stroke, current guidelines recommend prolonged outpatient cardiac rhythm monitoring for 30 days within 6 months of a stroke or TIA. In reality, that window should be a short as possible to prevent a recurrent stroke from undiagnosed atrial fibrillation. Working with your hospital or outpatient cardiology/ electrophysiology group to set up a streamlined process for outpatient monitoring can minimize gaps! Modern external loop recorders are small, wireless, and attach to the skin with adhesives, and patients should be able to shower with them on. Some centers are able to attach an external loop recorder to the patient on the day of discharge. Evidence also demonstrates that more extended monitoring beyond 30 days with implantable loop recorders (ILR) can substantially increase the rate of arrhythmia detection [13, 14]. ILRs are placed under the skin, have a battery life of several years, and can often be placed quickly during a stroke admission. Consider ILR placement over external loop recorders for patients with cognitive impairments (who might remove the monitor), latex/adhesive allergy, or significant cardiac history warranting more extended monitoring.

The Hematologic Evaluation in Ischemic Stroke

Hematologic conditions, both hereditary and acquired, can increase the risk of stroke by inducing a hypercoagulable state. Consider hematologic evaluations in patients <60 years old with suspected embolic stroke or venous thrombosis, otherwise healthy with normal vessels, prior history of venous or arterial thromboses including multiple miscarriages, other autoimmune conditions like lupus, or family history of clotting disorders. While the yield of a hematologic evaluation is usually low, it is higher in this subset of patients [15].

Deficiencies in coagulation inhibitors including antithrombin III, protein C, and protein S increase the risk of thrombosis due to decreased inhibition of the clotting cascade. While the risk for venous thromboembolism is higher than arterial thromboembolism in these conditions, ischemic stroke from paradoxical embolism, cerebral venous sinus thrombosis, or primary arterial thromboembolism have been reported. Consider an MRV of the pelvis in a patient with PFO and embolic stroke (in addition to lower extremity duplex ultrasound) to rule out pelvic vein thrombosis. While rare, conditions like May Thurner syndrome (compression of the left iliac vein by the right iliac artery) can be missed without pelvic imaging. Signs of pelvic vein thrombosis include leg pain or swelling.

Disorders such as thrombocytosis, polycythemia, paroxysmal nocturnal hemoglobinemia, and sickle-cell anemia cause ischemic strokes due to hyper-viscosity (thickening of blood) and decreased cerebral blood flow. Sickle-cell anemia can also lead to a Moya Moya-like syndrome with stenosis of intracranial vessels, causing further ischemic or hemorrhagic strokes. Several other conditions lead to increased arterial thrombosis through varying mechanisms, such as prothrombin gene mutation, factor V Leiden mutation, thrombotic thrombocytopenic purpura, disseminated intravascular coagulation, antiphospholipid antibody syndrome, and homocysteinemia [15, 16].

Malignancy Screening in Ischemic Stroke

Malignancy is another known cause of hypercoagulability. These patients tend to share common characteristics including fewer traditional stroke risk factors (other than tobacco use), more disabling strokes (though debility from the underlying malignancy can be confounding), and elevated rates of recurrent stroke, venous thromboembolism, morbidity, and mortality than their cancer-free counterparts. Adenocarcinomas of various organs are commonly associated with hypercoagulability. However, almost all cancer types, including solid tumors and hematologic malignancy from stages 1 through 4, have been associated with increased ischemic stroke risk [17].

Consider malignancy screening for patients with a history of tobacco or excessive alcohol use, family medical history of malignancy, review of systems concerning for "B symptoms" of night sweats, unexplained weight loss or fever, or those who are not up to date with age-appropriate cancer screening. Patients with recurrent unexplained strokes or strokes through anticoagulation may have underlying malignancies. Elevated D-dimer and inflammatory markers such as CRP tend to be elevated with cancer. Abnormally elevated white blood cells, red blood cells, or platelets without explanation should prompt an evaluation for hematological malignancy. A concerning history or abnormal blood work may prompt further imaging studies such as CT chest, abdomen, and pelvis with and without contrast and scrotal ultrasound in men [17].

Subspecialty Inpatient Consultation

There are times when a specialist's expertise is necessary. The need for specialty consultation will differ based on the experience and confidence of the treating provider and the resources available at the hospital where the patient is being treated. Timely specialist evaluations can avoid delays that come with outpatient referrals and could very well prevent a recurrent stroke. The following is a list of the most common specialties requested for stroke patients.

Cardiology: If during the inpatient cardiac evaluation, an intracardiac pathology such as severe valvular disease, endocarditis, new arrhythmia or heart failure, or intracardiac tumor is discovered, it is reasonable to consult a cardiologist to aid in management. Additionally, cardiac complications can occur after a stroke, including symptomatic arrhythmias, critical blood pressures (either hypertensive or hypotensive), myocardial injury, or heart failure, which often require the expertise of a cardiologist [18].

Ophthalmology: A STAT ophthalmology consult is warranted (if available) for patients with acute monocular visual loss to differentiate between vascular occlusion versus orbital injury. The consult is urgent because retinal artery occlusions can be treated with thrombolytics if diagnosed early. An ophthalmologic exam can also aid in diagnosing other systemic conditions like vasculitis or lymphoma. Patients with persistent diplopia or homonymous hemianopia should get close outpatient ophthalmology follow-up for visual field testing or consideration of prism lenses, especially before being cleared to drive.

Hematology: Hematologists are helpful when there is a suspicion of a hematologic source of stroke. Hematologists help interpret abnormal lab values and guide treatment options for patients with known conditions such as in cancer or antiphospholipid antibody syndrome, or acute management in patients with sickle cell crises needing urgent plasmapheresis. In the outpatient setting, hematologists can guide further hematologic workup for cryptogenic strokes.

Rheumatology: Rheumatology is often consulted on inpatient stroke patients when an inflammatory stroke pathology is suspected. Conditions such as autoimmune vasculitis and marantic endocarditis usually require a rheumatologist's expertise regarding options and duration of treatment. Consider rheumatology evaluation in stroke patients complaining of joint or muscle pain, skin changes, or headaches.

Infectious Disease: Infectious disease specialists are crucial in cases of infective endocarditis to guide treatment but also to determine the source of an infection. These conditions require targeted long-term antibiotic therapy, with treatment starting while inpatient and continuing after discharge requiring follow-up with an infectious disease expert outpatient.

Neurosurgery: Neurosurgeons may be asked to perform DSAs for either diagnostic or therapeutic purposes for stroke patients. Patients may need to undergo neurosurgical decompression and clot evacuation in the setting of a large intraparenchymal hemorrhage or hemicraniectomy for malignant cerebral edema associated with a large ischemic stroke. Those with symptomatic carotid stenosis often have their revascularization performed by a neurosurgeon.

Clinical Pearls
- An inpatient stroke workup aims to identify the mechanism of a stroke and guide appropriate secondary prevention plans.
- The TOAST criteria, while imperfect and not all-encompassing, helps characterize the mechanism of an ischemic stroke.
- Knowing the advantages and limitations of each brain and vessel imaging modality is helpful.
- Consider an MRI in a patient with a cardiac implantable electronic device only if it will impact diagnosis and decision-making. An MRI may be unnecessary if the infarct is visible on NCCT.
- A standard cardioembolic workup includes TTE and extended cardiac monitoring. TEE helps rule out specific conditions requiring unique and urgent treatment, such as endocarditis and left atrial appendage thrombus.
- Hematologic or malignancy evaluations are helpful when standard workup is unrevealing or if a patient's history raises concerns for prothrombotic conditions or cancer.
- Involving subspecialists early when warranted ensures timely completion of a thorough workup.

References

1. Adams HP Jr, Bendixen BH, Kappelle LJ, Biller J, Love BB, Gordon DL, Marsh EE 3rd. Classification of subtype of acute ischemic stroke. Definitions for use in a multicenter clinical trial. TOAST. Trial of Org 10172 in Acute Stroke Treatment. Stroke. 1993;24(1):35–41.
2. Latchaw RE, Alberts MJ, Lev MH, Connors JJ, Harbaugh RE, Higashida RT, Hobson R, Kidwell CS, Koroshetz WJ, Mathews V, Villablanca P, Warach S, Walters B, American Heart Association Council on Cardiovascular Radiology and Intervention, Stroke Council, and the Interdisciplinary Council on Peripheral Vascular Disease. Recommendations for imaging of acute ischemic stroke: a scientific statement from the American Heart Association. Stroke. 2009;40(11):3646–78.
3. Lansberg MG, Albers GW, Beaulieu C, Marks MP. Comparison of diffusion-weighted MRI and CT in acute stroke. Neurology. 2000;54(8):1557–61. https://doi.org/10.1212/wnl.54.8.1557. PMID: 10762493.
4. Allen L, Hasso A, Handwerker J, Farid H. Sequence-specific MR imaging findings that are useful in dating ischemic stroke. Radiographics. 2012;32(5):1285–97; discussion 1297.
5. Thurnher M. Imaging in acute stroke. Radiology Assistant. 2008. https://radiologyassistant.nl/neuroradiology/brain-ischemia/imaging-in-acute-stroke.
6. Knight-Greenfield A, Nario JJQ, Gupta A. Causes of acute stroke: a patterned approach. Radiol Clin North Am. 2019;57(6):1093–108.
7. Levine GN, Gomes AS, Arai AE, Bluemke DA, Flamm SD, Kanal E, Manning WJ, Martin ET, Smith JM, Wilke N, Shellock FS, American Heart Association Committee on Diagnostic and Interventional Cardiac Catheterization; American Heart Association Council on Clinical Cardiology; American Heart Association Council on Cardiovascular Radiology and Intervention. Safety of magnetic resonance imaging in patients with cardiovascular devices: an American Heart Association scientific statement from the Committee on Diagnostic and Interventional Cardiac Catheterization, Council on Clinical Cardiology, and the Council on Cardiovascular Radiology and Intervention: endorsed by the American College of

Cardiology Foundation, the North American Society for Cardiac Imaging, and the Society for Cardiovascular Magnetic Resonance. Circulation. 2007;116(24):2878–91.

8. Demchuk AM, Menon BK, Goyal M. Comparing vessel imaging: noncontrast computed tomography/computed tomographic angiography should be the new minimum standard in acute disabling stroke. Stroke. 2016;47:273–28.

9. Shaban S, Huasen B, Haridas A, et al. Digital subtraction angiography in cerebrovascular disease: current practice and perspectives on diagnosis, acute treatment and prognosis. Acta Neurol Belg. 2022;122:763–80.

10. Barras CD, Bhattacharya JJ. Current status of imaging of the brain and anatomical features. In: Grainger & Allison's diagnostic radiology, vol 53, pp 1351–1386.

11. Nakanishi K, Homma S. Role of echocardiography in patients with stroke. J Cardiol. 2016;68(2):91–9.

12. Vaziri SM, Larson MG, Benjamin EJ, Levy D. Echocardiographic predictors of nonrheumatic atrial fibrillation. The Framingham Heart Study. Circulation. 1994;89(2):724–30.

13. Kernan WN, Ovbiagele B, Black HR, et al. Guidelines for the prevention of stroke in patients with stroke and transient ischemic attack: a guideline for healthcare professionals from the American Heart Association/American Stroke Association. Stroke. 2014;45:2160–236.

14. Sanna T, Diener HC, Passman RS, Di Lazzaro V, Bernstein RA, Morillo CA, Rymer MM, Thijs V, Rogers T, Beckers F, Lindborg K, Brachmann J, CRYSTAL AF Investigators. Cryptogenic stroke and underlying atrial fibrillation. N Engl J Med. 2014;370(26):2478–86.

15. Tatlisumak T, Fisher M. Hematologic disorders associated with ischemic stroke. J Neurol Sci. 1996;140(1–2):1–11.

16. Cucchiara BL. Evaluation and management of stroke. Hematol Am Soc Hematol Educ Program. 2009;2009(1):293–301.

17. Navi BB, Kasner SE, Elkind MSV, Cushman M, Bang OY, DeAngelis LM. Cancer and embolic stroke of undetermined source. Stroke. 2021;52(3):1121–30.

18. Doehner W, Leistner DM, Audebert HJ, Scheitz JF. The role of cardiologists on the stroke unit. Eur Heart J Suppl. 2020;22(Suppl M):M3–M12.

Intracranial Atherosclerosis

18

Samantha Salas, Kun He Lee, and Adam De Havenon

Introduction

Intracranial atherosclerosis, or intracranial atherosclerotic disease (ICAD), is an important cause of ischemic strokes and perhaps the most common cause of strokes worldwide [1]. ICAD is atherosclerosis of the larger intracranial vessels, like the distal internal carotid artery, middle, anterior, and posterior cerebral arteries, and basilar artery. It differs from small vessel disease, discussed later in this chapter, in appearance on imaging and carries a higher recurrent stroke risk. One study estimates the prevalence of ICAD in individuals over 65 in the United States at 31% [2]. ICAD disproportionately affects non-white individuals, with 8% of white and 12% of Black individuals having stenosis ≥50% in the Atherosclerosis Risk in Communities Study [2, 3]. ICAD is believed to be the most common cause of strokes in the Asian population, with over 40% of ischemic strokes attributed to ICAD in both South Korea and China [4, 5]. However, there does not seem to be a difference in sex with respect to ICAD and strokes [6]. This chapter provides an overview

S. Salas
Stanford Health, Stanford, CA, USA

K. H. Lee
Temple Health, Philadelphia, PA, USA
e-mail: Kun.lee@yale.edu

A. De Havenon (✉)
Yale School of Medicine, New Haven, CT, USA
e-mail: adam.dehavenon@yale.edu

mechanisms of ischemic stroke, risk factors, appearance on imaging, acute management, and secondary stroke prevention in ICAD.

Risk Factors

Like any artery in the body, intracranial arteries are susceptible to forming cholesterol plaques. Older age, non-white race, higher systolic blood pressure (SBP), diabetes, metabolic syndrome, and higher low-density lipoprotein (LDL) levels are all associated with increased risk of developing ICAD [3, 7–9]. Higher high-density lipoprotein (HDL) levels and the use of cholesterol-lowering medications, on the other hand, are associated with a decreased risk [2]. Surprisingly, while there has been a wealth of literature supporting a link between smoking and the development of atherosclerotic disease in the carotid arteries, the link between smoking and the development of ICAD is weak [10, 11].

Imaging

The key feature of ICAD is that abnormal vessels are seen on vascular imaging (Fig. 18.1). Digital subtraction angiography (DSA) remains the gold standard because it provides the highest resolution for visualizing the stenotic artery. DSA also provides real-time flow assessment through the artery of interest. DSA also assesses collateral flow, or backup vessels that supply blood flow to areas downstream from a diseased vessel, similar to detours around a highway closure [12]. DSA, however, exposes the patient to CT radiation, requires iodinated contrast, and is an invasive catheter-based procedure carrying potential intra-procedural risks, such as arterial dissection, subarachnoid hemorrhage, and groin hematoma [13, 14]. Given the procedural risks, it is not appropriate as an initial screening study. Computed tomography angiography (CTA) is a noninvasive and fast imaging modality for assessing intracranial vessels and screening for ICAD. It is widely available with good inter-operator reliability (different people would interpret the scan in a similar way) but exposes the patient to radiation and requires iodinated contrast [15, 16]. Magnetic resonance angiography (MRA) can also screen for ICAD. The specific sequence used is time-of-flight (ToF), which does not require additional contrast, though it may overestimate the degree of stenosis [12, 17]. Newer magnetic resonance techniques called vessel wall MRI or black blood MRI that use gadolinium contrast have the potential to characterize the vessel walls of stenosed arteries better and rule out alternative causes of stenosis, such as vasculitis [18, 19]. Transcranial Doppler (TCD) ultrasound can provide real-time information on cerebral blood flow through the stenosed artery and microembolic signals (small free-floating plaque fragments suggesting an unstable plaque). However, one can't "visualize" the vessels with TCD in the same way as the other modalities, and other limitations include availability, variable quality depending on the technician's experience, and lack of inter-operator reliability [17, 20].

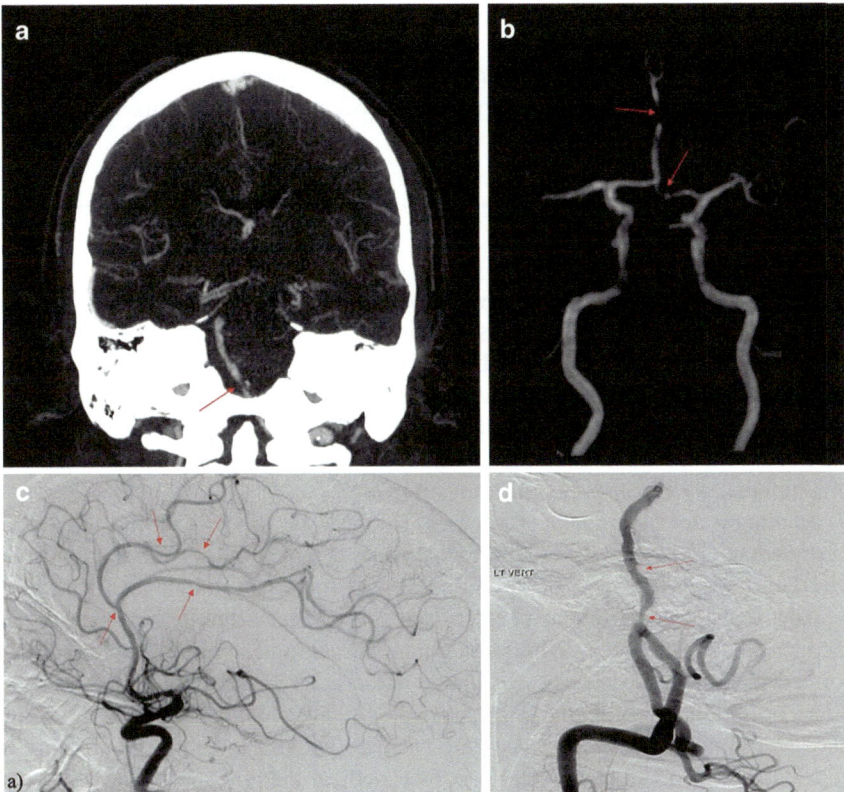

Fig. 18.1 (**a**) CTA of the head shows evidence of atherosclerotic plaques leading to irregular appearance and significant stenosis (arrow) of the basilar artery. (**b**) Magnetic resonance angiography time-of-flight three-dimensional reconstruction demonstrates the internal carotid, middle cerebral, and anterior cerebral arteries. There are multiple segments (arrow) of the anterior cerebral arteries with irregular caliber due to atherosclerosis. Digital subtraction angiography demonstrating multiple areas (arrows) of atherosclerosis causing stenosis in the segments of (**c**) both anterior cerebral arteries and (**d**) the proximal and mid basilar artery

How Does ICAD Lead to Stroke?

Several potential mechanisms can cause stroke in ICAD. In the Trial of Org 10172 in Acute Stroke Treatment (TOAST) classification of acute ischemic stroke subtypes, ICAD falls under "larger-artery atherosclerosis" [21]. The most common mechanism is thought to be a ruptured plaque leading to an artery-to-artery embolism (a piece of plaque or clot traveling from the source to occlude a vessel downstream), often leading to wedge-shaped or multifocal embolic-appearing infarcts [21, 22]. When the stenosis is so severe that it limits blood flow, hypoperfusion downstream to the artery can lead to border-zone, or watershed, strokes. Lastly, occlusion of the smaller branches of a diseased main artery, like the lenticulostriate arteries off the middle cerebral artery, can lead to stroke, like a highway closure blocking an exit. A mixed pattern of the three potential mechanisms is also possible [22, 23]. According to one study, the prevalence of the stroke patterns from ICAD was 61.8% artery-to-artery embolism, 23.4% perforator occlusion, 10.7% mixed, and 4.2% hypoperfusion [22].

Management

Antiplatelet therapy is the mainstay for the medical management of ICAD. While anticoagulation (e.g., warfarin) was used in the past, the WASID trial showed that anticoagulation was associated with a higher risk of intracranial hemorrhage without reducing recurrent stroke rates compared to aspirin [24, 25]. Guidelines recommend a course of dual antiplatelet therapy (DAPT) for secondary stroke prevention in ICAD. The optimal duration typically ranges from several weeks to a maximum of 3 months, with aspirin monotherapy afterward.

Stenting is not an option in most cases. The SAMMPRIS and VISSIT trials demonstrated an increased risk for recurrent strokes with angioplasty and stenting compared to intensive medical therapy [26, 27]. It is important to note that these trials aimed to evaluate the effectiveness of the surgical intervention, not the specific medical therapy regimen. While less common, angioplasty and stenting are performed in high-grade stenoses of major intracranial vessels, such as the basilar artery or middle cerebral artery, for patients who fail maximal medical therapy and have recurrent strokes [12]. Since outcomes are variable, stenting should only be considered if patients have failed maximal medical therapy, have a clearly symptomatic lesion, and even then, the location has to be suitable for stent placement. The medical management of ICAD also involves optimizing all vascular risk factors, including hypertension, diabetes, and dyslipidemia. Long-term SBP <140 mmHg is associated with lower rates of recurrent strokes in ICAD [24, 26]. Treatment with statins reduces the risk of recurrent strokes from ICAD in a dose-dependent manner [28]. Per the American Heart Association and American Stroke Association's 2021 guidelines, LDL goal <70 mg/dL, hemoglobin A1c goal ≤7%, and exercise are recommended for secondary prevention [29].

Clinical Pearls

- Strokes from ICAD disproportionately affect non-white patients.
- Risk factors for ICAD development include older age, non-white race, higher SBP and LDL, and diabetes.
- Three main types of strokes associated with ICAD are artery-to-artery embolism, hypoperfusion, and occlusion of perforating vessels.
- CTA or MRA are good first-line diagnostic tests for ICAD.
- A course of dual antiplatelet therapy, statins and managing risk factors remain the mainstay of secondary stroke prevention from ICAD. Ensure that patients stop DAPT when instructed.

Clinical Vignette 1

HPI: 62-year-old female with a history of smoking, hypertension, diabetes mellitus, hyperlipidemia, depression and poor medication adherence, who presented to the hospital with dysarthria, left facial droop and left arm weakness. Symptom onset was 5 h prior to arrival, so she was out of the thrombolytic window.

Exam: BP was 164/94, HR 87. NIHSS 6 for complete L homonymous hemianopia, left lower facial weakness, drift in L arm, and mild to moderate dysarthria. L leg was full strength and sensation was normal.

Workup: CTA revealed severe stenosis vs. occlusion of her R MCA (**a**, red arrow). Pt was taken for a diagnostic angiogram that showed high atherosclerotic high-grade stenosis of the R MCA M1 segment (**b**, blue arrow). Clot aspiration was attempted with minimal clot burden retrieved, making the diagnosis likely advanced intracranial atherosclerosis. MRI brain revealed multiple foci of restricted diffusion in the right MCA territory (**c**, **d**) and a chronic infarct in the right temporal lobe (**e**).

Management: The mechanism of her stroke was felt to be artery-to-artery embolism from intracranial plaque in her right MCA. She was started on dual antiplatelet therapy with aspirin and Plavix, high-intensity statin for plaque stabilization. Permissive HTN was allowed initially to avoid hypotension and extension of stroke with gradual reduction over time.

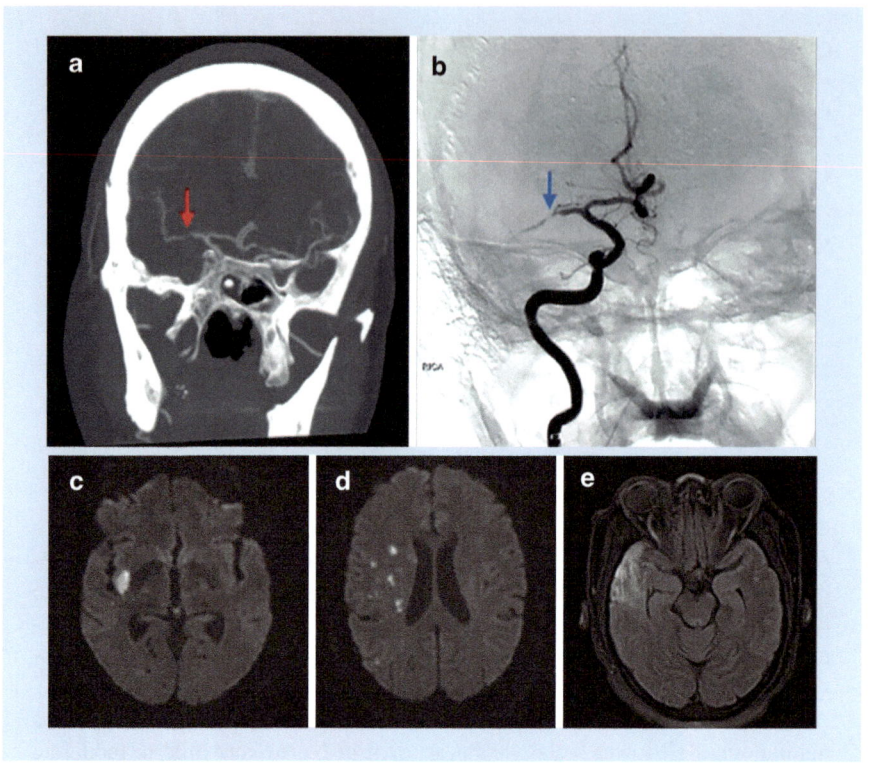

Clinical trials	Summary
Comparison of warfarin and aspirin for symptomatic intracranial artery stenosis (WASID)	A multicenter, double-blind, randomized controlled trial evaluating the effectiveness of either aspirin 1300 mg/day or warfarin titrated to international normalized ratio (INR) 2–3 in preventing recurrent strokes or death in patients with transient ischemic attack (TIA) or mild stroke (defined as modified Rankin Scale of <3) within 90 days and high-grade intracranial arterial stenosis (50–99%). There was no difference in recurrent ischemic or hemorrhagic stroke or death from non-stroke vascular causes between aspirin and warfarin, but there was an increased risk of death and major hemorrhage in the warfarin group [24]
Aspirin plus dipyridamole versus aspirin alone after cerebral ischemia of arterial origin (ESPIRIT)	A multicenter, randomized-controlled trial evaluating the effectiveness of aspirin, aspirin plus dipyridamole, and anticoagulation (vitamin K antagonist) in reducing vascular mortality, nonfatal stroke, nonfatal myocardial infarction, or nonfatal major bleeding in patients with TIAs and minor strokes (mRS <3) from an arterial origin. There was no difference between the groups for stroke, or myocardial infarction, but the warfarin group did have more bleeding complications [25]
Stenting versus Aggressive Medical Therapy for Intracranial Arterial Stenosis (SAMMPRIS)	A multicenter, randomized-controlled trial evaluating the effectiveness of either percutaneous transluminal angioplasty and stenting (PTAS) plus medical therapy vs. medical therapy alone in patients with TIA or ischemic strokes within 30 days due to 70–99% stenosis of a major intracranial artery. Medical therapy included aspirin 325 mg/day for the entire follow-up, clopidogrel 75 mg/day for 90 days, SBP <140 mmHg, LDL <70 mg/dL, and lifestyle coaching for smoking cessation, healthy eating, and exercise. Stroke, hemorrhage, and death were all higher in the PTAS group [26]
Effect of a Balloon-Expandable Intracranial Stent vs. Medical Therapy on Risk of Stroke in Patients With Symptomatic Intracranial Stenosis (VISSIT)	A multicenter, randomized-controlled trial evaluating the effectiveness of medical therapy (aspirin 81–325 mg/day for the entire study, clopidogrel 75 mg/day for the first 3 months, initiation of statin with LDL < 100 mg/dL, and SBP ≤ 140 mmHg) vs. intracranial stent plus medical therapy in reducing recurrent stroke or TIA. The medical group had lower rates of recurrent strokes and lower mean NIHSS at 12-month follow-up compared to the stent group
Wingspan Stent System Post Market Surveillance (WEAVE)	A post-market surveillance trial of the Wingspan stent system for treating ICAD in stroke. A total of 152 patients, with 70–99% stenosis of an intracranial artery, two or more strokes in the corresponding vascular territory while on medical therapy, and baseline mRS 3 or greater were included. 2.6% of patients had periprocedural stroke, hemorrhage, or death (lower than expected 4%). 97.4% were event-free at 72 h. This trial concluded that with careful selection of patients and with experienced interventionalists, the Wingspan stent system is safe and can potentially be beneficial in preventing strokes related to ICAD [30]

Clinical trials	Summary
Mechanisms of early Recurrence in Intracranial Atherosclerotic Disease (MyRIAD)	A prospective, multicenter observational study that enrolled patients with recent TIA or stroke due to ICAD with 50–99% stenosis to assess for recurrent strokes in the territory of the stenotic artery within one year. Patients were treated with aggressive medical therapy per the SAMMPRIS regimen. 8.8% had a stroke, while 5.9% had a TIA. In 24.7% of the patients, a new infarct was discovered within the first 6–8 weeks [31]
Vertebrobasilar Flow Evaluation and Risk of Transient Ischemic Attack and Stroke (VERiTAS)	A prospective, blinded, multicenter observational study evaluating patients with TIA or stroke secondary to 50% or greater atherosclerotic stenosis of extracranial or intracranial vertebral and basilar (VB) arteries. A total of 72 patients underwent measurement of blood flow measurement via MRA and were followed for 12 months to assess for any recurrent strokes in the VB territory. Those (25%) with low flow distal to the point of stenosis had a higher risk of subsequent stroke [32]

References

1. Gorelick PB, Wong KS, Bae HJ, Pandey DK. Large artery intracranial occlusive disease: a large worldwide burden but a relatively neglected frontier. Stroke. 2008;39:2396–9. https://doi.org/10.1161/strokeaha.107.505776.
2. Suri MF, Qiao Y, Ma X, Guallar E, Zhou J, Zhang Y, Liu L, Chu H, Qureshi AI, Alonso A, et al. Prevalence of intracranial atherosclerotic stenosis using high-resolution magnetic resonance angiography in the general population: the Atherosclerosis Risk In Communities Study. Stroke. 2016;47:1187–93. https://doi.org/10.1161/strokeaha.115.011292.
3. Rincon F, Sacco RL, Kranwinkel G, Xu Q, Paik MC, Boden-Albala B, Elkind MS. Incidence and risk factors of intracranial atherosclerotic stroke: the Northern Manhattan Stroke Study. Cerebrovasc Dis. 2009;28:65–71. https://doi.org/10.1159/000219299.
4. Wang Y, Zhao X, Liu L, Soo YO, Pu Y, Pan Y, Wang Y, Zou X, Leung TW, Cai Y, et al. Prevalence and outcomes of symptomatic intracranial large artery stenoses and occlusions in China: the Chinese Intracranial Atherosclerosis (CICAS) Study. Stroke. 2014;45:663–9. https://doi.org/10.1161/strokeaha.113.003508.
5. Kim JT, Yoo SH, Kwon JH, Kwon SU, Kim JS. Subtyping of ischemic stroke based on vascular imaging: analysis of 1,167 acute, consecutive patients. J Clin Neurol. 2006;2:225–30. https://doi.org/10.3988/jcn.2006.2.4.225.
6. Voigt S, van Os H, van Walderveen M, van der Schaaf IC, Kappelle LJ, Broersen A, Velthuis BK, de Jong PA, Kockelkoren R, Kruyt ND, et al. Sex differences in intracranial and extracranial atherosclerosis in patients with acute ischemic stroke. Int J Stroke. 2021;16:385–91. https://doi.org/10.1177/1747493020932806.
7. Bae HJ, Lee J, Park JM, Kwon O, Koo JS, Kim BK, Pandey DK. Risk factors of intracranial cerebral atherosclerosis among asymptomatics. Cerebrovasc Dis. 2007;24:355–60. https://doi.org/10.1159/000106982.
8. Rezaianzadeh A, Namayandeh SM, Sadr SM. National Cholesterol Education Program Adult Treatment Panel III versus International Diabetic Federation definition of metabolic syndrome, which one is associated with diabetes mellitus and coronary artery disease? Int J Prev Med. 2012;3:552–8.
9. Kim JS, Nah HW, Park SM, Kim SK, Cho KH, Lee J, Lee YS, Kim J, Ha SW, Kim EG, et al. Risk factors and stroke mechanisms in atherosclerotic stroke: intracranial compared with

extracranial and anterior compared with posterior circulation disease. Stroke. 2012;43:3313–8. https://doi.org/10.1161/strokeaha.112.658500.

10. Ritz K, Denswil NP, Stam OC, van Lieshout JJ, Daemen MJ. Cause and mechanisms of intracranial atherosclerosis. Circulation. 2014;130:1407–14. https://doi.org/10.1161/circulationaha.114.011147.

11. Bos D, van der Rijk MJ, Geeraedts TE, Hofman A, Krestin GP, Witteman JC, van der Lugt A, Ikram MA, Vernooij MW. Intracranial carotid artery atherosclerosis: prevalence and risk factors in the general population. Stroke. 2012;43:1878–84. https://doi.org/10.1161/strokeaha.111.648667.

12. Qureshi AI, Caplan LR. Intracranial atherosclerosis. Lancet. 2014;383:984–98. https://doi.org/10.1016/s0140-6736(13)61088-0.

13. Cloft HJ, Lynn MJ, Feldmann E, Chimowitz M. Risk of cerebral angiography in patients with symptomatic intracranial atherosclerotic stenosis. Cerebrovasc Dis. 2011;31:588–91. https://doi.org/10.1159/000324951.

14. Cloft HJ, Joseph GJ, Dion JE. Risk of cerebral angiography in patients with subarachnoid hemorrhage, cerebral aneurysm, and arteriovenous malformation: a meta-analysis. Stroke. 1999;30:317–20. https://doi.org/10.1161/01.str.30.2.317.

15. Bash S, Villablanca JP, Jahan R, Duckwiler G, Tillis M, Kidwell C, Saver J, Sayre J. Intracranial vascular stenosis and occlusive disease: evaluation with CT angiography, MR angiography, and digital subtraction angiography. AJNR Am J Neuroradiol. 2005;26:1012–21.

16. Lin E, Alessio A. What are the basic concepts of temporal, contrast, and spatial resolution in cardiac CT? J Cardiovasc Comput Tomogr. 2009;3:403–8. https://doi.org/10.1016/j.jcct.2009.07.003.

17. Nederkoorn PJ, van der Graaf Y, Eikelboom BC, van der Lugt A, Bartels LW, Mali WP. Time-of-flight MR angiography of carotid artery stenosis: does a flow void represent severe stenosis? AJNR Am J Neuroradiol. 2002;23:1779–84.

18. van den Wijngaard IR, Holswilder G, van Walderveen MA, Algra A, Wermer MJ, Zaidat OO, Boiten J. Treatment and imaging of intracranial atherosclerotic stenosis: current perspectives and future directions. Brain Behav. 2016;6:e00536. https://doi.org/10.1002/brb3.536.

19. Edjlali M, Qiao Y, Boulouis G, Menjot N, Saba L, Wasserman BA, Romero JM. Vessel wall MR imaging for the detection of intracranial inflammatory vasculopathies. Cardiovasc Diagn Ther. 2020;10:1108–19. https://doi.org/10.21037/cdt-20-324.

20. Pan Y, Wan W, Xiang M, Guan Y. Transcranial Doppler ultrasonography as a diagnostic tool for cerebrovascular disorders. Front Hum Neurosci. 2022;16:841809. https://doi.org/10.3389/fnhum.2022.841809.

21. Adams HP Jr, Bendixen BH, Kappelle LJ, Biller J, Love BB, Gordon DL, Marsh EE 3rd. Classification of subtype of acute ischemic stroke. Definitions for use in a multicenter clinical trial. TOAST. Trial of Org 10172 in Acute Stroke Treatment. Stroke. 1993;24:35–41. https://doi.org/10.1161/01.str.24.1.35.

22. López-Cancio E, Matheus MG, Romano JG, Liebeskind DS, Prabhakaran S, Turan TN, Cotsonis GA, Lynn MJ, Rumboldt Z, Chimowitz MI. Infarct patterns, collaterals and likely causative mechanisms of stroke in symptomatic intracranial atherosclerosis. Cerebrovasc Dis. 2014;37:417–22. https://doi.org/10.1159/000362922.

23. Wong KS, Gao S, Chan YL, Hansberg T, Lam WW, Droste DW, Kay R, Ringelstein EB. Mechanisms of acute cerebral infarctions in patients with middle cerebral artery stenosis: a diffusion-weighted imaging and microemboli monitoring study. Ann Neurol. 2002;52:74–81. https://doi.org/10.1002/ana.10250.

24. Chimowitz MI, Lynn MJ, Howlett-Smith H, Stern BJ, Hertzberg VS, Frankel MR, Levine SR, Chaturvedi S, Kasner SE, Benesch CG, et al. Comparison of warfarin and aspirin for symptomatic intracranial arterial stenosis. N Engl J Med. 2005;352:1305–16. https://doi.org/10.1056/NEJMoa043033.

25. Halkes PH, van Gijn J, Kappelle LJ, Koudstaal PJ, Algra A. Medium intensity oral anticoagulants versus aspirin after cerebral ischaemia of arterial origin (ESPRIT): a randomised controlled trial. Lancet Neurol. 2007;6:115–24. https://doi.org/10.1016/s1474-4422(06)70685-8.

26. Derdeyn CP, Chimowitz MI, Lynn MJ, Fiorella D, Turan TN, Janis LS, Montgomery J, Nizam A, Lane BF, Lutsep HL, et al. Aggressive medical treatment with or without stenting in high-risk patients with intracranial artery stenosis (SAMMPRIS): the final results of a randomised trial. Lancet. 2014;383:333–41. https://doi.org/10.1016/s0140-6736(13)62038-3.

27. Zaidat OO, Fitzsimmons BF, Woodward BK, Wang Z, Killer-Oberpfalzer M, Wakhloo A, Gupta R, Kirshner H, Megerian JT, Lesko J, et al. Effect of a balloon-expandable intracranial stent vs medical therapy on risk of stroke in patients with symptomatic intracranial steno-sis: the VISSIT randomized clinical trial. JAMA. 2015;313:1240–8. https://doi.org/10.1001/jama.2015.1693.

28. Zhou P, Cao Z, Wang P, Liu G, Yao X, Wang P, Li G, Zhang G, Gao P. The effect of inten-sive statin therapy on symptomatic intracranial arterial stenosis. Iran J Public Health. 2018;47:231–6.

29. Kleindorfer DO, Towfighi A, Chaturvedi S, Cockroft KM, Gutierrez J, Lombardi-Hill D, Kamel H, Kernan WN, Kittner SJ, Leira EC, et al. 2021 guideline for the prevention of stroke in patients with stroke and transient ischemic attack: a guideline from the American Heart Association/American Stroke Association. Stroke. 2021;52:e364–467. https://doi.org/10.1161/str.0000000000000375.

30. Alexander MJ, Zauner A, Chaloupka JC, Baxter B, Callison RC, Gupta R, Song SS, Yu W. WEAVE trial: final results in 152 on-label patients. Stroke. 2019;50:889–94. https://doi.org/10.1161/strokeaha.118.023996.

31. Romano JG, Prabhakaran S, Nizam A, Feldmann E, Sangha R, Cotsonis G, Campo-Bustillo I, Koch S, Rundek T, Chimowitz MI, et al. Infarct recurrence in intracranial atherosclero-sis: results from the MyRIAD study. J Stroke Cerebrovasc Dis. 2021;30:105504. https://doi.org/10.1016/j.jstrokecerebrovasdis.2020.105504.

32. Amin-Hanjani S, Pandey DK, Rose-Finnell L, Du X, Richardson D, Thulborn KR, Elkind MSV, Zipfel GJ, Liebeskind DS, Silver FL, et al. Effect of hemodynamics on stroke risk in symptom-atic atherosclerotic vertebrobasilar occlusive disease. JAMA Neurol. 2016;73:178–85. https://doi.org/10.1001/jamaneurol.2015.3772.

Small Vessel Disease

19

Samantha Salas, Kun He Lee, and Adam De Havenon

Introduction

"Small vessels" in the brain are commonly defined as perforating end arteries, originating from the larger intracranial vessels (anterior, middle, basilar, and posterior cerebral arteries). These end arteries do not have any more downstream branches, like a cul-de-sac or dead end, and perfuse subcortical brain territories like the basal ganglia, brainstem, and cerebellum. Damage to these arteries is called small vessel disease (SVD), and leads to a variety of changes on MRI. About 25% of all ischemic strokes are due to SVD. Hemorrhagic strokes can occur as well. Additionally, SVD is a leading cause of cognitive decline in older patients, accounting for 45% of dementia cases [1–3].

Risk Factors

There are modifiable and non-modifiable risk factors for SVD. Non-modifiable risk factors include age and sex. Modifiable risk factors include hypertension, smoking, diabetes, and high cholesterol [4].

Hypertension damages the endothelium of the vessel wall over time. Previous guidelines endorsed a systolic blood pressure goal of <140 mmHg, but recent studies have shown that <120 mmHg is associated with an 11% lower incidence of stroke in

S. Salas
Stanford Health, Stanford, CA, USA
e-mail: samanthasalas@stanfordhealthcare.org

K. H. Lee
Neurology, Temple Health, Philadelphia, PA, USA
e-mail: Kun.lee@yale.edu

A. De Havenon (✉)
Neurology, Yale School of Medicine, New Haven, CT, USA
e-mail: adam.dehavenon@yale.edu

patients at high risk for cardiovascular disease. In individuals with mild SVD, a systolic blood pressure goal of <130 mmHg is reasonable, and in those with severe SVD or cognitive impairment, a more aggressive goal of <120 mmHg is appropriate.

Diabetes type 1 and 2 can increase stroke risk through endothelial damage, vascular smooth muscle cell function, and thrombosis. Hyperglycemia causes oxidative stress and decreases endothelium-derived nitrous oxide, a substance used to maintain vascular homeostasis, ensure adequate blood flow, and prevent thrombosis. For diabetic patients, a hemoglobin A1C target of <7 mg/dL can help reduce the risk of a future lacunar stroke. Smoking is another modifiable risk factor that increases stroke risk. Observational studies have shown that smoking is associated with an increased burden of SVD. Smoking can increase viscosity in the blood, thereby increasing thrombotic risk [5].

The role of hyperlipidemia in small vessel disease remains unclear, unlike in large artery atherosclerosis or ICAD, where it is a clear risk factor. However, in the Stroke Prevention by Aggressive Reduction in Cholesterol Levels (SPARCL) study, patients with stroke or transient ischemic attack treated with atorvastatin had a significantly reduced risk of recurrent stroke. Therefore, statin therapy is still indicated with lacunar strokes with a target LDL <70.

Mechanism of Stroke in SVD

Long-term exposure to the risk factors mentioned above leads to fibrosis and wall thickening (lipohyalinosis). This is the leading cause of small vessel disease ischemic strokes in SVD. Long-term exposure to risk factors also causes the vessels to become elongated, tortuous, and inflexible, ultimately causing decreased cerebral blood flow causing stroke [1, 6].

SVD can also lead to intracerebral hemorrhage (ICH), usually seen in the basal ganglia, thalamus, brainstem, and cerebellum, similar to the locations of lacunar strokes [7–9]. Patients with long-standing HTN may also develop hypertensive microhemorrhages in those same locations, which are different from the microhemorrhages in cerebral amyloid angiopathy (CAA). Microbleeds do not represent *active* bleeding, but rather small deposits of blood products from damaged vessels. Microbleeds from hypertension tend to be confined to the subcortical structures, cerebellum and brainstem, unlike microbleeds with CAA which are in the frontal/parietal/occipital and temporal lobes. Microbleeds from hypertension are also not felt to pose the same risk of spontaneous hemorrhage like CAA microbleeds.

Imaging

Since the vessels affected in SVD are so small, they cannot be visualized on traditional vessel imaging. Diagnosis, therefore, requires brain imaging to depict parenchymal changes *caused by* SVD and chronic hypoperfusion. MRI is the most common and accurate imaging modality to detect SVD, manifesting on the T2 weighted and FLAIR sequences as white matter hyperintensities (WMH) (Fig. 19.1).

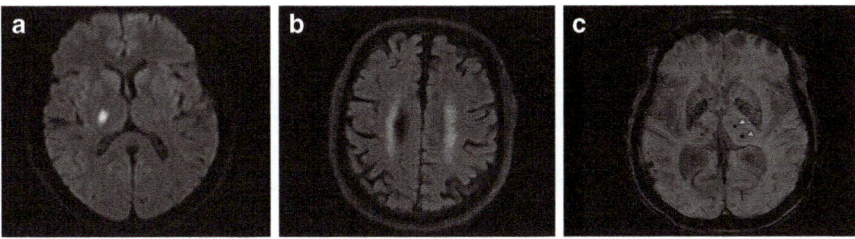

Fig. 19.1 SVD *appearance on neuroimaging*: (**a**) DWI sequence on MRI demonstrating an small, single acute lacunar infarct in the right posterior limb on the internal capsule; (**b**) axial FLAIR sequence on MRI showing white matter hyperintensities; and (**c**) SWI sequence on MRI showing subcortical cerebral microbleeds from hypertensive arteriopathy (white arrows)

Table 19.1 Comparison of ICAD and SVID

	ICAD	SVID
Brain imaging	White matter changes	White matter changes
Stroke type	Large and/or multifocal embolic (cortical) but in one vascular territory, or watershed	Lacunar (subcortical structures, brainstem, and cerebellum)
Vessel imaging	Irregular large intracranial vessels (distal ICA, MCA, ACA, PCA, Basilar)	Grossly normal (unless the patient also has ICAD!)
Risk factors	Traditional cardiovascular RF, age, and radiation	Same
Management	A course of DAPT followed by monotherapy. Stenting may be considered in refractory cases but high-risk Statin and RF control	Antiplatelet therapy, statin, and RF control
Likelihood of recurrent stroke	High	Lowest of all stroke subtypes

The white matter region of the brain is where most end arteries are. WMH usually appears bilateral and symmetric. If SVD causes a lacunar stroke, MRI will reveal a small, single lesion on diffusion-weighted imaging (DWI) sequence in the subcortical, brainstem, or cerebellar territories. The TOAST classification system defines a lacunar stroke as a single lesion less than 1.5 cm in diameter [4, 10, 11].

CT scan is the gold standard for detecting acute hemorrhage due to its high sensitivity, and will often demonstrate a hyperdense lesion with a surrounding rim of hypodense vasogenic edema. However, susceptibility-weighted imaging (SWI) or gradient recalled echo (GRE) sequence on MRI has the same sensitivity as CT to detect acute hemorrhage and can be more sensitive than CT for identification of prior hemorrhage. Microhemorrhages from HTN are only seen on SWI or GRE sequences on MRI and not on CT since they do not represent active bleeding [8, 9].

ICAD and SVID are similar diseases but at different points along the vascular "tree." Think of a carotid atherosclerosis as the tree trunk, followed by ICAD in the larger intracranial vessels (distal ICA, MCA, ACA, PCA or Basilar arteries) as the main branches of the trunk, and SVD as the smaller end twigs. The bigger the diseased vessel, the higher the risk of stroke. See Table 19.1 below for a side-by-side comparison of SVID and ICAD.

Management of SVD

The best way to prevent small vessel disease and stroke is to combine vascular risk factor control, lifestyle modification, and medical therapy. Primary care providers, including APCs, can often effectively manage these conditions, but referrals to cardiology or endocrinology may be warranted in advanced stages of HTN and diabetes.

Antiplatelet management with SVD reduces recurrent stroke compared to no antiplatelet therapy [3]. The SPS3 trial studied the benefit of dual antiplatelet therapy (DAPT) versus single antiplatelet therapy with aspirin. The results showed no significant difference in the stroke recurrence rate between either group. However, there were more bleeding complications in the DAPT group [12]. Therefore, aspirin monotherapy is the standard treatment for secondary stroke prevention. It remains uncertain, however, if antiplatelet therapy is beneficial in individuals with SVD but no clinical history of stroke. Such individuals would benefit from antiplatelet therapy if their atherosclerotic cardiovascular disease (ASCVD) Risk Score warrants it [13].

Clinical Pearls
- SVD results in lacunar strokes, which are single small strokes in the deep territories of the brain
- SVD is not visible on vessel imaging, unlike ICAD
- Standard treatment for patients with lacunar strokes is antiplatelet therapy, statin, and aggressive risk factor control

References

1. Adams HP, Bendixen BH, Kappelle LJ, Biller J, Love BB, Gordon DL, Marsh EE. Classification of subtype of acute ischemic stroke. Definitions for use in a multicenter clinical trial. TOAST. Trial of org 10172 in acute stroke treatment. Stroke. 1993;24(1):35–41. https://doi.org/10.1161/01.str.24.1.35.
2. Beckman J, Creager M, Lüscher T. Diabetes and vascular disease: pathophysiology, clinical consequences, and medical therapy: part I. Circulation. 2003; https://doi.org/10.1161/01.CIR.0000091257.27563.32.
3. Blair GW, Appleton JP, Flaherty K, Doubal F, Sprigg N, Dooley R, Richardson C, Hamilton I, Law ZK, Shi Y, Stringer MS, Thrippleton MJ, Boyd J, Shuler K, Bath PM, Wardlaw JM. Tolerability, safety and intermediary pharmacological effects of cilostazol and isosorbide mononitrate, alone and combined, in patients with lacunar ischaemic stroke: the LACunar Intervention-1 (LACI-1) trial, a randomised clinical trial. EClinicalMedicine. 2019;11:34–43. https://doi.org/10.1016/j.eclinm.2019.04.001.
4. Clancy U, Appleton JP, Arteaga C, Doubal FN, Bath PM, Wardlaw JM. Clinical management of cerebral small vessel disease. Chin Med J. 2020;134:127. Publish ahead of print. https://doi.org/10.1097/cm9.0000000000001177.
5. Benavente OR, et al. Effects of clopidogrel added to aspirin in patients with recent lacunar stroke. N Engl J Med. 2012;367(9):817–25. https://doi.org/10.1056/nejmoa1204133.

6. Hakim AM. Small vessel disease. Front Neurol. 2019;10 https://doi.org/10.3389/fneur.2019.01020.

7. Amarenco P, et al. High-dose atorvastatin after stroke or transient ischemic attack. N Engl J Med. 2006;355(6):549–59. https://doi.org/10.1056/nejmoa061894.

8. Joutel A, Faraci FM. Cerebral small vessel disease. Stroke. 2014;45(4):1215–21. https://doi.org/10.1161/strokeaha.113.002878.

9. McHutchison C, Blair GW, Appleton JP, Chappell FM, Doubal F, Bath PM, Wardlaw JM. Cilostazol for secondary prevention of stroke and cognitive decline. Stroke. 2020;51(8):2374–85. https://doi.org/10.1161/strokeaha.120.029454.

10. Pantoni L. Cerebral small vessel disease: from pathogenesis and clinical characteristics to therapeutic challenges. Lancet Neurol. 2010;9(7):689–701. https://doi.org/10.1016/s1474-4422(10)70104-6.

11. Unnithan AKA, Mehta P. Hemorrhagic stroke. StatPearls Publishing; 2020. https://www.ncbi.nlm.nih.gov/books/NBK559173/.

12. Dannenberg S, Scheitz JF, Rozanski M, Erdur H, Brunecker P, Werring DJ, Fiebach JB, Nolte CH. Number of cerebral microbleeds and risk of intracerebral hemorrhage after intravenous thrombolysis. Stroke. 2014;45(10):2900–5. https://doi.org/10.1161/strokeaha.114.006448.

13. de Havenon A, Meyer C, McNally JS, Alexander M, Chung L. Subclinical cerebrovascular disease: epidemiology and treatment. Curr Atheroscler Rep. 2019. https://pubmed.ncbi.nlm.nih.gov/31350593/. Accessed 1 Mar 2023.

Carotid Disease

20

Deonna Wissler and Karan Tarasaria

Epidemiology and Clinical Presentation

Carotid Artery disease accounts for approximately 20% of all ischemic strokes and is more common in men than women [1]. The estimated prevalence of carotid disease resulting in >50% stenosis increases with age, with approximately 2% in the 60–69 age group, increasing to 3–6% in the 70–79 age group to over 7.5% in patients over 80 years [2].

Atherosclerotic lesions in the vasculature tend to develop at bifurcations (splitting of one vessel into two, like a fork in the road). This is because blood likes to move in a linear, forward path. Bifurcations introduce turbulence in that path, causing local endothelial damage and leading to plaque development. So in the carotid system, atherosclerosis develops most often where the Common Carotid artery bifurcates into the Internal and External Carotid arteries. Contrast this with carotid dissections, which most often occur at the mid-segment of the internal carotid artery. Atherosclerotic plaque development is slow, starting initially with "fatty streaks" during adolescence and young adulthood, followed by plaque formation around the fourth decade. More significant atherosclerosis leading to stenosis or unstable plaques typically develops around the fifth decade [3].

In the initial stages of plaque development, lipids accumulate in the vessel wall, followed by an inflammatory response that drives atherosclerotic plaque progression [4]. Increased stenosis of the vascular lumen results in increased turbulence, further accelerating plaque growth. Increased turbulence and inflammatory activity eventually result in the rupture of the plaque surface, resulting in platelet clumping

D. Wissler
University of Arkansas for Medical Sciences, Little Rock, AR, USA
e-mail: dmwissler@uams.edu

K. Tarasaria (✉)
Neurology, Hartford HealthCare, Hartford, CT, USA
e-mail: Karan.Tarasaria@hhchealth.org

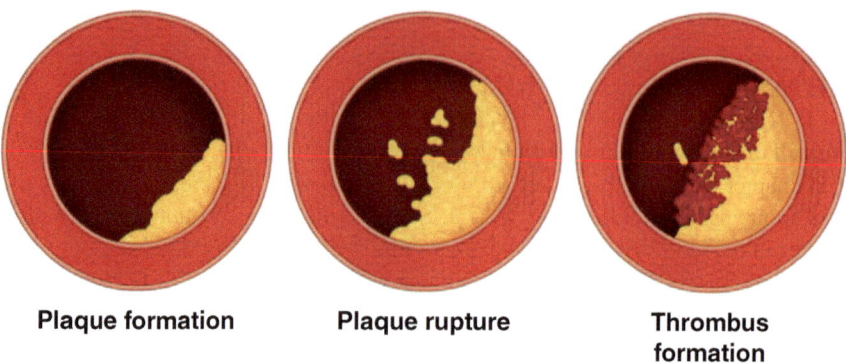

Plaque formation   **Plaque rupture**   **Thrombus formation**

Fig. 20.1 Carotid atherosclerosis

on the plaque surface (thrombus) formation (Fig. 20.1) [5, 6]. The most common mechanism of stroke or TIA from carotid disease is plaque rupture, resulting in a plaque fragment breaking off and traveling downstream to occlude a vessel in the brain, called atheroembolism. If imaging demonstrates a clear thrombus, it may also be a thromboembolism. Stenosis above 70% is considered high grade, but once stenosis reaches 80–90%, patients are at higher risk of hypoperfusion of the cerebral hemisphere resulting in cerebral ischemia.

Clinical Presentations of Carotid Disease

Transient ischemic attack (TIA): Amaurosis fugax (transient painless monocular blindness) or "hemispheric" TIAs result in transient motor, sensory, or speech symptoms. Limb-shaking TIAs are a rare form of TIAs that present as involuntary movements characterized by brief flailing or jerking movements of a leg or arm and are often confused with tremors or focal motor seizures. The clinical distinction is that these movements only occur on one side (contralateral to the stenosis), typically when the patient actively uses an extremity and not at rest. Imagine a patient is sawing a piece of wood with his right arm. This activity leads to increased metabolic demand in the left hemisphere. Suppose he has severe left carotid stenosis and cannot supply enough blood flow to the left motor cortex to meet the increased metabolic demand. In that case, he may develop shaking or jerking movements of the right arm while trying to use it. Other situations that can lead to similar situations include hypotension from medications, large meals, or vasodilation when in a hot bath [7]. This jerking is more pronounced than a typical tremor and has a clear onset and offset. Motor seizures occur at rest, are not as brief, and may have a post-ictal state not seen with limb-shaking TIA.

Cerebral ischemia: Atheroembolism causing central retinal artery occlusion (CRAO) or branch retinal artery occlusion (BRAO) will result in complete or partial monocular blindness. Carotid atheroembolism can also lead to single large embolic infarcts or multi-focal strokes confined to the ipsilateral hemisphere. Finally, infarcts due to hypoperfusion can occur at the border zones, also called watershed infarcts, between the vascular territories of the anterior and middle cerebral arteries or middle and posterior cerebral arteries. This can occur when a plaque ruptures into the lumen, limiting forward flow, or systemic hypotension in the setting of already present severe stenosis.

Vascular Risk Factors

Risk factors for carotid atherosclerosis are similar to atherosclerosis at other sites: hypertension, diabetes, cigarette smoking, coronary artery disease, increasing age, and, to some degree, hyperlipidemia. However, it is not uncommon for patients with reasonably normal lipid profiles to have focal significant atherosclerosis in their carotid arteries. It is also common for one carotid to be disproportionately more diseased than the other one. Smoking is strongly associated with carotid stenosis, likely due to endothelial exposure to chronic inflammation [8]. Additional risk factors include prior history of head and neck radiation, obstructive sleep apnea, coronary artery disease, and peripheral vascular disease. Young patients with disproportionate systemic vascular disease or a family history of early vascular disease may have elevated Lipoprotein (a), a very "sticky" form of cholesterol that, like LDL, builds up in the walls of blood vessels. High Lipoprotein (a) levels run in families.

Identifying Symptomatic Carotid Stenosis

A neck bruit can be detected in about 4–5% of the population aged 45–80 without prior stroke or TIA history [9]. Neck bruits have high specificity and relatively lower sensitivity, meaning the presence of a bruit is likely suggestive of carotid disease, but the absence of a bruit does not rule it out [10]. Many providers will order an outpatient carotid ultrasound (CUS) if a bruit is heard. Acute stroke patients often get CT or MR Angiography. CTA is preferred as MRA may overestimate the degree of stenosis. CUS can provide additional details about plaque morphology and degree of stenosis and is often performed as a complementary study to CTA or MRA in patients suspected of having symptomatic carotid disease [11]. For those interested, Fig. 20.2 illustrates the formulas used to measure the degree of stenosis.

Fig. 20.2 Carotid stenosis measurement based on the North American Symptomatic Carotid Endarterectomy Trial (NASCET) criteria [12]. A = normal lumen diameter distal to the stenosis. B = diameter at most stenotic segment

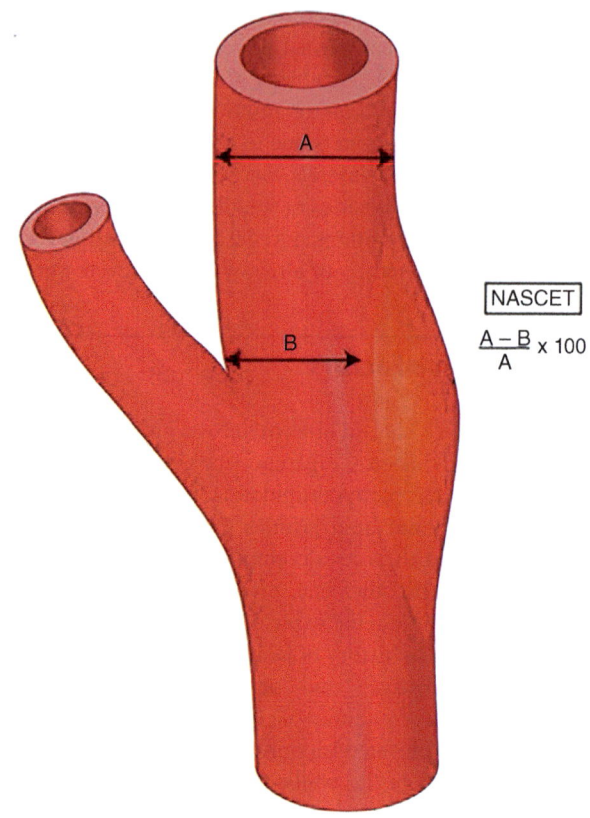

NASCET

$$\frac{A - B}{A} \times 100$$

Other High-Risk Features

In addition to the degree of stenosis, additional factors may impact the risk of recurrent TIA or ischemic stroke. Indeed, early studies have suggested that TIAs could be attributable to any degree of stenosis through microembolization from unstable but not stenotic plaques [13]. The NASCET and ECST trials demonstrated irregular or *ulcerated or ruptured plaque* surfaces as a significant predictor of stroke risk [14]. CTA and contrasted enhanced MR Angiography can help distinguish stable from ulcerated atherosclerotic plaques. Transcranial Doppler Ultrasound may also help identify *micro-emboli*, described as high-intensity signals (HITS), which can independently predict increased risk of ischemic events. HITS are detected by monitoring a vessel with an ultrasound probe for extended periods (15–60 min or longer). Carotid ultrasound can also detect plaque ulceration, *intraplaque hemorrhage*, and disruption of the luminal surface, all markers of an unstable and high-risk plaque. Intraplaque hemorrhage has been associated with a six to tenfold increase in risk of ipsilateral stroke compared to plaques without intraplaque hemorrhage [15]. Similarly, plaques with a disrupted luminal surface were found to have a 17-fold increased risk of stroke [16]. Identification of any of these features warrants consideration of carotid intervention, even with moderate stenosis.

Although carotid artery stenosis is a risk factor for stroke, not every carotid stenosis carries the same risk for future stroke. Key factors include the degree of stenosis and plaque appearance. Clinicians should work toward answering two questions: (1) Who requires revascularization and who is best managed with intensive medical therapy alone? and (2) For intervention, which mode of revascularization: CEA or carotid artery stenting?

Management of Carotid Artery Stenosis

Management of carotid artery stenosis includes both medical management and revascularization. All patients with carotid disease need maximal medical therapy. The challenge is identifying those that require revascularization.

Medical Management

Treatment of vascular risk factors, including dyslipidemia, hypertension, and diabetes mellitus, is of critical importance in the prevention and treatment of atherosclerotic disease. Statins are indicated to achieve LDL targets <70 for symptomatic carotids or patients with multiple risk factors. Hypertension is likely the strongest risk factor for carotid atherosclerosis. However, over-aggressive BP reduction can worsen stroke symptoms for patients depending on the degree of stenosis and the patient's ability to compensate via collateral circulation. If a patient demonstrates worsening symptoms when sitting up or standing, or if BP drops below a certain threshold, they have what is referred to as a "perfusion-dependent" exam. Allowing elevated BP and considering bed rest until symptoms stabilize and revascularization occurs is reasonable in those cases. All team members, including nurses, should be aware of the strict *lower-limit* BP threshold for perfusion-dependent patients, with instructions to notify providers if BP falls below. For example, if Mr. Jones develops worsening aphasia when his SBP is 135 mmHg, a lower SBP limit of 140 mmHg would be reasonable. If the BP falls below the target, the provider should examine the patient and identify any interventions that could keep SBP above target, such as IV fluids or removing anti-hypertensive medications. In rare cases, patients may require IV pressors for BP augmentation to avoid clinical worsening, which would necessitate ICU transfer. As such, blood pressure parameters should be decided on a case-by-case basis.

Antiplatelet agents, including aspirin or clopidogrel, are routinely used for primary and secondary stroke prevention for large artery atherosclerosis [17]. Since coated aspirin is less efficacious than uncoated aspirin in about 40% of individuals, uncoated aspirin is recommended [18]. Clopidogrel alone reduces stroke by only 1.7% more than aspirin and is thus only marginally better *except in patients with*

Table 20.1 Management of asymptomatic carotid disease

<50%	Do not require carotid revascularization.
51–69%	Revascularization is not recommended. Patients should be managed with intensive medical therapy alone and followed with interval surveillance carotid ultrasound imaging. If stenosis progresses over time, intervention should be considered.
70–99%	For medically stable patients with severe but asymptomatic carotid stenosis, either intensive medical therapy alone or intensive medical therapy plus carotid revascularization is reasonable. Modern-day medical management versus carotid revascularization is being evaluated in the ongoing CREST-2 study. For patients to potentially benefit from carotid revascularization, their life expectancy should be at least 5 years, and the combined perioperative risk of stroke and death should be ≤3%. A shared decision-making approach incorporating the patient's values and preferences is advised. Patients must understand that the risk of stroke with intensive medical therapy is relatively low for asymptomatic carotids (and that the benefits of carotid revascularization are limited).
Carotid occlusion	While it sounds scary, an asymptomatic patient with an occluded carotid has likely developed long-term collaterals that supply adequate blood flow to that hemisphere. For this reason, surgical intervention is not indicated.

peripheral arterial disease, whereas combined aspirin-dipyridamole (Aggrenox) is no better than clopidogrel [19].

Revascularization for *Asymptomatic* Extracranial Carotid Stenosis

Identifying high-grade stenosis in an asymptomatic patient presents a dilemma. Decision-making for asymptomatic atherosclerotic carotid stenosis intervention depends upon the severity of stenosis, comorbid conditions, surgical risk, and the patient's life expectancy. Detection of asymptomatic carotid stenosis is not an emergency, and outpatient referrals to vascular or neurosurgery and stroke clinics should be placed as long as the appointments can be scheduled in a reasonable timeframe. Stroke specialists can add further insight into the patient's neurological history and vasculature, educate the patient on risk factors to ensure comprehensive stroke prevention plans, and follow patients in the clinic if intervention is not warranted at the time. For patients with 60% or greater asymptomatic carotid stenosis, the 5-year risk of stroke is 11% with medical therapy and 5% with endarterectomy based on the ACAS study. Table 20.1 is a generally accepted framework on how to approach asymptomatic carotid disease.

Symptomatic Extracranial Carotid Stenosis

Patients with a clear TIA or minor ischemic stroke, good functional baseline, ipsilateral moderate to severe stenosis, and large territory at risk are appropriate for surgical revascularization. Numerous clinical trials have demonstrated the efficacy of revascularization for symptomatic carotid stenosis. The original method is carotid endarterectomy (CEA), a surgical approach with an incision in the neck and "cleaning out" the carotid directly. Three important trials include the European Carotid Surgery Trial (ESCT), the North American Symptomatic Carotid Endarterectomy Trial (NASCET), and the US Department of Veterans Affairs Cooperative Study Program (CSP) [12, 20, 21]. The NASCET study demonstrated that the 2-year stroke risk for symptomatic 70–99% stenosis was 26.1% in the medically treated patients compared to 12.9% in those who underwent endarterectomy (remember: 70 or more, one in four). For symptomatic 50–69% stenosis, the 5-year rate of any ipsilateral stroke was 15.7% in those surgically treated versus 22.2% in those medically treated. So, while there appears to be a benefit for presumed symptomatic moderate stenosis, it is not as great as for severe stenosis. Surgical intervention is not indicated for patients with less than 50% (mild) stenoses.

Carotid artery stenting is another option utilizing a catheter-based approach. Access is traditionally through the femoral artery in the groin. However, recent advances like Transcarotid Artery Revascularization (TCAR) allow access through the common carotid artery right above the clavicle, just before the ICA origin. TCAR is a much more direct approach with less distance for the catheter to travel through the body. Stenting will traditionally require dual antiplatelet therapy for 3–6 months, followed by monotherapy.

Revascularization is not indicated for patients who have had a complete holo-hemispheric stroke, are neurologically devastated, or have active critical medical issues making surgery unsafe.

Timing for Surgery

The optimal timing of carotid revascularization is within 2 weeks of the stroke if no contraindications exist. This window comes from data from the three trials mentioned earlier that demonstrated that the risk of recurrent stroke was highest in the first 2 weeks. Delaying surgery is reasonable for up to 6 months for patients with hemorrhagic transformation or other active medical issues, but those patients remain at high risk of a recurrent stroke. Discharging patients and bringing them back for surgery is not the best approach since these are high-risk situations; therefore, monitoring patients until the day of surgery is often the way to go.

Patients with clear TIA or punctate strokes from a symptomatic carotid could likely get revascularized within days, whereas larger strokes or medically complex patients may benefit from waiting closer to the 7 to 14-day window. That is because the perioperative intracerebral hemorrhage risk may be increased in patients with large cerebral infarctions, those with uncontrolled hypertension, or those undergoing early surgery. Reintroducing blood flow into a high-risk stroke could lead to hemorrhage or edema and can manifest as neurological worsening or seizures. Hypertension following surgery can lead to reperfusion injury (edema, hemorrhage, and seizures). For optimal blood pressure management before elective CEA, a systolic pressure of <160 mmHg should be targeted before surgery, and <140 mmHg afterward, but can be adjusted based on specific patient factors [22, 23]. Surgery can be considered up to 6 months after a stroke, but beyond 6 months, the risk of a recurrent event is felt to decrease significantly.

Clinical Vignette 1

HPI: 77-Year-old male with a past medical history of a saddle pulmonary embolism and deep venous thrombosis on full dose apixaban, coronary artery disease, hypertension, and hyperlipidemia who presented to the emergency room with new onset language deficits. The patient's last known normal was 24 h prior to arrival.

Exam: His blood pressure was 147/99 mmHg and blood glucose 106 mg/L. National Institute of Health Score (NIHSS) was 6 for answering neither orientation questions correctly, inability to follow commands, and severe receptive aphasia. He was otherwise moving all extremities normally.

Imaging: A CT head and CT angiogram of the head and neck were performed. CTA (a) demonstrated >70% stenosis of the left internal carotid artery (white arrow) with mixed-density plaque. MRI of the brain without contrast was completed (b), confirming stroke in the left superior temporal lobe.

Management: The patient was admitted to the stroke unit. The suspected etiology of this patient's stroke was large artery atherosclerosis. Care was taken not to lower his blood pressure below SBP 120, given his carotid stenosis and stroke. He underwent a left carotid artery endarterectomy approximately 1 week post-stroke.

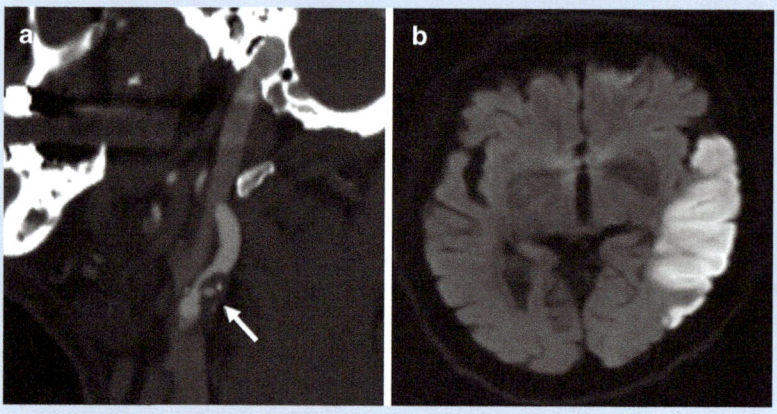

Case contributed by Dr. Amit Mehta

Deciding between the stenting and CEA is best left to surgeons and stroke neurologists. Factors favoring stenting include high cardiac or surgical risk, and factors favoring CEA include older age or high bleeding risk with DAPT (e.g., if the patient has atrial fibrillation and also needs anticoagulation) [24]. Table 20.2 compares the different modalities.

Table 20.2 Points to remember about different revascularization techniques

CEA	TF-CAS	TCAR
Low 30-day stroke risk	Higher 30-day stroke risk	Low 30-day stroke risk
High physiological stress avoid in high-risk cardiac patients	Long route to access carotid, higher risk of vessel injury, and stroke	Shorter route to access carotid
Does not require DAPT Consider for patients who also need long-term anticoagulation	Requires course of DAPT	Requires course of DAPT
Longer procedure, more likely to need general anesthesia	Shorter procedure time	Shorter procedure time
Possibility of cranial nerve injury	Risk of stent occlusion and migration	Risk of stent occlusion and migration
Longer recovery time	Shorter recovery time	Shorter recovery time

CEA carotid endarterectomy, *TF-CAS* trans-femoral carotid artery stent, *TCAR* transcarotid artery revascularization, *DAPT* dual antiplatelet therapy

Carotid Dissections

Cervical Carotid Artery Dissection (CAD) typically happens in young patients without atherosclerosis and occurs in the portion of the artery coursing through the neck [25]. Often due to trauma, CAD involves a tear of the innermost layer of the vessel that allows the development of an intramural hematoma between the tunica intima and media. This may lead to focal stenosis and thrombus formation, providing nidus of embolic stroke (Fig. 20.3) [26]. These may also result in the development of a "pseudoaneurysm" due to arterial dilatation from the extension of the tear through tunica media and adventitia [27].

Pathogenesis

CAD typically occurs at least 1–2 cm distal to the carotid bifurcation, compared to atherosclerotic disease, which affects the carotid siphon or the ICA origin. The pathogenesis of most spontaneous arterial dissections is idiopathic. They can be iatrogenic or due to severe trauma, in which case the causes are apparent, but most occur spontaneously or are associated with trivial antecedent triggers. Reported precipitant events include sudden head movement, coughing, vomiting, sneezing, chiropractic manipulation, yoga, and sexual intercourse [28, 29]. Predisposing conditions include arteriopathies such as fibromuscular dysplasia (FMD), cystic medial necrosis, Ehlers–Danlos syndrome type IV, Marfan's syndrome, Alpha-1 anti-trypsin

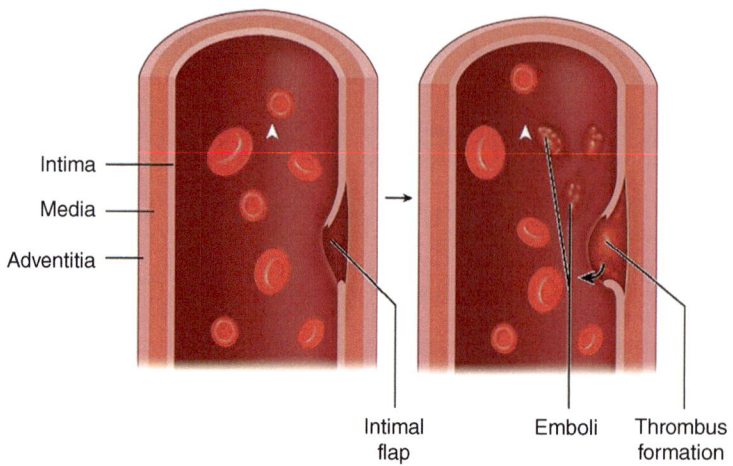

Fig. 20.3 Carotid dissection. Note the space created by the new intimal flap, also called a "false lumen," which is where thrombus formation can occur. Fragments of the thrombus can then break off, embolize downstream and occlude a distal vessel leading to stroke. The white arrows indicate direction of flow. (Source: Vascular Neurology Board Review. Amin, 2nd edition)

deficiency, Moya Moya disease, autosomal dominant polycystic kidney disease as well as migraine, family history of dissection, and Hyperhomocysteinemia [30–33].

Clinical Manifestations

Carotid dissection can result in cerebral ischemia due to hemodynamic compromise from luminal narrowing or occlusion, thromboembolism, or both. This is one of the few ischemic stroke processes that cause pain. Pain (in the head, face, or neck) is the most common overall symptom, seen in more than 80% of symptomatic cases. In addition to focal neurological symptoms, headache may be a preceding symptom in about two-thirds of patients. Headaches are often gradual in onset and non-throbbing in character, although sudden "thunderclap" headaches have also been reported. Unilateral neck pain may radiate to the ear, scalp, jaw, or face [34, 35].

In about one-third of cases, partial Horner's syndrome is present [35]. Horner's syndrome is characterized by partial oculo-sympathetic paresis resulting from the involvement of sympathetic fibers along the internal carotid artery. Ptosis (drooping of the eyelid) and miosis (narrowing of pupillary diameter) are seen, but facial sweating remains intact as these fibers travel along the external carotid artery. Lower cranial nerve palsies have been reported in about 10–15% of patients with carotid artery dissection. The most commonly affected cranial nerve is CN XII, followed by CN IX, X, XI, and V [36].

Ischemic symptoms: Most ischemic symptoms occur within 1–2 weeks of the dissection [37]. TIAs are common, reported in about 50% of patients, with half of them having recurrent symptoms. Transient monocular blindness is seen in one-fourth of cases. Dissections causing ischemic events are more often associated with occlusion or stenosis greater than 80%. In contrast, dissections that do not cause ischemic symptoms are more often associated with Horner's syndrome and lower cranial nerve palsies [38]. In summary, focal ischemic symptoms along with local symptoms such as neck pain, headache, or Horner's syndrome in a young patient should raise concern for a dissection.

Imaging

Non-invasive vessel imaging modalities such as computerized tomography angiography (CTA) and magnetic resonance angiography with T1-weighted fat suppression (MRA) are typically used to evaluate for dissection [39]. Conventional angiography remains the gold standard for accurately defining the level and territory of dissection but is invasive and seldom required to make the diagnosis. Carotid Doppler combined with transcranial Doppler imaging to evaluate for microemboli can also be utilized as an alternative imaging modality [40]. Imaging findings on CTA and MRA include the "Flame sign," referring to the characteristic tapering of the carotid artery sparing the bulb, as well as the "String sign," referring to long tapering stenosis distal to the carotid bulb (Fig. 20.4).

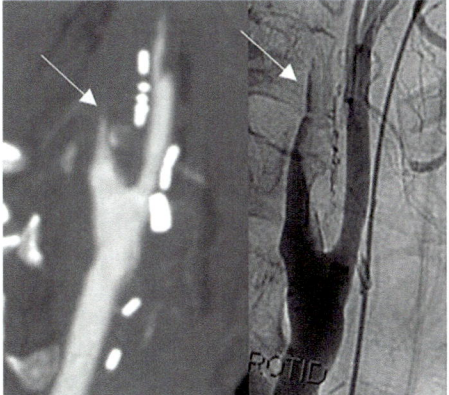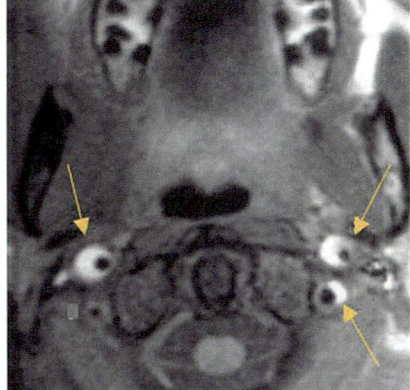

Fig. 20.4 (**a**) CT Angiography and conventional angiography depicting occlusion of ICA due to carotid dissection resulting in "flame sign" (white arrows). (**b**) MR Angiography with T1 fat-sat imaging demonstrating dissection in bilateral internal carotid arteries and left vertebral artery. Hyperintense T1 signal in bilateral internal carotid arteries and left vertebral artery demonstrating acute blood products from intramural hematoma due to arterial dissection (yellow arrows)

Medical Management

Acute thrombolysis with tissue plasminogen activator (tPA has been safely administered after a dissection-related stroke) [41]. Anti-thrombotic treatment of extracranial cervical artery dissection remains debatable, with large randomized clinical trials lacking. However, the treatment is based on preventing artery-to-artery embolism. Most recent AHA guidelines for secondary stroke prevention (2021) recommend treatment with anti-thrombotic therapy for at least 3 months (Class 1; Level C). It is reasonable to use either aspirin or warfarin to prevent recurrent stroke or TIA (Class 2a; Level B) [42]. A 2011 Cochrane review on the use of anti-thrombotic drugs for carotid dissection found no evidence that anticoagulants were better than aspirin for the treatment of extracranial carotid dissection, and a 2012 meta-analysis found no evidence of the superiority of anticoagulants over anti-platelet agents.

The Cervical Artery Dissection in Stroke Study (CADISS) and Aspirin versus Anticoagulation in Cervical Artery Dissection (TREAT-CAD) found no significant difference in stroke recurrence between the two treatments [43, 44]. Factors that would influence the potential benefit of anticoagulation include the presence of intramural thrombus, small infarct size, and absence of systemic bleeding risk factors. In patients with larger infarct size, hemorrhagic transformation, intracranial extension of dissection, or the presence of intracranial aneurysm, antiplatelet therapy may be a better option. Follow-up vascular imaging study in 3–6 months is typically recommended to re-evaluate the dissection and guide long-term anti-thrombotic therapy. The transition from anticoagulation to longer-term antiplatelet therapy can be considered if a persistent dissection flap is seen on follow-up imaging. In general, the prognosis following carotid dissection remains favorable, with an approximate 2% rate of recurrent ischemic stroke or death reported in the CADISS trial, with the highest risk being within the first 2 weeks. Angiographic stenosis improves or resolves in 80–90% of cases, with a complete resolution rate averaging approximately 50–65% in published case series [45].

Endovascular intervention by balloon angioplasty or stenting is considered in patients who have (1) recurrent ischemic symptoms, (2) contraindications to anticoagulation, (3) limited cerebrovascular reserve due to involvement of other vessels, or (4) persistent or expanding dissecting aneurysm [46]. Endovascular treatment can re-establish hemodynamic flow in severely stenotic or completely occluded lumen, and extracranial and intracranial components of dissection can be addressed simultaneously.

Carotid Webs

Carotid webs are a variant of fibromuscular dysplasia that results in the thin, linear membrane that extends into the lumen of the carotid artery due to hyperplasia of the intimal layer [47]. While carotid webs are less common, they are probably underdiagnosed and comprise an important cause of cryptogenic stroke. A retrospective study has demonstrated a prevalence of 2.5% in patients with acute ischemic stroke due to large vessel occlusion, being more common in females [48]. Carotid webs typically present with recurrent TIAs or ischemic stroke are detected on vessel imaging. CT Angiography (CTA) is used most commonly to detect and evaluate carotid webs, typically described as shelf-like, thin, linear, and smooth filling defects along the posterior wall of the internal carotid artery bulb (Fig. 20.5). Contrast-enhanced MR Angiography (MRA) of the neck can also be utilized, but carotid Doppler ultrasound may not be as reliable given the relatively small size of the lesion. Conventional angiography remains the gold standard, where contrast pooling in the venous phase and intraluminal thrombus can be detected.

Carotid webs are highly thrombogenic and cause stasis of blood and platelet activation, resulting in thrombus formation, which may then embolize distally. Medical management typically includes antithrombotic medications. However, there is a lack of data regarding single versus dual antiplatelet agents versus anticoagulation. The presence of an intraluminal thrombus may be a consideration for short-term anticoagulation. Endovascular treatment with stenting is typically considered in patients with recurrent ischemic events. Carotid endarterectomy can also be considered in patients who would not be candidates for endovascular intervention [49].

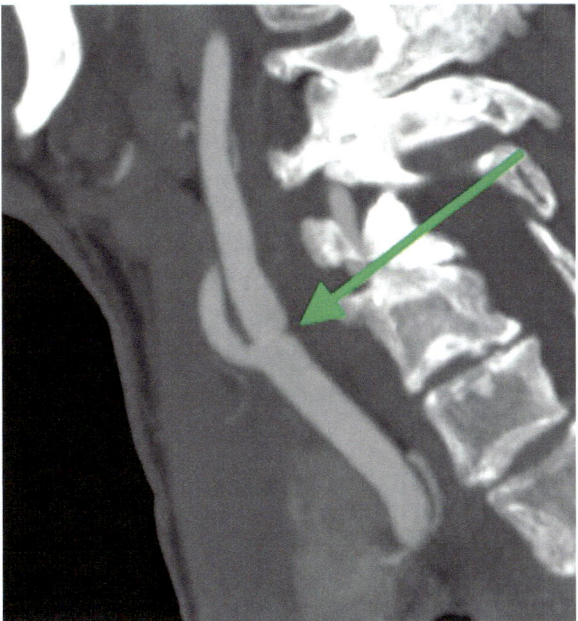

Fig. 20.5 CT Angiography with sagittal view of the Internal Carotid Artery demonstrating a carotid web (green arrow), often seen on the posterior wall of the proximal internal carotid artery

Clinical Vignette 2

HPI: 32-Year-old male with a history significant for cognitive delay and HTN presented to the ED for acute onset dizziness, headache, and gait ataxia, which he noticed when he woke up. He had received a neck and back massage the day prior.

Exam: BP was elevated to 157/113 with normal blood glucose. The exam was notable for right hemi face numbness, upgaze and bidirectional nystagmus, RUE ataxia, and gait imbalance. His strength appeared normal.

Imaging: The patient underwent CT head (bottom left), which was notable for the large hypodense region within the right cerebellum with partial effacement of the fourth ventricle. His CTA head and neck revealed a dissection of the right distal V3 and V4 with probable vessel wall hematoma and occlusion of the R PICA.

MRI brain confirmed the right cerebellar infarct in the distribution of the PICA territory with associated mass effect on the cerebellar vermis with partial effacement of the fourth ventricle. MRA head and neck with asymmetry in the right V2 and V3 segments of the right vertebral artery, as well as asymmetric increased T1 signal in the distal right V3 and proximal V4 segments (bottom right, red arrow). The constellation of findings is most concerning for subacute dissection/intramural hematoma.

Management: The patient was admitted to NICU to monitor for swelling due to his large cerebellar stroke and risk for herniation and hydrocephalus. He was started on aspirin 81 mg daily with a blood pressure goal of <180 SBP (to lower the risk of hemorrhage). Repeat imaging 3 days later was stable without progression of edema. The dissection was felt to be due to neck manipulation and compression of the right vertebral artery at the C1–2 level during contralateral head rotation. Anticoagulation for the dissection was considered but was felt to be high risk given the large stroke and intracranial dissection. He was able to be discharged home on aspirin with home physical therapy with a plan for repeat CT/CTA in 3 months.

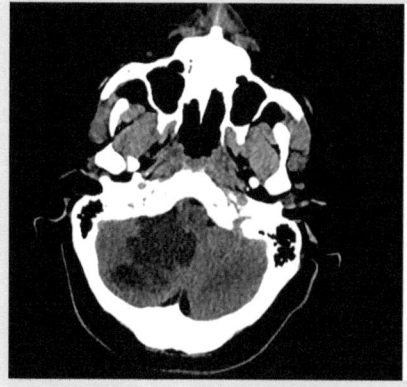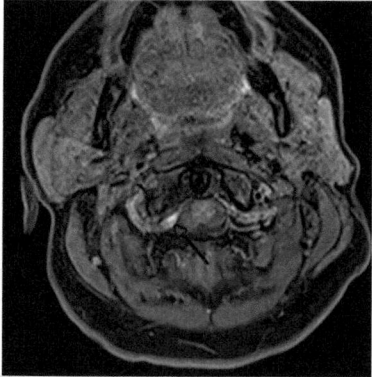

Case contributed by Dr. Melissa Mariscal

Noteworthy Clinical Trials

NASCET (1991, 1998): A two-part randomized trial comparing outcomes in patients with non-disabling recent stroke or TIA and ipsilateral carotid stenosis. Patients were randomized to surgical revascularization by endarterectomy or medical therapy. The first part evaluated severe stenosis and demonstrated that carotid endarterectomy for symptomatic high-grade carotid stenosis (70–99%) significantly reduced the risk of future stroke compared to medical therapy alone. The second part found a more modest risk reduction in patients with symptomatic moderate-grade stenosis (50–69%) compared to medical treatment alone. Patients with stenosis <50% did not benefit from surgery. This trial was conducted in the pre-statin era (NEJM, 1991 and 1998).

ECST (1991): A randomized European trial comparing outcomes in patients with recent non-disabling stroke or TIA with ipsilateral carotid stenosis. Patients were randomized to carotid endarterectomy or medical management alone. Grading stenosis followed a different formula than in NASCET. This study reported that surgical intervention is indicated in patients with non-disabling stroke and carotid stenosis greater than 80%. Similar criticism to NASCET that maximal medical therapy has changed since the trial (Lancet, 1991).

ACAS (1995): Multi-center randomized control trial comparing outcomes in patients with asymptomatic carotid stenosis treated with surgical revascularization versus medical management alone (aspirin). The trial demonstrated a 5-year risk of stroke or death reduction from 11% to 5.1%. There was a benefit of surgery for >60% stenosis in patients if the surgical risk was <3%. Most patients were not on optimum medical therapy. There is mounting evidence that surgical benefit in asymptomatic disease may be minimal compared to modern-day medical management. The ongoing CREST-2 trial compares modern-day medical therapy with revascularization for asymptomatic stenosis >70% (JAMA, 1995).

CADISS (2015): Multi-center, open-label, randomized control trial comparing antiplatelet vs. anticoagulation therapy in patients with extra-cranial carotid and vertebral artery dissection. Patients were given either antiplatelet treatment with ASA, dipyridamole, or clopidogrel alone or in combination with anticoagulation therapy with heparin followed by Coumadin within 7 days of symptom onset. There was no significant difference in ipsilateral stroke or death at 3 months (2% in the anti-platelet arm vs. 1% in the anticoagulation arm), with no significant differences in stroke, major bleeding, or death. Given the rare occurrences of stroke in this population, the authors estimated the study would have needed about 10,000 patients to be genuinely confident about which treatment option was superior. Unfortunately, the study only enrolled 250 patients. Additionally, the diagnosis of dissection could not be confirmed in about one in five patients (Lancet, 2015).

Clinical Pearls

Risk factor optimization with behavioral modifications and intensive medical therapy is critical for large artery atherosclerosis.

Carotid endarterectomy should only be considered for >70% asymptomatic carotid stenosis if surgical risk is <3%.

Detection of asymptomatic stenosis is not an emergency.

Patients with asymptomatic carotid stenosis should be prescribed daily aspirin and statin and screened for other treatable risk factors with appropriate medical therapies and lifestyle changes instituted.

Carotid intervention is warranted for patients with a transient ischemic attack or ischemic stroke within the past 6 months and ipsilateral severe (70–99%) carotid artery stenosis; for those with moderate (50–69%) carotid stenosis, carotid endarterectomy can be considered depending on patient-specific factors, such as age, sex, and comorbidities.

Carotid intervention is not indicated for less than 50% stenosis or complete occlusion.

The optimal timing of symptomatic carotid revascularization is within 2 weeks.

Carotid artery stenting has similar outcomes to CEA but may be higher risk in older patients or those with high bleeding risk since it requires DAPT.

References

1. Flaherty ML, Kissela B, Khoury JC, et al. Carotid artery stenosis as a cause of stroke. Neuroepidemiology. 2013;40(1):36–41. https://doi.org/10.1159/000341410.
2. de Weerd M, Greving JP, Hedblad B, et al. Prevalence of asymptomatic carotid artery stenosis in the general population: an individual participant data meta-analysis. Stroke. 2010;41(6):1294–7. https://doi.org/10.1161/STROKEAHA.110.581058.
3. Fisher CM, Gore I, Okabe N, White PD. Atherosclerosis of the carotid and vertebral arteries—extracranial and intracranial. J Neuropathol Exp Neurol. 1965. https://academic.oup.com/jnen/article-abstract/24/3/455/2612283. Accessed 26 Feb 2023.
4. Libby P, Ridker PM, Maseri A. Inflammation and atherosclerosis. Circulation. 2002;105(9):1135–43. https://doi.org/10.1161/hc0902.104353.
5. Shibata N, Glass CK. Regulation of macrophage function in inflammation and atherosclerosis. J Lipid Res. 2009;50(Suppl):S277–81. https://doi.org/10.1194/jlr.R800063-JLR200.
6. Dollery CM, Libby P. Atherosclerosis and proteinase activation. Cardiovasc Res. 2006;69(3):625–35. https://doi.org/10.1016/j.cardiores.2005.11.003.
7. The natural history of amaurosis fugax. https://pubmed.ncbi.nlm.nih.gov/5723016/. Accessed 26 Feb 2023.
8. Mathiesen EB, Joakimsen O, Bønaa KH. Prevalence of and risk factors associated with carotid artery stenosis: the Tromsø study. Cerebrovasc Dis (Basel, Switzerland). 2001;12(1):44–51. https://doi.org/10.1159/000047680.
9. Heyman A, Wilkinson WE, Heyden S, et al. Risk of stroke in asymptomatic persons with cervical arterial bruits a population study in Evans County, Georgia. N Engl J Med. 1980;302(15):838–41. https://doi.org/10.1056/NEJM198004103021504.

10. McColgan P, Bentley P, McCarron M, Sharma P. Evaluation of the clinical utility of a carotid bruit. QJM. 2012;105(12):1171–7. https://doi.org/10.1093/qjmed/hcs140.
11. King A, Markus HS. Doppler embolic signals in cerebrovascular disease and prediction of stroke risk: a systematic review and meta-analysis. Stroke. 2009;40(12):3711–7. https://doi.org/10.1161/STROKEAHA.109.563056.
12. North American Symptomatic Carotid Endarterectomy Trial. Methods, patient characteristics, and progress. Stroke. 1991;22(6):711–20. https://doi.org/10.1161/01.str.22.6.711.
13. Moore WS, Hall AD. Importance of emboli from the carotid bifurcation in the pathogenesis of cerebral ischemic attacks. Arch Surg (Chicago, IL: 1960). 1970;101(6):708–711 passim. https://doi.org/10.1001/archsurg.1970.01340300064012.
14. Rothwell PM, Eliasziw M, Gutnikov SA, Warlow CP, Barnett HJM, Carotid Endarterectomy Trialists Collaboration. Endarterectomy for symptomatic carotid stenosis in relation to clinical subgroups and timing of surgery. Lancet (London, England). 2004;363(9413):915–24. https://doi.org/10.1016/S0140-6736(04)15785-1.
15. Hosseini AA, Kandiyil N, Macsweeney STS, Altaf N, Auer DP. Carotid plaque hemorrhage on magnetic resonance imaging strongly predicts recurrent ischemia and stroke. Ann Neurol. 2013;73(6):774–84. https://doi.org/10.1002/ana.23876.
16. Takaya N, Yuan C, Chu B, et al. Association between carotid plaque characteristics and subsequent ischemic cerebrovascular events: a prospective assessment with MRI-initial results. Stroke. 2006;37(3):818–23. https://doi.org/10.1161/01.STR.0000204638.91099.91.
17. Taylor DW, Barnett HJ, Haynes RB, et al. Low-dose and high-dose acetylsalicylic acid for patients undergoing carotid endarterectomy: a randomised controlled trial. ASA and Carotid Endarterectomy (ACE) Trial Collaborators. Lancet (London, England). 1999;353(9171):2179–84. https://doi.org/10.1016/s0140-6736(99)05388-x.
18. Kalra K, Franzese CJ, Gesheff MG, et al. Pharmacology of antiplatelet agents. Curr Atheroscler Rep. 2013;15(12):371. https://doi.org/10.1007/s11883-013-0371-3.
19. CAPRIE Steering Committee. A randomised, blinded, trial of clopidogrel versus aspirin in patients at risk of ischaemic events (CAPRIE). CAPRIE Steering Committee. Lancet. 1996;348(9038):1329–39. https://doi.org/10.1016/s0140-6736(96)09457-3.
20. Randomised trial of endarterectomy for recently symptomatic carotid stenosis: final results of the MRC European Carotid Surgery Trial (ECST). Lancet. 1998;351(9113):1379–87. https://doi.org/10.1016/S0140-6736(97)09292-1.
21. Mayberg MR, Wilson SE, Yatsu F, et al. Carotid endarterectomy and prevention of cerebral ischemia in symptomatic carotid stenosis. Veterans Affairs Cooperative Studies Program 309 Trialist Group. JAMA. 1991;266(23):3289–94.
22. Biller J, Feinberg WM, Castaldo JE, et al. Guidelines for carotid endarterectomy. Circulation. 1998. https://www.ahajournals.org/doi/10.1161/01.CIR.97.5.501. Accessed 26 Feb 2023.
23. Stoneham MD, Thompson JP. Arterial pressure management and carotid endarterectomy. Br J Anaesth. 2009. https://academic.oup.com/bja/article/102/4/442/230836. Accessed 26 Feb 2023.
24. Davis SM, Donnan GA. Carotid-artery stenting in stroke prevention. N Engl J Med. 2010;363(1):80–2. https://doi.org/10.1056/NEJMe1005220.
25. Bassetti C, Carruzzo A, Sturzenegger M, Tuncdogan E. Recurrence of cervical artery dissection. A prospective study of 81 patients. Stroke. 1996;27(10):1804–7. https://doi.org/10.1161/01.str.27.10.1804.
26. Caplan LR, Baquis GD, Pessin MS, et al. Dissection of the intracranial vertebral artery. Neurology. 1988;38(6):868–77. https://doi.org/10.1212/wnl.38.6.868.
27. Mokri B, Sundt TM, Houser OW, Piepgras DG. Spontaneous dissection of the cervical internal carotid artery. Ann Neurol. 1986;19(2):126–38. https://doi.org/10.1002/ana.410190204.
28. Norris JW, Beletsky V, Nadareishvili ZG. Sudden neck movement and cervical artery dissection. The Canadian Stroke Consortium. CMAJ Can Med Assoc J. 2000;163(1):38–40.
29. Beatty RA. Dissecting hematoma of the internal carotid artery following chiropractic cervical manipulation. J Trauma. 1977;17(3):248–9. https://doi.org/10.1097/00005373-197703000-00014.

30. Brandt T, Morcher M, Hausser I. Association of cervical artery dissection with connective tissue abnormalities in skin and arteries. Front Neurol Neurosci. 2005;20:16–29. https://doi.org/10.1159/000088131.

31. North KN, Whiteman DA, Pepin MG, Byers PH. Cerebrovascular complications in Ehlers-Danlos syndrome type IV. Ann Neurol. 1995;38(6):960–4. https://doi.org/10.1002/ana.410380620.

32. Schievink WI, Prakash UB, Piepgras DG, Mokri B. Alpha 1-antitrypsin deficiency in intracranial aneurysms and cervical artery dissection. Lancet (London, England). 1994;343(8895):452–3. https://doi.org/10.1016/s0140-6736(94)92693-x.

33. Yuasa H, Tokito S, Izumi K, Hirabayashi K. Cerebrovascular moyamoya disease associated with an intracranial pseudoaneurysm. Case report. J Neurosurg. 1982;56(1):131–4. https://doi.org/10.3171/jns.1982.56.1.0131.

34. Schievink WI, Mokri B, Piepgras DG. Spontaneous dissections of cervicocephalic arteries in childhood and adolescence. Neurology. 1994;44(9):1607–12. https://doi.org/10.1212/wnl.44.9.1607.

35. Biousse V, D'Anglejan-Chatillon J, Massiou H, Bousser MG. Head pain in non-traumatic carotid artery dissection: a series of 65 patients. Cephalalgia. 1994;14(1):33–6. https://doi.org/10.1046/j.1468-2982.1994.1401033.x.

36. Guidetti D, Pisanello A, Giovanardi F, Morandi C, Zuccoli G, Troiso A. Spontaneous carotid dissection presenting lower cranial nerve palsies. J Neurol Sci. 2001;184(2):203–7. https://doi.org/10.1016/s0022-510x(01)00440-3.

37. Sturzenegger M. Spontaneous internal carotid artery dissection: early diagnosis and management in 44 patients. J Neurol. 1995;242(4):231–8. https://doi.org/10.1007/BF00919596.

38. Baumgartner RW, Arnold M, Baumgartner I, et al. Carotid dissection with and without ischemic events: local symptoms and cerebral artery findings. Neurology. 2001;57(5):827–32. https://doi.org/10.1212/wnl.57.5.827.

39. Kasner SE, Hankins LL, Bratina P, Morgenstern LB. Magnetic resonance angiography demonstrates vascular healing of carotid and vertebral artery dissections. Stroke. 1997;28(10):1993–7. https://doi.org/10.1161/01.str.28.10.1993.

40. Sturzenegger M, Mattle HP, Rivoir A, Baumgartner RW. Ultrasound findings in carotid artery dissection: analysis of 43 patients. Neurology. 1995;45(4):691–8. https://doi.org/10.1212/wnl.45.4.691.

41. Derex L, Nighoghossian N, Turjman F, et al. Intravenous tPA in acute ischemic stroke related to internal carotid artery dissection. Neurology. 2000;54(11):2159–61. https://doi.org/10.1212/wnl.54.11.2159.

42. Kleindorfer DO, Towfighi A, Chaturvedi S, et al. 2021 Guideline for the prevention of stroke in patients with stroke and transient ischemic attack: a guideline from the American Heart Association/American Stroke Association. Stroke. 2021. https://www.ahajournals.org/doi/10.1161/STR.0000000000000375. Accessed 26 Feb 2023.

43. Markus HS, Levi C, King A, et al. Antiplatelet therapy vs anticoagulation therapy in cervical artery dissection: the cervical artery dissection in stroke study (CADISS) randomized clinical trial final results. JAMA Neurol. 2019. https://jamanetwork.com/journals/jamaneurology/fullarticle/2725385. Accessed 26 Feb 2023.

44. Engelter ST, Traenka C, Gensicke H, et al. Aspirin versus anticoagulation in cervical artery dissection (TREAT-CAD): an open-label, randomised, non-inferiority trial. Lancet Neurol. 2021. https://www.thelancet.com/journals/laneur/article/PIIS1474-4422(21)00044-2/fulltext. Accessed 26 Feb 2023.

45. Engelter ST, Lyrer PA, Kirsch EC, Steck AJ. Long-term follow-up after extracranial internal carotid artery dissection. Eur Neurol. 2000;44(4):199–204. https://doi.org/10.1159/000008236.

46. Gomez CR, May AK, Terry JB, Tulyapronchote R. Endovascular therapy of traumatic injuries of the extracranial cerebral arteries. Crit Care Clin. 1999;15(4):789–809. https://doi.org/10.1016/s0749-0704(05)70088-9.

47. Choi PMC, Singh D, Trivedi A, et al. Carotid webs and recurrent ischemic strokes in the era of CT angiography. AJNR Am J Neuroradiol. 2015;36(11):2134–9. https://doi.org/10.3174/ajnr.A4431.
48. Compagne KCJ, van Es ACGM, Berkhemer OA, et al. Prevalence of carotid web in patients with acute intracranial stroke due to intracranial large vessel occlusion. Radiology. 2018;286:1000. Published online 16 Oct 2017. https://doi.org/10.1148/radiol.2017170094.
49. Zhang AJ, Dhruv P, Choi P, et al. A systematic literature review of patients with carotid web and acute ischemic stroke. Stroke. 2018. https://www.ahajournals.org/doi/10.1161/STROKEAHA.118.021907. Accessed 26 Feb 2023.

Cardioembolic Stroke

21

Jennifer Picagli, Yee Kuang Cheng, and Richa Sharma

Definition of Cardioembolic Stroke

An embolism is a small fragment or collection (blood clot, plaque, fat, air, amniotic fluid) that travels from one place in the body to another. The term embolism does not identify the source, which can be a clot in the heart, a DVT, plaque rupture, broken bone, injected air, or entry of amniotic fluid into the maternal bloodstream during childbirth. An embolic stroke implies that something from outside the brain traveled into the brain and occluded a blood vessel. Due to their size, emboli often lodge into the larger intracranial vessels, like the MCA, ACA, and basilar arteries. Clinical features pointing to an embolic stroke include sudden onset and maximal deficits at onset, aphasia, gaze deviation or neglect (i.e., cortical symptoms), or performing a Valsalva maneuver (straining, for example) at the time of stroke onset. Large or multifocal strokes on imaging, especially in different vascular distributions, should raise suspicion for an embolic stroke.

J. Picagli
Yale New Haven Hospital, New Haven, CT, USA
e-mail: Jennifer.picagli@yale.edu

Y. K. Cheng
St. Luke's Medical Center, Boise, ID, USA
e-mail: chengye@slhs.org

R. Sharma (✉)
Neurology, Yale School of Medicine, New Haven, CT, USA
e-mail: richa.sharma@yale.edu

H. P. Amin (ed.), *Stroke for the Advanced Practice Clinician*,
https://doi.org/10.1007/978-3-031-66289-8_21

Cardioembolic stroke implies that an embolism is suspected to have originated in the heart. Cardioembolism accounts for approximately 20–30% of all ischemic strokes and can result from various etiologies originating from the heart. Non-valvular atrial fibrillation accounts for 50% of these cases, followed by myocardial infarction, left ventricular thrombus, valvular heart disease, patent foramen ovale (PFO), or cardiac tumors.

Epidemiology

Similar to heart disease, the risk of cardioembolic stroke increases with age. One reason may be that older individuals are more likely to develop atrial fibrillation [1]. The ATRIA study estimated the overall prevalence of AF in the United States is about 1%, but in people >80 years old, prevalence increased to 10% [2]. The US Census Bureau projects that the percentage of the US population >85 years old will double between 2020 and 2050. Accordingly, the ATRIA study estimated that the overall prevalence of AF in the United States will increase from 2.3 million people in 2001 to 5.6 million by 2050 [3]! The risk of stroke among those with atrial fibrillation can be up to 12.2% per year per the CHADS-VASC2 scoring system (see below).

Sources of Cardioembolic Stroke

The Trial of Org 10172 in Acute Stroke Treatment, or TOAST classification system, devised in 1993, provides specific criteria for determining the causative mechanism of stroke [4]. Table 21.1 outlines the pathologies or anatomic abnormalities implicated in cardioembolism.

Table 21.1 TOAST classification of high- and medium-risk sources of cardioembolism [4]

High-risk sources	Medium-risk sources
1. Mechanical prosthetic valve	1. Mitral valve prolapse
2. Mitral stenosis with atrial fibrillation	2. Mitral annulus calcification
3. Atrial fibrillation	3. Mitral stenosis without atrial fibrillation
4. Left atrial/atrial appendage thrombus	4. Left atrial turbulence (smoke)
5. Sick sinus syndrome	5. Atrial septal aneurysm
6. Recent MI (<4 weeks)	6. Patent foramen ovale (PFO)
7. Left ventricular thrombus	7. Atrial flutter
8. Dilated cardiomyopathy	8. Lone atrial fibrillation
9. Akinetic left ventricular segment	9. Bioprosthetic cardiac valve
10. Atrial myxoma	10. Marantic endocarditis
11. Infective endocarditis	11. Congestive heart failure
	12. Hypokinetic left ventricular segment
	13. Myocardial infarction (>4 weeks, <6 months)

Severity of Cardioembolic Stroke

Cardioembolic strokes have a worse prognosis than other mechanisms. In the Framingham Study, patients with cardioembolic strokes experienced more severe symptoms and a higher mortality rate than patients with ischemic stroke from other causes [5]. The worse prognosis is not surprising when one considers that in addition to motor deficits, cardioembolic strokes can also include language, visual, and cognitive impairment. Cardiac embolism can also cause transient ischemic attack (TIA). Consider this if a patient presents with cortical symptoms like acute transient aphasia and normal appearing vessels.

Diagnostic Investigation

Patients with cardioembolic stroke may have abnormal heart structure, function, or heart rhythm discovered on focused testing. Embolic strokes with normal-appearing blood vessels in the territory of the stroke also suggest a cardioembolic process.

MRI Patterns of Infarcts

Cardioembolic infarcts can occur in various regions of the brain and are often cortical. Cortical strokes occur in the large lobes, and subcortical strokes involve the deeper structures. An MRI brain can demonstrate one or more wedge-shaped areas of ischemia involving multiple vascular territories and scattered infarcts.

Evaluation for Heart Structure/Function

Investigation of heart structure function typically begins with a transthoracic echocardiogram (TTE) with a bubble study. Left atrial dilation or low left ventricular ejection fraction on TTE is strongly associated with underlying atrial fibrillation (but do not automatically warrant anticoagulation) [6]. If TTE is unremarkable, but suspicion for intracardiac thrombus or valvular vegetation remains, it is reasonable to consider a transesophageal echocardiogram (TEE) or cardiac MRI, which are more sensitive ways to view the heart and valve structure. A comparison of the characteristics of TTE and TEE for identifying sources of stroke is provided in Table 21.2. A cardiac ischemic workup with cardiology consultation should be considered for recent myocardial infarction, newly reduced ejection fraction, or akinetic segment on TTE.

Table 21.2 TTE vs TEE (adapted from Carmen et al. 2020 [7])

	TTE	TEE
Advantages	• Readily available • Cheap • Non-invasive	• Excellent spatial and temporal resolution
Disadvantages	• Operator-dependent • Limited by patient characteristics (e.g., obesity, lung disease)	• Operator-dependent • Semi-invasive • Usually requires sedation
Cardiomyopathy	++	+
LV thrombus	++	+
PFO	++	+++[a]
Valvular disease, vegetation/thrombus	++	+++[a]
Cardiac tumors	+	++
LA/LAA thrombus	+	+++[a]
Aortic atheroma	−	++

CT computed tomography, *LA* left atrium, *LAA* left atrial appendage, *LV* left ventricle, *MRI* magnetic resonance imaging, *PFO* patent foramen ovale, *TEE* transesophageal echocardiography, *TTE* transthoracic echocardiography
[a] Diagnostic gold standard

Evaluation for Abnormal Heart Rhythm

Atrial fibrillation and atrial flutter are two of the most common arrhythmias associated with stroke. Symptoms include palpitations, dizziness, fatigue, shortness of breath, and chest pain, but most patients with AF are asymptomatic until they experience a stroke or TIA. AF is often described as paroxysmal (episodic), persistent (lasting >7 days at a time), or permanent, but for purposes of secondary stroke prevention, the subtype does not matter; all patients with stroke and AF require anticoagulation. Without a diagnosis of AF, however, anticoagulation should not be started.

Multiple ways exist to monitor for atrial fibrillation in patients with suspected cardioembolic stroke [8]. While the yield is often low, all stroke patients should have telemetry monitoring in the hospital. This is followed by outpatient monitoring with a 30-day external or long-term implantable loop recorder (ILR). Wearable devices like smartwatches have touted the ability to detect arrhythmias, though the technology is new, and evidence for wearables is still limited [9].

What is the optimal duration of cardiac monitoring? Anything less than 30 days is considered sub-optimal by modern-day standards, so many patients will receive a 30-day monitor. An ILR may be appropriate for patients with cognitive impairments who are unlikely to wear an external monitor for an entire month, concerning structural TTE findings, recurrent stroke, or if the initial 30-day monitor was negative but concern for AF remains. The CRYSTAL AF study compared AF detection rates in stroke patients with normal 24-h monitoring who were randomized to ILR placement vs. EKGs at the discretion of their doctors (control group) [10]. At the 1-year point, AF was detected in 12% of the ILR group vs. only 2% in the control group, and at 3 years, detection rates were 36% versus 3%, respectively. Higher detection rates led to significantly more patients starting oral anticoagulation in the ILR group. While many stroke clinics and all general cardiology offices should be able to arrange external 30-day monitoring, ILR placement requires referral to an electrophysiologist. The decision about monitoring modalities hinges on patient-provider discussions, considering efficacy and patient preference. Some centers start with an external 30-day monitor and then proceed with ILR; others prefer ILR placement from the outset.

Risk Assessment for Atrial Fibrillation

To stratify the risk of stroke with AF, the CHADS(2) score was published in 2001, and the CHA2DS2-VASc score in 2010 [11]. These scores were developed with data from primarily European cohorts to estimate the risk of future stroke or thromboembolism without anticoagulation attributable to AF. CHADS2 noted increased risks for patients with congestive heart failure, hypertension, age >75, diabetes, and prior stroke or TIA. CHA2DS2-VASc included more "moderate" risk factors, including a slightly lower age group, female gender, and history of other vascular diseases such as prior myocardial infarction, peripheral arterial disease, or known aortic plaque (Table 21.3). The components of the CHA2DS2-VASc score are presented in Table 21.3. Higher scores suggest a higher risk of future stroke in untreated atrial fibrillation. The annual risk of stroke associated with a particular CHA2DS2-VASc score can inform discussions between provider and patient as they weigh the risks and benefits of treatment.

If a patient has a stroke with a history of AF, calculating the CHA2DS2-VASc may be a moot point since they automatically qualify for anticoagulation. A truly "low-risk" patient who does not require anticoagulation is a male with a score of 0 or a female with a score of 1 (by default since female sex gives one point). For patients without a history of stroke, consider anticoagulation if they have ≥1 additional risk factor.

Table 21.3 CHA2DS2-VASc score in calculating the risk of stroke or systemic thromboembolism without anticoagulation (adapted from Lip et al. 2010 [11])

Risk factor	Score
Congestive heart failure/LV dysfunction	1
Hypertension	1
Age ≥75 years	2
Diabetes mellitus	1
Stroke/TIA/TE	2
Vascular disease (prior myocardial infarction, peripheral artery disease, or aortic plaque)	1
Age 65–74 years	1
Sex **c**ategory (female gender)	1

LV left ventricular, *TE* thromboembolism. Give points if patients meet each individual criteria.

Anticoagulation Options

Warfarin, the primary vitamin K antagonist (VKA) in the United States, is an established drug with generic formulations available. Warfarin must be monitored via the international normalized ratio (INR) blood test to ensure therapeutic effect. Frequent blood draws, therefore, are necessary for patients, especially during the initiation period, which adds cost, transportation time, and discomfort. Frequent dose adjustments to maintain INR and interactions with food and other medications are common. The newer direct-acting oral anticoagulants (DOACs) have the benefit of not requiring serum monitoring, rarely needing dose adjustment, and have demonstrated superior efficacy and safety profile compared to Warfarin [12]. However, these newer drugs can be costly for many patients, even with insurance coverage. The most common DOACs are apixaban (Eliquis), dabigatran (Pradaxa), and rivaroxaban (Xarelto). Additionally, DOACs are only FDA-approved for non-valvular AF (patients without mechanical valves), whereas Warfarin is approved for both valvular and non-valvular AF.

When counseling patients on DOACs, it is important to stress a few key points. Compared to Warfarin, DOACs have a much shorter life span in the body. Generally, if the patient misses 2 days of their DOAC, the drug is out of their system, and their stroke risk shoots back up. It is therefore critical to ensure no gaps in refills, enough pills while traveling, and minimize time off medication for any procedures. The peri-procedural management of DOACs is covered in another chapter. While the lack of lab monitoring is seen as a "plus," it makes it difficult for clinicians to confirm adherence. Therefore, patients with a history of medication non-adherence might not be suitable candidates for these medications. Discussing co-pays might also identify patients at risk of non-adherence since patients may try to stretch out prescriptions if co-pays are high. A real-world clinical conundrum occurs when patients prescribed a DOAC come to the emergency room with stroke symptoms. Suppose the patient is aphasic, and the stroke team cannot confirm whether they took their DOAC within the past 48 h. In that case, the patient is not eligible for thrombolytics even if they present within the time window. There is currently no standardized test that can be done quickly to confirm whether a patient has recently taken a DOAC or not.

Anticoagulation After Stroke

All patients with AF and ischemic stroke need to start anticoagulation. However, starting a potent blood thinner too soon after an ischemic stroke can risk hemorrhage into the injured stroke area (called hemorrhagic transformation). Given the competing risks of recurrent thromboembolism and hemorrhagic transformation, determining when to start oral anticoagulation after ischemic stroke is a major decision point for clinicians and patients and is best left to stroke specialists. Current AHA/ASA guidelines recommend 4–14 days post-infarct for initiating or resuming anticoagulation (following a stability CT scan). However, a further delay may be indicated in cases of spontaneous hemorrhagic transformation. TIA patients with untreated AF might be able to start treatment immediately since there is no stroke to develop hemorrhagic conversion!

Patients with intracranial hemorrhage from trauma can likely resume anticoagulation after 1–2 months after follow-up imaging and neurosurgery clearance. Patients with hemorrhages clearly due to uncontrolled hypertension (basal ganglia) and not due to anticoagulation can also be restarted after 1–2 months after clearance from a stroke specialist. Unprovoked hemorrhages (either due to possible cerebral amyloid angiopathy or no other reason besides anticoagulation) are a separate, higher risk group and are best managed by a stroke specialist.

Assessing the Risk of Bleeding

Anticoagulants, in general, are safe with a low risk of bleeding if taken correctly. Certain patients, however, have higher bleeding risks. The HAS-BLED score incorporates features of medical history that might increase the risk of bleeding with Warfarin, such as uncontrolled hypertension, advanced kidney or liver disease, abnormal coagulation tests, advanced age, alcohol abuse, or prior bleeding history. The score translates to a 1-year percent risk of major bleeding while on Warfarin. *The score itself should not be the only determining factor in deciding the appropriateness of anticoagulation; rather, it should be a data point in the overall conversation in a medically complex patient. The risk of bleeding with the highest score is still lower than that of ischemic stroke without anticoagulation.* A high score may warrant considering DOACs as they have lower bleeding risks than coumadin.

Age, risk of bleeding, risk of falls, comorbidities including alcohol use, cognitive impairment, and other reasons for non-compliance are cited by physicians as the rationale for not prescribing anticoagulation for patients with atrial fibrillation. While some reasons (prior spontaneous ICH, thrombocytopenia) may be justified, many other potential "risks" require a more thoughtful approach. The "fall risk" designation is a particularly overused and misguided reason to avoid anticoagulation. Many studies have shown that the benefit of anticoagulation far outweighs bleeding risks in patients who occasionally fall, and one study reported that to justify withholding anticoagulation, a patient must fall more than 250 times a year. In reality, the average number of falls is less than 2 per year in the elderly population; thus, there is a distortion in the perception of bleeding risk with falls while on anticoagulation. Reflexively stopping anticoagulation for a patient who presents with a fall only increases their risk of future stroke and death and does nothing to treat the actual reason for falling. A more thoughtful approach would be to investigate and address the reason for falling to prevent future injury *while continuing anticoagulation*. Some reasons include orthostasis, neuropathy, arthritis, poor vision, progressive neurodegenerative conditions, or even abuse. Patients might require medication adjustment, a prescription for a cane or walker, a proper vision exam, a neurology or physical therapy referral, or a social work and home safety evaluation.

High Bleeding Risk Patients

The left atrial appendage is a small extension of the left atrium, shaped like a wind-sock, and is the location of about 80–90% of clots in patients with AF. For AF patients with a valid contraindication to anticoagulation, surgically occluding the left atrial appendage can remove the need for long-term anticoagulation. Two large studies (PROTECT AF and PREVAIL) have demonstrated non-inferiority (in other words, just as effective) of left atrial appendage closure using "the Watchman'" device compared to warfarin therapy in stroke risk reduction. Patients need a short course of post-closure anticoagulation to prevent thrombosis around the device, fol-lowed by dual antiplatelet therapy and, ultimately, single antiplatelet treatment going forward [13]. This procedure requires a referral to electrophysiology.

Left Ventricular Thrombus

Anticoagulation is recommended if a thrombus is detected in the left ventricle (LV) by TTE, TEE, cardiac MRI, or cardiac CTA. The 2021 AHA/ASA guidelines rec-ommend that in patients with stroke or TIA and an LV thrombus, anticoagulation with Warfarin for at least 3 months is warranted to reduce the risk of recurrent stroke [14]. The guidelines also state that the safety of anticoagulation using a direct oral anticoagulant to reduce recurrent stroke risk is uncertain, so the current recommen-dation is Warfarin with an INR goal of 2–3 [15]. Guidelines might change in the future as new data emerge for DOACs.

Endocarditis

Endocarditis is a collection of material on a heart valve, such as bacteria due to a bloodstream infection (called bacterial or infective endocarditis) or a thrombus in the setting of cancer or autoimmune disease (called Libman-Sacks, sterile or maran-tic endocarditis). Approximately 1.7% of all strokes are associated with endocardi-tis, but it is seen more in younger patients [16]. Bacterial endocarditis is associated with both ischemic and hemorrhagic stroke through various mechanisms. Transthoracic echocardiogram is moderately sensitive for valvular endocarditis, but TEE is the gold standard to view valve disease.

It is crucial, and often challenging, to distinguish infectious endocarditis (IE) from non-infectious endocarditis as the workup and treatment are vastly different. IE occurs when bacteria or fungus enter the bloodstream, leading to a systemic infection (bacteremia or fungemia), ultimately infecting the heart valves and form-ing clumps or vegetations. These vegetations then embolize (septic emboli) through-out the body (including the brain) to occlude a downstream vessel. Septic emboli can go anywhere in the body, not just the brain. Bacteria can also weaken the blood

Fig. 21.1 Sagittal view of the diagnostic angiogram demonstrates the right M4 segment mycotic aneurysm (yellow arrow). Notice the distal location along a branch, not at a bifurcation like a traditional intracranial aneurysm

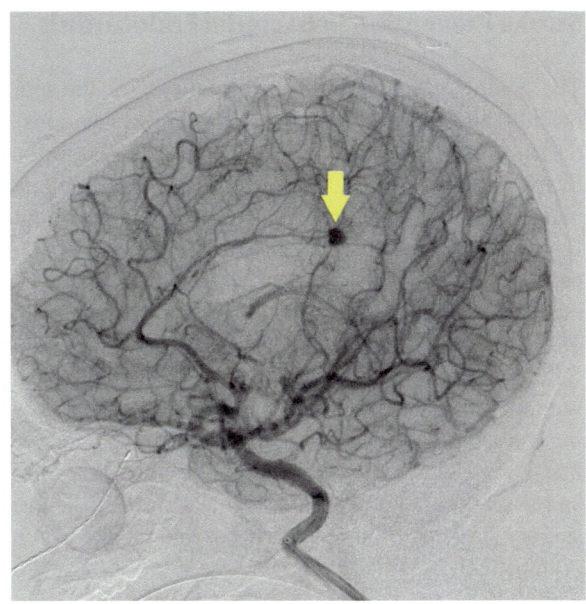

vessel walls, leading to mycotic (infectious) aneurysms and subarachnoid or intra-parenchymal hemorrhage. Mycotic aneurysms are best seen on formal angiography but may also be detected on a high-quality CTA or MRA. All patients with endocarditis and stroke require at least a CTA or MRA to evaluate for mycotic aneurysms; some might require an invasive formal angiogram (Fig. 21.1). If one or more aneurysms are detected, neurosurgery consultation is needed to determine if they must be treated as they pose a significant risk of intracerebral hemorrhage.

Sources of infection include dental abscess, skin puncture from intravenous drug use, skin wounds, infected central access lines or hardware, and rarely GI malignancy. A patient presenting with neurologic change, fever, and clinical signs suggestive of infection with a history of recent surgery, known intravenous drug use, or dental procedure or infection should have blood cultures drawn before empiric antibiotic coverage. Treatment for IE is at least 6 weeks of IV antibiotics or antifungal therapy.

In non-infectious endocarditis, thrombus formation occurs on the valve or cardiac hardware due to the deposition of platelets, fibrin, and related blood components. Since these emboli are not infectious, they do not cause mycotic aneurysms or pose a high risk of hemorrhage. Treatment in this case is anticoagulation, and the workup should include screening for cancer and autoimmune or hematological conditions. Thrombus on a mechanical valve is likely due to subtherapeutic anticoagulation. Blood cultures should still be drawn and should be negative, and both Infectious Disease and Cardiology consultants should agree that the process is not infectious.

Stroke Prevention in Bacterial Endocarditis

The goal of treating valvular vegetations (or thrombi) is to prevent emboli from reaching the brain. In addition to forming vegetations, IE can penetrate heart valve tissue, leading to regurgitation, perforation, or ultimately rupture. Antimicrobial therapy is the mainstay of infectious endocarditis treatment, but nearly half of all patients require valve surgery. The usual course of antibiotic therapy is 2–6 weeks for most bacterial infections, with surgery indicated in "complicated IE." These cases include patients with injury to the valve or valve root (often presenting with heart failure or severe regurgitation), conduction abnormalities, or those with large or antimicrobial-resistant vegetations leading to recurrent embolization. The need for surgery is typically categorized as emergent (unstable patient, surgery usually within 24 h or the patient is unlikely to survive), urgent (surgery should occur during the same hospitalization with some time to address other active medical issues first), and elective (a period soon after a course of antibiotic therapy, if warranted and the risk is low) [17]. Despite these broad categories, optimal timing for valve surgery has not been standardized and requires multidisciplinary discussion for each patient.

Alteplase, tenecteplase, and other forms of anticoagulation are contraindicated in infective endocarditis due to the risk of intracerebral hemorrhage. One exception might be a patient with a mechanical valve awaiting replacement surgery; however, that is a very high-risk situation requiring a heparin drip that should be closely monitored in an ICU level of care. Thrombectomy remains an option for patients with acute stroke symptoms due to large vessel occlusion from a septic embolism.

Stroke specialists are often asked to comment on the risk of hemorrhage when a patient with endocarditis and a recent stroke requires valve surgery. Valve surgery typically requires intraoperative heparin, which raises the risk of hemorrhage. If the patient has a valve rupture and will die without emergent surgery, then there is no point in discussing bleeding risk. Post-op CT scans and neurological assessment [16]. In reality, most cases are less clear-cut and fall into the "urgent" or closer to the "elective" category. Some factors that increase the risk of bleeding include the size of the stroke, the presence of acute blood, mycotic aneurysms, and positive blood cultures. These are complex cases without straightforward algorithms. A generally accepted principle is that waiting several weeks for surgery significantly lowers the risk of bleeding. With the help of cardiology and cardiothoracic surgery to determine the urgency of valve surgery, stroke specialists can estimate the risk of perioperative hemorrhage.

Treatment for Severely Reduced Ejection Fraction

Severely reduced left ventricular ejection fraction (EF), even without a left ventricular thrombus, is an established risk factor for ischemic stroke, but its optimal treatment is uncertain [18]. Multiple trials, including WARCEF, WATCH, and HELAS, demonstrated no benefit of Warfarin compared to Aspirin with respect to a recurrent stroke or death among patients with reduced ejection fraction and sinus rhythm. However, there was a heightened risk of hemorrhage [19, 20]. In the COMMANDER-HF trial, anticoagulation with low-dose rivaroxaban versus placebo did not result in any net benefit [21]. Current guidelines state that the effectiveness of anticoagulation compared with antiplatelet therapy is uncertain, but antiplatelet therapy is reasonable unless there is an indication for anticoagulation.

Mechanical and Bioprosthetic Valves

There are two types of heart valve replacements: mechanical and bioprosthetic valves. Mechanical valves are artificial valves made from metallic alloys or plastic materials. Bioprosthetic valves are constructed from porcine heart valves or bovine pericardium [22]. Both mechanical and bioprosthetic valve replacements are associated with thrombus formation [23]. The risk of thromboembolism is higher in the mechanical valve population, and mechanical mitral valves are at higher risk than aortic. Patients with mechanical valves require long-term anticoagulation (AC) with Warfarin. DOACs have not been adequately studied in this context.

Patients with bioprosthetic valves do not require long-term anticoagulation; however, short-term anticoagulation for 3–6 months is recommended to reduce the risk of bioprosthetic valve thrombosis, followed by long-term antiplatelet therapy.

INR Goals for Mechanical Valves and Bioprosthetic Valves

- **Mechanical aortic valve:** Target INR 2.5 (range 2.0–3.0)
- **Mechanical mitral valve:** Target INR 3.0 (range 2.5–3.5)
- **Bioprosthetic valve (first 3–6 months):** Target INR 2.5 (range 2.0–3.0)

Clinical Pearls

- Cardioembolic strokes are larger, wedge-shaped, and/or multifocal in different vascular territories
- Atrial fibrillation accounts for about half of all cardioembolic strokes
- Evidence does not support empirically starting anticoagulation embolic stroke of undetermined source (ESUS)
- Thirty days is considered to be the minimum duration for cardiac monitoring. Monitoring is indicated for all embolic appearing strokes and TIAs with normal vessel imaging.
- ILRs may be preferred over external loop recorders in some cases
- Anticoagulation is contraindicated for bacterial endocarditis

---

References

1. Kornej J, Börschel CS, Benjamin EJ, Schnabel RB. Epidemiology of atrial fibrillation in the 21st century. Circ Res. 2020;127(1):4–20.
2. Go AS, Hylek EM, Phillips KA, Chang Y, Henault LE, Selby JV, Singer DE. Prevalence of diagnosed atrial fibrillation in adults: national implications for rhythm management and stroke prevention: the AnTicoagulation and Risk Factors in Atrial Fibrillation (ATRIA) Study. JAMA. 2001;285(18):2370–5. https://doi.org/10.1001/jama.285.18.2370.
3. https://www.census.gov/data/tables/2017/demo/popproj/2017-summary-tables.html.
4. Adams HP Jr, Bendixen BH, Kappelle LJ, Biller J, Love BB, Gordon DL, Marsh EE 3rd. Classification of subtype of acute ischemic stroke. Definitions for use in a multicenter clinical trial. TOAST. Trial of Org 10172 in Acute Stroke Treatment. Stroke. 1993;24(1):35–41. https://doi.org/10.1161/01.str.24.1.35.
5. Lin HJ, Wolf PA, Kelly-Hayes M, Beiser AS, Kase CS, Benjamin EJ, D'Agostino RB. Stroke severity in atrial fibrillation. The Framingham Study. Stroke. 1996;27:1760–4.
6. Seko Y, Kato T, Haruna T, Izumi T, Miyamoto S, Nakane E, Inoko M. Association between atrial fibrillation, atrial enlargement, and left ventricular geometric remodeling. Sci Rep. 2018;8(1):6366. https://doi.org/10.1038/s41598-018-24875-1.
7. Camen S, Haeusler KG, Schnabel RB. Cardiac imaging after ischemic stroke or transient ischemic attack. Curr Neurol Neurosci Rep. 2020;20(8):36. https://doi.org/10.1007/s11910-020-01053-3.
8. Baker AD, Sharma R. Cardiac testing in search for occult atrial fibrillation after ischemic stroke. Curr Treat Options Cardiovasc Med. 2021;23:30. https://doi.org/10.1007/s11936-021-00908-3.
9. Perez MV, et al. Large-scale assessment of a smartwatch to identify atrial fibrillation. N Engl J Med. 2019;381:1909. https://www.nejm.org/doi/full/10.1056/nejmoa1901183.
10. Sanna T, Diener HC, Passman RS, Di Lazzaro V, Bernstein RA, Morillo CA, Rymer MM, Thijs V, Rogers T, Beckers F, Lindborg K, Brachmann J, CRYSTAL AF Investigators. Cryptogenic stroke and underlying atrial fibrillation. N Engl J Med. 2014;370(26):2478–86.

11. Lip GY, Nieuwlaat R, Pisters R, Lane DA, Crijns HJ. Refining clinical risk stratification for predicting stroke and thromboembolism in atrial fibrillation using a novel risk factor-based approach: the euro heart survey on atrial fibrillation. Chest. 2010;137(2):263–72.
12. Granger CB, Alexander JH, McMurray JJ, Lopes RD, Hylek EM, Hanna M, Al-Khalidi HR, Ansell J, Atar D, Avezum A, Bahit MC, Diaz R, Easton JD, Ezekowitz JA, Flaker G, Garcia D, Geraldes M, Gersh BJ, Golitsyn S, Goto S, Hermosillo AG, Hohnloser SH, Horowitz J, Mohan P, Jansky P, Lewis BS, Lopez-Sendon JL, Pais P, Parkhomenko A, Verheugt FW, Zhu J, Wallentin L, ARISTOTLE Committees and Investigators. Apixaban versus Warfarin in patients with atrial fibrillation. N Engl J Med. 2011;365(11):981–92.
13. Reddy VY, Akehurst RL, Armstrong SO, Amorosi SL, Brereton N, Hertz DS, Holmes DR Jr. Cost effectiveness of left atrial appendage closure with the Watchman device for atrial fibrillation patients with absolute contraindications to warfarin. Europace. 2016;18(7):979–86.
14. Kleindorfer DO, Towfighi A, Chaturvedi S, Cockroft KM, Gutierrez J, Lombardi-Hill D, Kamel H, Kernan WN, Kittner SJ, Leira EC, Lennon O, Meschia JF, Nguyen TN, Pollak PM, Santangeli P, Sharrief AZ, Smith SC Jr, Turan TN, Williams LS. 2021 Guideline for the prevention of stroke in patients with stroke and transient ischemic attack: a guideline from the American Heart Association/American Stroke Association. Stroke. 2021;52(7):e364–467. https://doi.org/10.1161/STR.0000000000000375. Epub 2021 May 24. Erratum in: Stroke. 2021 Jul;52(7):e483–4.
15. Dalia T, Lahan S, Ranka S, et al. Warfarin versus direct oral anticoagulants for treating left ventricular thrombus: a systematic review and meta-analysis. Thrombosis J. 2021;19:7. https://doi.org/10.1186/s12959-021-00259-w.
16. Sotero FD, Rosário M, Fonseca AC, Ferro JM. Neurological complications of infective endocarditis. Curr Neurol Neurosci Rep. 2019;19(5):1–8.
17. Venn RA, Ning MM, Vlahakes GJ, Wasfy JH. Surgical timing in infective endocarditis complicated by intracranial hemorrhage. Am Heart J. 2019;216:102–12.
18. Sharma R, Silverman S, Patel S, et al. Frequency, predictors and cardiovascular outcomes associated with transthoracic echocardiographic findings during acute ischaemic stroke hospitalization. Stroke Vasc Neurol. 2022;7:10.1136/svn-2021-001170.
19. Homma S, Thompson JL, Pullicino PM, Levin B, Freudenberger RS, Teerlink JR, Ammon SE, Graham S, Sacco RL, Mann DL, Mohr JP, Massie BM, Labovitz AJ, Anker SD, Lok DJ, Ponikowski P, Estol CJ, Lip GY, Di Tullio MR, Sanford AR, Mejia V, Gabriel AP, del Valle ML, Buchsbaum R, WARCEF Investigators. Warfarin and aspirin in patients with heart failure and sinus rhythm. N Engl J Med. 2012;366(20):1859–69. https://doi.org/10.1056/NEJMoa1202299. Epub 2012 May 2.
20. Cokkinos DV, Haralabopoulos GC, Kostis JB, Toutouzas PK, HELAS Investigators. Efficacy of antithrombotic therapy in chronic heart failure: the HELAS study. Eur J Heart Fail. 2006;8(4):428–32. https://doi.org/10.1016/j.ejheart.2006.02.012. Epub 2006 Jun 5.
21. Mehra MR, Vaduganathan M, Fu M, Ferreira JP, Anker SD, Cleland JGF, Lam CSP, van Veldhuisen DJ, Byra WM, Spiro TE, Deng H, Zannad F, Greenberg B. A comprehensive analysis of the effects of rivaroxaban on stroke or transient ischaemic attack in patients with heart failure, coronary artery disease, and sinus rhythm: the COMMANDER HF trial. Eur Heart J. 2019;40(44):3593–602. https://doi.org/10.1093/eurheartj/ehz427.
22. Anticoagulation for valvular heart disease. American College of Cardiology. 18 May 2015. https://www.acc.org/latest-in-cardiology/articles/2015/05/18/09/58/anticoagulation-for-valvular-heart-disease. Accessed 9/12/2023.
23. Verstraete A, Herregods MC, Verbrugghe P, Lamberigts M, Vanassche T, Meyns B, Oosterlinck W, Rega F, Adriaenssens T, Van Hoof L, Keuleers S, Vandenbriele C, Sinnaeve P, Janssens S, Dubois C, Meuris B, Verhamme P. Antithrombotic treatment after surgical and transcatheter heart valve repair and replacement. Front Cardiovasc Med. 2021;8:702780. https://doi.org/10.3389/fcvm.2021.702780.

Hypercoagulable States

22

Allison Lewandowski and Jennifer L. Dearborn-Tomazos

Thrombophilias

A thrombophilia is a disorder that promotes clotting in both the arterial and venous systems, and can be inherited (courtesy of parents) or acquired (develops spontaneously or due to specific circumstances). Screening for inherited or acquired thrombophilia is reasonable in younger patients with a cryptogenic stroke (Table 22.1), a prior history of clotting, recurrent stroke, venous thrombosis, or women with multiple miscarriages [1]. The decision to test for thrombophilia depends on the index of suspicion that a stroke is attributable to thrombophilia and whether the results of testing would affect management [1].

Table 22.1 Hematological disorders causing stroke

– Protein C or S deficiency	– Polycythemia vera
– Factor V Leiden	– Thrombotic thrombocytopenic purpura
– Antiphospholipid syndrome	– Heparin-induced thrombocytopenia
– Sickle cell disease	– Nephrotic syndrome
– Leukemia	– Pregnancy
– Antithrombin III deficiency	– Malignancy
– Prothrombin gene mutation	– Oral contraceptives
– Essential thrombocytosis	

A. Lewandowski
Department of Anesthesia, Beth Israel Deaconess Medical Center, Boston, MA, USA
e-mail: alewando@bidmc.harvard.edu

J. L. Dearborn-Tomazos (✉)
Department of Neurology, Beth Israel Deaconess Medical Center, Harvard Medical School, Boston, MA, USA
e-mail: jtomazos@bidmc.harvard.edu

© The Author(s), under exclusive license to Springer Nature Switzerland AG 2024
H. P. Amin (ed.), *Stroke for the Advanced Practice Clinician*,
https://doi.org/10.1007/978-3-031-66289-8_22

Table 22.2 Diagnosis of antiphospholipid antibody syndrome [2]

Criteria		
Laboratory	Lupus anticoagulant, anti-cardiolipin, beta-2 glycoprotein antibodies	Two positive tests at least 12 weeks apart
Vascular	Thrombosis in any tissue or organ, venous or arterial	Confirmed by imaging or histopathology
Pregnancy	Multiple early or at least one late pregnancy loss	Excluded anatomic, hormonal, or chromosomal abnormalities

Common Thrombophilias

A common thrombophilia is antiphospholipid syndrome (APLS). In this autoimmune condition, lupus anticoagulant, beta-2 glycoprotein, and anti-cardiolipin antibodies disrupt and damage the endothelium (innermost lining) of blood vessels, promoting clot formation. This leads to thrombosis, or a blood clot at a site of vessel injury, which can then embolize and occlude another vessel downstream. Diagnosing APLS requires meeting multiple clinical and lab criteria outlined in Table 22.2 [3].

Antiphospholipid antibodies can increase the risk of clotting veins and arteries, leading to deep vein thrombosis, miscarriages, myocardial infarction, or ischemic stroke. Anticoagulation with Warfarin is recommended in patients with APLS based on large studies that support the use of Warfarin over DOACs [4].

Two inherited thrombophilias that increase the level of natural procoagulants include Factor V Leiden (FVL) and prothrombin gene mutation. Under normal conditions, protein C (a natural anticoagulant) binds to factor V (a clotting agent) to inactivate it, as a means to regulate its activity. In FVL, a mutation in the gene that produces factor V prevents protein C from binding normally to factor V, leading to an unchecked pro-clotting state. Patients with FVL have an increased risk of DVT or pulmonary embolism. Patients in this condition inherit one copy of the gene from each parent. If a patient has one copy carrying the mutation and one normal copy, they are called heterozygotes for FVL and have a 4–5× increased risk of developing blood clots. If both copies carry the mutation, the patient is homozygous for FVL, and the risk of developing clots jumps to 25–50×! Prothrombin gene mutation leads to increased production of prothrombin (factor II), a blood clotting protein needed to form fibrin [5]. Too much prothrombin protein increases the venous clotting risk by 2–5× in heterozygotes, and a much higher risk in homozygous individuals.

Decreased levels of natural anticoagulants like protein C, S, and antithrombin also increase the risk of clotting. Deficiencies in these proteins can be inherited or acquired, and testing is not recommended during an acute thrombotic event or while on anticoagulation like Warfarin, as the levels can be falsely affected. Testing should be performed after the patient has recovered from the acute event and not on anticoagulation to improve accuracy. Evidence suggests that for patients with antithrombin, protein C, and S deficiencies plus a history of thrombosis, the likelihood of recurrence is 19% at 2 years, 40% at 5 years, and 55% at 10 years [6].

Acquired states with a high risk of developing blood clots include critical illness, prolonged immobility, dehydration, injury or recent surgery, pregnancy, and certain medications. Estrogen-containing oral contraceptives are known to increase the risk of thrombosis. Pregnancy, especially around the peri-partum stage, is associated with a higher risk of thrombosis. This is primarily due to the body preparing for childbirth and increasing the production of clotting proteins. Studies have demonstrated that the risk of thrombus formation can linger several months after childbirth.

Cerebral Venous Sinus Thrombosis

Recall that arteries are "high flow" blood vessels bringing oxygenated blood to the brain, like clean water pipes to a house. Veins are "slow flow" vessels that drain used-up blood away from the brain, like a septic system. Slow-flow areas are where thrombophilias are most likely to cause clots.

The venous system has several large central veins called "sinuses" and many smaller cortical veins that drain blood into them. A Cerebral Venous Thrombosis (CVT) is a blood clot that causes complete or partial occlusion of a cerebral vein or sinus. Although thrombi can occur within any vein in the brain, the most common locations include the superior sagittal sinus, the transverse sinus, and the sigmoid sinus [7]. Like a blocked septic tank, a CVT may lead to outflow obstruction over several days or more, which can manifest in several different ways (headache, nausea/vomiting, papilledema, focal deficits).

Unlike traveling emboli, that occlude arteries and cause symptoms instantly, venous occlusions are caused by a thrombus that slowly grows *within the vein itself.* Therefore, arterial occlusions result in acute focal symptoms, whereas symptoms from venous occlusions can be slowly progressive and often accompanied by headaches. A venous occlusion leads to congestion and fluid collecting in the brain tissue (edema), similar to overflowing water in a clogged sink. Arterial thrombus can embolize, sending smaller fragments to occlude a vessel downstream. CVT is not known to embolize, but a DVT in the legs or pelvis can. A thromboembolism from a pelvic or leg DVT can lead to a pulmonary embolism as it returns to the lungs through the venous system. It can also be shunted through a patent foramen ovale (if present) and enter the arterial circulation, causing an ischemic stroke.

Epidemiology

The epidemiology for CVT is lacking, in part due to the underrepresentation of lower and middle-income countries where the incidence of CVT may be higher due to higher pregnancy rates and higher incidence rates of infection and nutritional deficiencies [8]. Still, compared to arterial stroke, CVT is a relatively rare condition that can affect patients of any age, but it is more commonly seen in young patients (mean age of 33) and women (three times more common in women than men) [8].

Table 22.3 Risk factors for CVT [7, 9]

Younger age	Mean age of 33
Female sex	Likely related to pregnancy, puerperium, and the use of estrogen-containing oral contraceptives
Hypercoagulable conditions	Discussed further below. Notably, thrombophilia and malignancy.
Inflammatory conditions	Systemic autoimmune conditions (lupus, inflammatory bowel disease)
Infection	i.e., Bacterial meningitis, abscess, or empyema
Head trauma	Result of direct injury to the vein or sinus (skull fracture that extends to the vessel, dissection, penetrating injury)

The female preponderance is likely related to pregnancy, puerperium, and use of estrogen-containing oral contraceptives, the latter of which is the number one risk factor for this condition (Table 22.3) [7, 9]. This is discussed in more detail below. Other notable risk factors are listed below.

Manifestations

Clinical manifestations of CVT can differ based on the location of the thrombus and the degree of surrounding tissue damage (Table 22.4). Symptom onset may be slow if the occlusion is gradual and collateral blood vessels have developed in response. Outflow obstruction of blood can lead to elevated intracranial pressure and intracranial hypertension. Symptoms may include headache (present in 70–90% of cases), typically subacute in onset and progressive [10], vomiting, papilledema, blurred or double vision, or coma. Monitoring for vision loss is crucial for patients with increased intracranial pressure. Patients can also develop focal neurological deficits such as cranial nerve palsy, aphasia, weakness, or numbness. Seizures occur more commonly with CVT (30–40% of patients) than with arterial strokes or intracerebral hemorrhage [7, 10]. Given the wide range of clinical manifestations, CVT should be on the differential for new neurological symptoms, especially those presenting with headache.

One result of CVT is a venous infarct. Venous infarcts differ from arterial infarcts because the ischemia does not occur in an arterial distribution. Venous infarcts also tend to have more edema than arterial infarcts and as a result have both areas of ischemia (compression of surrounding tissue from edema) and hemorrhage (rupture of draining veins that) [10, 12]. Another differentiating factor is the type of edema. Venous infarcts often have more vasogenic edema, whereas arterial infarcts typically have cytotoxic edema [12]. Vasogenic edema occurs as fluid accumulates outside the cells due to blood-brain barrier disruption. Cytotoxic edema occurs as cells enlarge as a result of an increase in intracellular water. Since the arteries remain open, the area of brain tissue affected by vasogenic edema still receives adequate blood flow and oxygenation. Symptoms may improve as the edema resolves. Therefore, venous infarcts typically have less irreversible tissue damage and a more favorable prognosis than arterial infarcts [12]. Venous hemorrhage occurs when engorged draining veins rupture due to outflow obstruction (Fig. 22.1).

Table 22.4 Clinical manifestations of CVT [7, 10, 11]

Signs of intracranial hypertension	Headache (present in 70–90% of cases, typically subacute in onset and progressive), vomiting, papilledema, blurred or double vision, or coma.
Headache	Varied presentations, ranging from thunderclap, throbbing, band-like, migraine-like. An association between the location of the pain and the site of thrombosis has not been found.
Focal neurological deficits	Cranial nerve palsy, aphasia, weakness, or numbness.
Seizures	Occur more commonly with CVT (30–40% of patients) than with arterial strokes or intracerebral hemorrhage.

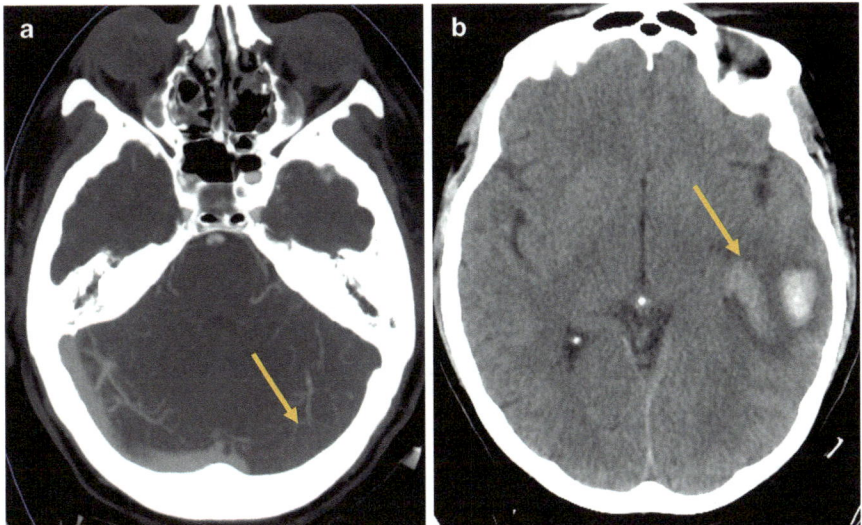

Fig. 22.1 Venous hemorrhage. Note occluded left transverse sinus (**a**, yellow arrow) leading to outflow obstruction of draining veins. This leads to increased venous pressure and hemorrhage (**b**, yellow arrow). Despite the presence of hemorrhage, the treatment in this case is still anticoagulation because the underlying problem is venous thrombosis

Imaging

Various modalities of neuroimaging are utilized in the diagnosis of CVT. Non-contrast head CT (NCHCT) is a common study utilized in the initial workup of many of the above signs or symptoms. The sensitivity of NCHCT in detecting CVT is low (about 30%) [6]. In some cases of CVT, an NCHCT may reveal a hyperdensity in a vein or sinus (see clinical vignette), an intraparenchymal hemorrhage surrounded by edema, or evidence of ischemia that does not follow an arterial distribution [6]. Intraparenchymal, subarachnoid, or subdural hemorrhage from CVT can be seen on NCHCT and is due to increased pressure in the venous system, causing rupture of the blood vessels [13]. A CT angiogram of the head may be performed as one of the initial studies. Most CTAs also adequately assess the venous

Fig. 22.2 Empty delta sign (yellow arrow) of the superior sagittal sinus, with contrast outlining a filling defect (triangular, hence delta), representing a thrombus

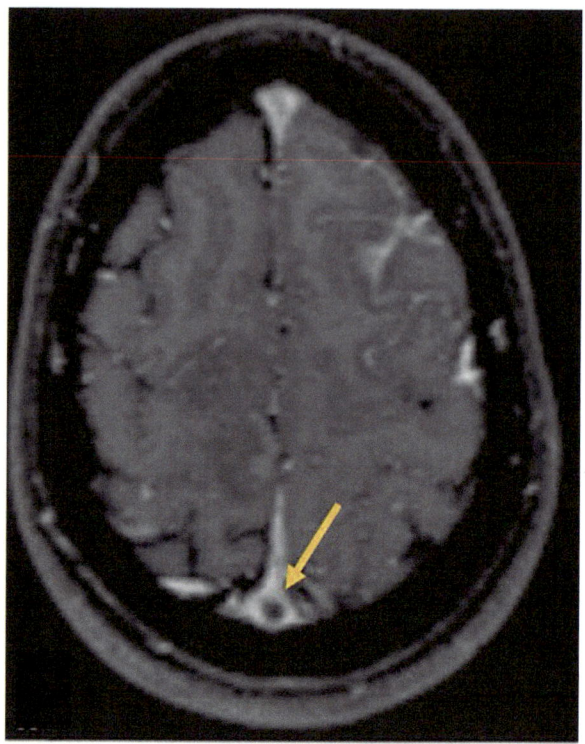

system and may reveal a filling defect (i.e., an area of the vessel where contrast does not flow because of the occlusion) in the affected sinus. The "**empty delta sign**" in the superior sagittal sinus is an example of a filling defect with high sensitivity in detecting CVST (Fig. 22.2) [6, 14]. A dedicated CT venogram is also an option and is as accurate as an MR venogram in diagnosing CVT, and both require contrast [15]. An MRI brain is the most sensitive imaging modality for venous infarct [6, 16].

Ancillary Testing

Testing for hypercoagulability is recommended for patients without an identifiable precipitating cause for their CVT. Hematology consultation is warranted to guide workup and long term management. Laboratory workup should include lupus anticoagulant, prothrombin mutation, factor V Leiden, proteins C and S, antithrombin III, and beta-2 glycoprotein. It could also include ANA and ANCA. Patients should be referred to hematology if abnormalities are identified in these tests or if there is a concerning history. Guidelines recommend testing for the deficiencies (protein C, S, antithrombin) at least 6 weeks after a thrombotic event and 2–4 weeks after completion of anticoagulation therapy. So, testing for thrombophilia has the highest yield after a patient has completed a several-month course of anticoagulation. Antibodies in APLS are also called "acute phase reactants," meaning they can be elevated in the setting of an acute illness but do not necessarily imply underlying APLS. It is important not to over-interpret abnormal APLS labs if drawn early after CVT diagnosis, and follow-up confirmatory testing is required 12 weeks later.

Common Pitfalls

Sometimes, imaging will demonstrate a hypoplastic (anatomically small) sinus, which may be incidental and not clinically significant. When scans are ordered for nonspecific dizziness, headaches, or other neurological symptoms, knowing if an abnormal venous finding is related to the presenting symptoms can be challenging. To determine if a venous abnormality is clinically relevant, look at the adjacent brain tissue on MRI for evidence of outflow obstruction. Outflow obstruction manifests as ischemia on DWI, edema on FLAIR, and dilated or engorged cortical draining veins going toward the sinus or hemorrhage on SWI. Normal brain tissue without any signs of outflow obstruction is a strong clue that the venous finding is incidental, that blood is draining through collateral (bypass) veins, and that the presenting symptoms are due to another process.

Another common reason for delay in diagnosis is not considering CVT as a source for hemorrhage on CT. It is prudent to obtain venous imaging if a patient has a prolonged headache prodrome, hemorrhage, or edema in bilateral hemispheres or a history of a hypercoagulable state.

Although useful in the workup for underlying hypercoagulable state once a CVT is identified (discussed further below), laboratory studies are not of major clinical significance in the initial workup and management of CVT. D-dimer is a marker of blood clotting with a sensitivity of 97.1% and a specificity of 91.2% [17]. An elevated D-dimer may also suggest underlying malignancy. Imaging is the gold standard if CVT is suspected, and hypercoagulable labs are only helpful in determining the underlying cause.

Management

Anticoagulation is the mainstay of treatment of CVT. Anticoagulation reduces the chance of clot expansion, alleviating venous pressure that can lead to significant complications such as ischemia or hemorrhage. Therapeutic dosages of IV unfractionated heparin or low-molecular-weight heparin are typically used for initiation of anticoagulation for CVT [6, 15]. IV unfractionated heparin is preferred initially in the hospital setting as it can be stopped and reversed immediately if there are any complications. *Intracranial hemorrhage from CVT is not a contraindication to anticoagulation because the underlying problem is a thrombus.* The hemorrhage occurs due to increased venous pressure, and anticoagulation is the treatment of choice to reduce clot expansion. Following initial treatment and once stability is observed, patients can switch to an oral vitamin K antagonist (i.e., Warfarin) with a target INR of 2–3 [10]. Despite being used in clinical practice, there is little evidence for direct oral anticoagulants in this setting [6, 15]. Duration of anticoagulation depends on whether the CVT was provoked (3–6 months) or unprovoked (3–12 months). Indefinite anticoagulation is indicated for patients with diagnosed thrombophilias or recurrent thrombus [18].

Severe CVT can lead to malignant cerebral edema and is a life-threatening condition. Severe cerebral edema and hemorrhagic infarcts can lead to herniation, coma, and death. Early recognition and intervention in an ICU with timely medical and surgical interventions is crucial in managing these patients [19]. Decompressive craniectomy may be a life-saving measure and may result in improved functional outcomes in this population [20]. More invasive treatments, such as direct catheter thrombolysis and endovascular thrombectomy for CVT, may be considered in severe cases with continued clinical deterioration despite anticoagulation. However, no randomized controlled studies have investigated these interventions, so careful consideration should be taken when recommending these therapies [6].

Other life-threatening conditions associated with CVT include seizures, hydrocephalus, and intracranial hypertension. Anti-seizure medications should only be initiated if the patient experiences a seizure [21]. Communicating and obstructive hydrocephalus can both occur in association with CVT, the former due to impaired CSF absorption and the latter as a result of hemorrhage in the ventricular system [6]. In cases of hydrocephalus, emergency neurosurgery consultation should be requested for CSF diversion via ventriculostomy. Intracranial hypertension results from venous congestion and impaired CSF absorption. A common manifestation of intracranial hypertension is severe headache and vision loss. If left untreated, intracranial hypertension can result in permanent vision loss. Management of intracranial hypertension and its effects may involve serial lumbar punctures, acetazolamide, and ophthalmology consultation to consider optic nerve fenestration [6]. Decompressive craniectomy is a common consideration for large arterial ischemic stroke and could be considered if all other options are exhausted.

Long-Term Management

A follow-up CTV or MRI/MRV can be performed at 3–6 months following initiation of anticoagulation to assess for recanalization [6]. Most CVTs will recanalize by 3 months, but about 15% may remain stenotic or occluded. Continuing or stopping anticoagulation is the main long-term decision. However, there is a lack of well-designed studies to determine whether recanalization is associated with improved functional outcomes [18]. For cryptogenic CVT, or CVT during critical illness, the overall risk of recurrence is low. However, patients with diagnosed thrombophilias, cancer, or a history of recurrent thromboses would be at higher risk of recurrent CVT. In those cases, long-term anticoagulation is certainly a consideration with guidance from hematology.

Clinical Vignette 1

HPI: A 68-year-old male presents with a new left-sided weakness that started while showering at 7:00 AM. Later in the morning, he called his wife, who noted his speech was slurred and called the ambulance. He arrived at the ED at 10:30 AM.

Exam: Blood pressure and glucose were normal. His exam was notable for dysarthria, mild left facial droop, and LUE drift.

Imaging: He underwent a CT and CT angiogram per stoke protocol. CTA was normal; CT demonstrated a possible hyperdense vein of Galen and straight sinus (white arrow), suggesting thrombosis. MRV confirmed filling defects within the straight sinus extending anteriorly to the vein of Gallen and internal cerebral veins and posteriorly to the confluence of sinuses and medical aspect of the left transverse sinus (orange arrow represents the absence of signal). MRI revealed a non-hemorrhagic venous infarct involving the right greater than left thalamus (blue arrows) secondary to dural venous sinus thrombosis within straight sinus (along with the vein of Gallen and internal cerebral veins) extending to the confluence of sinus and left transverse sinus.

Management: A hypercoagulable panel was sent, after which he was started on intravenous heparin. Hypercoagulable workup was unremarkable. CT of his body revealed mild colonic thickening of unclear significance. He was transitioned to oral anticoagulation with Eliquis after tolerating IV heparin for 48 h (no hemorrhage on follow-up CT) with outpatient follow-up with hematology and plan for colonoscopy.

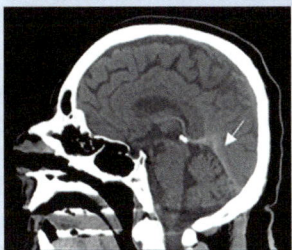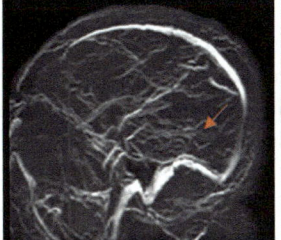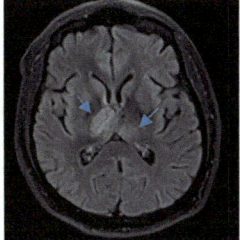

Case contributed by Dr. Ahmed Elmashad

Hypercoagulability of Malignancy

Stroke and cancer are common conditions that carry a significant burden of morbidity and mortality in the United States [22]. Cancer patients are especially high risk because they can have strokes from traditional risk factors and cancer-associated hypercoagulability. It is important, however, to emphasize that the most common causes of stroke in cancer patients are still traditional causes, such as atrial fibrillation, hypertension, diabetes, or smoking. Cancer-related causes of stroke can include hypercoagulability induced by the cancer itself or by the cancer treatment, leading to both arterial occlusions and CVT [23]. Occasionally, a cryptogenic stroke in a patient not otherwise known to have cancer can result in a new diagnosis of malignancy.

Thrombosis in cancer occurs when a tumor secretes proteins that contribute to a hypercoagulable state. Adenocarcinoma is a type of cancer that can occur in various organs and is associated with a high rate of hypercoagulability [24]. Adenocarcinoma produces a substance called mucin that activates platelets leading to hypercoagulable state. Other procoagulant molecules, such as tissue factor and cancer procoagulant, can be secreted directly into the bloodstream.

Cancer can cause both arterial and venous thrombi by the hypercoagulability mentioned above. The presence of venous clots, or deep venous thrombosis, may increase the risk of stroke by causing paradoxical embolism through a PFO, if present. Another mechanism by which cancer can contribute to stroke risk is through nonbacterial thrombotic endocarditis (NBTE) [23]. In NBTE, sterile (noninfectious) vegetations develop on the heart valves, providing a source of emboli that can cause stroke. The treatment for the causes mentioned above is anticoagulation with low-molecular-weight heparin or oral factor Xa inhibitors in addition to cancer treatment.

Some cancer treatments, such as cisplatin, methotrexate, and L-asparaginase, are associated with both venous and arterial thromboembolic events [25, 26]. Bevacizumab, a monoclonal antibody against VEG-F receptors, is associated with ischemic and hemorrhagic stroke [27]. There is no consensus as to when it is appropriate to screen for cancer in a patient with a stroke. If a patient has a cryptogenic stroke, it is reasonable to ask for a detailed review of systems to isolate any symptoms that may raise suspicion of an underlying malignancy. For example, a history of unexplained weight loss, night sweats, or systemic signs/symptoms may raise concern for malignancy. Occupational exposures and social history, especially smoking, may raise cancer risk. Asking patients about age-appropriate routine health screening for cancer, such as mammograms or colonoscopies, is also essential. In select circumstances, it may be appropriate to consider imaging modalities such as CT chest, abdomen, and pelvis for patients with high clinical suspicion [23].

Stroke in Women

As previously mentioned, oral contraceptives increase the risk of thrombosis. Women with a history of VTEs are advised not to use estrogen-containing contraceptives. There are no studies on progestin-only contraceptives in patients with prior CVT, but progestin is generally less hypercoagulable than estrogen [28]. Nonhormonal forms of birth control may be safest in this population.

Pregnancy and the puerperium are major risk factors for stroke in women of childbearing age [29], and occur in approximately 30 of 100,000 pregnancies [30]. The increased risk of stroke in pregnancy is multifactorial. Stroke can occur at any point in pregnancy, but the incidence is highest in the third trimester, the puerperium phase, or the first 6 weeks following childbirth. The risk of stroke in pregnancy is highest in those of advanced maternal age, African American race, those with pre-existing cardiac conditions, thrombophilia, rheumatological disorders, pregnancy-related hypertensive disorders, diabetes, and cesarean delivery [30].

Hemorrhagic strokes are the most common type of stroke in pregnancy. They can be associated with rupture of cerebral aneurysm, arteriovenous malformation, pregnancy-related hypertension (preeclampsia/eclampsia), pregnancy-related HELLP syndrome, posterior reversible leukoencephalopathy syndrome (PRES), or other rare vascular disorders [29, 30]. Management of hemorrhagic strokes in this population is similar to the general population overall. Hypertension in HELLP and PRES should be treated per obstetric guidelines with medications that are safe for the pregnant/postpartum woman [31].

Arterial ischemic strokes in pregnancy and the puerperium can present with atypical symptoms, so it is important to keep on the differential when caring for this high-risk population. Etiologies can include carotid or vertebral artery dissection, reversible cerebral vasoconstriction syndrome, embolism related to hypercoagulable state with or without patent foramen ovale, amniotic fluid embolism, cardiac remodeling or cardiomyopathy resulting in cardioembolism, among others [30]. *Pregnant patients with stroke are still eligible for thrombolytics and thrombectomy if they meet all other criteria* [32].

CVT can occur in pregnancy or the puerperium due to the hypercoagulable state and venous stasis. It can also be associated with dehydration, epidural catheter placement, or CNS or systemic infection due to increased inflammation [30, 33]. Unfractionated heparin (UFH) does not cross the placenta and can be used safely to initiate anticoagulation in pregnant patients [34]. The preferred long-term agent for anticoagulation for CVT in pregnant and breastfeeding women is LMWH, as it does not cross the placenta and is not considered teratogenic [33, 34]. Both UFH and LMWH can continue while breastfeeding [34].

Diagnosis of stroke in pregnancy can be challenging, and the risks and benefits of imaging studies should be weighed carefully. MRI is considered safe in pregnancy [35]; however, a CT scan would be the preferred imaging modality in certain emergent situations as it takes significantly less time to complete. As per the American College of Obstetrics and Gynecology recommendations, if a CT is a more appropriate study, it should be performed given that the radiation dosage is typically lower than the dose associated with harm to the fetus. Gadolinium (MRI) contrast should be limited in pregnant women unless it will significantly improve the diagnostic utility of the study and if the benefits outweigh the risks. Iodinated (CT) contrast can cross the placenta; however, studies have not demonstrated harm to the fetus. Breastfeeding can continue after both gadolinium and iodinated contrast administration [35].

Clinical Pearls

- Thrombophilia can be inherited or acquired and can cause cryptogenic stroke or CVST. The decision to test for thrombophilia, such as antiphospholipid antibody syndrome, should depend on the clinical suspicion (i.e., pretest probability) that the stroke or CVST could be attributable to a thrombophilic cause. Other more common causes should still be ruled out.
- Cerebral venous thrombosis could be suspected in a patient who presents with unexplained headaches, focal neurological deficits, or seizures.
- Cancer can cause both arterial and venous hypercoagulability and lead to stroke via several mechanisms. The most common causes of stroke in patients with cancer would still be traditional risk factors such as hypertension, diabetes, and atrial fibrillation.
- The highest of stroke during pregnancy is in the third trimester and puerperium.

Summary of Important Clinical Trials

1. An important paper by Kamel et al. used claims data of over 1.6 million U.S. women to examine the thrombotic risk in 6-week intervals after pregnancy compared to a 6-week interval 1 year later. The authors measured thrombotic risk by reviewing cases of stroke, myocardial infarction, and venous thromboembolism. The authors found that the risk of events in the first 6 weeks after delivery was markedly higher compared to 1 year later (411 events vs. 38 events). There was a modest and significant risk of events from 6 to 12 weeks post-delivery compared to the interval 1 year later (95 vs 44 events). After 12 weeks, the risk of thrombotic events was not increased. The authors concluded that the highest risk period for thrombotic events after pregnancy was in the first 6 weeks, with a modest risk continuing up to 12 weeks [36].
2. The TRAPS trial was a randomized, open-label, blinded endpoint trial that enrolled patients with antiphospholipid antibody syndrome (APLAS) to compare treatment with rivaroxaban with warfarin for the prevention of thromboembolic events, major bleeding, or vascular death. Patients with triple-positive APLAS were included, defined by the presence of lupus anticoagulant, anticardiolipin antibodies, and beta-2 glycoprotein antibodies. Rivaroxaban 20 mg was compared to warfarin with an INR target of 2.5. The study was stopped prematurely when an excess of events occurred in the rivaroxaban arm. The use of rivaroxaban was associated with increased thrombotic events in the patient population with APLAS [4].

References

1. Salehi Omran S, Hartman A, Zakai NA, Navi BB. Thrombophilia testing after ischemic stroke. Stroke. 2021;52(5):1874–84. https://doi.org/10.1161/STROKEAHA.120.032360.
2. Sammaritano LR. Antiphospholipid syndrome. Best Pract Res Clin Rheumatol. 2020;34(1):101463. https://doi.org/10.1016/j.berh.2019.101463.
3. Miyakis S, Lockshin MD, Atsumi T, et al. International consensus statement on an update of the classification criteria for definite antiphospholipid syndrome (APS). J Thromb Haemost. 2006;4(2):295–306. https://doi.org/10.1111/j.1538-7836.2006.01753.x.
4. Pengo V, Denas G, Zoppellaro G, et al. Rivaroxaban vs warfarin in high-risk patients with antiphospholipid syndrome. Blood. 2018;132(13):1365–71. https://doi.org/10.1182/blood-2018-04-848333.
5. Varga EA, Moll S. Prothrombin 20210 mutation (factor II mutation). Circulation. 2004;110(3):e15–8. https://doi.org/10.1161/01.CIR.0000135582.53444.87.
6. Saposnik G, Barinagarrementeria F, Brown RD, et al. Diagnosis and management of cerebral venous thrombosis. Stroke. 2011;42(4):1158–92. https://doi.org/10.1161/STR.0b013e31820a8364.
7. Ferro JM, Canhão P, Stam J, Bousser MG, Barinagarrementeria F. Prognosis of cerebral vein and dural sinus thrombosis: results of the International Study on Cerebral Vein and Dural Sinus Thrombosis (ISCVT). Stroke. 2004;35(3):664–70. https://doi.org/10.1161/01.Str.0000117571.76197.26.
8. Ferro JM, Aguiar de Sousa D. Cerebral venous thrombosis: an update. Curr Neurol Neurosci Rep. 2019;19(10):74. https://doi.org/10.1007/s11910-019-0988-x.
9. Ulivi L, Squitieri M, Cohen H, Cowley P, Werring DJ. Cerebral venous thrombosis: a practical guide. Pract Neurol. 2020;20(5):356–67. https://doi.org/10.1136/practneurol-2019-002415.
10. Ropper AH, Klein JP. Cerebral venous thrombosis. N Engl J Med. 2021;385(1):59–64. https://doi.org/10.1056/NEJMra2106545.
11. Wasay M, Kojan S, Dai AI, Bobustuc G, Sheikh Z. Headache in cerebral venous thrombosis: incidence, pattern and location in 200 consecutive patients. J Headache Pain. 2010;11(2):137–9. https://doi.org/10.1007/s10194-010-0186-3.
12. Capecchi M, Abbattista M, Martinelli I. Cerebral venous sinus thrombosis. J Thromb Haemost. 2018;16(10):1918–31. https://doi.org/10.1111/jth.14210.
13. Gajurel BP, Shrestha A, Gautam N, Rajbhandari R, Ojha R, Karn R. Cerebral venous sinus thrombosis with concomitant subdural hemorrhage and subarachnoid hemorrhages involving cerebral convexity and perimesencephalic regions: a case report. Clin Case Rep. 2021;9(10):e04919. https://doi.org/10.1002/ccr3.4919.
14. Linn J, Ertl-Wagner B, Seelos KC, et al. Diagnostic value of multidetector-row CT angiography in the evaluation of thrombosis of the cerebral venous sinuses. AJNR Am J Neuroradiol. 2007;28(5):946–52.
15. Ferro JM, Bousser MG, Canhão P, et al. European Stroke Organization guideline for the diagnosis and treatment of cerebral venous thrombosis—endorsed by the European Academy of Neurology. Eur J Neurol. 2017;24(10):1203–13. https://doi.org/10.1111/ene.13381.
16. van Dam LF, van Walderveen MAA, Kroft LJM, et al. Current imaging modalities for diagnosing cerebral vein thrombosis—a critical review. Thromb Res. 2020;189:132–9. https://doi.org/10.1016/j.thromres.2020.03.011.
17. Talbot K, Wright M, Keeling D. Normal d-dimer levels do not exclude the diagnosis of cerebral venous sinus thrombosis. J Neurol. 2002;249(11):1603–4. https://doi.org/10.1007/s00415-002-0893-z.
18. Alimohammadi A, Kim DJ, Field TS. Updates in cerebral venous thrombosis. Curr Cardiol Rep. 2022;24(1):43–50. https://doi.org/10.1007/s11886-021-01622-z.

19. Soriano-Navarro E, Cano-Nigenda V, Menéndez-Manjarrez F, et al. Bilateral decompressive craniectomy in malignant cerebral venous thrombosis. Eur J Case Rep Intern Med. 2020;7(7):001560. https://doi.org/10.12890/2020_001560.

20. Ferro JM, Crassard I, Coutinho JM, et al. Decompressive surgery in cerebrovenous thrombosis: a multicenter registry and a systematic review of individual patient data. Stroke. 2011;42(10):2825–31. https://doi.org/10.1161/strokeaha.111.615393.

21. Ferro JM, Canhão P, Bousser MG, Stam J, Barinagarrementeria F. Early seizures in cerebral vein and dural sinus thrombosis: risk factors and role of antiepileptics. Stroke. 2008;39(4):1152–8. https://doi.org/10.1161/strokeaha.107.487363.

22. Xu J, Murphy SL, Kochanek KD, Arias E. Mortality in the United States, 2021. https://www.cdc.gov/nchs/products/databriefs/db456.htm#section_4. Accessed 15 Feb 2023.

23. Dearborn JL, Urrutia VC, Zeiler SR. Stroke and cancer—a complicated relationship. J Neurol Transl Neurosci. 2014;2(1):1039.

24. Varki A. Trousseau's syndrome: multiple definitions and multiple mechanisms. Blood. 2007;110(6):1723–9. https://doi.org/10.1182/blood-2006-10-053736.

25. Grisold W, Oberndorfer S, Struhal W. Stroke and cancer: a review. Acta Neurol Scand. 2009;119(1):1–16. https://doi.org/10.1111/j.1600-0404.2008.01059.x.

26. Foreman NK, Mahmoud HH, Rivera GK, Crist WM. Recurrent cerebrovascular accident with L-asparaginase rechallenge. Med Pediatr Oncol. 1992;20(6):532–4. https://doi.org/10.1002/mpo.2950200608.

27. Scappaticci FA, Skillings JR, Holden SN, et al. Arterial thromboembolic events in patients with metastatic carcinoma treated with chemotherapy and bevacizumab. J Natl Cancer Inst. 2007;99(16):1232–9. https://doi.org/10.1093/jnci/djm086.

28. Durmuş B, Yperzeele L, Zuurbier SM. Cerebral venous thrombosis in women of childbearing age: diagnosis, treatment, and prophylaxis during a future pregnancy. Ther Adv Neurol Disord. 2020;13:1756286420945169. https://doi.org/10.1177/1756286420945169.

29. Yoshida K, Takahashi JC, Takenobu Y, Suzuki N, Ogawa A, Miyamoto S. Strokes associated with pregnancy and puerperium: a nationwide study by the Japan Stroke Society. Stroke. 2017;48(2):276–82. https://doi.org/10.1161/strokeaha.116.014406.

30. Miller EC, Leffert L. Stroke in pregnancy: a focused update. Anesth Analg. 2020;130(4):1085.

31. Zambrano MD, Miller EC. Maternal stroke: an update. Curr Atheroscler Rep. 2019;21(9):33. https://doi.org/10.1007/s11883-019-0798-2.

32. Demaerschalk BM, Kleindorfer DO, Adeoye OM, et al. Scientific rationale for the inclusion and exclusion criteria for intravenous alteplase in acute ischemic stroke: a statement for healthcare professionals from the American Heart Association/American Stroke Association. Stroke. 2016;47(2):581–641. https://doi.org/10.1161/str.0000000000000086.

33. Gao H, Yang BJ, Jin LP, Jia XF. Predisposing factors, diagnosis, treatment and prognosis of cerebral venous thrombosis during pregnancy and postpartum: a case-control study. Chin Med J (Engl). 2011;124(24):4198–204.

34. Kalaitzopoulos DR, Panagopoulos A, Samant S, et al. Management of venous thromboembolism in pregnancy. Thromb Res. 2022;211:106–13. https://doi.org/10.1016/j.thromres.2022.02.002.

35. Committee Opinion No. 723: guidelines for diagnostic imaging during pregnancy and lactation. Obstet Gynecol. 2017;130(4):e210–6. https://doi.org/10.1097/AOG.0000000000002355.

36. Kamel H, Navi BB, Sriram N, Hovsepian DA, Devereux RB, Elkind MS. Risk of a thrombotic event after the 6-week postpartum period. N Engl J Med. 2014;370(14):1307–15. https://doi.org/10.1056/NEJMoa1311485. Epub 2014 Feb 13. PMID: 24524551; PMCID: PMC4035479.

Patent Foramen Ovale

23

Amberlea Elliott and Andrew Huffer

What Is a PFO?

Let us start with some dense anatomy, shall we? In normal blood flow through the heart, deoxygenated blood (blood that has delivered oxygen to the body and ready to pick up more) returns to the right atrium via the superior and inferior vena cava, dumps into the right ventricle, and then travels to the pulmonary circulation via the pulmonary arteries. The lungs provide oxygen to the red blood cells, but they also catch and break down small blood clots floating in the bloodstream, and protect the systemic circulation from inhaled toxins. Oxygenated blood returns to the left atrium from the lungs via the pulmonary veins, passes through the left ventricle, and is pumped into the systemic circulation through the aorta, ready to deliver oxygen throughout the body again (Fig. 23.1).

In a typical situation, an intact interatrial septum (a wall of heart tissue) separates the right and left atria and prevents any direct shunting from the right to the left side. Now, imagine how blood would flow if there was a connection between the right and left atria, also called a Patent Foramen Ovale (PFO). A PFO refers to a persistent remnant of the fetal circulation between the right and left atrium of the heart and is present in a surprisingly high 25–30% of the healthy adult population.

Blood flow in the fetal circulation is very different compared to post-birth. The umbilical vein carries oxygenated blood from the placenta to the right atrium of the fetal heart. Blood entering the right atrium is shunted through the foramen ovale into the left atrium. Think of it as a one-way door that opens only into the left atrium (not typically bi-directional). In the first minutes to hours after birth, expansion of

A. Elliott
Mercy Hospital, Oklahoma City, OK, USA
e-mail: Amberlea.Bradford-Elliott@Mercy.Net

A. Huffer (✉)
Neurology, University of Washington, Seattle, WA, USA
e-mail: Andrew.huffer@va.gov

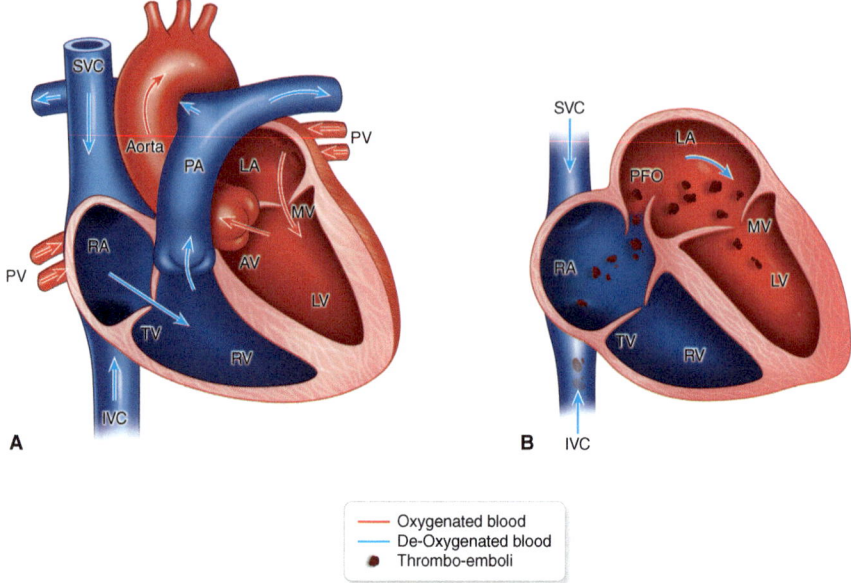

Fig. 23.1 Blood flow through normal heart structure (**a**) and PFO (**b**). Deoxygenated blood is marked by blue, and oxygenated blood is marked by red. Note in image (**a**), deoxygenated blood returning from the inferior vena cava (IVC) and superior vena cava (SVC) enters the right atrium (RA), then the right ventricle (RV) through the tricuspid valve (TV), travels into the lungs via the pulmonary arteries (PA) for filtration and oxygenation. Oxygenated and filtered blood returns to the heart via the pulmonary veins (PV) into the left atrium (LA), then the left ventricle (LV) through the mitral valve (MV), and into the systemic circulation via the aortic valve (AV) and aorta. In image (**b**), deoxygenated blood returns from the IVC carrying thromboemboli from a deep vein thrombosis (DVT) and, in the presence of a PFO, bypasses filtration in the lungs and instead is shunted directly into the LA, then LV, and the systemic circulation. The emboli then have direct access to the brain and other organs

the lungs leads to a drop in pulmonary arterial resistance. These changes result in higher pressure in the left atrium than the right, abruptly closing the shunt (think of a draft slamming a door closed). Eventually, the foramen ovale flaps fuse shut to form an intact atrial septum (usually within the first few months of life). This fusion remains incomplete in roughly 25% of the adult population, leaving a *patent* foramen ovale (PFO). The PFO, while largely irrelevant to cardiac function, can allow passage of de-oxygenated blood (carrying clots and other debris) to flow from the right to the left atrium, bypassing the pulmonary circulation [1].

It is important to know that blood is not constantly shunted if a PFO is present. Since the pressure in the left atrium is higher than in the right atrium under normal conditions, the "one-way door" remains closed, and blood flows along the normal route. The PFO swings open when the right atrium pressure exceeds that of the left atrium. Conditions that increase right heart pressures include vomiting, heavy coughing or Valsalva (forced expiration against a closed glottis with heavy lifting/pulling/pushing), Mueller's maneuver (inspiring against a closed airway during obstructive sleep apnea), pulmonary hypertension, or pulmonary embolism. Even a brief swing in the pressure gradient can open a PFO, allowing unfiltered and deoxygenated blood (or emboli) into the left atrium and the arterial circulation.

PFO and Stroke

A PFO is an incidental finding in most people and does not impact heart function or health. However, suppose an embolism from a deep vein thrombosis (DVT) in the legs or pelvis floats back toward the heart. In the 70% or so of people *without* a PFO, that embolism will take the normal route of blood and go into the lungs via the pulmonary arteries. Depending on the size, the embolism may get broken down by enzymes or, if big enough, might cause a symptomatic pulmonary embolism by occluding a vessel and impairing oxygen delivery (potentially fatal). With a PFO, that embolism can go from the right atrium directly into the left atrium (bypassing the lung filters), and into the circulation where it can travel anywhere in the body, including the brain. We call this process paradoxical embolism because the source of the clot is a vein, but the downstream occlusion is in an artery. Alternatively, the PFO itself might be a location for thrombus formation. Patients with cryptogenic strokes, meaning no clear cause is evident after a thorough risk factor evaluation, have a higher prevalence of PFOs than the general population (up to 40% vs 25%, respectively) [2]. In these cases, the team must determine if a PFO is just an innocent bystander or a participant in the crime. The discovery of a PFO should not raise panic, nor should it lead to a sense of self-satisfaction that the mystery is solved. Remember, since the prevalence of PFO is already high in the general population, it is widely considered an anatomical variation, not an "abnormality." One should think, "OK, the patient has a PFO, but first let's rule out other more common stroke risk factors that are higher risk before considering closure." How, then, is a provider expected to know if a PFO should be treated in a stroke patient?

Evidence for PFO Closure

Early Trials

Given the high prevalence of PFO in the general population, particularly in patients with cryptogenic strokes, there has been considerable interest in the efficacy of percutaneous PFO closure to prevent recurrent stroke. The CLOSURE I enrolled adult patients ≤60 years old with a PFO and cryptogenic stroke or TIA and randomized them to PFO closure or medical therapy [3]. Over 2 years of follow-up, there was no significant difference in recurrent stroke, TIA, or mortality. The PC [4] and RESPECT [5] trials randomized a similar population of patients to device closure vs medical therapy. Over 4 and 2.6 years of mean follow-up, respectively, there was no significant difference in death, non-fatal stroke, TIA, or peripheral embolism. Serious procedural complications were rare in all trials, but new-onset atrial fibrillation (AF) in the peri-procedural period was seen in the closure groups, raising a conundrum…was the AF there before the stroke, or did the device cause it [6]?

Several important observations emerged from these trials. First, the risk of recurrent embolic stroke over the follow-up period was relatively low regardless of the group, ranging from 0.12–1.45% per year for the device closure groups to 0.59–1.55% per year for the medical management groups. However, a more detailed analysis of the RESPECT trial suggested that patients with a large shunt size had a more than five-fold reduction in stroke risk after PFO closure. Patients with PFO associated with an atrial septal aneurysm also had a significant risk reduction with PFO closure. These findings suggested more careful selection for patients with clearly embolic strokes and high-risk PFO features, and a more extended follow-up period might be necessary to conclusively demonstrate the benefit of PFO closure in secondary stroke prevention.

Recent Trials

The RESPECT trial published more long-term data about 4 years later, with a follow-up of almost 6 years demonstrating that in high-risk PFO, closure significantly reduced fatal and non-fatal ischemic stroke and early death by roughly 45% [7]. The CLOSE trial enrolled patients with recent cryptogenic embolic stroke and PFO with either an atrial septal aneurysm or a larger-size shunt [8]. After a mean of 5.3 years of follow-up, no recurrent strokes had occurred among the 238 patients randomized to PFO closure, compared to 14 out of 235 patients in the antiplatelet-only medical arm. In the larger REDUCE trial, symptomatic ischemic strokes and clinically silent radiographic infarctions were both significantly reduced in the PFO closure group over a median follow-up of 3.2 years [9]. Similar to prior trials, new-onset atrial fibrillation rates were higher in each study's closure arms. Other complications, although rare, included device migration, erosion, embolization, and pericardial effusion or cardiac tamponade. These results suggest a role for PFO closure in preventing recurrent cryptogenic strokes in appropriately selected patients with appropriate workups (see section on "Diagnostic Evaluation" below).

Data consistently demonstrate that PFOs are more likely to be implicated in stroke for younger patients (<60) with no other risk factors. A PFO is usually not much of a consideration in older patients unless a DVT is also found. When discussing a PFO with patients, the first thing to stress is that it is a *normal* anatomical variant and has no impact on heart function. The concept of a "hole in the heart" can be scary to patients, and rightfully so! Explain that while the PFO may have played a role in the stroke, it is much less common, and more common causes of stroke must be ruled out first. The workup can take several months (cardiac monitoring, hematological labs), but recall that for true PFO-related strokes, the risk of a recurrent stroke over the following 2 years is very low. Other conditions with higher risks need to be ruled out first. If no other identifiable cause is found, then PFO closure may be discussed in the outpatient setting.

Diagnostic Evaluation

How can we determine which patients are likely to benefit from PFO closure? The most important thing is to have a methodical, stepwise approach to the workup while knowing that the PFO is not dangerous and can be closed later if the embolic evaluation is otherwise negative (Table 23.1). Historical clues that could implicate a

Table 23.1 Cryptogenic stroke checklist

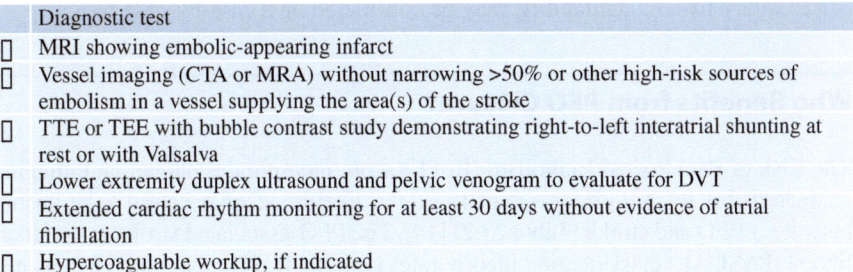

Diagnostic test
☐ MRI showing embolic-appearing infarct
☐ Vessel imaging (CTA or MRA) without narrowing >50% or other high-risk sources of embolism in a vessel supplying the area(s) of the stroke
☐ TTE or TEE with bubble contrast study demonstrating right-to-left interatrial shunting at rest or with Valsalva
☐ Lower extremity duplex ultrasound and pelvic venogram to evaluate for DVT
☐ Extended cardiac rhythm monitoring for at least 30 days without evidence of atrial fibrillation
☐ Hypercoagulable workup, if indicated

PFO include pronged immobility, prior venous thromboembolism (VTE) or known hypercoagulable states, factors promoting increased right-to-left shunting such as coughing, heavy lifting/pulling/pushing, Valsalva (during vomiting or a bowel movement), and sleep apnea should all be elicited in the history. Magnetic resonance imaging (MRI) should demonstrate an embolic pattern of infarction characterized by wedge-shaped cortical or subcortical infarcts or multifocal infarcts within multiple vascular territories. All patients should have head and neck vascular imaging to exclude atherosclerotic stenosis >50% in an ipsilateral vessel.

Transthoracic echocardiogram (TTE) is routinely used to assess for structural or functional abnormalities in the heart, such as focal or global ventricular wall hypokinesis, intracardiac thrombus or tumor, or valvular vegetations. For younger stroke patients with PFO, transesophageal echocardiogram (TEE) can provide the best view of the interatrial septum and allow direct visualization of a PFO to assess size and other high-risk features. A bubble contrast study identifies a PFO on either TTE or TEE, in which agitated saline with tiny bubbles is injected intravenously. The ultrasound then looks for a mobile flap or the passage of microbubbles from the right atrium to the left atrium, indicating a shunt. This test is performed at rest and with Valsalva, where the patient is asked to take a deep breath, then try to breathe out while holding their mouth and nose closed for 15–20 s. The inflated lungs increase intrathoracic pressure, reducing venous return to the heart with blood accumulating in the superior and inferior vena cava. Note that the pressure gradient at this point is still higher in the left atrium, so the PFO would remain closed. However, when the patient breathes out, all that accumulated blood surges back to the right atrium, leading to a transient increase in right atrial pressure, swinging the PFO open.

Once a PFO is identified, workup for a venous thrombus with lower extremity Doppler ultrasound and pelvic venous angiography is warranted. Patients with unilateral leg swelling, erythema, or pain are more likely to have an underlying DVT. Although the detection rate of deep vein thrombosis (DVT) without other clinical findings is low, a positive finding would lead to consideration of anticoagulation (AC) therapy and make paradoxical embolism more likely [10, 11].

The American Heart Association/American Stroke Association guidelines recommend obtaining a 12-lead electrocardiogram and, at minimum, 24-hour Holter or telemetry monitoring for all patients with embolic strokes [12]. You, however, know that extended cardiac rhythm monitoring for 30 days is the standard of care and dramatically increases the detection rate of paroxysmal atrial fibrillation [13].

Additional testing to exclude uncommon causes of embolic stroke, such as acquired or hereditary hypercoagulability, may be considered on a case-by-case basis.

Who Benefits from PFO Closure?

The Risk of Paradoxical Embolism (RoPE) score incorporates patient and imaging characteristics to provide an estimate of the likelihood of a causal relationship between a PFO and stroke (Table 23.2) [14]. The PFO-associated stroke causal likelihood (PASCAL) classification incorporates both the RoPE score and the presence of high-risk features such as concomitant venous VTE, a straddling thrombus, large shunt, or associated atrial septal aneurysm to stratify patients into low, medium, high, or very high-risk categories (Table 23.3) [15]. A general approach for evaluating patients ≤60 years of age for PFO closure would first confirm the presence of an embolic stroke (no lacunes!) without evident cause despite thorough evaluation, exclude patients with a lifelong indication for anticoagulation or a contraindication to the procedure and apply the RoPE/PASCAL score to determine patients with a possible, probable, or definite likelihood that the stroke was related to the PFO. However, the Society for Cardiovascular Angiography and Interventions (SCAI) recommends PFO closure even in patients who require lifelong AC due to high thrombosis risk (not AF) because of the potential for anticoagulation interruption. A vascular neurologist should guide conversations about the risks and benefits of PFO closure, ideally in conjunction with an interventional cardiologist [16]. Once a patient has a comprehensive workup with vessel imaging, cardiac monitoring, and hematological workup, a direct provider-provider discussion between vascular neurology and cardiology, or a multidisciplinary conference setting, can help patients move forward with PFO closure in a streamlined way.

In the real world, some patients may get put on a path to PFO closure without a stroke neurologist evaluation. This simplistic approach bypasses the expertise that a stroke neurologist provides about the true stroke mechanism, completeness of workup, and whether closure is warranted. Without a thoughtful approach, closing

Table 23.2 Risk of paradoxical embolism (RoPE) score (range 0–10)

Factor	Points
No history of hypertension	1
No history of diabetes	1
Nonsmoker	1
Cortical infarct on imaging	1
Age, 18–29	5
Age, 30–39	4
Age, 40–49	3
Age, 50–59	2
Age, 60–69	1
Age, ≥70	0

Scores >6 indicate a higher likelihood of a causative link

Table 23.3 PFO-associated stroke causal likelihood (PASCAL) classification

Risk source	Features	RoPE score low (0–6)	RoPe score high (≥7)
Very high	PFO with straddling thrombus	Definite	Definite
High	Concomitant VTE and PFO with either (a) atrial septal aneurysm or (b) large shunt	Probable	Highly probable
Medium	PFO with either (a) atrial septal aneurysm or (b) large shunt	Possible	Probable
Low	Small shunt PFO without atrial septal aneurysm	Unlikely	Possible

a PFO may do nothing to lower future stroke risk and only expose that patient to surgical risk.

Percutaneous PFO Closure and Follow-Up Care

It is important to remember that the risk of recurrent stroke is low, even in patients who do not undergo PFO closure, so there is no urgent need to pursue closure within the first weeks or months after an incident stroke. PFO closure, if indicated, is often performed several months after a stroke, after a thorough evaluation of other possible causes, and requires informed decision-making by the neurologist, cardiologist, and patient/family.

PFO closure is performed by inserting a catheter into the right atrium via the right femoral vein. A guide catheter is passed across the interatrial septum before the left-sided and right-sided occluders are deployed sequentially, "sandwiching" the septal defect. Device placement is confirmed by either TEE or intracardiac echocardiography. Patients are maintained on an antiplatelet agent before, during, and after the procedure, usually indefinitely. Specific regimens are variable, but dual antiplatelet therapy is often used for several months, followed by single-agent therapy.

Clinical Pearls
- A PFO is a connection between the right and left atrium caused by incomplete fusion of the interatrial septum at birth, and it is found in almost one-third of the general population.
- Increased right atrial pressures can promote right-to-left shunting across a PFO that can lead to paradoxical embolism.
- Early trials of PFO closure did not show a significant reduction in secondary strokes, partly because of low rates of recurrent strokes and short follow-up windows. Later trials with extended follow-up periods demonstrated reduced recurrent stroke risk for specific patient groups.
- All patients should see a stroke neurologist before PFO closure. Patients <60 years of age with embolic strokes, PFO, and a negative comprehensive workup should be considered for percutaneous PFO closure.

Summary of Trials

CLOSURE I (2012): Randomized 909 patients ≤60 years old with PFO and cryptogenic stroke or TIA to PFO closure with STARFlex closure device or medical management at the discretion of treating providers. At 2 years, there was no difference in the composite of stroke or TIA plus 30-day mortality and neurologic mortality beyond 30 days.

PC (2013): Randomized 414 patients ≤60 years old with PFO and stroke, TIA, or systemic embolization to PFO closure with Amplatzer closure device or medical management. At 4 years, there was no difference in the composite of death, non-fatal stroke, TIA, or systemic embolism.

RESPECT (2013): Randomized 980 patients ≤60 years old with PFO and cryptogenic stroke to PFO closure with Amplatzer closure device or medical management. At 2.6 years, there was no difference in the composite of recurrent non-fatal stroke, fatal stroke, or early death.

RESPECT long-term follow-up (2017): Followed the same cohort as the original RESPECT trial for a median of 5.9 years and found a significant reduction in recurrent ischemic stroke in the closure compared to the medical therapy group.

CLOSE (2017): Randomized 473 patients ≤60 years old with PFO and cryptogenic stroke and an associated atrial septal aneurysm or large interatrial shunt to PFO closure with Amplatzer closure device or medical management with antiplatelet therapy. At 5.3 years, recurrent strokes were significantly reduced in the closure group. A separate arm of the study found a non-significant reduction in medically-managed patients who received anticoagulation vs antiplatelet therapy.

REDUCE (2017): Randomized 664 patients ≤60 years old with PFO and cryptogenic stroke to PFO closure with either the HELIX or CARDIOFORM septal closure device or medical management at a 2:1 ratio. At 5 years, there was a significant reduction in clinical ischemic stroke in the closure group.

References

1. Hagen PT, Edwards WD, et al. Incidence and size of patent foramen ovale during the first 10 decades of life: an autopsy study of 965 normal hearts. Mayo Clin Proc. 1984;59(1):17.
2. Mazzucco S, Rothwell PM, Oxford Vascular Study Phenotyped Cohort. Prevalence of patent foramen ovale in cryptogenic transient ischemic attack and non-disabling stroke at older ages; a population-based study, systematic review, and meta-analysis. Lancet Neurol. 2018;17(7):609–17.
3. Furlan AJ, Wechsler L, CLOSURE I Investigators. Closure or medical therapy for cryptogenic stroke with patent foramen ovale. N Engl J Med. 2012;366(11):991–9.
4. Meieer B, Jüni P, PC Trial Investigators. Percutaneous closure of patent foramen ovale in cryptogenic embolism. N Engl J Med. 2013;368(12):1083–91.
5. Carroll JD, Tirschwell DL, RESPECT Investigators. Closure of patent foramen ovale versus medical therapy after cryptogenic stroke. N Engl J Med. 2013;368(12):1092–100.

6. De Rosa S, Indolfi C, et al. Percutaneous closure versus medical treatment in stroke patients with patent foramen ovale: a systematic review and meta-analysis. Ann Intern Med. 2018;168(5):343–50.
7. Saver JL, Tirchwell DL, RESPECT Investigators. Long-term outcomes of patent foramen ovale closure or medical therapy after stroke. N Engl J Med. 2017;377:1022–32.
8. Mas JL, Chatellier G, CLOSE Investigators. Patent foramen ovale closure or anticoagulation vs antiplatelets after stroke. N Engl J Med. 2017;377(11):1011–21.
9. Søndergaard L, Thomassen L, Gore REDUCE Investigators. Patent foramen ovale closure or antiplatelet therapy for cryptogenic stroke. N Engl J Med. 2017;377(11):1033–42.
10. Lethan H, Hanrath P, et al. Frequency of deep vein thrombosis in patients with patent foramen ovale and ischemic stroke or transient ischemic attack. Am J Cardiol. 1997;80(8):1066–9.
11. Cramer SC, Longstreth WT Jr, et al. Increased pelvic vein thrombi in cryptogenic stroke: the result of the Paradoxical Emboli from Large Veins in Ischemic Stroke (PELVIS) study. Stroke. 2004;35(1):46–50.
12. Powers WJ, Tirschwell DL, American Heart Association Stroke Council. Guidelines for the early management of patients with acute ischemic stroke. Stroke. 2019;50(12):e344.
13. Sanna T, Brachmann J, CRYSTAL AF Investigators. Cryptogenic stroke and underlying atrial fibrillation. N Engl J Med. 2014;370(26):2478–86.
14. Kent DM, Ruthazer R, et al. An index to identify stroke-related vs incidental patent foramen ovale in cryptogenic stroke. Neurology. 2013;81(7):619–25.
15. Elgendy AY, Saver JL, et al. Proposal for updated nomenclature and classification of potential causative mechanism in patent foramen ovale-associated stroke. JAMA Neurol. 2020;77(7):878–86.
16. Kavinsky CJ, Szerlip M, et al. SCAI guidelines for the management of patent foramen ovale. JSCAI. 2022;1:100039. Available online on 19 May 2022. https://doi.org/10.1016/j.jscai.2022.100039.

Stroke and COVID

24

Jennifer Picagli, Kun He Lee, and Adam S. Jasne

Epidemiology and Clinical Context

While infection is associated with stroke, COVID-19 infection has been associated with at least a three-fold increased risk of ischemic stroke [1–3]. COVID-19 infection is linked not to just arterial stroke but also hemorrhagic strokes and cerebral venous thrombosis [4, 5].

In addition to the pathological effects of the virus, many other factors impacted stroke care during the pandemic. Fewer Emergency Medical Services (EMS) calls and delays in seeking medical care were associated with increased deaths from stroke in the United States and internationally. The pandemic influenced individual and population-level decisions to seek medical care, prehospital and hospital services, stroke interventions and inpatient care, the availability and logistics of post-stroke rehabilitation, and accessibility and organization of home environments [6–8].

Patient characteristics associated with increased mortality from COVID-19 include older age, male gender, pre-existing hypertension, diabetes, and coronary artery disease. While the typical patient with COVID-19 and stroke most often fit this profile, the overall age of patients with stroke and COVID-19 skewed younger than those without COVID-19 infection. Combined COVID-19 and stroke were associated with higher National Institutes of Health Stroke Scale (NIHSS) and higher inpatient mortality [9–11].

J. Picagli
Yale New Haven Hospital, New Haven, CT, USA
e-mail: Jennifer.picagli@yale.edu

K. H. Lee
Neurology, Temple Health, Philadelphia, PA, USA
e-mail: Kun.lee@yale.edu

A. S. Jasne (✉)
Neurology, Yale School of Medicine, New Haven, CT, USA
e-mail: adam.jasne@yale.edu

© The Author(s), under exclusive license to Springer Nature Switzerland AG 2024   271
H. P. Amin (ed.), *Stroke for the Advanced Practice Clinician*,
https://doi.org/10.1007/978-3-031-66289-8_24

Suggested Pathophysiology

Most COVID-associated ischemic strokes occured within days up to 2 weeks of COVID-19 symptom onset. Most were due to large vessel occlusions (LVO), stenoses, or multifocal strokes without large vessel stenosis. In some cases, patients who have severe COVID-19 illness may also have watershed (low-flow) infarcts, possibly due to critical illness leading to poor cerebral perfusion [10, 12, 13].

Multiple potential mechanisms increase the risk for ischemic strokes in those with COVID-19, including hypercoagulability, endotheliopathy (damage to the inner lining of blood vessels), systemic inflammation, platelet activation leading to clotting, arterial dissection, and cardiac pathologies (Fig. 24.1). Compared to patients with influenza and many other coronaviruses, COVID-19 patients had evidence of increased microthrombi in the pulmonary vasculature, disrupted endothelial architecture, and viral particles in the endothelial cells themselves [14, 15].

Additionally, most studies have indicated that risk factors for stroke are often multiplicative; patients with more pre-existing stroke risk factors are more at risk for stroke with COVID-19 infection than those with fewer [5, 16, 17].

Inflammation leading to cytokine and acute phase protein release are associated with a higher risk of thrombosis, endotheliopathy, and the potential for vascular dissection. Injury and inflammation in the endothelium lead to the release of more inflammatory components, which then increase inflammation at the endothelial

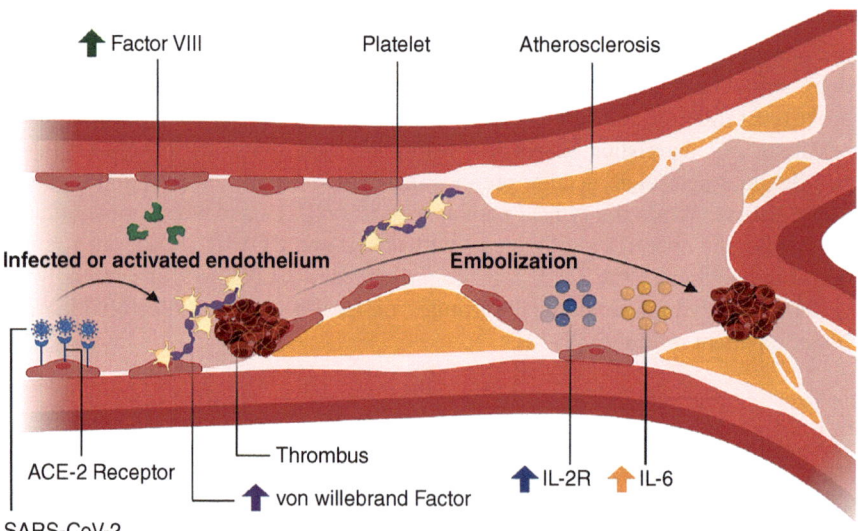

Fig. 24.1 Potential mechanisms of COVID-19 endotheliopathy and stroke. COVID-19 infection leads to von Willebrand factor (vWF) and Factor VIII release from activated endothelium, resulting in platelet aggregation and thrombus formation. A thrombus can occlude the vessel locally or embolize distally, leading to cerebral ischemia. (Reprinted with permission from McAlpine et al., Stroke, 2021 [25])

wall, leading to a cycle of injury and thrombosis [15, 18, 19, 20]. Massive release of cytokines appears to be associated with hemorrhagic posterior reversible encephalopathy syndrome, hemorrhagic conversion of ischemic strokes, and vasculitis [15, 21].

Evidence also demonstrated that COVID-19 disrupts the balance of pro- and anti-thrombotic proteins involved in the coagulation cascade [22, 23]. Elevated markers of clot formation and other serum tests suggesting global prothrombotic states are common findings in COVID-19 infection. D-dimer, a product of fibrin linkage breakdown commonly serving as a marker of thrombus formation, for example, in pulmonary embolism and DVT, is often elevated in COVID-19 patients. Antiphospholipid antibody titers (e.g., anticardiolipin antibody), which are associated with increased risk for both arterial and venous clot formation, were also shown to be elevated acutely in COVID-19 patients [24]. Of particular interest in COVID-19 is the virus's affinity to ACE-2 receptors, which appears to contribute to infectivity and blood pressure dysregulation [2, 25–28]. ACE-2 is a multi-functional protein with receptors in organs throughout the body and the endothelium of blood vessels. In COVID-19, the ACE-2 receptor was found to be a receptor for COVID-19 viral particles, allowing their entry into human cells.

COVID-19 infection can lead to cardiac embolism from direct and indirect damage to the heart itself. Post-viral cardiomyopathy can be triggered by COVID-19 infection by respiratory failure from pulmonary manifestations of infection and, in rare cases, by vaccination. This increases the risk of akinesis and arrhythmia, which are implicated in thrombus formation in the heart itself [29–31].

Media attention has focused on the potential thrombogenicity of vaccination, specifically cerebral venous sinus thrombosis after vaccination. Retrospective analysis suggests that adenovirus vector vaccines have an increased risk of central venous sinus thrombosis via vaccine-induced immune thrombotic thrombocytopenia (ITP) [32]. A consistent presentation of cerebral venous thrombosis due to vaccination included a very low platelet count from immune-mediated destruction. How might someone with low platelets develop a thrombosis? The dwindling platelets send out little vesicles called Platelet-derived Microparticles (PMPs), which are prothrombotic and promote clotting in someone with low platelets. High levels of circulating PMPs in patients with ITP are associated with an increased risk of developing venous thrombosis. As a result of this known risk, authorization has expired for the adenovirus vector vaccine in the United States, and limitations for administration have been issued in some countries [33, 34].

Evaluation

Some patients may present with moderate to severe COVID-19 and are also found to have pre-existing and un- or under-treated metabolic or cardiac comorbidities requiring management. Clinicians evaluating a patient with moderate-to-severe COVID-19 disease should be aware of the pre-existing comorbidities of the patient and ensure ongoing treatment of these conditions.

In many cases, laboratory testing for an individual with COVID-19 and stroke will include (1) stroke-specific risk-management testing, such as fasting lipid panels and hemoglobin A1c and (2) COVID-19 labs and D-dimer, based on the severity of illness. The initial presentation should dictate the need for laboratory testing and the severity of illness, such as oxygen requirement, signs of sepsis, or criticality of stroke. Other COVID-19 investigative labs have been studied but are not routinely recommended for guiding clinical management [35].

In COVID-19 patients with stroke, who are young have minimal cardiovascular risk factors, or have a milder infection, additional studies beyond traditional stroke labs may be considered, including a hypercoagulable panel. Abnormal hypercoagulable labs should be repeated as an outpatient several weeks after the infection resolves. Standard timeframes are 12+ weeks for antiphospholipid antibodies and 4–12+ weeks for von Willebrand factor panel labs.

Cardiovascular evaluation is an essential part of the workup of the patient with COVID-19 requiring hospitalization, given that cardiac involvement is common with COVID-19 infection. Trending troponin measurements, usually a series of three initially, are recommended. An electrocardiogram (ECG) is recommended due to the potential for arrhythmia; patients on nirmatrelvir and ritonavir (Paxlovid) in combination with medications metabolized through the Cytochrome P450 3A4 pathway may also have an increased risk of QT prolongation. The rate of newly discovered arrhythmia can range from 8% to 18% in hospitalized COVID-19 patients, leading to embolic stroke [36]. Extended telemetry (48 h or longer) is recommended for patients with COVID-19. Finally, a transthoracic echocardiogram is recommended, given the increased incidence of heart failure, myocardial ischemia, and myocarditis in COVID-19. For the stroke patient, a transthoracic echocardiogram demonstrating intracardiac thrombus likely confirms a cardioembolic process; left atrial dilation might indicate underlying arrhythmia [37–39].

Acute Stroke in COVID-19

The patient who presents initially with stroke or transient ischemic attack (TIA) should be triaged per stroke guidelines based on clinical impression, including NIHSS score and time since onset of symptoms. It is important to note that patients with known active or recent COVID-19 infection are not excluded from stroke thrombolysis or thrombectomy; however, it may be appropriate to use a streamlined process with more limited personnel to limit exposure [40].

COVID-19 patients should still receive all acute stroke treatments they would otherwise meet the criteria for. In a review of 111 cases in Germany, outcomes at 90 days were statistically worse in the COVID-19-positive stroke patients, primarily due to comorbidities from severe COVID-19. There was also a higher incidence of re-occlusion or re-stenosis [41]. Heparinization to treat acute thrombus is appropriate but may require closer laboratory and clinical monitoring.

Carotid stenosis is preferentially treated after acute inflammatory markers improve. A multidisciplinary discussion with vascular or neurovascular surgery will be necessary to risk-stratify for individual patient needs [39].

In the outpatient setting, patients who have recovered from COVID-19 infection continue to have an increased risk of cardiac arrhythmia, heart failure, pulmonary embolism (PE), deep vein thrombosis (DVT), and superficial thrombosis. Those patients who previously had these comorbidities are at elevated risk for progression of their chronic disease. Some evidence exists that the risk for stroke continues to remain elevated for a prolonged period after initial infection for anywhere from 1 to 12 weeks [17, 21, 36, 42].

Management

COVID-19 is an active area of study, and the virus itself has undergone mutation, affecting treatment and side-effect profile since its emergence in late 2019. Ongoing studies, such as the large international Call to Action: SARS-CoV-2 and CerebrovAscular DisordErs (CASCADE) study, and multicenter registries, such as the American Heart Association COVID-19 Cardiovascular Disease Registry, are continuing to refine the treatment recommendations for patients [36, 43]. In most cases, the standard of care for neurovascular disease should remain without significant modification. Current considerations for the neurovascular patient with COVID-19 include:

Initiating prophylactic anticoagulation for all hospitalized COVID-19-positive patients or continuing home anticoagulation.

It is acceptable to initiate aspirin or P2Y12 inhibitor(s) for neurovascular indications for antiplatelet therapy [19].

It is acceptable to initiate statin therapy if there is no contraindication. Some antiviral treatments may interact with statin therapy. In this case, documentation about medication holds, resumption, and reinitiation must be clearly documented. These should be held and resumed per individual guidelines [44].

Consider monitoring anticoagulation, factor activity, and platelets more closely, as these may vary during critical illness.

Local and current guidelines for COVID-19 laboratory monitoring and standards for cerebrovascular disease should be followed [19].

Heparin-induced thrombocytopenia (HIT) and disseminated intravascular coagulation (DIC) are rare but possible complications of COVID-19 [45].

Clinical Pearls
- The risk of stroke appears to be the highest within two weeks of COVID-19 symptom onset, but a higher risk can linger well after the infection has resolved.
- Multiple mechanisms, notably a widespread inflammatory state, contribute to clot development in COVID-19 patients.
- Venous thrombosis after vaccine is tied to immune-mediated platelet destruction and thrombocytopenia on lab testing.
- COVID-19 infection is not a contraindication to interventional or pharmaceutical stroke treatment.
- All COVID-19 patients with stroke still warrant a complete stroke evaluation, especially those few other risk factors for stroke.

References

1. World Health Organization. WHO COVID-19 dashboard. 2020. https://covid19.who.int/.
2. Amruta N, Chastain WH, Paz M, Solch RJ, Murray-Brown IC, Befeler JB, Gressett TE, Longo MT, Engler-Chiurazzi EB, Bix G. SARS-CoV-2 mediated neuroinflammation and the impact of COVID-19 in neurological disorders. Cytokine Growth Factor Rev. 2021;58:1–15.
3. Belani P, Schefflein J, Kihira S, Rigney B, Delman BN, Mahmoudi K, Mocco J, Majidi S, Yeckley J, Aggarwal A, Lefton D, Doshi AH. COVID-19 is an independent risk factor for acute ischemic stroke. AJNR Am J Neuroradiol. 2020;41(8):1361–4.
4. Shahjouei S, Naderi S, Li J, Khan A, Chaudhary D, Farahmand G, Male S, Griessenauer C, Sabra M, Mondello S, Cernigliaro A, Khodadadi F, Dev A, Goyal N, Ranji-Burachaloo S, Olulana O, Avula V, Ebrahimzadeh SA, Alizada O, et al. Risk of stroke in hospitalized SARS-CoV-2 infected patients: a multinational study. EBioMedicine. 2020;59:102939.
5. Fatima N, Saqqur M, Qamar F, Shaukat S, Shuaib A. Impact of COVID-19 on neurological manifestations: an overview of stroke presentation in pandemic. Neurol Sci. 2020;41(10):2675–9.
6. Dula AN, Gealogo Brown G, Aggarwal A, Clark KL. Decrease in stroke diagnoses during the COVID-19 pandemic: where did all our stroke patients go? JMIR Aging. 2020;3(2):e21608.
7. Sharma R, Kuohn LR, Weinberger DM, Warren JL, Sansing LH, Jasne A, Falcone G, Dhand A, Sheth KN. Excess cerebrovascular mortality in the United States during the COVID-19 pandemic. Stroke. 2021;52(2):563–72.
8. Nawabi NLA, Duey AH, Kilgallon JL, Jessurun C, Doucette J, Mekary RA, Aziz-Sultan MA. Effects of the COVID-19 pandemic on stroke response times: a systematic review and meta-analysis. J Neurointerv Surg. 2022;14(7):642–9.
9. Parohan M, Yaghoubi S, Seraji A, Javanbakht MH, Sarraf P, Djalali M. Risk factors for mortality in patients with coronavirus disease 2019 (COVID-19) infection: a systematic review and meta-analysis of observational studies. Aging Male. 2020;23(5):1416–24.
10. Nannoni S, de Groot R, Bell S, Markus HS. Stroke in COVID-19: a systematic review and meta-analysis. Int J Stroke. 2021;16(2):137–49.
11. Rashedi J, Mahdavi Poor B, Asgharzadeh V, Pourostadi M, Samadi Kafil H, Vegari A, Tayebi-Khosroshahi H, Asgharzadeh M. Risk factors for COVID-19. Infez Med. 2020;28(4):469–74.
12. Lersy F, Benotmane I, Helms J, Collange O, Schenck M, Brisset J-C, Chammas A, Willaume T, Lefebvre N, Solis M, Hansmann Y, Fabacher T, Caillard S, Mertes PM, Pottecher J, Schneider F, Meziani F, Fafi-Kremer S, Kremer S. Cerebrospinal fluid features in patients with coronavirus disease 2019 and neurological manifestations: correlation with brain magnetic resonance imaging findings in 58 patients. J Infect Dis. 2021;223(4):600–9.
13. Tan Y-K, Goh C, Leow AST, Tambyah PA, Ang A, Yap E-S, Tu T-M, Sharma VK, Yeo LLL, Chan BPL, Tan BYQ. COVID-19 and ischemic stroke: a systematic review and meta-summary of the literature. J Thromb Thrombolysis. 2020;50(3):587–95.
14. Varga Z, Flammer AJ, Steiger P, Haberecker M, Andermatt R, Zinkernagel AS, Mehra MR, Schuepbach RA, Ruschitzka F, Moch H. Endothelial cell infection and endotheliitis in COVID-19. Lancet (London, England). 2020;395(10234):1417–8.
15. Wang H, Tang X, Fan H, Luo Y, Song Y, Xu Y, Chen Y. Potential mechanisms of hemorrhagic stroke in elderly COVID-19 patients. Aging. 2020;12(11):10022–34.
16. Pilato F, Profice P, Dileone M, Ranieri F, Capone F, Minicuci G, Tagliente D, Florio L, Di Iorio R, Plantone D, Tonali PA, Di Lazzaro V. Stroke in critically ill patients. Minerva Anestesiol. 2009;75(5):245–50.
17. Chavda V, Chaurasia B, Fiorindi A, Umana GE, Lu B, Montemurro N. Ischemic stroke and SARS-CoV-2 infection: the bidirectional pathology and risk morbidities. Neurol Int. 2022;14(2):391–405.
18. Escher R, Breakey N, Lämmle B. Severe COVID-19 infection associated with endothelial activation. Thromb Res. 2020;190:62.

19. Gu SX, Tyagi T, Jain K, Gu VW, Lee SH, Hwa JM, Kwan JM, Krause DS, Lee AI, Halene S, Martin KA, Chun HJ, Hwa J. Thrombocytopathy and endotheliopathy: crucial contributors to COVID-19 thromboinflammation. Nat Rev Cardiol. 2021;18(3):194–209.

20. Huang C, Wang Y, Li X, Ren L, Zhao J, Hu Y, Zhang L, Fan G, Xu J, Gu X, Cheng Z, Yu T, Xia J, Wei Y, Wu W, Xie X, Yin W, Li H, Liu M, et al. Clinical features of patients infected with 2019 novel coronavirus in Wuhan, China. Lancet (London, England). 2020;395(10223):497–506.

21. Katz JM, Libman RB, Wang JJ, Filippi CG, Sanelli P, Zlochower A, Gribko M, Pacia SV, Kuzniecky RI, Najjar S, Azhar S. COVID-19 severity and stroke: correlation of imaging and laboratory markers. AJNR Am J Neuroradiol. 2021;42(2):257–61.

22. Davidson SJ. Inflammation and acute phase proteins in haemostasis. In: Janciauskiene S, editor. Acute phase proteins. InTech; 2013.

23. Mantovani A, Garlanda C. Humoral innate immunity and acute-phase proteins. N Engl J Med. 2023;388(5):439–52.

24. Benjamin LA, Paterson RW, Moll R, Pericleous C, Brown R, Mehta PR, Athauda D, Ziff OJ, Heaney J, Checkley AM, Houlihan CF, Chou M, Heslegrave AJ, Chandratheva A, Michael BD, Blennow K, Vivekanandam V, Foulkes A, Mummery CJ, et al. Antiphospholipid antibodies and neurological manifestations in acute COVID-19: a single-centre cross-sectional study. EClinicalMedicine. 2021;39:101070.

25. McAlpine LS, Zubair AS, Maran I, Chojecka P, Lleva P, Jasne AS, Navaratnam D, Matouk C, Schindler J, Sheth KN, Chun H, Lee AI, Spudich S, Sharma R, Sansing LH. Ischemic stroke, inflammation, and endotheliopathy in COVID-19 patients. Stroke. 2021;52(6):e233–8.

26. Spence JD, de Freitas GR, Pettigrew LC, Ay H, Liebeskind DS, Kase CS, Del Brutto OH, Hankey GJ, Venketasubramanian N. Mechanisms of stroke in COVID-19. Cerebrovasc Dis (Basel, Switzerland). 2020;49(4):451–8.

27. Yeahia R, Schefflein J, Chiarolanzio P, Rozenstein A, Gomes W, Ali S, Mehta H, Al-Mufti F, McClelland A, Gulko E. Brain MRI findings in COVID-19 patients with PRES: a systematic review. Clin Imaging. 2022;81:107–13.

28. Zhang S, Liu Y, Wang X, Yang L, Li H, Wang Y, Liu M, Zhao X, Xie Y, Yang Y, Zhang S, Fan Z, Dong J, Yuan Z, Ding Z, Zhang Y, Hu L. SARS-CoV-2 binds platelet ACE2 to enhance thrombosis in COVID-19. J Hematol Oncol. 2020;13(1):120.

29. Patone M, Mei XW, Handunnetthi L, Dixon S, Zaccardi F, Shankar-Hari M, Watkinson P, Khunti K, Harnden A, Coupland CAC, Channon KM, Mills NL, Sheikh A, Hippisley-Cox J. Risks of myocarditis, pericarditis, and cardiac arrhythmias associated with COVID-19 vaccination or SARS-CoV-2 infection. Nat Med. 2022;28(2):410–22.

30. Mele D, Flamigni F, Rapezzi C, Ferrari R. Myocarditis in COVID-19 patients: current problems. Intern Emerg Med. 2021;16(5):1123–9.

31. Yaghi S, Ishida K, Torres J, Mac Grory B, Raz E, Humbert K, Henninger N, Trivedi T, Lillemoe K, Alam S, Sanger M, Kim S, Scher E, Dehkharghani S, Wachs M, Tanweer O, Volpicelli F, Bosworth B, Lord A, Frontera J. SARS-CoV-2 and stroke in a New York healthcare system. Stroke. 2020;51(7):2002–11.

32. Sharifian-Dorche M, Bahmanyar M, Sharifian-Dorche A, Mohammadi P, Nomovi M, Mowla A. Vaccine-induced immune thrombotic thrombocytopenia and cerebral venous sinus thrombosis post COVID-19 vaccination; a systematic review. J Neurol Sci. 2021;428:117607.

33. CDC. Janssen (Johnson & Johnson) COVID-19 vaccine. Administration overview for Johnson & Johnson's Janssen COVID-19 vaccine. CDC; 2023. https://www.cdc.gov/vaccines/covid-19/info-by-product/janssen/index.html. Accessed 8 Aug 2023.

34. European Medicines Agency. COVID-19 medicines. 2024. https://www.ema.europa.eu/en/human-regulatory/overview/public-health-threats/coronavirus-disease-covid-19/covid-19-medicines. Accessed 8 Aug 2023.

35. Jarius S, Pache F, Körtvelyessy P, Jelčić I, Stettner M, Franciotta D, Keller E, Neumann B, Ringelstein M, Senel M, Regeniter A, Kalantzis R, Willms JF, Berthele A, Busch M, Capobianco M, Eisele A, Reichen I, Dersch R, et al. Cerebrospinal fluid findings in COVID-19: a multi-center study of 150 lumbar punctures in 127 patients. J Neuroinflammation. 2022;19(1):19.

36. Shakil SS, Emmons-Bell S, Rutan C, Walchok J, Navi B, Sharma R, Sheth K, Roth GA, Elkind MSV. Stroke among patients hospitalized with COVID-19: results from the American Heart Association COVID-19 Cardiovascular Disease Registry. Stroke. 2022;53(3):800–7.
37. Li P, Lee Y, Jehangir Q, Lin C-H, Krishnamoorthy G, Sule AA, Halabi AR, Patel K, Poisson L, Nair GB. SARS-COV-ATE risk assessment model for arterial thromboembolism in COVID-19. Sci Rep. 2022;12(1):16176.
38. Oates CP, Bienstock SW, Miller M, Giustino G, Danilov T, Kukar N, Kocovic N, Sperling D, Singh R, Benhuri D, Beerkens F, Camaj A, Lerakis S, Croft L, Stein LK, Goldman ME. Using clinical and echocardiographic characteristics to characterize the risk of ischemic stroke in patients with COVID-19. J Stroke Cerebrovasc Dis. 2022;31(2):106217.
39. Schwartzmann Y, Leker RR, Filioglo A, Molad J, Cohen JE, Honig A. Covid-19 associated free hanging clots in acute symptomatic carotid stenosis. J Neurol Sci. 2023;444:120515.
40. Khosravani H, Rajendram P, Notario L, Chapman MG, Menon BK. Protected code stroke: hyperacute stroke management during the coronavirus disease 2019 (COVID-19) pandemic. Stroke. 2020;51(6):1891–5.
41. Styczen H, Maus V, Goertz L, Köhrmann M, Kleinschnitz C, Fischer S, Möhlenbruch M, Mühlen I, Kallmünzer B, Dorn F, Lakghomi A, Gawlitza M, Kaiser D, Klisch J, Lobsien D, Rohde S, Ellrichmann G, Behme D, Thormann M, et al. Mechanical thrombectomy for acute ischemic stroke in COVID-19 patients: multicenter experience in 111 cases. J Neurointerv Surg. 2022;14(9):858–62.
42. Xie Y, Xu E, Bowe B, Al-Aly Z. Long-term cardiovascular outcomes of COVID-19. Nat Med. 2022;28(3):583–90.
43. Abootalebi S, Aertker BM, Andalibi MS, Asdaghi N, Aykac O, Azarpazhooh MR, Bahit MC, Barlinn K, Basri H, Shahripour RB, Bersano A, Biller J, Borhani-Haghighi A, Brown RD, Campbell BC, Cruz-Flores S, De Silva DA, Di Napoli M, Divani AA, et al. Call to action: SARS-CoV-2 and CerebrovAscular DisordErs (CASCADE). J Stroke Cerebrovasc Dis. 2020;29(9):104938.
44. UpToDate, Inc. Lexicomp online, pediatric and neonatal lexi-drugs online [database]. 2021. https://online.lexi.com. https://doi.org/10.1016/S0140-6736(20)30937-5. Accessed 8 Aug 2023.
45. Fragkou PC, Palaiodimou L, Stefanou MI, Katsanos AH, Lambadiari V, Paraskevis D, Andreadou E, Dimopoulou D, Zompola C, Ferentinos P, Vassilakopoulos TI, Kotanidou A, Sfikakis PP, Tsiodras S, Tsivgoulis G. Effects of low molecular weight heparin and fondaparinux on mortality, hemorrhagic and thrombotic complications in COVID-19 patients. Ther Adv Neurol Disord. 2022;15:17562864221099472.

Vasculitis

25

Ryan L. Orie, Islam Zaydan, and Hardik P. Amin

Introduction

Vasculitis is a rare condition that is often difficult to understand and describe. In essence, it combines "vascular" (blood vessels) and "itis," implying inflammation, so vasculitis is considered inflammation of the blood vessels. Inflammation damages the arterial walls, changing their appearance. Therefore, on imaging, vasculitis leads to an abnormal appearance of blood vessels and can lead to hemorrhage or occlusion and ischemia [1].

Vasculitis can occur spontaneously (primary vasculitis) or in the context of another illness (secondary vasculitis). There are a variety of ways to describe vasculitides, either based on organ involvement or vessel involvement, but we will try to keep things simple for now and focus on central nervous system (CNS) vasculitis [2, 3].

R. L. Orie
University of Pittsburgh Medical Center, Pittsburgh, PA, USA
e-mail: orierl@upmc.edu

I. Zaydan (✉)
Neurology and Ophthalmology, University of Pittsburgh Medical Center, Pittsburgh, PA, USA
e-mail: islam.zaydan@va.gov

H. P. Amin
Neurology, Hartford Hospital, Hartford, CT, USA
e-mail: hardik.amin@hhchealth.org

© The Author(s), under exclusive license to Springer Nature Switzerland AG 2024
H. P. Amin (ed.), *Stroke for the Advanced Practice Clinician*,
https://doi.org/10.1007/978-3-031-66289-8_25

When to Consider Vasculitis

Compared to other mechanisms of stroke, both primary and secondary forms of CNS Vasculitis are rare and difficult to diagnose due to the lack of widespread recognition of the disease. The median age of onset is approximately 50 years, with males more commonly affected, but it can affect at any age. The clinical presentation is highly variable, but a typical patient would be a younger patient with some "prodrome" (heralding symptoms) before actually developing stroke symptoms. The most common prodromal symptom is headache. Headache is not common in most cases of acute ischemic stroke unless there is a dissection, so the presence of a headache should raise a concern for the inflammatory process (Table 25.1). Patients may also report confusion, disorientation, or seizures. Systemic prodromal symptoms may include weight loss, night sweats, fevers, and skin rash.

Vessel imaging with CTA or MRA may demonstrate multifocal irregular, tortuous, or kinked-appearing vessels. MRI can demonstrate strokes in various vascular territories of varying ages.

Differential Diagnosis Any time you see abnormal vessels (vasculopathy), you should determine whether you think the underlying process is inflammatory or noninflammatory.

See Chap. 26 for a more in-depth review of *noninflammatory* conditions. In brief, noninflammatory conditions with irregular appearing intracranial vessels include intracranial atherosclerosis (which can also lead to irregular, kinked, or tortuous intracranial vessels, but no prodrome since it is non-inflammatory) and Reversible Cerebral Vasoconstriction Syndrome (which presents with a sudden thunderclap headache similar to subarachnoid hemorrhage, but on CT you will see irregular vessels, with focal stroke symptoms). A sudden, thunderclap headache is unusual for vasculitis. Vasculitis usually has unrelenting, progressive headaches for days or weeks.

Now, we will review two forms of primary brain vasculitis you should be familiar with.

Table 25.1 Features suggesting vasculitis

- Cerebral ischemia in different vascular territories, usually separated by time
- Cerebral ischemia in young patients lacking cerebrovascular risk factors
- Unexplained headache or other prodromal symptoms, perhaps altered sensorium or cognitive changes
- Unexplained focal and diffuse neurologic dysfunction

Primary CNS Vasculitis Also called Primary Angiitis of the Central Nervous System (PACNS). This condition is restricted to the CNS and not associated with other systemic illnesses. Brain vessel imaging with CTA, MRA, or digital subtraction angiography will demonstrate multifocal areas of stenosis, representing inflammation of small and medium-sized vessels. A higher level of imaging called vessel wall imaging (not available in most places) may help differentiate inflammation vs atherosclerosis, although this is still being studied. MRI of brain (with contrast) can show multifocal strokes of various sizes in multiple territories and enhancement within the stroke and the meninges. Spinal fluid analysis will show elevated protein and white blood cell count. A leptomeningeal biopsy (the definitive diagnostic test) will demonstrate that inflammatory infiltrates have entered the blood vessels. Notably, serum inflammatory markers (Erythrocyte Sedimentation Rate (ESR), C-reactive protein (CRP)) are not elevated because they are in the serum, and the disease is restricted to the CNS.

Amyloid Beta-Related Angiitis (ABRA) Consider this the angry cousin of cerebral amyloid angiopathy (CAA). CAA, discussed in Chap. 28, is a noninflammatory condition localized to the brain, characterized by the deposition of abnormal $\alpha\beta$ protein in the walls of blood vessels. This leads to fragile blood vessel walls in and around the brain, the accumulation of cortical microbleeds (CMB), and increases the risk of spontaneous lobar hemorrhages. In some patients, those abnormal protein deposits trigger an immune response and a cascade of events thereafter. Both CAA and ABRA have CMB and a higher risk of ICH. In CAA, an ICH will occur without warning, whereas with ABRA, patients may have unrelenting headaches before an ICH, dramatic cognitive or behavioral changes, or seizures. MRI will show the typical CMB and perhaps lobar hemorrhage, but what separates it from CAA is the presence of significant, asymmetric, white matter FLAIR changes representing inflammation and edema, typically in the symptomatic areas of the brain. You will not see much edema in traditional non-inflammatory CAA. While lumbar puncture is often performed, no standard Cerebrospinal fluid (CSF) profile is used to diagnose ABRA. Clinical and radiographic criteria primarily make the diagnosis, and the confirmation test is a follow-up MRI after several months of steroids that shows the resolution of the FLAIR changes. Despite resolution, though, ABRA episodes can recur and are associated with a poor prognosis overall.

Clinical Vignette

81-Year-old male who presented to the hospital with whole-body convulsions, incontinence, and tongue bite suggestive of new-onset seizure activity. MRI revealed confluent T2 FLAIR signal abnormality involving the white matter of R cerebral hemisphere (a), with microhemorrhages surrounding the vessels (b). MRA was negative for underlying vascular lesion. He was started on IV solumedrol for 5 days, followed by oral prednisone 60 mg daily and Keppra for seizure control. A repeat MRI 2 months later demonstrated significant improvement in the FLAIR abnormalities (c) and stable microhemorrhages (d) making inflammatory CAA the most likely diagnosis.

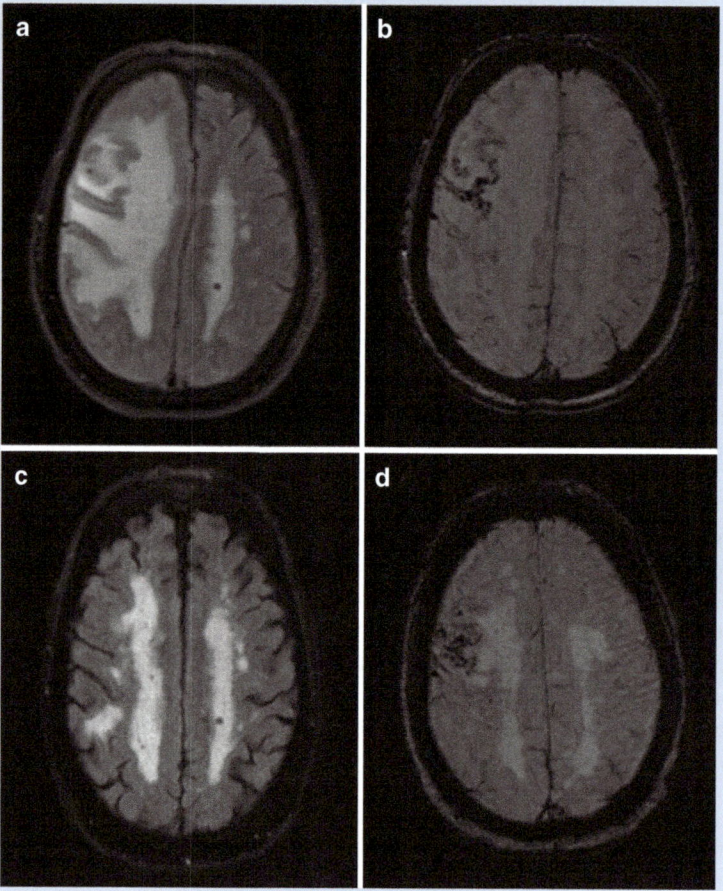

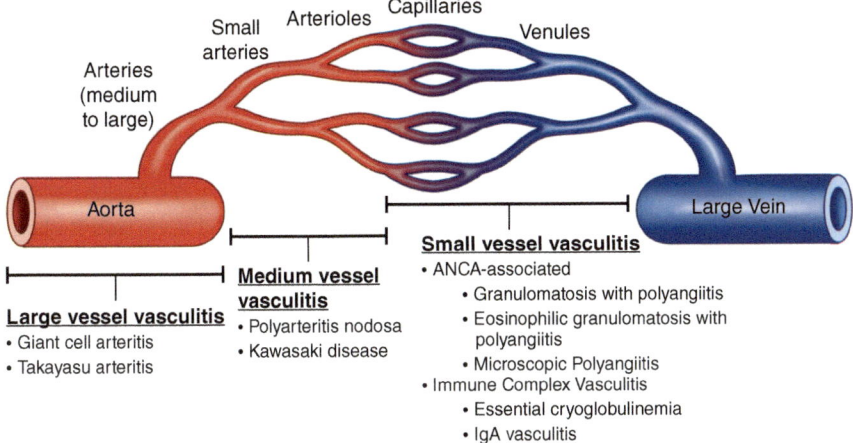

Fig. 25.1 Flow of blood: from the heart, blood flows into the aorta, large arteries (carotids, larger proximal intracranial vessels, large muscular arteries in the body), medium arteries, small vessels (small arteries, arterioles, capillaries, venules), and finally, large draining veins. Notice the transition from red to blue as oxygenated blood (red) becomes deoxygenated (blue) as it enters the venous system

Now, let us discuss vasculitides associated with systemic conditions. Strokes are less common in this group (certainly not as a first manifestation), but they are still worth knowing since patients with established diagnoses may present with stroke. They are typically organized by the type of blood vessels they affect (small, medium, or large). This is not an exhaustive list, but we will highlight some more commonly known conditions. Recall that blood flows from arteries to veins, with gradually shrinking branches between, as seen in Fig. 25.1.

Large Artery Vasculitis

Giant cell (Temporal) arteritis (GCA) is a large vessel vasculitis typically affecting the extracranial vessels of the head and neck and, less commonly, intracranial vessels. It affects older patients in their 70s or above (rarely less than 50) and women more than men. There is a strong association between GCA and polymyalgia rheumatica.

The most common form is temporal arteritis involving the superficial temporal artery, a branch of the external carotid artery. Patients present with headaches and vision loss. Other symptoms indicating soft tissue ischemia of the head include jaw claudication (jaw fatigue and pain with chewing), tongue claudication, and occasionally tongue infarctions. Asking the patient to chew gum (one chew per second) for a few minutes should elicit symptoms (immediate pain on chewing suggests possibly a dental issue). Palpation of the superficial temporal artery with GCA should demonstrate an artery that does not compress but instead feels like a "firm cord," as described by C. Miller Fisher.

Labs are notable for an elevated erythrocyte sedimentation rate (usually >50 mm/h). GCA should be confirmed with a temporal artery biopsy (unilateral or bilateral), if suspected. Still, even a biopsy can be negative in true GCA cases, if the sample is too short or does not include an affected segment. Biopsy, therefore, should not delay immediate treatment with steroids if GCA is suspected. Delayed or untreated GCA can result in CNS and systemic ischemia, with permanent vision loss, aortitis, arm claudication, and gangrene.

Takayasu arteritis is a large vessel vasculitis affecting the aorta and its large branches, leading to progressive large vessel occlusive disease. It primarily affects women between 10 and 40 and can be considered the "younger" version of GCA. Fatigue, weight loss, and fevers are common presenting symptoms, followed by muscle and joint pain. Orthostatic changes, hypertension, and atypical chest pain are common due to aortic involvement. The hallmark findings are absent or weak peripheral pulses (which is why it has been called the "pulseless disease"), often asymmetric between limbs. Imaging of the vasculature by MRA, CTA, or conventional angiogram will demonstrate smooth tapering of large vessels.

Medium Artery Vasculitis

Polyarteritis nodosa (PAN) is a necrotizing type of vasculitis, which means it actually leads to necrosis and death of the cell wall. PAN affects small and medium-sized arteries typically associated with infections (hepatitis B or C), also reported with connective tissue diseases, especially rheumatoid arthritis. Specific symptoms could include new onset (typically profound) hypertension, a distinct reddish purple, net-like skin pattern called livedo reticularis, or renal failure. The most common symptoms, however, include fatigue, weight loss, fever, and joint pains.

Kawasaki disease is more common in infants and children <4 years old, Kawasaki disease presents with conjunctival injection, erythema of the palms and soles, rash, a swollen red "strawberry" tongue, and fever. It can also affect the coronary arteries, making it one of the leading causes of acquired heart disease in kids in Japan and the USA. Diagnosis is usually made by tissue biopsy.

Small Vessel Vasculitis

Antineutrophil cytoplasmic antibodies (ANCA) are autoimmune antibodies that target neutrophils (normal white blood cells that fight infection). P-ANCA and C-ANCA are two different groups of antibodies that target different proteins. The presence of these antibodies can indicate certain types of vasculitides.

- **Granulomatosis with polyangiitis**: A necrotizing vasculitis affecting small and medium-sized blood vessels. Its hallmark is necrotizing granulomas in the upper and lower respiratory tract (seen on chest X-ray) and kidneys, leading to shortness of breath, hematuria, rash, and joint pains. 95% of these patients will be c-ANCA positive. Formerly called Wegener's granulomatosis, the name change was largely prompted following the discovery of Wegener's Nazi associations.

- **Eosinophilic granulomatosis with polyangiitis**: Another necrotizing vasculitis affecting small and medium vessels, but this one is more often seen in patients with a history of airway allergic hypersensitivity, asthma, sinusitis, and rash. It is p-ANCA positive, and as suggested by the name, abnormally high numbers of eosinophils on WBC testing. It was formerly called Churg-Strauss syndrome.
- **Microscopic polyangiitis**: A necrotizing vasculitis (see a theme?) affecting capillaries and venules. It is mainly associated with kidney disease, skin changes, and neuropathy, among other constitutional symptoms.

Immune complexes are adjoined pairs of antibodies and antigens, often seen with a hypersensitivity response, systemic lupus erythematosus, and rheumatoid arthritis. They form in the circulation and deposit into blood vessel walls, joints, and tissues, leading to inflammation.

- **Essential cryoglobulinemia**: Cryoglobulins are proteins that normally circulate in the serum and are typically a combination of immunoglobulins and complement components (immune complexes). In healthy individuals, cryoglobulins are present at lower levels but can be seen at much higher levels in patients with hematological disorders or hepatitis. In an autoimmune response, these immune complexes deposit in the blood vessels, leading to hyperviscosity (thicker blood) and organ damage. 90% of cryoglobulinemia vasculitis is associated with Hepatitis C infections, but is also associated with Hepatitis B, HIV, and other autoimmune conditions like Systemic Lupus Erythematosus (SLE) and Sjogren's syndrome.
- **IgA vasculitis (Henoch-Shonlein Purpura)**: Deposition of IgA immune complexes into the skin and GI tract leads to a purpura-type rash and abdominal symptoms. CNS manifestations occur with severe disease, including ischemic stroke, venous thrombosis, seizure, and hemorrhage.

Other Triggers for Vasculitis

Inflammatory bowel diseases like ulcerative colitis (UC) flares are associated with systemic inflammation and vasculitis. UC patients are at a three to four-fold increased risk of thromboembolism. They are also at risk of elevated homocysteine levels due to malabsorption, which can cause further endothelial injury.

Drug-induced vasculitis: Commonly associated with chronic use of CNS stimulants (cocaine, amphetamines) as well as the use of heroin.

Infectious vasculitis: It can be seen in the broader context of bacterial, viral, or fungal meningitis, which leads to inflammation of the subarachnoid space, which in turn leads to vessel inflammation and occlusion. Singles (varicella-zoster virus, VZV) eruption in the face is also associated with a delayed VZV vasculopathy that can occur 2–6 weeks later as the virus infiltrates the trigeminal nerve and gains access to the arterial wall.

Diagnosis

Diagnostic criteria for CNS vasculitis have been proposed but not validated, given the rarity of the disease. Criteria should include a clinical history of neurological deficits with a prodrome, neurological and physical exam including ophthalmologic, musculoskeletal, skin, and cardiac, imaging with multifocal strokes without any other attributable cause, and ancillary testing suggesting an underlying inflammatory process [4].

Lab studies for inflammatory markers and acute phase reactants such as ESR, C-reactive protein, Antinuclear Antibodies (ANA), and ANCA can identify systemic vasculitis or inflammatory process, but recall that serum markers are generally normal in patients with primary CNS vasculitis. Infectious etiology should be ruled out with the appropriate cultures, serology, and molecular testing (Fig. 25.2). Cerebrospinal fluid (CSF) evaluation by lumbar puncture is critical to rule out CNS vasculitis and infection. CSF panels in patients with vasculitis will usually demonstrate lymphocytic pleocytosis (elevated white blood cells with lymphocyte

Labs for suspected CNS vasculitis

CBC	RVVT
UA	Protein C/S
Urine/Serum tox	Prothrombin mt
LFT's	Anti-cardiolipin
CK	Beta-2 glycoprotein
ESR	Factor V Leiden
CRP	Mixing studies
Rheumatoid factor	Complement 3/4
ANA	ACE
SPEP	PPD
ANCA	
ENA	
Anti-SSA (Ro)	
Anti-SSB (La)	
Anti-RNP	
Anti-Sm	
Anti-Scl-70	
Anti-Jo-1	
Anti-DS DNA	
Anti-Histone	
Hepatitis panel	
HIV	
Cryoglobulins	
Lyme titer	

Fig. 25.2 Vasculitis labs

Table 25.2 CSF values for inflammatory and infectious processes

	Appearance	Opening pressure (mmHg)	WBCs (μL)	Protein (mg/dL)	Glucose (mg/dL)
Normal	Clear	Normal	<5	15–45	40–70
Vasculitis	Clear		Elevated, lymphocyte predominance	Elevated	Normal
Viral meningitis	Clear	Normal	Elevated but <300 lymphocyte predominance	Elevated but <200	Normal
Bacterial meningitis	Turbid	Elevated	>1000–2000	>200	Low (<40)
Fungal meningitis	Clear	Normal–elevated	Elevated but <500	>200	Normal–low

predominance) and elevated protein with normal glucose. Patients with CNS infections often have elevated WBC count with neutrophil predominance and elevated opening pressure (Table 25.2) [5]. No lab tests will diagnose PACNS. Additional labs to consider sending are outlined in Fig. 25.2.

Brain and vessel imaging are helpful in the evaluation. Imaging findings suggestive of CNS vasculitis include multifocal strokes of varying size and age (usually smaller), leptomeningeal enhancement, stenoses or occlusions in multiple vessels, parenchymal hemorrhages, and rarely tumor-like lesions. Small vessel or microcirculation vasculitides may have normal vessel imaging, however. Those cases universally required histologic confirmation [6].

In addition to the detailed evaluation, all patients with presumed CNS vasculitis presenting with ischemic manifestation should undergo routine stroke evaluation with echocardiogram, stroke risk stratification (diabetes, lipids, EKG, etc.), cardiac monitoring, and toxic and metabolic etiologies.

Brain and leptomeningeal biopsy, while considered the gold standard for diagnosing CNS vasculitis, has limited sensitivity and up to 25% false-negative rates [7]. However, it can serve a very important role in ruling out mimics and secondary causes of vasculitis. Special stains and cultures, as well as a review by a pathologist, should be performed.

Treatment

No controlled, randomized, prospective studies are available to guide therapeutic decision making for primary CNS vasculitis. Retrospective observational studies and expert opinion form the basis of treatment guidelines. The mainstay of treatment is using glucocorticoids as a monotherapy or in combination with immune suppression such as cyclophosphamide. Treatment should be initiated with the guidance of neurology/immunology and, for systemic conditions, rheumatology. Typically, glucocorticoids are started at a higher dose of 1 mg/kg and tapered over months, depending on the response and the severity of the neurologic symptoms.

Other immunosuppression agents may be added in cases of severe neurologic symptoms or as a steroid-sparing agent. If immunosuppression is used, whether orally or intravenously, close monitoring of the renal, liver, and bone marrow function and prophylaxis against opportunistic infections should be incorporated into the treatment plan. Cyclophosphamide is typically used between 3 and 6 months and stopped if there is no evidence of clinical or radiographic progression of the disease.

Response to treatment is variable, but in a French Cohort of patients with primary vasculitis of the CNS (PVCNS), 95% of cases had improved survival with (remission after initial immunosuppressive induction treatment and prolonged remission without relapse in two-thirds after a mean of 57 months follow-up [8].

Follow-Up

Patients should be closely followed in a stroke or neuro-immunology clinic, and a rheumatology clinic if systemic conditions are present.

Assessment of disease activity, as a patient's course evolves, is an ongoing challenge for clinicians following patients with CNS vasculitis. Patients may have a recurrence or a progressive disease or may only experience a monophasic (one-time) bout of vasculitis. While a monophasic course is ideal, many of these patients have residual neurologic deficits, including cognitive symptoms. Monitoring for new neurological symptoms, paired with serial brain imaging with MRI for new parenchymal lesions or leptomeningeal enhancement, can be very helpful in following patients with CNS vasculitis.

Abnormal vasculature might not resolve completely, so routine vessel imaging without new symptoms is of little utility. Serial lumbar punctures and CSF analysis might demonstrate improvement in patients undergoing therapy, but this has not been confirmed in the large-scale series.

Clinical Pearls
- Vasculitis typically presents younger patients with prodromal symptoms, most often headaches, and strokes in multiple distributions.
- CSF analysis can help confirm inflammation with elevated white blood cell count and protein.
- Leptomeningeal biopsy is the gold standard for diagnosing vasculitis.
- Treatment typically requires a long duration of steroids, possibly in combination with immune suppression therapy.

References

1. Younger DS. Epidemiology of neurovasculitis. Neurol Clin. 2016;34:887–917.
2. Younger DS. Epidemiology of the vasculitides. Neurol Clin. 2019;37:201–17.

3. de Boysson H, et al. Primary angiitis of the central nervous system. Arthritis Rheum. 2012;64:1665.
4. Ho M-L. Neuroradiology signs. McGraw Hale Education; 2014.
5. Calabrese LH, et al. Primary angiitis of the CNS: diagnostic criteria and clinical approach. Cleve Clin J Med. 1992;59:293.
6. Russo RAG, et al. Takayasu arteritis. Front Pediatr. 2018;6:265.
7. Chen SH, et al. Utility of diagnostic cerebral angiography in the management of suspected central nervous system vasculitis. J Clin Neurosci. 2019;64:98–100.
8. Newman W, Wolf A. Noninfectious granulomatous angiitis involving the central nervous system. Trans Am Neurol Assoc. 1952;56:114.

Noninflammatory Vasculopathies

26

Nicole Veltri and Hardik P. Amin

Cerebral Dysautoregulation Syndromes: RCVS and PRES

Reversible Cerebral Vasoconstriction Syndrome (RCVS)

Vasculopathies can be due to structural changes or fluctuations in blood pressures (Table 26.1). Cerebral autoregulation is the ability of the intracranial blood vessels to dilate or constrict in response to fluctuations in systemic blood pressure to maintain normal blood flow. In normal circumstances, drops in blood pressure lead to vaso*dilation* of the brain vasculature (larger vessel diameter means more blood is delivered), and elevations in pressure lead to vaso*constriction* (smaller diameter because high pressures need less blood flow). To recap: drop in pressure → wider lumen, rise in pressure → smaller lumen. Autoregulation, therefore, allows people to keep humming along without noticing these changes in pressure. However, this dynamic process only occurs if the BP stays within a specific range (autoregulatory threshold). If BP falls below the lower limit of the threshold, insufficient blood flow reaches the brain, leading to ischemia. If BP exceeds the threshold, dysregulation leads to vasospasm, RCVS/PRES, edema, and hemorrhage (Table 26.1).

RCVS is an acute condition that involves the abrupt narrowing of one or more cerebral vessels due to dysregulated increased pressure in the cerebral vasculature. The classic clinical presentation is a sudden "thunderclap" headache, which can be accompanied by focal neurological deficits due to ischemia. Given the headache, the differential diagnosis also includes aneurysmal subarachnoid or intracerebral

N. Veltri
Yale New Haven Hospital, New Haven, CT, USA
e-mail: Nicole.veltri@yale.edu

H. P. Amin (✉)
Neurology, Hartford Hospital, Hartford, CT, USA
e-mail: hardik.amin@hhchealth.org

Table 26.1 Noninflammatory vasculopathies

Noninflammatory vasculopathies	Clinical features	Imaging
Atherosclerosis	Classic stroke symptoms	Calcified and noncalcified plaque in large vessels Irregular appearing intracranial vessels
Arterial dissection	Headache, Horner syndrome Marfan syndrome, Ehlers Danlos Trauma, neck manipulation, or high-pressure maneuvers (vomiting, coughing)	Abrupt tapering, flame shape lesion Intraluminal flap Intramural hematoma
Fibromuscular dysplasia	Headache	Beading of cervical carotids
Moyamoya disease and syndrome	Known genetic syndrome (MMS), hyperventilation	Severe stenosis of distal ICA, proximal MCA, ACA Unilateral or bilateral
Vasospasm	Headache Post SAH Recent intravascular procedure	Transcranial Dopplers with elevated velocities
Cerebral amyloid angiopathy	Cognitive symptoms	Lobar hemorrhage MRI-SWI with cerebral microhemorrhages or superficial siderosis
CADASIL	Cognitive, psychiatric symptoms, stroke at early age Migraines Family history of early strokes	Diffuse symmetric bilateral FLAIR white matter changes, lacunar infarcts FLAIR hyperintensities in anterior temporal lobes and external capsules
Posterior reversible encephalopathy syndrome	Encephalopathy, seizure Hypertension	Cerebral edema in one or more hemispheres
Reversible cerebral vasoconstriction syndrome	Thunderclap headache Vasoactive substances/ medications	Abrupt stenosis of otherwise normal-looking vessel(s)
Sickle cell disease	Many strokes can be silent	Moyamoya type vasculopathy

MMS Moyamoya syndrome, *ICA* internal carotid artery, *MCA* middle cerebral artery, *ACA* anterior cerebral artery, *SAH* subarachnoid hemorrhage, *MRI-SWI* magnetic resonance imaging-susceptibility weighted imaging, *CADASIL* Cerebral Autosomal Dominant Arteriopathy with Subcortical Infarcts and Leukoencephalopathy, *FLAIR* fluid attenuated inversion recovery

hemorrhage, carotid dissection, or venous thrombosis. RCVS tends to affect females more than males and usually middle-aged patients.

Workup and Management

Patients present with the "worst headache of life." The initial diagnostic study should be a CT brain, which may appear normal, but has the potential to reveal hemorrhage or signs of ischemia. A CT angiogram (head and neck) done simultaneously should detect any narrowing (vasoconstriction) of cerebral vessels (or other vascular lesions) in one or more affected areas. Vasoconstriction leads to

Table 26.2 Triggers for RCVS and PRES

RCVS	PRES
Medications	Hypertension
• Selective serotonin reuptake inhibitors (SSRIs)	• Essential hypertension
	• Renal disease
• Serotonin-noradrenaline reuptake inhibitors (SNRIs)	• Drug withdrawal
	• Stimulants
• Triptans	Immuno/chemotherapy agents
• Tacrolimus	• Cyclosporin A, tacrolimus, sirolimus, methotrexate, interferon alpha, gemcitabine, cisplatin, bevacizumab, intravenous immunoglobulin, rituximab, vincristine
• Cyclophosphamide	
• Nicotine patches	
• Nasal decongestants	Pregnancy
Illicit drugs	• Eclampsia and preeclampsia
• Marijuana	Autoimmune disease
• Cocaine	• Systemic lupus erythematosus
• Ecstasy	• Thrombotic thrombocytopenic purpura
• Amphetamines	• Vasculitis
• Lysergic acid diethylamide (LSD)	Post-carotid endarterectomy
	Sepsis
Pregnancy	
• Eclampsia and preeclampsia	
Miscellaneous	
• Diet pills/caffeine	
• Licorice	
• Sexual activity	
• High altitude	
• Sudden cold water exposure	

hypoperfusion and puts patients at risk of ischemic stroke. Subarachnoid hemorrhage in RCVS is due to the rupture of small blood vessels along the brain's surface, but a ruptured intracranial aneurysm (a completely different disease and treatment) should certainly be ruled out.

Common triggers for RCVS include vasoactive medications, illicit drugs, and pregnancy (Table 26.2). Removal of the offending medication is necessary in the acute setting. Most patients who present with RCVS get a lumbar puncture to rule out evidence of inflammation, infection, or blood. CSF findings in RCVS are normal, whereas in vasculitis, CSF will demonstrate an increased white blood cell count and elevated protein. A formal diagnostic angiogram (DSA) could be obtained for more detailed visualization of the vessels and may help differentiate between RCVS, vasculitis, and intracranial atherosclerosis. Strokes can occur in both the posterior and anterior circulations. In RCVS of anterior circulation vessels, MRIs will often demonstrate borderzone (watershed) strokes instead of scattered or lacunar strokes seen in other conditions.

RCVS, for most patients, has a self-limiting course with a good prognosis. Headache control is the most common management issue. One can use NSAIDs, Tylenol, or more potent agents such as opioids, but do not give triptans or ergots since they are vasoconstrictors. Avoid steroids as they can worsen the condition [1]. In the case of severe preeclampsia or eclampsia, delivery of the fetus is typically warranted. Calcium channel blockers (CCBs) often treat vasoconstriction and may help with headaches. The typical course of CCBs is 3–6 months. Around that time, repeat imaging will demonstrate the resolution of the vasoconstriction seen on the initial scans. If vascular abnormalities persist, consider alternative diagnoses (intracranial atherosclerosis, vasculitis) because RCVS is, by name, reversible.

Counseling patients on avoiding triggers is critical, especially in cases of drug use. For patients taking antidepressants, consider other options such as tricyclics or bupropion. Since the risk of recurrence is low, SSRI and SNRI could be considered again if no other options are effective. Patients have been restarted on these agents without recurrence of RCVS.

Posterior Reversible Encephalopathy Syndrome (PRES)

PRES is an awkwardly named syndrome that involves headaches, confusion or altered sensorium, visual symptoms, and seizures in the setting of significantly elevated blood pressure. Symptoms can progress over several hours to days (unlike RCVS, which occurs more acutely). Typical triggers for PRES include uncontrolled hypertension, renal disease, immunotherapy, and some chemotherapies.

Workup and Management

A STAT CT scan is required, which can show evidence of edema in the bilateral parietooccipital lobes. Other areas of involvement include watershed (border-zone) areas, frontal, temporal, brainstem, and cerebellar regions. Symmetric, bilateral hyperintense FLAIR signal on MRI represents vasogenic edema in the affected areas. Other conditions with similar imaging findings include progressive multifocal leukoencephalopathy (PML), demyelinating disease, infection of the brain tissue (encephalitis), or infiltrative tumors. PRES can lead to ischemic stroke or hemorrhage in about 10–30% of patients, leading to lasting deficits. Hence the awkward name, as, it is neither always "posterior" nor "reversible." Vessel imaging does not typically show multifocal areas of constriction like RCVS, but more often, a single vessel with a segment of narrowing that accounts for the patient's symptoms. A lumbar puncture is typically normal since it is not an infectious or inflammatory process.

Management of PRES focuses on the treatment of hypertension and seizures, and severe cases require ICU level of care. Blood pressure should be reduced gradually, as rapid overcorrection can precipitate or worsen cerebral ischemia. In the case of severe preeclampsia or eclampsia, delivery of the fetus is typically warranted, and magnesium is used to treat seizures. EEG is indicated for patients with altered sensorium to evaluate for subclinical seizures. Management of ongoing seizures or status epilepticus should involve a seizure specialist.

Clinical Vignette 1: RCVS

HPI: 58-Year-old female with a history of anxiety presents with acute onset of severe headache and bilateral vision changes.

Exam: Blood pressure was elevated at 185/87, HR 88. On exam, she was awake but uncomfortable appearing due to a severe headache. She had a right lower quadrant field deficit, and her left visual fields appeared intact. Normal speech and strength.

Workup: Axial FLAIR image (a) shows T2 hyperintense lesions in the bilateral parieto-occipital and right frontal lobes. Time of flight MRA (b) showed multifocal areas of irregularity and narrowing (blue arrows). Urine toxicology was positive for cannabinoids. LP was normal. Serum inflammatory markers were normal.

Management: Given acute headache and urine tox positive for cannabinoids, a presumed diagnosis of RCVS was made. She was started on calcium channel blockers for headaches and advised to stop smoking marijuana. Headaches subsided over the next 2 months, and her vision improved but did not recover completely. Repeat CTA 3 months later showed resolution of her vasculopathy.

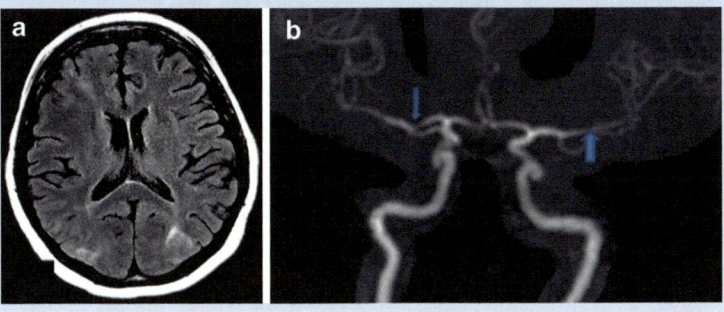

Prophylactic anti-seizure medication is typically not indicated if the patient has no seizure activity and has a normal EEG. Like RCVS, steroids may worsen the condition, so it is best to avoid them. In that same vein, treat hyperglycemia aggressively in both situations. If an immunotherapy or chemotherapy agent has been identified as a probable trigger, it should be held acutely, and consideration should be given to alternative treatments if possible.

Like RCVS, PRES is a self-limiting condition with a good prognosis (unless the patient suffers a stroke). Edema resolves in weeks with aggressive blood pressure and seizure control. To confirm resolution, a follow-up MRI should be performed within 1–3 months (Fig. 26.1). If the abnormal FLAIR signal persists, consider an alternative diagnosis.

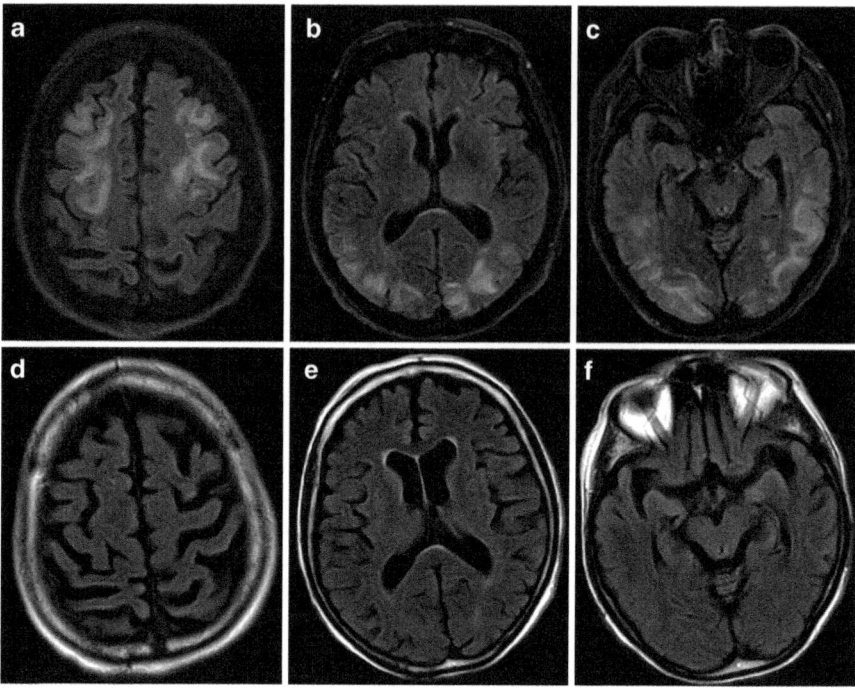

Fig. 26.1 Posterior reversible encephalopathy syndrome. MRI demonstrating FLAIR hyperintensities in bilateral frontal, temporal, and occipital lobes (**a–c**) representing edema. Repeat MRI 2 months later (**d–f**) reveals complete resolution of FLAIR hyperintensities. (Images courtesy of Dr. Ajay Malhotra)

Moyamoya Disease and Syndrome

Moyamoya is a vasculopathy characterized by progressive stenosis in very specific locations: the distal internal carotid artery (after it enters the head) and proximal middle and anterior cerebral arteries. It was first described in the Japanese population in the 1950s. Moyamoya means "puff of smoke" in Japanese, which you see on the angiogram representing the dilated lenticulostriate blood vessels. Why are they dilated? The lenticulostriate arteries branch off the middle cerebral artery and supply the basal ganglia. In Moyamoya, the stenosis is just before the lenticulostriate arteries branch off, cutting off not only their blood flow but also flow to the entire hemisphere. As a result, blood flow to the ipsilateral hemisphere is often redirected through collateral vessels, such as the external carotid artery (ECA) or posterior circulation. This retrograde blood flow enters the brain through small collateral vessels and eventually travels backwards through the lenticulostriates, leading to dilation. Instead of flowing in the normal direction from the MCA into the lenticulostriates to supply the basal ganglia, blood now flows in the opposite direction through the hypertrophied lenticulostriates and collateral vessels toward the affected hemisphere (Fig. 26.2).

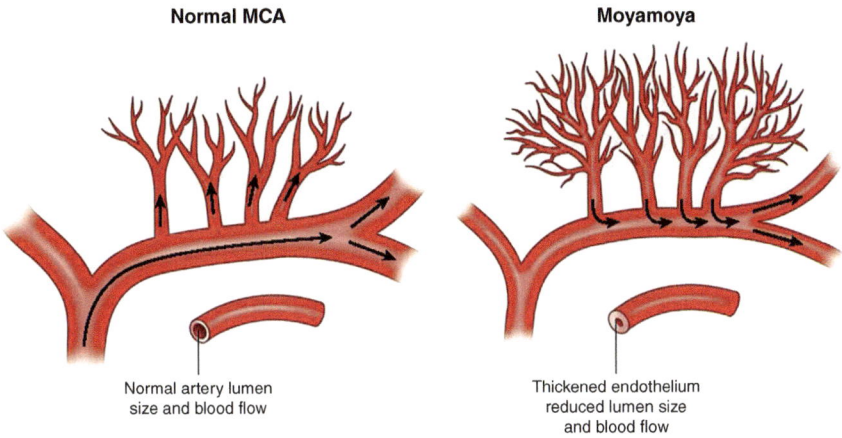

Fig. 26.2 Normal vs. Moyamoya vessels. Note the increased collateralization of the lenticulostriates in the Moyamoya vessels

How does Moyamoya happen? The etiology is not clear, but there are genetic elements. It is not atherosclerosis, but rather a thickening of the innermost layer of the vessel wall, the intima. Genetic conditions associated with Moyamoya vasculopathy include Neurofibromatosis 1, Trisomy 21, and Sickle cell anemia. If Moyamoya is associated with a known genetic condition, it is called Moyamoya *Syndrome*. If it is idiopathic (no associated condition), it is called Moyamoya *Disease*.

Moyamoya has a "bimodal" peak for symptom onset and is associated with both ischemic and hemorrhagic strokes. The first peak occurs in childhood, and the second peak in mid-life. One concept to remember is that hyperventilation leads to vasoconstriction of blood vessels in the brain. Therefore, hyperventilation during crying or running in children with Moyamoya can bring about stroke symptoms because it leads to hypoperfusion. Ischemia is more common during the first peak in children, and hemorrhage is more common during the second peak in adults.

A CT scan can demonstrate hemorrhage or ischemia, and a CT angiogram shows the classic pattern of stenosis described above. A diagnostic angiogram may be necessary to visualize the "puff of smoke" more clearly and better evaluate specific flow patterns. On MRI, one might see the "Ivy sign," a pattern of snakelike hyperintensities in the subarachnoid spaces representing engorged collateral vessels carrying extra blood supply towards the lenticulostriates.

Aspirin can be helpful for Moyamoya patients with symptoms related to ischemia, but the definitive treatment of Moyamoya involves surgical bypass of the areas of stenosis. The "direct" approach refers to a surgical procedure with a direct graft between the superficial temporal artery, which can be felt over the temples, and the middle cerebral artery downstream from the stenosis. The "indirect" approach involves trying to stimulate the growth of extra blood vessels by placing various types of tissue over the surface of the symptomatic hemisphere. Direct bypass is an immediate supply of extra blood flow to that hemisphere, whereas the indirect approach can take months or longer to develop. These procedures (described in an almost offensively simplistic manner) should only be performed by an experienced neurosurgeon specializing in neurovascular conditions.

Helpful consults: Neurosurgery and neurogenetics.

Fibromuscular Dysplasia (FMD)

FMD is a vasculopathy that leads to multifocal arterial stenosis and tortuosity. It is almost always diagnosed by imaging, with a classic "beading" pattern, like a string of pearls. Other patterns are also seen but are rare. It can affect the renal arteries, cervical carotid arteries, vertebral arteries, and iliac arteries.

Workup and Management

FMD might lead to stroke or TIA by several mechanisms. Patients may present with severe headaches, neck pain, tinnitus, TIA, or stroke. FMD may also be an incidental finding unrelated to the presenting symptoms. If the stenosis is severe enough, hypoperfusion could lead to ischemia. FMD is associated with carotid dissections, which lead to occlusions or thromboembolism. Aneurysms can also be seen in patients with FMD. A careful evaluation of the vessel is essential to rule out severe stenosis, dissection, and aneurysms. If there is an ipsilateral Horner syndrome (ptosis and miosis), there is a higher likelihood of an underlying internal carotid artery dissection.

CTA is preferred for FMD evaluation. MRA is an alternative but may miss milder cases. Invasive diagnostic angiograms are typically not performed because FMD usually does not require interventional treatment, except in cases of severe symptomatic stenosis or large aneurysms. The key differentiating factor between FMD and carotid atherosclerosis is that atherosclerosis typically develops at the carotid bifurcation/proximal ICA. In contrast, FMD involves longer middle and distal cervical ICA segments. Whereas Moyamoya is a singular extended length of stenosis at the distal ICA, proximal MCA, or ACA, FMD is typically in the neck vessels and is multifocal.

Antiplatelet therapy is generally used for patients with a cerebrovascular event, but evidence of future risk reduction is lacking. In the event of a dissection, anticoagulation can be considered. Controlling other cardiovascular risk factors and lifestyle modification are also warranted.

FMD generally is not felt to be a progressive disease. Therefore, long-term surveillance imaging may not be necessary.

Helpful consults: Neurosurgery or vascular surgery (for severe stenosis).

Clinical Vignette 2: Moyamoya Disease

HPI: 47-Year-old woman with a history of recently diagnosed hypertension who presented with 3 days of dysfluent speech that was getting progressively worse.

Exam: BP was elevated to 173/99 with normal blood glucose. The exam was notable for mild word-finding difficulty with paraphasic errors, with preserved comprehension and naming, but difficulty with repeating longer phrases. Otherwise, no facial droop, full strength.

Workup: CT head was unremarkable, but CTA head and neck near occlusion of the A1 segments of the anterior cerebral and M1 segments of bilateral middle cerebral arteries. MRI brain (a, b) demonstrated numerous punctate acute infarcts in the left temporal, parietal, and frontal lobes in an MCA distribution. A diagnostic angiogram (c) revealed the absence of flow through the left ICA with extensive collateralization via the lenticulostriate arteries (i.e., a puff of smoke, red arrow). CSF analysis was normal, and serum labs were negative for inflammatory or hypercoagulable process. Her genetic testing was completely normal.

Management: She was diagnosed with Moyamoya disease, and ultimately underwent indirect bypass surgery (EDAS) 6 months after her stroke and maintained on aspirin. She continues to do well without recurrent stroke 6 years later, with recent MRI/A imaging demonstrating stable EDAS collateral vessels.

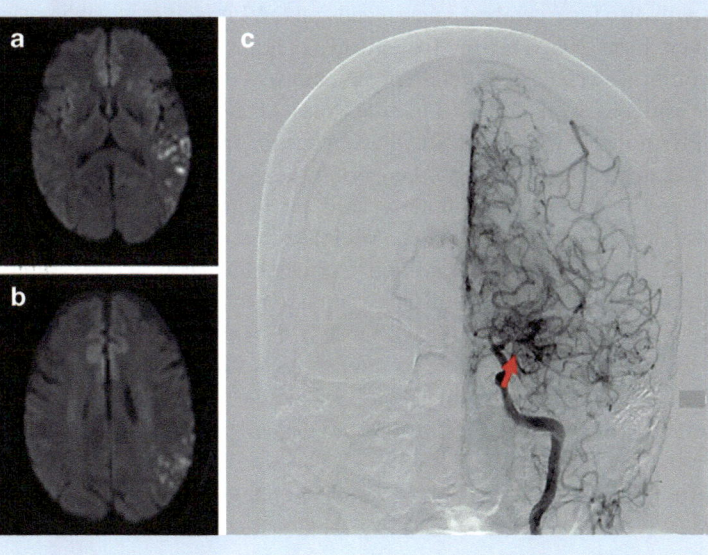

Cerebral Autosomal Dominant Arteriopathy with Subcortical Infarcts and Leukoencephalopathy (CADASIL)

The full name is a mouthful, but luckily, the acronym is easier to say. CADASIL is a hereditary *autosomal dominant* condition that can be passed down from parents to children. Autosomal dominant means that if one parent has the condition, their children have a 50% chance of inheriting it as well, regardless of gender. CADASIL is a noninflammatory vasculopathy that primarily affects small arteries and capillaries. CADASIL should be considered when a younger patient (typically in their 40s) has subcortical (not embolic appearing) strokes. Before a stroke, many patients may have a history of migraines with aura and cognitive or psychiatric symptoms.

Workup and Management

Because it is a small vessel arteriopathy, a CT or MR angiogram can be normal. MRI of the brain, however, will demonstrate diffuse white matter disease (also called leukoaraiosis) surrounding the ventricles, subcortical lacunar infarcts, or symmetrical FLAIR hyperintensities in the external capsules and anterior temporal lobes. The MRI findings are variable, however. Some patients may have less dramatic imaging findings if they are caught earlier in the course. White matter disease is also seen in older patients with long-standing hypertension, diabetes, smoking, and hyperlipidemia. Consider CADASIL if the degree of white matter disease is disproportionate to the patient's age or risk factors. About a third of CADASIL patients will also have cerebral microbleeds on SWI imaging, which may suggest a more severe form of CADASIL. To confirm a diagnosis of CADASIL, genetic analysis to confirm a *NOTCH3* mutation or skin biopsy demonstrating the characteristic granular osmophilic material within blood vessel walls is necessary.

There is no cure for CADASIL, but management typically involves low-dose aspirin and aggressive control of other cardiovascular risk factors. Vasoactive medications like triptans are not routinely used for migraines in CADASIL patients. Referrals to cognitive and psychiatric specialties may be required.

CADASIL is a progressive condition, but the clinical course can vary drastically between patients. Patients typically develop cognitive symptoms in their 50s, and their life expectancy is 60–70 years. Once a CADASIL diagnosis is confirmed, referral for genetic counseling for asymptomatic adult family members should be considered. Asymptomatic family members should get genetic counseling before tests such as MRI or genetic testing are performed. Genetic testing for children is not recommended.

Helpful consults: Neurogenetics, cognitive and psychiatry.

Sickle Cell Disease (SCD)

Patients with SCD are at risk of both ischemic and hemorrhagic strokes, with almost 1 in 4 patients having an ischemic stroke by age 45. SCD is the most common cause of strokes in children. Ischemic stroke is often due to stenosis or occlusion of intracranial vessels, often in border zone (watershed) territories. The mechanism by which a vasculopathy occurs in sickle cell patients is complex.

One mechanism involves sickled red blood cells abnormally adhering to the endothelium and causing vaso-occlusive events. Adhesion also leads to the release of pro-inflammatory molecules, leading to platelet clumping and increased vessel wall thickening, which in turn leads to stenosis and occlusion. This thickening is most commonly seen in the distal internal carotid, middle cerebral, and anterior cerebral arteries and is similar to a Moyamoya-type vasculopathy.

The American Society of Hematology Guidelines suggests that children and young adults with SCD and no history of clinical stroke should undergo an MRI of the brain to screen for silent infarcts. Silent infarcts are considered a separate risk factor for future strokes.

In children with SCD, transcranial dopplers showing elevated velocities in the distal ICA and MCA vessels mean a high risk of stroke [2]. Elevated velocities are a marker of severe stenosis (think of water coming out of a narrow hose opening). Transcranial Doppler monitoring in adults has not yet been established.

The Stroke Prevention Trial in Sickle Cell Anemia (STOP) Trial demonstrated that chronic transfusion therapy effectively prevents stroke in SCD [3]. Transfusions improve the oxygen-carrying ability of red blood cells, reduce sickling, and reduce arterial wall thickening. Regular transfusion therapy can reduce the risk of stroke by 80% or more [4]. However, iron overload is a known complication of regular transfusion therapy, which can be managed through iron chelation therapy. There is no evidence to support antiplatelet therapy for patients for secondary stroke prevention in patients with SCD.

Patients should have close hematology follow-ups to coordinate transfusion therapy and other treatments. For SCD patients who have acute strokes, emergent exchange transfusion therapy should be considered, and a stat consult to hematology should be placed. The goal of exchange transfusion therapy in patients with acute stroke is to lower the <u>Hemoglobin S fraction to <30%.</u> In patients with anemia and hemoglobin less than 5 g/dL, simple transfusions can raise <u>hemoglobin levels to a target of 10 g/dL</u>. However, simple transfusions do not effectively lower the hemoglobin S fraction. Thrombolytic therapy in SCD patients is less clear. Expert opinion is that if a patient has other risk factors for stroke (i.e., atrial fibrillation), thrombolytic therapy can be considered in addition to the SCD therapies mentioned above. SCD is *not* a contraindication to tPA.

Clinical Vignette 3

HPI: 57-Year-old male with a history of bipolar disease, migraines, and chronic vertigo, brought to the hospital for confusion. His wife had called him on the phone and noticed he was making odd statements about Santa Claus and random movies and thought his speech was slurred. His brother, mother, and maternal grandmother all had strokes at an early age. He also has multiple family members with psychiatric illnesses.

Exam: Blood pressure 128/76, HR 66. The exam was only notable for disorientation to date and day of the week; he knew the month and year. His speech was clear, he had full strength and sensation.

Workup: MRI demonstrated extensive patchy and confluent areas of T2/FLAIR signal hyperintensity in periventricular and subcortical white matter (a), notably in the anterior temporal lobes (b) and bilateral external capsules (c). Vessel imaging was normal.

Management: Given his strong family history of early stroke and MRI demonstrating extensive white matter disease without a significant cardiovascular history, a diagnosis of CADASIL was suspected. This was confirmed on both genetic testing for NOTCH3 mutation and skin biopsy with typical features of CADASIL. He was treated with aspirin and statin. Unfortunately, he had a rapid cognitive and psychiatric decline over the next 3 years, leading to severe dementia, and ultimately died 4 years after his diagnosis. His two children were offered genetic counseling but ultimately declined.

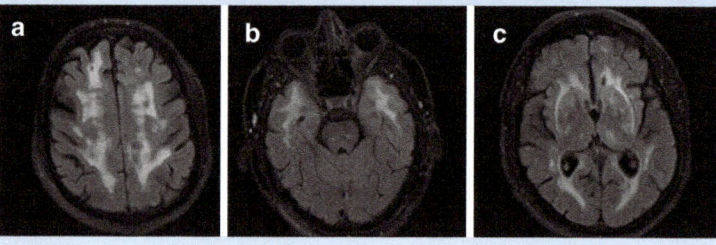

Helpful consults: Hematology.

Clinical Pearls
- Vasculopathy is a nonspecific term implying diseased blood vessels. The key is determining whether the disease is due to inflammation (vasculitis) or not.
- Diagnostic uncertainty is common. In addition to brain and noninvasive vessel imaging, lumbar puncture, diagnostic angiograms, and discussions between multiple specialties can help determine the underlying diagnosis.
- In some cases, steroids can harm patients with noninflammatory vasculopathies.
- Noninflammatory vasculopathies all have specific treatments and should be comanaged with a stroke specialist plus any other condition-specific specialists.

References

1. Singhal AB, Topcuoglu MA. Glucocorticoid-associated worsening in reversible cerebral vasoconstriction syndrome. Neurology. 2017;88(3):228–36. https://doi.org/10.1212/WNL.0000000000003510. Epub 2016 Dec 9.
2. Adams R, McKie V, Nichols F, Carl E, Zhang DL, McKie K, Figueroa R, Litaker M, Thompson W, Hess D. The use of transcranial ultrasonography to predict stroke in sickle cell disease. N Engl J Med. 1992;326(9):605–10. https://doi.org/10.1056/NEJM199202273260905.
3. Lee MT, Piomelli S, Granger S, Miller ST, Harkness S, Brambilla DJ, Adams RJ, STOP Study Investigators. Stroke prevention trial in sickle cell anemia (STOP): extended follow-up and final results. Blood. 2006;108(3):847–52. https://doi.org/10.1182/blood-2005-10-009506.
4. Fullerton HJ, Adams RJ, Zhao S, Johnston SC. Declining stroke rates in Californian children with sickle cell disease. Blood. 2004;104(2):336–9. https://doi.org/10.1182/blood-2004-02-0636. Epub 2004 Mar 30.

Pediatric Stroke

27

Kathleen E. Walsh, Natalie L. Ullman, and Lauren A. Beslow

Epidemiology

The term "stroke" encompasses arterial ischemic stroke (AIS), hemorrhagic stroke (HS), and cerebral sinovenous thrombosis (CSVT). AIS accounts for about half of all pediatric strokes. Newborns are at the highest risk, with AIS rates six times those of their childhood counterparts, occurring in about 1 in 3500–4000 newborns versus 1–3 per 100,000 per year in older children [1, 2]. About 80% of perinatal strokes are ischemic [1]. Spontaneous, nontraumatic hemorrhagic stroke (HS) encompasses about half of all strokes in the pediatric population, occurring with an incidence of about 1 per 6300 live births, and 1.7 per 100,000 per year in older children [1]. CSVT refers to the presence of a thrombus in the draining veins of the brain. The incidence (the number of new cases per unit of time) of CSVT is lower than AIS but the true incidence is unknown [3]. CSVT is covered in great depth in a prior chapter [1].

Large epidemiologic studies have shown that strokes of all subtypes have increased an estimated 35% globally since 1990 [4]. Interestingly, the prevalence

K. E. Walsh
Division of Neurology, Children's Hospital of Philadelphia, Philadelphia, PA, USA
e-mail: WalshKE@chop.edu

N. L. Ullman
Division of Neurology, Children's Hospital of Philadelphia, Philadelphia, PA, USA

Department of Neurology, The Hospital of the University of Pennsylvania, Philadelphia, PA, USA
e-mail: ULLMANN@chop.edu

L. A. Beslow (✉)
Division of Neurology, Children's Hospital of Philadelphia, Philadelphia, PA, USA

Departments of Neurology and Pediatrics, Perelman School of Medicine at the University of Pennsylvania, Philadelphia, PA, USA
e-mail: BESLOW@chop.edu

© The Author(s), under exclusive license to Springer Nature Switzerland AG 2024
H. P. Amin (ed.), *Stroke for the Advanced Practice Clinician*,
https://doi.org/10.1007/978-3-031-66289-8_27

(the total number of cases at a point in time) of all strokes was significantly higher in developed versus developing countries. However, it is unclear if this overall increase and higher prevalence in developed countries is due to an actual increase in incidence versus improved diagnostic methods and availability of imaging [2]. Conversely, death and disability rates were lower in developed versus developing countries, indicating disparities in diagnosis, treatment, and long-term care of pediatric stroke patients [4].

A 2013 multicenter retrospective cohort study of hospitalized children with neurologic diagnoses estimated an overall stroke mortality rate of 10.6%, with HS as the highest case mortality percentage at 14.3%, followed by AIS ranging from 2.6 to 9.9%, and CSVT from 2.2 to 4.39% [5–7].

Presentation

Stroke should be suspected in any child with acute onset of focal neurologic deficits. Similar to adults, the most common presentation of AIS includes hemiparesis and hemifacial weakness, followed by changes in speech, language, vision, and ataxia [1]. Non-localizing symptoms, including altered mental status and SEIZURES may also occur in any subtype. Headache and cranial nerve palsies are the most common presenting symptoms of CSVT [1]. Briefly, CSVT results in venous congestion and consequent intracranial pressure (ICP) elevations. High ICP can cause headaches that are often positional and exacerbated when lying down. Cranial nerve VI palsy can occur because elevated ICP results in downward displacement of the brainstem, stretching and damaging the nerve, leading to ipsilateral lateral gaze palsy (left CN VI palsy = can't move eyes to left) [8]. A clot in the cavernous sinus can lead to palsies of cranial nerves III, IV, the ophthalmic (V1) and maxillary (V2) branches of cranial nerve V, and VI [9, 10]. In addition to focal deficits, hemorrhagic stroke is often associated with severe headache, emesis, and alteration in consciousness. In subarachnoid hemorrhage (SAH), children may present with days to even weeks of headaches, possibly indicating a phenomenon known as a "sentinel bleed" or "warning leak" before a larger SAH. It is believed that experiencing a "sentinel" headache may signal an increased risk of rebleeding [11].

It is important to recognize that children presenting with focal deficits are more likely to be experiencing a stroke mimic than a stroke. As a result, pediatric providers may think of alternative diagnoses first, which can potentially delay a stroke diagnosis [3]. Common stroke mimics include seizure, mass lesion, migraine, meningitis, functional neurologic disorders, medication toxicity (methotrexate), demyelinating disorders, posterior reversible encephalopathy syndrome (PRES), and metabolic stroke-like syndromes [3]. See the chapter on stroke mimics for a detailed review. Timely imaging is necessary to differentiate these entities and guide treatment.

Clinical Evaluation and Imaging

Initial evaluation of a child with suspected stroke should start with determination of time of last know well (which notably is not time that symptoms are recognized but time that the child was last seen at their baseline). In some reports the median time to stroke diagnosis was 15 to 24 hours [1]. This is important, as later presentation or diagnosis limits acute treatment options.

A pertinent medical history, including any stroke risk factors, should be obtained. Stroke risk factors in children include vasculopathies like moyamoya, congenital cardiac disease, sickle cell disease, recent trauma, and thrombophilias or coagulation disorders. A Pediatric National Institutes of Health Stroke Scale (PedNIHSS) score, performed by a pediatric neurologist or personnel trained in neurologic assessment, should be completed to assess stroke severity. The PedNIHSS was modified from the adult NIHSS for children aged 2–18, keeping the same 15 core items with modifications for developmental appropriateness [12]. The PedNIHSS has excellent inter-rater reliability and is often assessed serially to monitor for stroke progression or improvement of deficits [12, 13].

After initial stabilization, including securing the airway and treating seizures, neuroimaging should be obtained to differentiate stroke subtypes and rule out stroke mimics. Imaging choice may differ depending on the institutional level of care/experience with pediatric strokes, the child's clinical stability for transport, and the need for sedation. While magnetic resonance imaging (MRI) is the gold standard for diagnosis AIS in the pediatric population, non-contrast CT head is often obtained initially. CT is sensitive for diagnosing acute hemorrhage but 47–84% of acute AIS will be missed on CT, and like in adults, it should not be relied on to rule out AIS [14, 15]. Vascular imaging of the head and neck is also needed to detect large vessel occlusion, dissection, or arterial stenosis [16]. CT/CTA should be obtained when large vessel occlusion is suspected but MR-based imaging is not rapidly available due to incompatible medical devices like a ventricular assist device or extracorporeal membrane oxygenation (ECMO), or difficulty providing timely sedation if required [16]. Shorter MRI protocols with diffusion imaging and MRA are available at some institutions to minimize the need for sedation.

Contrast-enhanced MR is often the most sensitive sequence for detecting CSVT. Magnetic resonance venography (MRV) or CT Venography (CTV) can be performed, though normal vessel variants leading to slow or irregular flow can mimic thrombosis (Fig. 27.1).

Brain and vascular imaging are also required for hemorrhagic stroke to evaluate for a source of the hemorrhage, including underlying vascular malformations like arteriovenous malformations, arteriovenous fistulas, or aneurysms. Note that cavernous malformations are not seen on vascular imaging due to their low flow state and relatively small size. Identification of these lesions is best achieved through contrast MRI and SWI, with a characteristic "popcorn" like appeerence [17].

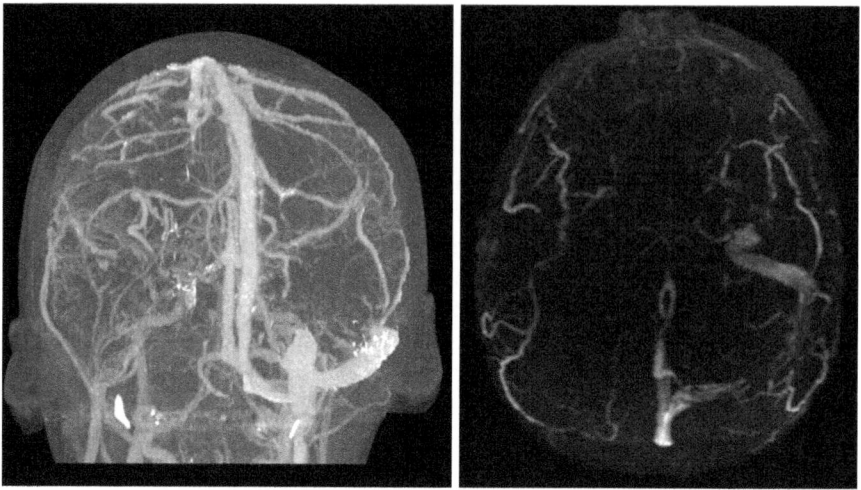

Fig. 27.1 Left: Coronal view CTV noting non-opacification (no contrast visible) indicating complete obstruction of the right transverse and sigmoid sinuses and right internal jugular vein. Right: Axial view MRV of the same patient, re-demonstrating the absence of flow in the right transverse and sigmoid sinus. In each scan, note the lack of symmetry in the sinuses

Laboratory Screening

General laboratory studies for all stroke patients include complete blood count (CBC), prothrombin time (PT), international normalized ratio (INR), activated partial thromboplastin time (aPTT), and basic metabolic panel (BMP) [3]. In some cases, especially if infection or systemic inflammation is suspected, inflammatory markers such as erythrocyte sedimentation rate (ESR) and C-reactive protein (CRP) may be helpful. While thrombophilia screening is indicated in all children with AIS or CSVT, interpretation in neonates should be performed in conjunction with a hematologist. Protein C, S, and antithrombin deficiencies are established hypercoagulable states in children and adults. In neonates, however, their levels are normally lower and only approach their adult levels later in childhood. Low levels of these proteins might be misinterpreted without an experienced hematologist [1]. If vasculitis (inflammation of cerebral vessels) or CNS infections are suspected, CSF analysis with lumbar puncture is warranted for diagnosis and to guide treatment [3]. Table 27.1 below lists labs to consider in pediatric stroke.

Table 27.1 Suggested laboratory workup

Initial labs in ER	Thrombophilia labs	Special cases
CBC	Protein C	*Suspected infection*: CRP,
BMP	Protein S	ESR
Coagulation studies: PT, PTT,	Antithrombin III	*Suspected ingestion*:
INR Toxicology screen	Factor VIII level	toxicology screen
	Homocysteine level	*Family history of*
	Lipoprotein(a)	*hyperlipidemia*: fasting lipid
	Anticardiolipin antibodies	screen
	Anti-β2 glycoprotein Ib	
	antibodies	
	DRVVT factor V Leiden	
	gene mutation (*G1691A*)	
	Prothrombin gene mutation	
	(*G20210A*)	

Acute Treatment

Unlike in adult patients for whom numerous clinical trials demonstrate the safety and efficacy of mechanical thrombectomy and intravenous (IV) tissue plasminogen activator (tPA) and tenecteplase, no randomized clinical trials have evaluated these interventions in pediatrics. The Thrombolysis in Pediatric Stroke (TIPS) trial was designed to determine the safety, optimal dose, and feasibility of treatment with tPA in children with AIS. However, this trial closed due to low patient recruitment [18]. There were no reported cases of symptomatic intracerebral hemorrhage in the subsequent retrospective review of 26 children with AIS treated with IV tPA at prior TIPS sites (TIPSTER study) [19]. The FDA has not yet approved tPA for childhood stroke. However, American Heart Association guidelines state that tPA can be used in carefully selected pediatric patients based on expert consensus [1]. An important consequence of the TIPS trial was the establishment of pediatric stroke centers equipped with multidisciplinary teams to care for children with acute stroke. TIPS led to the institution of stroke triage protocols, the use of stroke alerts, and stroke order sets [20].

The Save ChildS study was a large multicenter, international cohort study that included 73 children who underwent endovascular recanalization between 2000 and 2018. This study showed that the risks of thrombectomy in pediatric patients did not differ from those in adult thrombectomy trials. Furthermore, most children had a favorable neurologic outcome, with the median NIHSS score decreasing from 14 on admission to 4 on day seven [21]. The American Heart Association recommendation for consideration of thrombectomy in children includes radiologically confirmed large artery occlusion, persistent disabling neurologic deficit (PedNIHSS ≥6), and consideration of patient/vessel size in relation to instruments and contrast/radiation exposure. If offered, such intervention should be recommended by experienced pediatric neurology professionals and performed by an endovascular surgeon experienced in adult and pediatric populations [1]. Regardless of acute treatment, all children with acute stroke require admission to an intensive care unit for at least 24 h for close monitoring and evaluation for potential complications.

Antithrombotics

The primary strategy for secondary AIS and CSVT prevention is medical management with antithrombotic medications. Based on the mechanism, medical management consists of either antiplatelet therapy with aspirin or anticoagulation with warfarin or low molecular weight heparin (LMWH) for thrombophilia or CSVT [22]. The newer direct oral anticoagulants (DOACs) have been approved for stroke prevention in atrial fibrillation in adults, but have not yet been studied in pediatric AIS. However, some children with CSVT are transitioned to rivaroxaban based on studies that included pediatric CSVT patients [23]. In pediatric stroke, aspirin or anticoagulation can be initiated while the workup is ongoing. No trials or guidelines suggest that antiplatelet versus anticoagulants are superior for AIS, and local practices and stroke risk factors often determine treatment. However, anticoagulation should be used cautiously in higher-risk situations, such as larger strokes or when there is already evidence of hemorrhagic transformation. Cervical dissection is often treated with anticoagulation, though some use aspirin. Aspirin is typically favored for intracranial dissection since intracranial dissection may carry a higher risk of subarachnoid hemorrhage. For most other stroke risk factors, children are usually placed on 3–5 mg/kg/day of aspirin for at least 2 years post-stroke [1]. More research is required to identify antithrombotic therapy's optimal type and duration for various stroke risk factors. The choice of antithrombotic agent is best made through a multidisciplinary approach, including stroke neurologists, hematologists, and cardiologists for patients with cardiac disease. Antithrombotics are not typically indicated in perinatal stroke because of the low risk of recurrent stroke, except in the rare cases due to thrombophilia, neonatal arteriopathy, or congenital heart disease [1].

Focal cerebral arteriopathy (FCA) is an entity that is a common cause of pediatric stroke. FCA is defined as unifocal and unilateral stenosis/irregularity of the large intracranial arteries of the anterior circulation (distal internal carotid artery or its proximal branches, Fig. 27.2) [24]. FCA is thought to be driven by focal inflammation, as evidenced by enhancement of the vessel wall on vessel wall MRI. FCA is commonly reported following viral infections such as varicella-zoster and herpes viruses [24, 25]. For this reason, it is hypothesized that steroids may be helpful by suppressing the inflammatory process and preventing further vessel wall narrowing. However, there is currently no clinical trial data to support this practice. There is also concern that steroids could worsen an underlying infection. A recent Delphi panel recognized steroid use for FCA as the most important and feasible clinical trial in pediatric stroke, and other trials are ongoing investigating the efficacy of steroids in this condition [26].

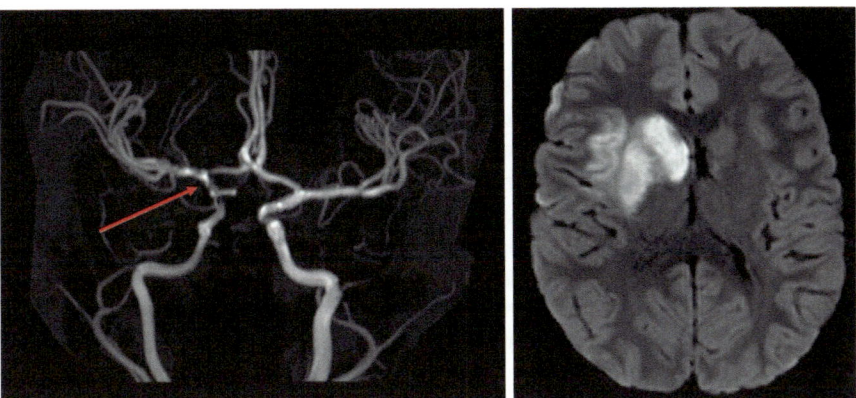

Fig. 27.2 MRA shows focal cerebral arteriopathy (FCA) involving the right internal carotid artery and the M1 segment of the right MCA (arrow). DWI shows a corresponding right MCA infarct involving primarily the right basal ganglia

Supportive Management and Neuroprotection

Neuroprotective strategies including normothermia and normoglycemia, avoidance of hypotension, and avoidance of significant hypertension are essential to ensure consistent cerebral perfusion, particularly in children with arteriopathies such as moyamoya. Patients are often hypertensive after an acute stroke, and the BP will usually slowly normalize over the subsequent days. Permissive hypertension may be allowed in some cases, and any blood pressure treatment should be done slowly to avoid overcorrection. Hypotension can worsen stroke size and symptoms. Seizures occur in an estimated 20% of children with ischemic stroke and should be treated aggressively in the acute period. Rarely, decompressive hemicraniectomies are required for children with large territory strokes and significant edema, typically MCA or posterior circulation strokes, to prevent herniation [1].

Presentation, and Acute Management of Perinatal Stroke

Stroke should be in the differential diagnosis for any neonate presenting within hours to days after birth with seizures, particularly focal motor seizures, or in neonates with encephalopathy. Encephalopathy is also seen with hypoxic-ischemic injury, and neuroimaging is imperative for distinguishing perinatal stroke from hypoxic-ischemic injury [1]. The most common location of AIS in this population is infarct in the MCA territory, disproportionately affecting the left MCA [1] for reasons that are not well understood.

Presumed perinatal AIS is often diagnosed weeks to months after birth. Neonates are typically asymptomatic after birth and first present at 4–6 months of age when asymmetric motor development (i.e., handedness) becomes apparent or when focal motor seizures or other seizure types develop [3]. Neuroimaging then reveals a chronic infarction.

If suspected during the neonatal period, the initial imaging study is often a head ultrasound (US), as this can be done quickly and at the bedside. Head US can identify AIS, intraparenchymal, and intraventricular hemorrhage. US with Doppler can also evaluate for CSVT. However, head US is not sensitive for early or small AIS and can miss small hemorrhages, particularly those in the posterior fossa. MRI is the imaging of choice to differentiate perinatal stroke from other entities. Arterial or venous imaging can be added if hemorrhage or CSVT is suspected.

The management of acute perinatal stroke is primarily focused on controlling seizures. Thrombolytics and thrombectomy are not used in this population for many reasons. It is impossible to determine a stroke time of onset as infants do not typically show focal weakness, and seizure does not indicate stroke onset. In most cases, perinatal AIS is caused by placental thrombi entering the fetal circulation, which suggests that these strokes occur before delivery. Endovascular devices have not been designed or validated for neonates, and there is a risk of damage to vessel walls, resulting in vasospasm, dissection, and intracranial hemorrhage [27].

Arterial Ischemic Stroke Workup

The workup after childhood stroke should focus on determining the underlying etiology to mitigate the risk for future stroke. The TOAST classification is a system developed for standardized categorizing AIS etiology in adults [28]. As pediatric stroke often has different risk factors than adult stroke, the CASCADE (Childhood AIS Standardized Classification and Diagnostic Evaluation) criteria were developed by a working group of investigators from the International Pediatric Stroke Study (IPSS) as a comprehensive classification system for childhood AIS. CASCADE consists of 7 major classification categories based on anatomic location of disease: small vessel arteriopathy, unilateral focal cerebral arteriopathy of childhood (FCA), bilateral cerebral arteriopathy of childhood (for example, moyamoya disease, fibromuscular dysplasia), aortic/cervical arteriopathy (e.g., dissection), cardioembolic, other (undetermined, hypercoagulable state), or multifactorial [29]. Cerebral arteriopathies account for about half of AIS in children, whereas cardiac disease, either congenital or acquired, accounts for about 30% [3].

Vessel imaging of the head and neck should be completed to evaluate for cerebral arteriopathy and cervical arteriopathy. CTA or MRA is usually first-line. However, MRA is preferred since it avoids radiation exposure and should include both the head and neck. Vessel wall imaging, a post-contrast sequence on an MRI brain, can be performed to assess for inflammation in the vessel wall, though enhancement is not specific for inflammation. T1 fat-saturated images on MRA neck help further evaluate for cervical dissection. This sequence can highlight vessel wall injury and associated intramural hemorrhage (blood within the vessel wall), as seen in dissection [30]. Furthermore, dissection and FCA may not be visualized on initial imaging. They can progress over time, so serial vessel imaging is recommended within the first year and potentially longer if vessel abnormalities persist [1].

All children with AIS should undergo an echocardiogram with contrast to evaluate for cardiac disease (such as valve disease, endocarditis, or decreased left-ventricular function), PFO that could allow paradoxical embolism, ventricular septal defect, or other structural heart disease. Children on ventricular assist devices or ECMO are also at risk for cardioembolic events. In patients with a PFO with right-to-left shunting, single ventricle physiology, or other structural cardiac abnormality that would permit a paradoxical venous embolism, four-extremity dopplers should be considered to evaluate for venous clots. The role of PFO in childhood AIS is not well understood. In one study, PFO with right-to-left shunt has been reported to be more prevalent in children with cryptogenic stroke, but unclosed PFO was not associated with increased risk for recurrent stroke [2]. Finally, while arrhythmia, particularly atrial fibrillation, is a common and well-described cause of AIS in adults, the role of arrhythmia in childhood stroke is less clearly defined. Nevertheless, it is recommended that children with AIS undergo an electrocardiogram (ECG) and be monitored on telemetry while admitted for poststroke care [1]. The role of longer-term arrhythmia monitoring (for example, with a Holter) is not well defined.

Thrombophilia can either be acquired or inherited. In most pediatric AIS and CSVT cases, a thrombophilia workup should be pursued even when another known stroke risk factor exists. The presence of thrombophilia may increase stroke recurrence risk and treatment choice or duration. Initial laboratory testing typically includes antiphospholipid antibodies, lupus anticoagulant, anti-β2 glycoprotein Ib antibodies, protein C, protein S, homocysteine level, antithrombin III, factor V Leiden gene mutation (G1691A), prothrombin gene mutation (G20210A), and lipoprotein(a). It is recommended that thrombophilia workup abnormalities be interpreted by a hematologist who can direct follow-up testing if indicated, as many of these results can be falsely elevated immediately following AIS. A thorough family history of unprovoked blood clots and strokes in children and young adults should also be completed. Thrombophilia workup is typically unnecessary for perinatal AIS cases without active thrombosis, congenital heart disease, or strong family history due to minimal recurrence risk.

A fasting lipid profile should be considered in adolescents and those with a family history of hyperlipidemia. Illicit substance use in adolescents/young adults also increases stroke risk. A drug toxicology screen should be considered to screen for substances such as amphetamines, marijuana, phencyclidine, cocaine, and opiates, as both AIS and HS have been reported in such cases [31]. After a thorough evaluation, about 9–16% of individuals with AIS still will not have any identifiable risk factors and will be classified as cryptogenic [32, 33].

Cerebral Sinovenous Thrombosis Workup

In cases of clinical suspicion of CSVT, patients should undergo MRI and MR venography (MRV) to confirm the diagnosis. If MR imagining cannot be obtained, a CT with CT venography (CTV) is also adequate. Imaging will show a lack of flow within one or multiple cerebral veins. MRI will be more sensitive in detecting acute associated infarct if present.

Risk factors for neonatal CSVT include dehydration, perinatal complications (e.g., premature rupture of membranes, maternal infection, placental abruption, and gestational diabetes), sepsis or other infections, prothrombotic disorders, ECMO treatment, intubation at birth, congenital heart disease, congenital diaphragmatic hernia, polycythemia, and meconium aspiration [34–36]. In addition to infection, dehydration, and prothrombotic disorders, other risk factors for CSVT in older children include head and neck trauma, otitis media, mastoiditis, meningitis, sinusitis, and upper respiratory tract infections [34]. In one large study of Canadian children and neonates with CSVT, the most common prothrombotic disorder was the presence of anticardiolipin antibodies, followed by deficiencies in protein C, antithrombin III, and protein S [36].

Hemorrhagic Stroke Workup

In children, hemorrhagic stroke (HS) is caused by structural lesions in about 75% of cases, most commonly arteriovenous malformations (AVMs, Fig. 27.3) [1]. This is in contrast to HS in adults, which is more often the result of chronic hypertension or cerebral amyloid angiopathy. Therefore, workup for hemorrhagic stroke in children should focus on detecting an underlying vascular lesion. Brain MRI with and without gadolinium can detect AVMs, cavernous malformations, or brain tumors. Vascular imaging is helpful for the evaluation of AVMs, arteriovenous fistulas (AVFs), or aneurysms. MRA is often preferred since it avoids radiation exposure. Acute hemorrhage can obscure underlying lesions; thus, a conventional angiogram is often required and is considered the gold standard for detecting and characterizing vascular lesions [1]. Even if a lesion is identified on CTA or MRA, a conventional angiogram may help define the lesion better or for intervention. Repeat imaging should be performed in a delayed fashion (1–3 months later) if initial imaging did not reveal an underlying vascular lesion.

Less commonly, hemorrhagic stroke can result from inherited (e.g., hemophilia, von Willebrand disease), acquired coagulopathies (idiopathic thrombocytopenic purpura, neoplasm), or anticoagulation use. Hematologic workup should be pursued when coagulopathy or thrombocytopenia is suspected or when vascular imaging is normal [1].

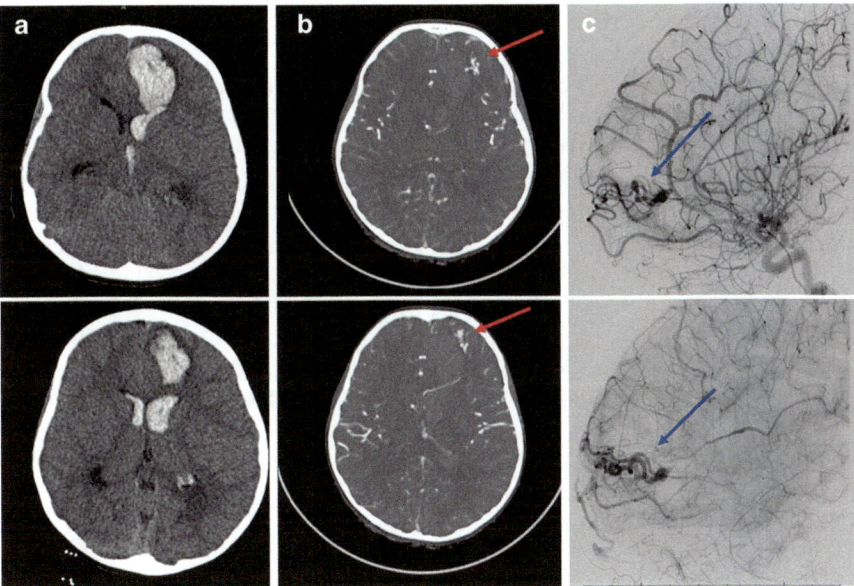

Fig. 27.3 (a) Non-contrast head CT showing left frontal intraparenchymal hemorrhage with extension into bilateral lateral and third ventricles. (b) CTA showing a cluster of abnormal blood vessels next to intraparenchymal hemorrhage (red arrow). (c) DSA left internal carotid artery injection showing left frontal AVM with arterial supply from left ACA feeders (top) and early venous filling (bottom)

Perinatal Stroke Workup

Since perinatal stroke is usually related to placental pathology or maternal factors, it does not translate to a higher risk of future stroke. Thus, workup for perinatal ischemic stroke is not nearly as extensive as childhood ischemic stroke. MRI should be performed to confirm stroke, and MRV should be considered if venous thrombosis is suspected (Fig. 27.4) [1]. However, vessel imaging with MRA or CTA is not typically necessary for perinatal AIS. Based on findings from a prospective case-control study, routine thrombophilia is also not recommended in neonates unless there is a strong family history of thrombosis or evidence of thrombosis in other organs [37]. In cases of perinatal hemorrhage, testing for mutations in COL4A1 and COL4A2 should be considered, especially in neonates with hemorrhage and porencephaly, glaucoma, or cataracts. Of note, COL4A1/2 can also cause ischemic stroke and hemorrhage in older children and adults. It should be considered in younger patients with new stroke and imaging showing leukoaraiosis, prior lacunar infarcts, or prior hemorrhage [38, 39]. Acquired or congenital coagulopathy may also lead to HS in newborns, with the most common coagulopathic cause worldwide being lack of vitamin K administration at birth.

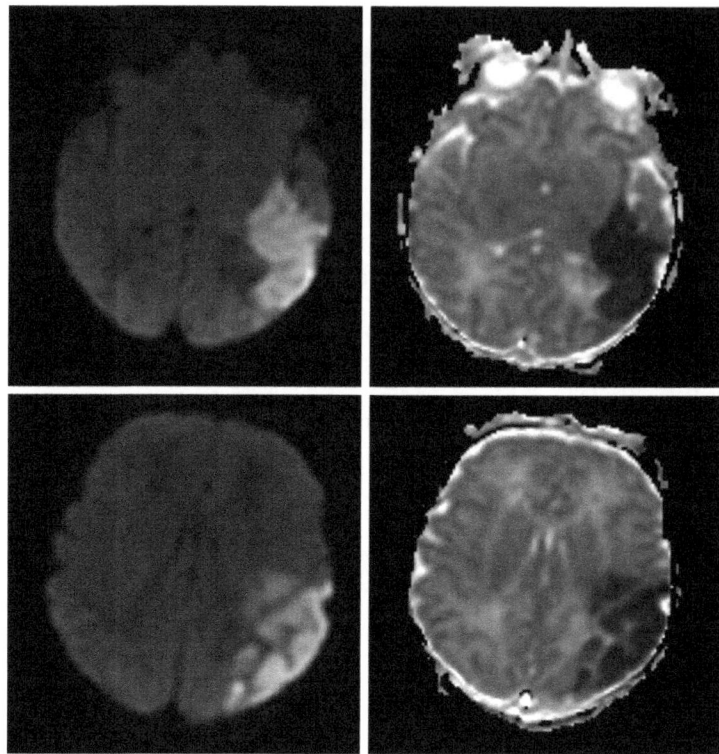

Fig. 27.4 MRI of a 3-day-old infant who developed seizures, showing restricted diffusion in left posterior MCA territory consistent with acute arterial ischemic stroke. Acute stroke appears bright on DWI (left upper and lower) and dark on ACD (right upper and lower)

Long-Term Considerations for Pediatric Stroke Patients

Mortality after AIS ranges from 4 to 28%, for hemorrhagic stroke from 6 to 54%, and for CSVT from 5.6 to 14% [3, 8, 9]. Survivors of stroke are at risk for lifelong disability. Long-term sequelae after stroke depend on the patient's age, location, and stroke severity. All pediatric stroke patients are at risk for motor deficits, cognitive and language deficits, and epilepsy. Children who suffer a stroke require close neurodevelopmental follow-up to allow for early detection of any developmental delays and engagement in appropriate therapies (physical, occupational, speech, behavioral) and school supports.

Motor Deficits and Spasticity

About 40–70% of children with perinatal stroke will have consequent hemiplegic cerebral palsy [40, 41]. Motor impairment is also common after childhood stroke and can range from mild clumsiness to significant hemiparesis, depending on the size and location of the injury [42]. Children with weakness from stroke often require physical and occupational therapy and may also benefit from orthotics. Severe weakness can result in spasticity that may require medications, casting, or botulinum toxin injections, often managed by physical medicine and rehabilitation (PM&R) physicians.

Cognitive and Learning Difficulties

Cognitive outcomes vary significantly across studies, likely due to different methodologies and measures of cognitive function [42]. However, stroke survivors are at risk for cognitive deficits that may impact learning and activities of daily living. Cognitive, speech, and behavioral difficulties have been reported in 31–59% of children with perinatal AIS and up to 50% in HS [40–42].

Epilepsy

Epilepsy is observed in roughly 47% of children who have experienced perinatal stroke and 15–20% of patients with childhood AIS. The risk increases in patients with larger cortical lesions [41, 42]. In a prospective cohort of 72 children with HS, 4% developed epilepsy at 1 year and 13% at 2 years [43]. If a neonate or child experiences seizures during the acute stroke period, a period of seizure freedom may occur after the acute injury occurs when the patient can be successfully weaned off anti-seizure medications. However, patients who suffered a prior stroke (either hemorrhagic or ischemic) are at risk for developing epilepsy at any point in their lifetime. Children with epilepsy have worse cognitive outcomes and quality of life compared to stroke survivors who do not develop epilepsy [42].

Stroke Recurrence

While perinatal stroke recurrence is low, the recurrence rate for childhood AIS ranges from 6 to 35%, with the greatest risk closest to the time of initial stroke [44, 45]. One prospective cohort of 355 children with AIS identified the greatest predictor of recurrence to be the presence of an arteriopathy (e.g., moyamoya, FCA, dissection), which increased the risk fivefold compared to idiopathic AIS [45]. Between 10 and 20% of children with CSVT will experience recurrent symptomatic venous thrombosis, although only about half are cerebral, with the remainder being systemic thromboses [34, 46]. Like ischemic stroke, the risk for recurrent HS also depends on the underlying etiology. While there is generally less data on risk factors for recurrent HS in children, one large cohort study demonstrated an overall 5-year recurrent rate of 10% [47]. In this study, no patients with idiopathic HS had a recurrent hemorrhage, while 13% with a structural pathology (AVM, tumor) had a recurrent hemorrhage. The majority of recurrences (64%) occurred within the first 6 months [47]. The annual rate of rupture of cerebral AVMs is estimated to be between 2–4%55, but has be reported as high as 17% in the year following initial hemorrhage [48, 49]. The most important secondary stroke prevention in children with hemorrhagic stroke is to surgically treat the underlying lesion if possible.

Special Population: Sickle Cell Disease

Patients with sickle cell disease are at risk for both AIS and HS, with AIS being more common in childhood and HS occurring more often in the second and third decade of life. Several important randomized clinical trials have evaluated AIS prevention in sickle cell disease (SCD) patients. The Stroke Prevention Trial in Sickle Cell Anemia (STOP) was a randomized controlled trial that demonstrated that in patients with risk for stroke (identified by elevated velocities on transcranial Doppler studies), reducing sickle hemoglobin (HgbS) to 30% or less with periodic blood transfusions led to a 92% reduction in stroke risk [50]. Furthermore, discontinuing transfusion therapy raised the risk of stroke to pretreatment levels [51]. SIT was another randomized controlled trial demonstrating that regular transfusion prevented stroke recurrence or new silent infarcts in patients with prior silent infarcts [52]. The STOP protocol is followed in many parts of world, including the United States. However, regular transfusion therapy may not be feasible in all parts of the world, especially more resource-limited settings The SPRING trial evaluated the efficacy of low- versus moderate-dose hydroxyurea for primary stroke prevention in children in Nigeria with SCD and abnormal transcranial Doppler velocities. There was no difference in stroke incidence rate between participants in the two groups. This study supports the use of low-dose hydroxyurea to decrease stroke risk in children with SCD and abnormal TCDs when transfusions are not possible [53]. In patients with moyamoya syndrome (e.g., from SCD, neurofibromatosis, trisomy 21, idiopathic), neurosurgical revascularization reduces recurrent stroke and TIA [54].

Clinical Pearls
- Stroke should be on the differential for any child presenting with focal neurologic deficits (including those with seizures and focal deficits before or after the seizure) or any neonate with new-onset seizures.
- CT may not detect AIS in the pediatric population. MRI should be used to evaluate pediatric patients with suspected stroke if CT is negative.
- Acute interventions (tPA, tenecteplase, thrombectomy) may be safe and improve outcomes in children with AIS, but randomized clinical trials are lacking. The use of Tenecteplase in children has yet to be reported.
- Pediatric stroke has different causes and risk factors than adult stroke. Children with stroke should have a diagnostic workup that reflects these differences.
- Pediatric stroke patients are at risk for motor deficits, learning difficulties, mood disorders, behavioral challenges, and epilepsy. They should be monitored closely and connected with appropriate therapies and support to maximize developmental potential.

Notable Trials

"EINSTEIN-Jr CVT" (2020): Children with CSVT were randomized to treatment with rivaroxaban or standard anticoagulants (continued on heparin or switched to vitamin K antagonist). None of the 73 rivaroxaban recipients and 1 of the 41 standard anticoagulant recipients had symptomatic, recurrent VTE after 3 months. Clinically relevant bleeding occurred in 5 rivaroxaban recipients and in 1 standard anticoagulant recipient. Complete or partial sinus recanalization occurred in 18 (25%) and 39 (53%) rivaroxaban recipients and in 6 (15%) and 24 (59%) standard anticoagulant recipients, respectively. The authors concluded that children with CSVT treated with rivaroxaban or standard anticoagulation had a low risk of recurrent VTE and clinically relevant bleeding [23].

"Save ChildS" (2020): A large multicenter cohort study that included 73 children who underwent endovascular recanalization between 2000 and 2018. This study showed that the safety profile of thrombectomy in pediatric patients did not differ from that reported in adult thrombectomy trials. Furthermore, most children had a favorable neurologic outcome, with median NIHSS dropping from a score of 14 on admission to 4 on day 7 [21].

"SIT"—Controlled Trial of Transfusions for Silent Cerebral Infarcts in Sickle Cell Anemia (2014): Randomized clinical trial assigned 196 children with sickle cell anemia and one or more silent infarcts on MRI to receive regular blood transfusions (transfusion group) or standard care (observation group). In the transfusion group, 6 of 99 children (6%) had an end-point event (1 had a stroke, and 5 had new or enlarged silent cerebral infarcts). In the observation group, 14 of 97 children (14%) had an end-point event (7 had strokes, and 7 had new or enlarged silent cerebral infarcts). Authors concluded that regular blood transfusion therapy significantly reduced the incidence of the recurrence of cerebral infarct in children with sickle cell anemia [52].

"SPRING"—Hydroxyurea for primary stroke prevention in children with sickle cell anemia in Nigeria (2022): A double-blind, multicenter, randomized, phase 3 trial evaluating moderate-dose versus low-dose hydroxyurea for stroke prevention in children with SCD and abnormal transcranial Doppler velocities. They enrolled 220 Nigerian children from August 2016 to June 2018. In the low-dose hydroxyurea group, 3 (3%) had strokes, with an incidence rate of 1.19 per 100 person-years. In the moderate-dose hydroxyurea group, 5 (5%) had strokes with an incidence rate of 1.92 per 100 person-years. There was no significant difference between these groups, providing evidence for using low-dose hydroxyurea therapy. Of note, there was a decrease in the hospitalization rate for any reason in a moderate-dose group [53].

"STOP"—Stroke Prevention Trial in Sickle Cell Anemia (1998): STOP 1 was a randomized clinical trial evaluating whether chronic transfusion prevents first-time stroke in sickle cell patients with elevated peak velocities (>200 cm/s) on transcranial Doppler. Patients were randomized to standard of care or transfusion therapy. Transfusion therapy aimed to lower hemoglobin S fraction to <30%. Transfusion therapy led to a 92% reduction in stroke risk [50]. In the subsequent STOP 2 trial, discontinuation of chronic transfusions raised the risk of stroke to pretreatment levels [51].

"TIPS"—Thrombolysis in Pediatric Stroke Trial (closed 2013): Safety and dose-finding study of IV tPA in children 2–17 years treated within 4.5 h of last seen well with partial or complete vessel occlusion and Pediatric NIH Stroke Scale score of 4–25. The study was closed in 2013 due to poor recruitment [18].

"TIPSTER"—Thrombolysis in Pediatric Stroke Extended Results (2019): Retrospective study that reported on safety and outcomes of children treated with IV tPA after TIPS closure at the 16 former TIPS sites and included 26 children treated with IV tPA. None had symptomatic intracranial hemorrhage, and two developed epistaxis. The authors concluded that the overall risk of symptomatic intracranial hemorrhage is low [19].

References

1. Ferriero DM, Fullerton HJ, Bernard TJ, et al. Management of stroke in neonates and children: a scientific statement from the American Heart Association/American Stroke Association. Stroke. 2019;50(3):E51–96. https://doi.org/10.1161/STR.0000000000000183.
2. Agrawal N, Johnston SC, Wu YW, Sidney S, Fullerton HJ. Imaging data reveal a higher pediatric stroke incidence than prior us estimates. Stroke. 2009;40(11):3415–21. https://doi.org/10.1161/STROKEAHA.109.564633.
3. Amlie-Lefond C. Evaluation and acute management of ischemic stroke in infants and children. Continuum (Minneap Minn). 2018;24(1):150–70. https://doi.org/10.1212/CON.0000000000000559.

4. Krishnamurthi RV, Deveber G, Feigin VL, et al. Stroke prevalence, mortality and disability-adjusted life years in children and youth aged 0–19 years: data from the global and regional burden of stroke 2013. Neuroepidemiology. 2015;45(3):177–89. https://doi.org/10.1159/000441087.

5. Moreau JF, Fink EL, Hartman ME, et al. Hospitalizations of children with neurological disorders in the United States. Pediatr Crit Care Med. 2013;14(8):801. https://doi.org/10.1097/PCC.0B013E31828AA71F.

6. Beslow LA, Dowling MM, Hassanein SMA, et al. Mortality after pediatric arterial ischemic stroke. Pediatrics. 2018;141(5):e20174146. https://doi.org/10.1542/PEDS.2017-4146/37938.

7. Haghighi AB, Edgell RC, Cruz-Flores S, et al. Mortality of cerebral venous-sinus thrombosis in a large national sample. Stroke. 2012;43(1):262–4. https://doi.org/10.1161/STROKEAHA.111.635664.

8. Reid JE, Reem RE, Aylward SC, Rogers DL. Sixth nerve palsy in paediatric intracranial hypertension. Neuro-Ophthalmology. 2016;40(1):23. https://doi.org/10.3109/01658107.2015.1117498.

9. Straub J, Magistris MR, Delavelle J, Landis T. Facial palsy in cerebral venous thrombosis: transcranial stimulation and pathophysiological considerations. Stroke. 2000;31(7):1766–9. https://doi.org/10.1161/01.STR.31.7.1766.

10. Byju N, Jose J, Saifudheen K, Gafoor VA, Jithendranath P. Cerebral venous thrombosis presenting as multiple lower cranial nerve palsies. Indian J Crit Care Med. 2012;16(4):213. https://doi.org/10.4103/0972-5229.106505.

11. Beck J, Raabe A, Szelenyi A, et al. Sentinel headache and the risk of re-bleeding after aneurysmal subarachnoid hemorrhage. Stroke. 2006;37(11):2733–7. https://doi.org/10.1161/01.STR.0000244762.51326.e7.

12. Ichord RN, Bastian R, Abraham L, et al. Interrater reliability of the Pediatric National Institutes of Health Stroke Scale (PedNIHSS) in a multicenter study. Stroke. 2011;42(3):613–7. https://doi.org/10.1161/STROKEAHA.110.607192.

13. Lehman LL, Khoury JC, Taylor JM, et al. Pediatric stroke rates over 17 years: report from a population-based study. J Child Neurol. 2018;33(7):463–7. https://doi.org/10.1177/0883073818767039.

14. McGlennan C, Ganesan V. Delays in investigation and management of acute arterial ischaemic stroke in children. Dev Med Child Neurol. 2008;50(7):537–40. https://doi.org/10.1111/J.1469-8749.2008.03012.X.

15. Srinivasan J, Miller SP, Phan TG, Mackay MT. Delayed recognition of initial stroke in children: need for increased awareness. Pediatrics. 2009;124(2):e227. https://doi.org/10.1542/PEDS.2008-3544.

16. Tierradentro-García LO, Zandifar A, Ullman NL, et al. Imaging of suspected stroke in children, from the AJR Special Series on Emergency Radiology. AJR Am J Roentgenol. 2022;31:330. https://doi.org/10.2214/AJR.22.27816.

17. Zyck S, Gould GC. Cavernous venous malformation. Radiopaedia.org. 2022. https://doi.org/10.53347/rid-22603.

18. Rivkin MJ, De Veber G, Ichord RN, et al. Thrombolysis in pediatric stroke (TIPS) study. Stroke. 2015;46(3):880. https://doi.org/10.1161/STROKEAHA.114.008210.

19. Amlie-Lefond C, Shaw DWW, Cooper A, et al. Risk of intracranial hemorrhage following intravenous tPA (tissue-type plasminogen activator) for acute stroke is low in children. Stroke. 2020;51:542–8. https://doi.org/10.1161/STROKEAHA.119.027225.

20. Bernard TJ, Rivkin MJ, Scholz K, et al. Emergence of the primary pediatric stroke center: impact of the thrombolysis in pediatric stroke trial. Stroke. 2014;45(7):2018–23. https://doi.org/10.1161/STROKEAHA.114.004919.

21. Sporns PB, Sträter R, Minnerup J, et al. Feasibility, safety, and outcome of endovascular recanalization in childhood stroke: the Save ChildS Study. JAMA Neurol. 2020;77(1):25–34. https://doi.org/10.1001/JAMANEUROL.2019.3403.

22. Shlobin NA, LoPresti MA, Beestrum M, Lam S. Treatment of pediatric cerebral venous sinus thromboses: the role of anticoagulation. Childs Nerv Syst. 2020;36(11):2621–33. https://doi.org/10.1007/S00381-020-04829-7.

23. Connor P, van Kammen MS, Lensing AWA, et al. Safety and efficacy of rivaroxaban in pediatric cerebral venous thrombosis (EINSTEIN-Jr CVT). Blood Adv. 2020;4(24):6250. https://doi.org/10.1182/BLOODADVANCES.2020003244.

24. Wintermark M, Hills NK, De Veber GA, et al. Clinical and imaging characteristics of arteriopathy subtypes in children with arterial ischemic stroke: results of the VIPS study. AJNR Am J Neuroradiol. 2017;38(11):2172–9. https://doi.org/10.3174/AJNR.A5376.

25. Fullerton HJ, Hills NK, Elkind MSV, et al. Infection, vaccination, and childhood arterial ischemic stroke: results of the VIPS study. Neurology. 2015;85(17):1459. https://doi.org/10.1212/WNL.0000000000002065.

26. Steinlin M, O'callaghan F, Mackay MT. Planning interventional trials in childhood arterial ischaemic stroke using a Delphi consensus process. Dev Med Child Neurol. 2017;59(7):713–8. https://doi.org/10.1111/DMCN.13393.

27. Kirton A, Jordan LC, Orbach DB, Fullerton HJ. The case against endovascular thrombectomy in neonates with arterial ischemic stroke. Clin Neuroradiol. 2022;32(2):581–2. https://doi.org/10.1007/S00062-022-01153-2.

28. Adams HP, Bendixen BH, Kappelle LJ, et al. Classification of subtype of acute ischemic stroke definitions for use in a multicenter clinical trial. Stroke. 1993;24(1):35–41. https://doi.org/10.1161/01.STR.24.1.35.

29. Bernard TJ, Manco-Johnson MJ, Lo W, et al. Towards a consensus-based classification of childhood arterial ischemic stroke. Stroke. 2012;43(2):371–7. https://doi.org/10.1161/STROKEAHA.111.624585/-/DC1.

30. Cuvinciuc V, Viallon M, Momjian-Mayor I, et al. 3D fat-saturated T1 SPACE sequence for the diagnosis of cervical artery dissection. Neuroradiology. 2013;55(5):595–602. https://doi.org/10.1007/S00234-013-1141-1.

31. Sloan MA, Kittner SJ, Feeser BR, et al. Illicit drug-associated ischemic stroke in the Baltimore-Washington Young Stroke Study. Neurology. 1998;50(6):1688–93. https://doi.org/10.1212/WNL.50.6.1688.

32. MacKay MT, Wiznitzer M, Benedict SL, Lee KJ, Deveber GA, Ganesan V. Arterial ischemic stroke risk factors: the International Pediatric Stroke Study. Ann Neurol. 2011;69(1):130–40. https://doi.org/10.1002/ANA.22224.

33. Shih EK, Beslow LA, Natarajan SS, Falkensammer CB, Messé SR, Ichord RN. Prevalence of patent foramen ovale in a cohort of children with cryptogenic ischemic stroke. Neurology. 2021;97(21):E2096–102. https://doi.org/10.1212/WNL.0000000000012892.

34. Dlamini N, Billinghurst L, Kirkham FJ. Cerebral venous sinus (sinovenous) thrombosis in children. Neurosurg Clin N Am. 2010;21(3):511–27. https://doi.org/10.1016/J.NEC.2010.03.006.

35. Mandel-Shorer N, Sabapathy CA, Krishnan P, et al. Cerebral sinovenous thrombosis in infants and children: a practical approach to management. Semin Pediatr Neurol. 2022;44:100993. https://doi.org/10.1016/j.spen.2022.100993.

36. deVeber G, Andrew M, Adams C, et al. Cerebral sinovenous thrombosis in children. N Engl J Med. 2001;345(6):417–23. https://doi.org/10.1056/NEJM200108093450604.

37. Curtis C, Mineyko A, Massicotte P, et al. Thrombophilia risk is not increased in children after perinatal stroke. Blood. 2017;129(20):2793–800. https://doi.org/10.1182/BLOOD-2016-11-750893.

38. Lanfranconi S, Markus HS. COL4A1 mutations as a monogenic cause of cerebral small vessel disease: a systematic review. Stroke. 2010;41(8):e513–8. https://doi.org/10.1161/STROKEAHA.110.581918.

39. Rannikme K, Sivakumaran V, Millar H, et al. COL4A2 is associated with lacunar ischemic stroke and deep ICH: meta-analyses among 21,500 cases and 40,600 controls. Neurology. 2017;89(17):1829. https://doi.org/10.1212/WNL.0000000000004560.

40. Grunt S, Mazenauer L, Buerki SE, et al. Incidence and outcomes of symptomatic neo-natal arterial ischemic stroke. Pediatrics. 2015;135(5):e1220–8. https://doi.org/10.1542/PEDS.2014-1520.
41. Golomb MR, Saha C, Garg BP, Azzouz F, Williams LS. The Association of Cerebral Palsy with other disability in children with perinatal arterial ischemic stroke. Pediatr Neurol. 2007;37(4):245. https://doi.org/10.1016/J.PEDIATRNEUROL.2007.06.003.
42. Greenham M, Gordon A, Anderson V, MacKay MT. Outcome in childhood stroke. Stroke. 2016;47(4):1159–64. https://doi.org/10.1161/STROKEAHA.115.011622.
43. Beslow LA, Abend NS, Gindville MC, et al. Pediatric intracerebral hemorrhage: acute symptomatic seizures and epilepsy. JAMA Neurol. 2013;70(4):448. https://doi.org/10.1001/JAMANEUROL.2013.1033.
44. Uohara MY, Beslow LA, Billinghurst L, et al. Incidence of recurrence in posterior circulation childhood arterial ischemic stroke. JAMA Neurol. 2017;74(3):316. https://doi.org/10.1001/JAMANEUROL.2016.5166.
45. Fullerton HJ, Wintermark M, Hills NK, et al. Risk of recurrent arterial ischemic stroke in childhood: a prospective international study. Stroke. 2016;47(1):53. https://doi.org/10.1161/STROKEAHA.115.011173.
46. Kenet G, Kirkham F, Niederstadt T, et al. Risk factors for recurrent venous thromboembolism in the European collaborative paediatric database on cerebral venous thrombosis: a multicentre cohort study. Lancet Neurol. 2007;6(7):595. https://doi.org/10.1016/S1474-4422(07)70131-X.
47. Fullerton HJ, Wu YW, Sidney S, Johnston SC. Recurrent hemorrhagic stroke in children: a population-based cohort study. Stroke. 2007;38(10):2658–62. https://doi.org/10.1161/STROKEAHA.107.481895.
48. Jordan LC, Jallo GI, Gailloud P. Recurrent intracerebral hemorrhage from a cerebral arterio-venous malformation undetected by repeated non-invasive neuroimaging in a 4-year-old boy. J Neurosurg Pediatr. 2008;1(4):316. https://doi.org/10.3171/PED/2008/1/4/316.
49. Fults D, Kelly DL. Natural history of arteriovenous malformations of the brain: a clinical study. Neurosurgery. 1984;15(5):658–62. https://doi.org/10.1227/00006123-198411000-00003.
50. Adams RJ, McKie VC, Hsu L, et al. Prevention of a first stroke by transfusions in children with sickle cell anemia and abnormal results on transcranial Doppler ultrasonography. N Engl J Med. 1998;339(1):5–11. https://doi.org/10.1056/NEJM199807023390102.
51. Adams RJ, Brambilla D. Discontinuing prophylactic transfusions used to prevent stroke in sickle cell disease. N Engl J Med. 2005;353(26):2769–78. https://doi.org/10.1056/NEJMOA050460.
52. DeBaun MR, Gordon M, McKinstry RC, et al. Controlled trial of transfusions for silent cerebral infarcts in sickle cell anemia. N Engl J Med. 2014;371(8):699–710. https://doi.org/10.1056/NEJMOA1401731/SUPPL_FILE/NEJMOA1401731_DISCLOSURES.PDF.
53. Abdullahi SU, Jibir BW, Bello-Manga H, et al. Hydroxyurea for primary stroke preven-tion in children with sickle cell anaemia in Nigeria (SPRING): a double-blind, multicentre, randomised, phase 3 trial. Lancet Haematol. 2022;9(1):e26–37. https://doi.org/10.1016/S2352-3026(21)00368-9.
54. Scott RM, Smith JL, Robertson RL, Madsen JR, Soriano SG, Rockoff MA. Long-term outcome in children with moyamoya syndrome after cranial revascularization by pial syn-angiosis. J Neurosurg. 2004;100(2 Suppl Pediatrics):142-149:142. https://doi.org/10.3171/PED.2004.100.2.0142.

Workup of ICH

28

Michael Levien, Yee Kuang Cheng, and Teng J. Peng

ICH can be classified as primary or secondary based on identifying the underlying mechanism [1]. Primary ICH constitutes 70-88% of all ICH cases and is caused by the rupture of small vessels due to longstanding hypertension-related degenerative vascular changes or the deposition of beta-amyloid protein in small to medium-sized blood vessels in the brain called Cerebral Amyloid Angiopathy (CAA) [1]. Secondary ICH refers to ICH caused by tumors, aneurysms, venous malformations, or coagulopathy. While anticoagulant and antiplatelet medications are associated with an increased risk of ICH, it is often unclear whether the medication directly caused the ICH or merely compounded another risk factor.

Diagnostic Workup for ICH

A non-contrast computed tomographic (CT) scan of the head is often the first and most sensitive method to view the brain tissue, establish the presence of ICH, and estimate hematoma volume. CT angiography (CTA) scan is necessary to visualize the patient's arterial blood vessels and rule out secondary causes of ICH, such as underlying aneurysms or arteriovenous malformations (Fig. 28.1a, b). Similarly, a CT venogram (CTV) can evaluate for cortical vein or cerebral sinus venous thrombosis, a less common but known cause of ICH. Pursuing digital subtraction

M. Levien
Yale New Haven Hospital, New Haven, CT, USA
e-mail: michael.levien@yale.edu

Y. K. Cheng
St. Luke's Medical Center, Boise, ID, USA
e-mail: yeekuang.cheng@yale.edu

T. J. Peng (✉)
University of Florida School of Medicine, Gainesville, FL, USA
e-mail: teng.peng@neurology.ufl.edu

© The Author(s), under exclusive license to Springer Nature Switzerland AG 2024
H. P. Amin (ed.), *Stroke for the Advanced Practice Clinician*,
https://doi.org/10.1007/978-3-031-66289-8_28

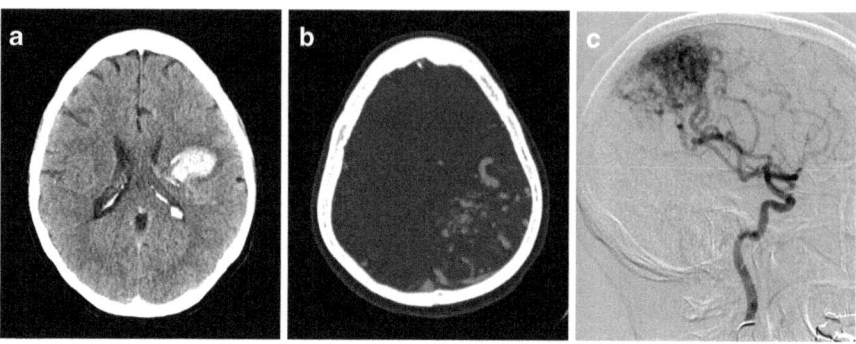

Fig. 28.1 The patient presents to the hospital with a headache and right-sided weakness. (**a**) The CT scan shows a left-sided ICH. (**b**) CTA shows a left-sided AVM close to the ICH. (**c**) A digital subtraction angiography study allows for better visualization of the AVM. *CT* computed tomographic, *CTA* computed tomographic angiogram, *AVM* arteriovenous malformation

angiography may be necessary to further evaluate, confirm, or treat vascular abnormalities, but not as a first-line imaging method (Fig. 28.1c).

Magnetic resonance imaging (MRI) offers additional information about ICH etiology and is more sensitive than CT scans at detecting underlying tumors and arterial or venous infarcts [2]. Petechial (spotty or patchy) hemorrhage within a broader area of infarct suggests that the ICH is secondary to hemorrhagic transformation of an ischemic stroke (secondary bleeding into an area of ischemia) rather than a primary hemorrhage. Other MRI sequences, such as susceptibility-weighted imaging (SWI) or gradient echo (GRE), enable the visualization of tiny cerebral microbleeds (CMB), which are asymptomatic deposits of hemosiderin and other blood products. CMBs do not represent active bleeding and are rarely symptomatic, but can point to an underlying disease process. CMBs in the brainstem and basal ganglia may indicate longstanding hypertension. In contrast, cortical CMBs in the frontal, parietal, temporal, and occipital lobes may be more suggestive of CAA or, less commonly, other conditions like CADASIL or connective tissue diseases (Fig. 28.2).

The location of hemorrhage can also point to an underlying process. Primary hemorrhages in the deep brain structures of the basal ganglia and brainstem are often due to hypertension because small perforating "end arteries" reside here and are most affected by longstanding hypertension. In contrast, larger cortical bleeds in the frontal, parietal, occipital, and temporal lobes may be due to impaired blood vessels from CAA. In some cases, the etiology may still be inconclusive despite neuroimaging. In these circumstances, guidelines suggest repeating MRI with intracranial vessel imaging in 3–6 months to rule out underlying tumors or vascular malformations that may be obscured by the initial blood or perihematomal edema. If there is a strong suspicion of a primary tumor or metastatic lesion, it may be reasonable to pursue a contrast-enhanced CT scan of the chest, abdomen, and pelvis to evaluate for malignancy that could have spread to the brain.

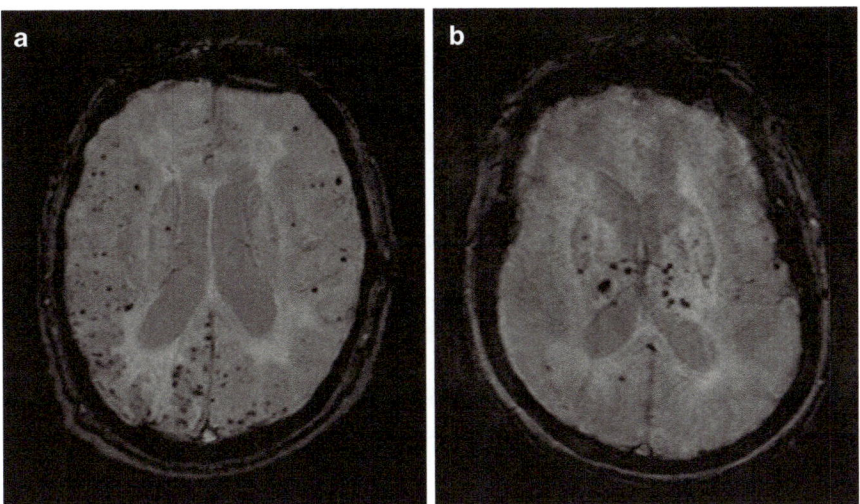

Fig. 28.2 SWI MRI images demonstrating microhemorrhages in (**a**) cerebral cortex consistent with CAA and in (**b**) basal ganglia consistent with hypertension. The underlying mechanism of the two types is different, which is why CAA microhemorrhages carry a higher risk of spontaneous hemorrhage vs microhemorrhages from hypertension

Laboratory Studies

All patients with ICH should get a complete blood count to evaluate for platelet count, as less than 50,000 platelets per microliter may increase the risk of spontaneous hemorrhage. A coagulation panel with partial thromboplastin time and prothrombin time should be obtained to calculate the International Normalized Ratio (INR), as elevated values indicate prolonged clotting times, sometimes due to the use of anticoagulant medications. Patients with elevated INR but not taking blood thinners may have liver disease. Other laboratory studies to consider include inflammatory markers such as erythrocyte sedimentation rate or C-reactive protein to evaluate for vasculitis, hemoglobin electrophoresis to evaluate for hemophilia, hemolysis labs to evaluate for diffuse intravascular coagulation, and urine toxicology studies for sympathomimetic drugs to evaluate for cocaine or amphetamine-associated vasculopathy.

Primary ICH

Hypertensive vasculopathy is the most common cause of ICH and results from long-standing hypertension, resulting in weakened vessel walls that can rupture and cause bleeding into the brain parenchyma. ICH caused by hypertensive vasculopathy occurs in areas of the brain supplied by small penetrating arteries, such as the thalamus, putamen, caudate, brainstem, and deep cerebellar nuclei. These small penetrating arteries are the same as those affected by lacunar stroke and diabetic vasculopathy.

MRI may show evidence of CMBs in the subcortical region (caudate, internal capsule, lentiform nucleus, thalamus) and signs of microvascular ischemic disease in patients with ICH due to hypertensive vasculopathy. Patients will often have other signs of end-organ damage from longstanding uncontrolled hypertension, such as chronic kidney disease or heart failure due to concentric left ventricular hypertrophy. Fortunately, hypertension is a modifiable risk factor for ICH and can be treated with medications and lifestyle changes. Adequate treatment of HTN should reduce the risk of ICH recurrence. If hypertension is refractory to multiple blood pressure agents, consider workup for secondary hypertension such as renal artery stenosis, primary aldosteronism, and obstructive sleep apnea.

Cerebral Amyloid Angiopathy (CAA) is more commonly diagnosed in individuals over the age of 60. It results from an accumulation of misfolded amyloid beta proteins within the walls of small and medium-sized blood vessels in the brain and meninges. This accumulation leads to necrosis of the vessel wall and an increased risk of bleeding. The most common location for CAA-related ICH is near the cerebral cortex, often termed lobar hemorrhage. Figure 28.3 compares hemorrhages from hypertension and CAA. MRI with CAA can also demonstrate cortical CMBs, superficial siderosis (small snake-like deposits of blood on the surface indicating slow oozing), or frank subarachnoid hemorrhage. Accumulation of CMBs may also lead to cognitive impairment as deposition of the same amyloid beta protein in brain tissue (instead of the blood vessels) is strongly linked to Alzheimer's disease (AD). The Modified Boston Criteria (Table 28.1) is a validated clinical tool used to diagnose CAA [3, 4]. The definitive diagnosis of CAA is through brain

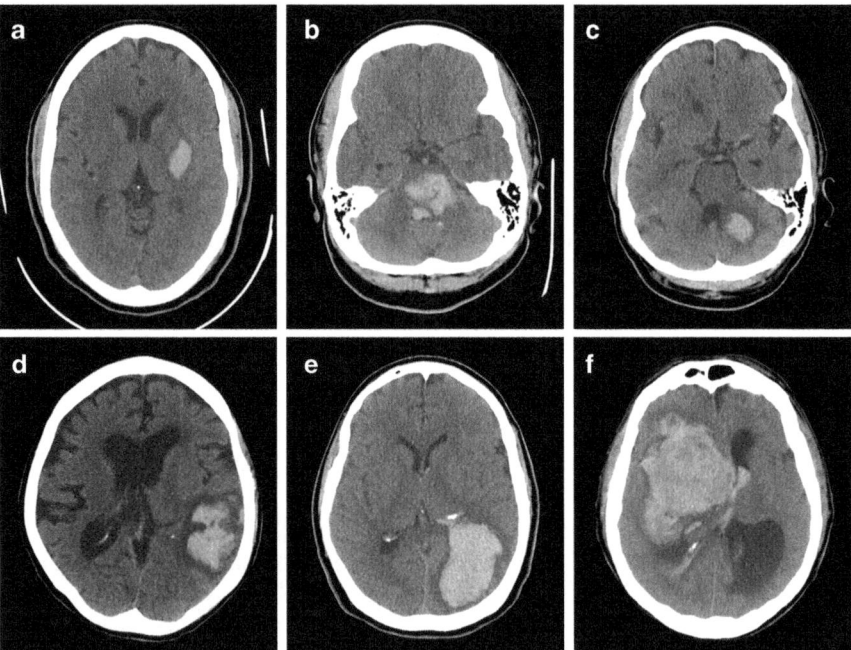

Fig. 28.3 CT scan of hypertensive hemorrhages in the putamen (**a**), brainstem (**b**), and cerebellum (**c**). Lobar hemorrhages from presumed Cerebral Amyloid Angiopathy in the parietal lobe (**d**), occipital lobe (**e**), and frontal lobe with significant midline shift and edema (**f**)

Table 28.1 Modified Boston Criteria version 2.0 for sporadic CAA

Definite CAA

Complete brain postmortem examination demonstrating:

- Spontaneous intracerebral hemorrhage, transient focal neurological episodes, convexity subarachnoid hemorrhage, cognitive impairment, or dementia
- Severe CAA with vasculopathy
- Absence of another lesion

Probable CAA with supporting pathology

Clinical data and pathological tissue (from evacuated hematoma or cortical biopsy) demonstrating:

- Presentation with spontaneous intracerebral hemorrhage, transient focal neurological episodes, convexity subarachnoid hemorrhage, cognitive impairment, or dementia
- Some degree of CAA in pathological tissue
- Absence of another lesion

Probable CAA

Pathological tissue is not required. MRI required. For patients aged 50 years and older:

- Presentation with spontaneous intracerebral hemorrhage, transient focal neurological episodes, convexity subarachnoid hemorrhage, cognitive impairment, or dementia
- MRI should demonstrate either:
  - **TWO** lobar hemorrhagic lesions on T2-weighted MRI in any combination: intracerebral hemorrhage, cerebral microbleed, foci of cortical superficial siderosis (multiple foci counted as independent lesions), or convexity subarachnoid hemorrhage (multiple distinct foci counted as independent lesions)

OR

  - **ONE** lobar hemorrhagic lesion on T2-weighted MRI (intracerebral hemorrhage, cerebral microbleed, foci of cortical superficial siderosis or convexity subarachnoid hemorrhage) **PLUS ONE** white matter feature (severe perivascular spaces in centrum semiovale or white matter hyperintensities in a multifocal pattern)
- MRI should have the absence of:
  - Any deep hemorrhagic lesion on T2-weighted MRI (this includes both intracerebral hemorrhage and cerebral microbleeds). A hemorrhagic lesion in the cerebellum is not counted as either lobar or deep
  - Other causes of hemorrhagic lesions

Possible CAA

Pathological tissue is not required. MRI required. For patients aged 50 years and older:

- Presentation with spontaneous intracerebral hemorrhage, transient focal neurological episodes, convexity subarachnoid hemorrhage, cognitive impairment, or dementia
- MRI should demonstrate either:
  - **ONE** lobar hemorrhagic lesion on T2-weighted MRI in any combination: intracerebral hemorrhage, cerebral microbleed, foci of cortical superficial siderosis (multiple foci counted as independent lesions), or convexity subarachnoid hemorrhage (multiple distinct foci counted as independent lesions)

OR

  - **ONE** white matter feature: severe perivascular spaces in centrum semiovale or white matter hyperintensities in a multifocal pattern
- MRI should have the absence of the following:
  - Any deep hemorrhagic lesion on T2-weighted MRI (this includes both intracerebral hemorrhage and cerebral microbleeds). A hemorrhagic lesion in the cerebellum is not counted as either lobar or deep
  - Other causes of hemorrhagic lesions

(Adapted from Charidimou et al. [4])

biopsy, which is not typically performed due to the lack of a cure. Instead, radiographic evidence of CMB accumulation, lobar hemorrhage, superficial siderosis, and cognitive impairment can aid in diagnosis.

In patients with probable CAA with a lobar hemorrhage, the annual risk of spontaneous rebleeding is around 10%. For possible CAA patients with CMBs but without prior lobar hemorrhage, the risk of a first-time ICH is lower (closer to 5%), but difficult to define due to other possible etiologies of the CMBs. Studies show that more CMBs translate to a higher risk of spontaneous bleeding.

Since there is no cure for CAA, treatment aims to manage high bleeding-risk comorbidities such as hypertension and smoking, avoid NSAIDs, and carefully monitor patients who need anticoagulation. Blood pressure should be ideally controlled to a goal of <130/80 to reduce the risk of future hemorrhage.

A patient who needs anticoagulation and has CAA presents a difficult challenge. While not studied in randomized trials, anticoagulation likely increases the risk of spontaneous bleeding. Indications for anticoagulation include (1) cancer-related thrombophilia, (2) hypercoagulable conditions such as antiphospholipid syndrome, (3) mechanical heart valve replacement, (4) or atrial fibrillation with a high risk of ischemic stroke. For patients with AF, consider left atrial appendage closure, discussed in the Cardioembolic Stroke chapter.

Secondary ICH

Secondary ICH accounts for less than 30% of all ICH. It is diagnosed when a traumatic, pathological, or structural cause is identified, such as vascular abnormalities, venous thrombus, hemorrhagic transformation of an ischemic stroke, or mass lesion.

Cerebral cavernous malformations, sometimes called cavernomas, are single or multiple abnormally dilated blood vessels found in the brain or spinal cord, ranging from ¼ inch up to 4 inches in size. These can occur sporadically as single lesions, or in 20% of patients and can be hereditary and multifocal. Most cavernomas do not cause any symptoms and are found incidentally on brain imaging. Incidental cavernomas should be referred to neurosurgery for outpatient monitoring. The 5-year bleeding risk of an incidentally found cavernoma is around 4%, except in the brainstem, where the risk doubles.

An individual with a symptomatic cavernoma with intracerebral hemorrhage may experience headaches, seizures, or focal neurological deficits. Risk factors for hemorrhage include prior cavernoma-associated hemorrhage and brainstem location. Increased risk of hemorrhage has been reported in females, those with multiple cavernomas, and larger size [5]. Symptomatic cavernomas that have bled can carry up to a 29% yearly risk of rebleeding [6]. Resection of a cavernoma can be high risk, especially if the lesion is in an "eloquent" area of the brain responsible for an important function like speech or movement. Surgical indications include multiple hemorrhages from the same lesion or seizures that do not respond to traditional anti-seizure medications. A neurosurgeon will determine if a cavernoma is resectable.

Brain imaging should be completed as soon as possible following the discovery of the hemorrhage. MRI with contrast is the testing of choice to visualize the cavernoma, with near-perfect sensitivity and great specificity [5]. Cavernomas have a characteristic "popcorn" or "berry" -like appearance with a rim of signal loss due to hemosiderin on T2 FLAIR, sometimes with surrounding edema. Importantly, cavernomas are not detected on vessel imaging as they are isolated lesions not attached to main blood vessels.

An **Arteriovenous malformation (AVM)** is an abnormal connection between arteries and veins that bypasses the capillary network, leading to higher pressures in veins and increasing the risk of rupture. The most common clinical presentation of an AVM is hemorrhage (60%), followed by seizure (10–30%). Bleeding from an AVM will typically be parenchymal (within the brain tissue). AVMs are identified via noninvasive vessel imaging like CTA or MRA. However, a diagnostic angiogram performed by a neurosurgeon is typically required to diagnose and treat an AVM. If incidentally found, the risk of AVM bleeding is estimated at around 2% yearly. For a symptomatic AVM, the risk of rebleeding is around 4–5% yearly. Other factors that increase risk are advanced age and deep brain location.

Brain tumors can occasionally bleed and cause symptomatic ICH. Primary hemorrhagic brain tumors include high-grade glioma or glioblastoma multiforme. Metastatic tumors with high bleeding rates include melanoma, choriocarcinoma, renal cell carcinoma, and thyroid papillary carcinomas. The cause of bleeding in tumors is believe to be due to dilated and thin-walled vessels supplying the malignant tissue and tumor necrosis [7]. A hemorrhagic mass may be considered for patients with a history of cancer, smoking, or unexplained weight loss. For patients with intraparenchymal hemorrhage with suspicion of tumor, clinicians may consider repeat imaging, typically MRI with contrast gadolinium in 2–3 months after the bleeding event, to allow time for the hemorrhage to get reabsorbed back into the brain tissue and then evaluate for underlying mass. If a suspicious-looking hemorrhage is present, it may be helpful to consult with a neuro-oncologist to expedite further investigation.

Cerebral Venous Sinus Thrombosis (CVST) leads to obstruction of the venous outflow of the brain's blood supply and can cause ICH due to increased pressure on upstream draining vessels leading to rupture. Think of it as a blocked septic tank causing significant backup. A thrombosis is a blood clot that begins at and is adhered to the endothelium of a blood vessel (as opposed to an embolism that travels from elsewhere and blocks an artery). Dehydration, oral contraceptives, pregnancy, puerperium, trauma, external compression, surgery, or systemic prothrombotic conditions such as malignancy and infection can all cause a CVST. Still, in approximately 30% of cases, no underlying cause can be found [8]. Patients with CVST commonly have headaches and other features of increased intracranial pressure, including reduced visual acuity, papilledema, nausea, seizures, cranial nerve palsies, and other focal neurological findings. CT angiography is sometimes sufficient for diagnosis to identify filling defects within the venous system. However, a dedicated CT Venogram has been shown to have up to 95% sensitivity for diagnosing CVST [9]. The treatment of CVST consists of anticoagulation therapy, even when the patient has an acute hemorrhage. This may seem counter-intuitive, but the root of the problem is a thrombus blocking a vein and causing an outflow obstruction, rather than a primary hemorrhage. Patients with CVST and no hemorrhage can be started on oral anticoagulation. However, patients with CVST and associated hemorrhage should be initiated on a heparin drip, and they must be monitored in the ICU to assess hematoma expansion.

Vasculopathy, Vasculitis, and Reversible Cerebral Vasoconstriction Syndrome

Pathologic inflammation of blood vessels can lead to both ICH and ischemic stroke through vasoconstriction and vessel damage. Specific causes of pathologic vessel constriction include exogenous substances such as cocaine or amphetamine, viruses such as varicella-zoster virus or herpes simplex virus, or autoimmune diseases such as lupus vasculitis. Reversible cerebral vasoconstriction syndrome (RCVS) is a vasculopathy characterized by sudden onset of severe or "thunderclap" headache followed by focal neurological symptoms such as ischemic stroke or ICH; it is associated with vasoactive substances like serotonergic medications, stimulants, or marijuana [10].

Spontaneous Hemorrhage in Anticoagulated Patients

Although very effective at reducing the risk of ischemic stroke, anticoagulants carry an increased risk of hemorrhage. Warfarin (Coumadin) is an older but widely used oral anticoagulant. Compared to Warfarin, newer direct oral anticoagulants (DOACs) such as apixaban, rivaroxaban, and dabigatran have lower risk of ICH [11]. In patients with anticoagulation-related ICH, brain imaging may show a "blood-fluid level", seen in Fig. 28.4. This happens when red blood cells settle to the bottom of the hematoma and plasma rises to the top, separated by a clear horizontal line. Essentially, the red blood cells pool into the cavity created by the hemorrhage when the patient lies flat for the scan. In patients without a coagulopathy, a hemorrhage will solidify into a "clot" quicker and, therefore, will not have this CT finding when the patient lies flat.

The decision to resume anticoagulation following intracerebral hemorrahge is challenging and requires a stroke specialist to determine future bleeding risk and consider clinical trials or alternative treatments. It is important to note that not all types of intracranial hemorrhage imply that future anticoagulation is prohibited. Patients with intracranial hemorrhage from trauma, vascular lesions, and hypertension can usually resume anticoagulation. For high-risk patients, the HAS-BLED score (Tables 28.2 and 28.3) can help assess the risk of first-time bleeding from Warfarin [12, 13]. This score has not been studied with DOACs and should not be the sole factor in deciding to start anticoagulation since the risk of stroke usually outweighs bleeding. Instead, a high HAS-BLED score should lead to consideration of a DOAC.

Fig. 28.4 A case of a 74-year-old male on Warfarin who presented with left-sided weakness. INR was 6.5. CT demonstrated a right frontal hemorrhage with a blood fluid level, commonly associated with patients who have a coagulopathy or are on anticoagulation

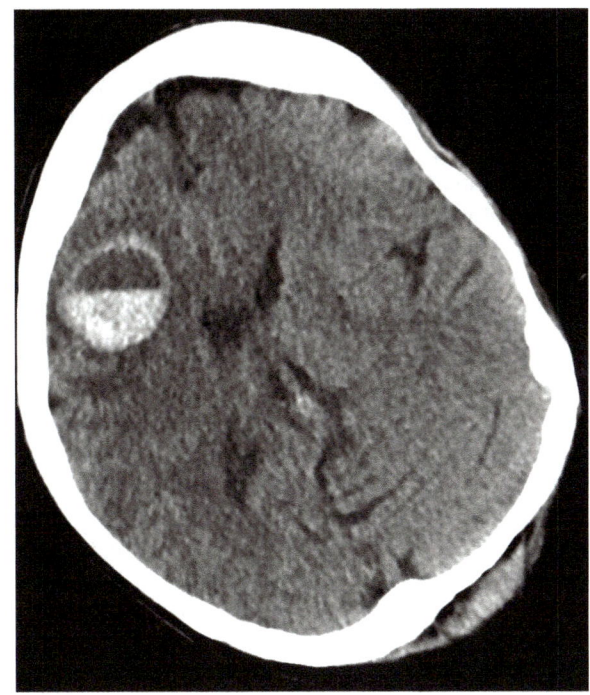

Table 28.2 HAS-BLED score

Parameter	Score
Hypertension	1
Renal disease (dialysis, transplant, creatinine >2.26 mg/dL or 200 µmol/L)	1
Liver disease (cirrhosis or bilirubin >2 times normal with AST/ALT >3times normal)	1
Stroke history	1
Prior major bleeding or predisposition to bleeding	1
Labile INR (unstable/high INR, time in therapeutic range of <60%)	1
Age >65	1
Medication usage predisposing to bleeding (aspirin, clopidogrel, NSAIDs)	1
Alcohol use (8 or more drinks per week)	1

(Adapted from Lip et al. and Pisters et al. [12, 13])

Table 28.3 HAS-BLED scoring: the maximum score is 9

HAS-BLED score	1-Year risk of major bleeding	Risk group
0	0.9%	Low
1	3.4%	
2	4.1%	Moderate
3	5.8%	
4	8.9%	High
5	9.1%	
Five or more	Greater than 10%	

A higher score indicates a higher risk of bleeding

Hemorrhagic Transformation of Ischemic Stroke

Ischemic strokes that are large, from a cardioembolic source, or treated with thrombolytics are at higher risk of hemorrhagic transformation (HT). HT should be monitored with repeat imaging, ensuring tight BP control. In most cases, HT is asymptomatic and self-resolves. Significant HT is less common but can cause mass effect and neurological decline, in which case urgent neurosurgical evaluation is critical. For patients with atrial fibrillation and HT, waiting until HT resolves on a follow-up CT scan before starting or resuming AC is prudent. Antiplatelet therapy is typically felt to be safe in this period. Close post-discharge contact, timely follow-up imaging, and clinic follow-up are necessary due to the higher risk of recurrent cardioembolic stroke during this period.

Clinical Pearls
- The etiology of a hemorrhage is often deduced by the patient's risk factors and imaging (Table 28.4).
- CT or MRI helps diagnose an ICH, and CTA or MRA can identify an underlying vascular lesion.
- While initial imaging helps diagnose an ICH, a follow-up MRI at 3–6 months can help to rule out underlying masses or vascular malformations that the initial blood or peri-hematomal edema may obscure.
- Primary ICH is often due to hypertension or cerebral amyloid angiopathy.
- Treatment of hypertensive ICH should be focused on blood pressure management, while management of cerebral amyloid angiopathy involves mitigating factors that further increase bleeding risk.
- Secondary ICH has various causes, including cavernous malformations, arteriovenous malformations, brain tumors, cerebral venous sinus thrombosis, vasculopathy, vasculitis, and reversible cerebral vasoconstriction syndrome.
- DOACs have a lower risk of ICH than Warfarin. Before initiating therapy, it is important to counsel patients and families about the potential risks and benefits. Usually, the benefit of ischemic stroke prevention outweighs the risk of hemorrhage.
- The HAS-BLED can calculate the risk of ICH with Warfarin but should not be used in isolation to determine the appropriateness of anticoagulation therapy.

Table 28.4 Causes, risk factors, and imaging findings for primary and secondary ICH

Cause of primary ICH	Risk factors	Imaging findings
Hypertensive vasculopathy	– Hypertension – Heart failure	– ICH in basal ganglia, cerebellum, brainstem, or intraventricular system – Prior microbleeds or ischemic strokes in basal ganglia, brainstem, or cerebellum
Cerebral amyloid angiopathy	– Older age – Family history of hemorrhages in older people – No hypertension	– Large lobar ICH – Microbleeds in cerebral hemispheres – Superficial siderosis – Cortical subarachnoid hemorrhages

Cause of secondary ICH	Risk factors	Imaging findings
Cavernous malformations	– Genetic	– On MRI, it can have a "popcorn" appearance with a rim of signal loss
Arteriovenous malformations	– Genetic	– Cone-shaping lesions at periphery +/– calcification – CTA shows
Brain tumors	– Primary brain tumors like glioblastoma multiforme – Metastatic cancers, especially melanoma, renal cell carcinoma, papillary thyroid carcinoma, choriocarcinoma	– Besides bleed, the patient may have other areas of enhancement suggestive of tumors
Cerebral venous sinus thrombosis	– Hypercoagulable state (pregnancy, postpartum, autoimmune, or inherited coagulopathy) – Dehydration	– The location of hemorrhage is typically adjacent to the venous sinus – Dilated draining veins on SWI and edema out of proportion to the size of the hemorrhage on FLAIR sequences (both suggesting outflow obstruction) – Hyperdense venous sinuses on head CT, filling defect on CT venogram (empty delta sign)

(continued)

Table 28.4 (continued)

Cause of secondary ICH	Risk factors	Imaging findings
Coagulopathy	– Patient on blood thinners – Coumadin has a higher risk of ICH than direct oral anticoagulants such as apixaban and rivaroxaban – Acquired coagulopathy (uremia, liver failure, bone marrow dysfunction) – Hemophilia	– Possible blood-fluid level, irregular shape, and blood of varying ages
Hemorrhagic conversion of ischemic stroke	– Large ischemic strokes – Patients with coagulopathy, such as low platelets or elevated INR from liver failure – Concurrent use of anticoagulants	– Large areas of hypodensity (CT scan) or diffusion restriction (MRI) surrounding bleed
Pharmacologic agents or drugs	– Cocaine – Stimulants – Phenylpropanolamine	– Similar to hypertensive vasculopathy

References

1. Greenberg SM, Ziai WC, Cordonnier C, Dowlatshahi D, Francis B, Goldstein JN, Hemphill JC, Johnson R, Keigher KM, Mack WJ, et al. 2022 Guideline for the management of patients with spontaneous intracerebral hemorrhage: a guideline from the American Heart Association/American Stroke Association. Stroke. 2022;53:e282–361.
2. Wijman CAC, Venkatasubramanian C, Bruins S, Fischbein N, Schwartz N. Utility of early MRI in the diagnosis and management of acute spontaneous intracerebral hemorrhage. Cerebrovasc Dis. 2010;30:456–63.
3. Greenberg SM, Charidimou A. Diagnosis of cerebral amyloid angiopathy: evolution of the Boston criteria. Stroke. 2018;49:491–7.
4. Charidimou A, Boulouis G, Frosch MP, Baron J-C, Pasi M, Albucher JF, Banerjee G, Barbato C, Bonneville F, Brandner S, et al. The Boston criteria version 2.0 for cerebral amyloid angiopathy: a multicentre, retrospective, MRI-neuropathology diagnostic accuracy study. Lancet Neurol. 2022;21:714–25.
5. Akers A, Al-Shahi Salman R, Awad IA, Dahlem K, Flemming K, Hart B, Kim H, Jusue-Torres I, Kondziolka D, Lee C, et al. Synopsis of guidelines for the clinical management of cerebral cavernous malformations: consensus recommendations based on systematic literature review by the Angioma Alliance Scientific Advisory Board Clinical Experts Panel. Neurosurgery. 2017;80:665–80.
6. Horne MA, Flemming KD, Su I-C, Stapf C, Jeon JP, Li D, Maxwell SS, White P, Christianson TJ, Agid R, et al. Clinical course of untreated cerebral cavernous malformations: a meta-analysis of individual patient data. Lancet Neurol. 2016;15:166–73.
7. Lieu AS, Hwang SL, Howng SL, Chai CY. Brain tumors with hemorrhage. J Formos Med Assoc. 1999;98:365–7.
8. Saadatnia M, Fatehi F, Basiri K, Mousavi SA, Mehr GK. Cerebral venous sinus thrombosis risk factors. Int J Stroke. 2009;4:111–23.
9. Poon CS, Chang J-K, Swarnkar A, Johnson MH, Wasenko J. Radiologic diagnosis of cerebral venous thrombosis: pictorial review. Am J Roentgenol. 2007;189:S64–75.

10. Calabrese LH, Dodick DW, Schwedt TJ, Singhal AB. Narrative review: reversible cerebral vasoconstriction syndromes. Ann Intern Med. 2007;146:34–44.
11. Umashankar K, Mammi M, Badawoud E, Tang Y, Zhou M, Borges JC, Liew A, Migliore M, Mekary RA. Efficacy and safety of direct oral anticoagulants (DOACs) versus warfarin in atrial fibrillation patients with prior stroke: a systematic review and meta-analysis. Cardiovasc Drugs Ther. 2022;37:1225.
12. Pisters R, Lane DA, Nieuwlaat R, de Vos CB, Crijns HJGM, Lip GYH. A novel user-friendly score (HAS-BLED) to assess 1-year risk of major bleeding in patients with atrial fibrillation: the euro heart survey. Chest. 2010;138:1093–100.
13. Lip GYH, Frison L, Halperin JL, Lane DA. Comparative validation of a novel risk score for predicting bleeding risk in anticoagulated patients with atrial fibrillation: the HAS-BLED (hypertension, abnormal renal/liver function, stroke, bleeding history or predisposition, labile INR, elderly, drugs/alcohol concomitantly) score. J Am Coll Cardiol. 2011;57:173–80.

Subarachnoid Hemorrhage

29

Susan Wilson and Ryan Hebert

Quick Anatomy Review

Let's start by reviewing the anatomy of the brain's surface. The meninges are a set of protective layers of membranes that surround and safeguard the brain and spinal cord against damage and injury. The Pia mater is the innermost layer that adheres to the brain, following the sulci and gyri. The next layer is the Arachnoid mater, followed by the outermost layer called the Dura mater. Together, they form a PAD, which cushions the brain against injury. The subarachnoid space is between the pia and arachnoid layers containing cerebrospinal fluid and blood vessels that can form aneurysms (Fig. 29.1). When blood enters this space from a ruptured aneurysm, it is called an aneurysmal subarachnoid hemorrhage (aSAH).

aSAH is a neurosurgical emergency that carries a high risk of death, so it requires a collaborative approach to treatment within specialized medical centers.

S. Wilson
University of North Carolina School of Medicine, Chapel Hill, NC, USA
e-mail: WilsonS@neurology.unc.edu

R. Hebert (✉)
Yale School of Medicine, New Haven, CT, USA
e-mail: ryan.hebert@yale.edu

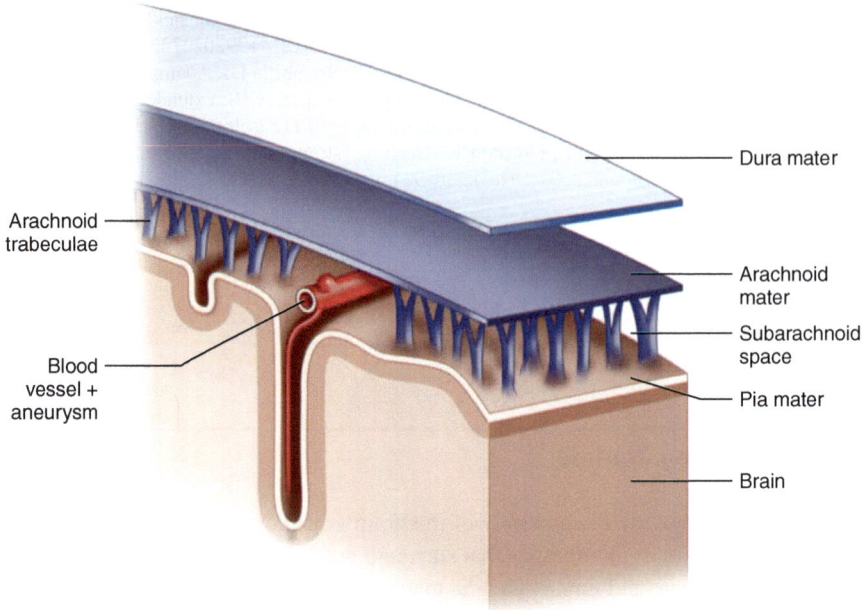

Fig. 29.1 Meningeal layers around the brain

Epidemiology and Risk Factors

Unruptured intracranial aneurysms (UIAs) occur in nearly 3% of the general population. Approximately 20–30% of those patients will have multiple UIAs [1, 2]. Morbidity and mortality are high, with 15% dying before reaching the hospital and a 30-day mortality rate of approximately 45%. 50% of survivors report not returning to baseline, 25% require some form of assistance, and 35% report decreased quality of life associated with depression, anxiety, post-traumatic stress, and memory loss [3].

The most common risk factors associated with aSAH include female gender, advanced age, smoking, hypertension, alcohol abuse, first-degree family history of aneurysms, use of sympathomimetic drugs (stimulants, cocaine), and genetic conditions, such as autosomal dominant polycystic kidney disease and type IV Ehlers-Danlos syndrome [4, 5]. A population-based study examining inpatient hospitalizations from 2007 to 2017 in New York and Florida found that the mean age for aSAH was 61.4 years, and also highlighted racial differences in aSAH incidence, with a higher incidence in Black patients compared to non-Hispanic White patients and other races [6].

Up to 85% of SAH cases are caused by ruptured saccular aneurysms, which primarily occur within the anterior circulation and at bifurcating arteries [1]. The most common location of an intracranial aneurysm is at the bifurcation of the A1 and anterior communicating artery segments (Fig. 29.2). Aneurysms may be saccular,

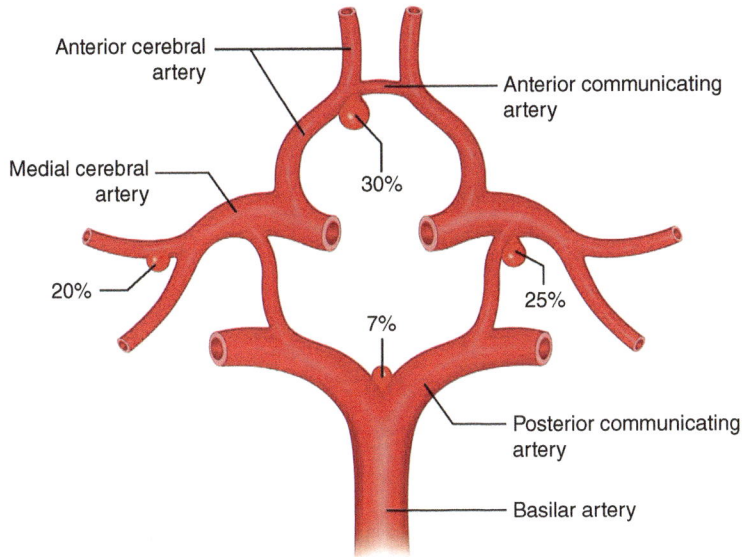

Fig. 29.2 Common locations of intracranial aneurysms. (Source: Vascular Neurology Board Review)

bulging on one side and involving a portion of the circumference of the vessel wall, or fusiform, bulging on both sides and involving the entire circumference of the vessel wall. Although aneurysms occur less frequently in the vertebrobasilar (posterior) circulation, they carry a greater risk of rupture and poor outcomes [1]. Other causes of SAH include trauma, cerebral amyloid angiopathy, and endocarditis.

How Does an Aneurysm Form?

Intracranial arteries are structurally composed of three distinct layers. The innermost layer is called the intima (endothelial cells), followed by the media (smooth muscle with elastin and collagen fibers), and the outermost layer is called the adventitia (collagen fibers and fibroblasts) [1]. Hemodynamic stress (the force of blood flow against the vascular wall) triggers inflammatory responses, weakening the vessel wall and destroying elasticity between the intima and media, thus leading to aneurysm formation [1, 4].

Clinical Presentation and Management

It is helpful to approach aSAH as a three-phase condition: acute (0–24 h), subacute (24–72 h), and chronic or delayed (>72 h) (Fig. 29.3). Each phase requires specific evaluation and management strategies. In acute aneurysmal rupture, the release of

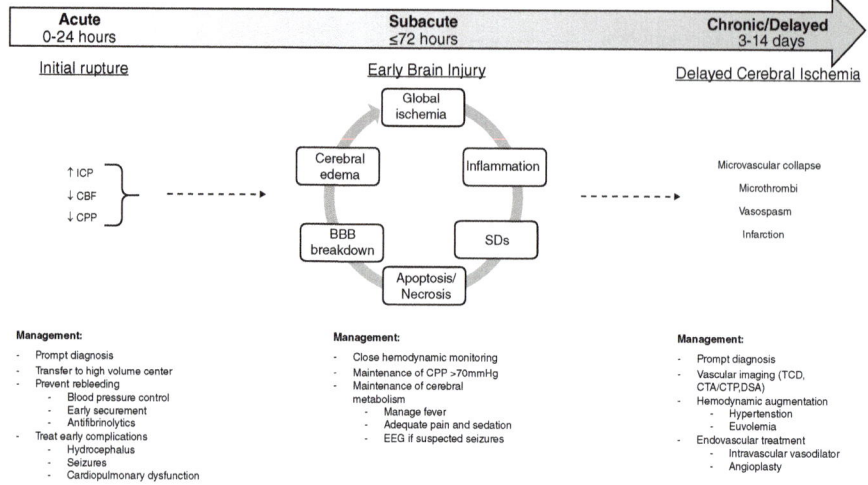

Fig. 29.3 aSAH as a disease process with three phases, (reprinted with permission from Osgood et al. [3])

Table 29.1 Common symptoms associated with aSAH [3, 5, 7]

Symptom	Percent of occurrence (%)
Severe headache	90
Nausea and vomiting	77
Loss of consciousness	53
Terson syndrome (intraocular hemorrhage)	40
Meningismus (neck stiffness, photophobia, headache)	35
Seizure	26
Focal neurological deficits	10

blood into the subarachnoid space results in increased intracranial pressure (ICP), decreased cerebral blood flow (CBF), and ischemia. During the acute phase, the patient may experience significant complications like aneurysm rebleeding, hydrocephalus, seizures, and cardiopulmonary collapse [3].

The most common clinical presentation of aSAH is a sudden onset, severe, rapidly escalating headache occurring in approximately 90% of patients, often described as "the worst headache of life" [7, 8]. Approximately 10–43% of patients report experiencing a sentinel or warning headache 2–8 weeks before the acute event, which represents an early aneurysm leak [5, 9, 10]. Additional presenting symptoms include nausea, vomiting, loss of consciousness, meningismus (neck stiffness, photophobia, and headache that occurs roughly 6 h post-SAH), seizure, focal neurological deficits, and cardiac arrhythmias (Table 29.1) [5].

Vasospasm (abrupt arterial narrowing) following aSAH is an important cause of delayed cerebral ischemia (DCI). It can be diagnosed with transcranial Doppler and typically occurs between days three and 14 following aSAH. DCI occurs in 30–40% of patients and is clinically identified by new focal neurological deficits following aSAH or decrease in GCS of ≥2 points, lasting at least 1 h, and cannot be ascribed to another cause [1]. Nimodipine, a calcium channel blocker, is started during acute hospitalization to prevent vasospasm and DCI. The current recommended dosage is 60 mg every 4 h for 21 days. Because hypotension is a common side effect, the provider should instruct the patient to monitor for dizziness, lightheadedness, irregular heartbeat, and blood pressure [10].

Diagnosis and Workup

Diagnosis of aSAH is based on key clinical characteristics, with history, physical exam, and diagnostic imaging occurring as quickly as possible [10]. Since the most common symptom is headache, history should focus on the acuity of headache onset, characteristics, duration, and severity to assist in determining benign versus emergent etiology and ruling out associated trauma.

The initial diagnostic imaging is non-contrast computed tomography (CT) of the head. CT sensitivity for detecting SAH is 99% within 12 h, decreasing to 93% after 24 h and <60% after 5 days. Magnetic resonance imaging (MRI) detects subarachnoid blood after several days (94–100% sensitivity) [11]. The location of the hemorrhage can help predict the aneurysm location, but vessel imaging is needed to find the aneurysm itself. CT angiography (CTA) can detect aneurysms larger than 4 mm at 100% sensitivity and is comparable to digital subtraction angiography, which is the gold standard [5, 12]. MR angiography (MRA) can detect aneurysms larger than 3 mm with an 89% sensitivity rate [13].

Vessel imaging with CTA and MRA is recommended for the initial screening for aneurysms in suspected aSAH. If an aneurysm is detected on CTA, neurosurgery will determine the next steps of imaging and treatment. Digital subtraction angiography (DSA) is the gold standard for aneurysm visualization and treatment, using IV contrast for 3D views of cerebral arteries.

Sometimes, CT scans may miss a small sentinel bleed. If there is a high suspicion of aSAH after a negative CT, and MRI is not an option, a lumbar puncture (LP) may be performed. The LP should be performed within 12 h of symptom onset. CSF with xanthochromia (yellow discoloration of cerebrospinal fluid from the breakdown of hemoglobin in red blood cells) is diagnostic of SAH. However, with the availability of advanced imaging modalities like MRI, LPs to detect SAH are not always needed [8].

Clinical Vignette

HPI: A 68-year-old woman presented after developing the worst headache of her life while at the gym and had episodes of unresponsiveness and possible seizures in the ambulance on the way to the ED. She was noted to have episodic left gaze deviation and urinary incontinence. She was intubated on arrival. No history of smoking, alcohol or drug use.

Workup: NCCT demonstrated diffuse SAH without midline shift (a, b). CTA revealed a ruptured 4mm anterior communicating artery saccular aneurysm (c, white arrow). EEG negative for seizures.

Management: She underwent successful coiling of the aneurysm 2 days later (d, blue arrow). Her course was notable for central fevers (infectious workup negative) due to central temperature dysregulation, and sinus tachycardia felt to be a possible stress reaction and sympathetic upregulation (pulmonary embolism ruled out). She was eventually extubated with a nonfocal exam.

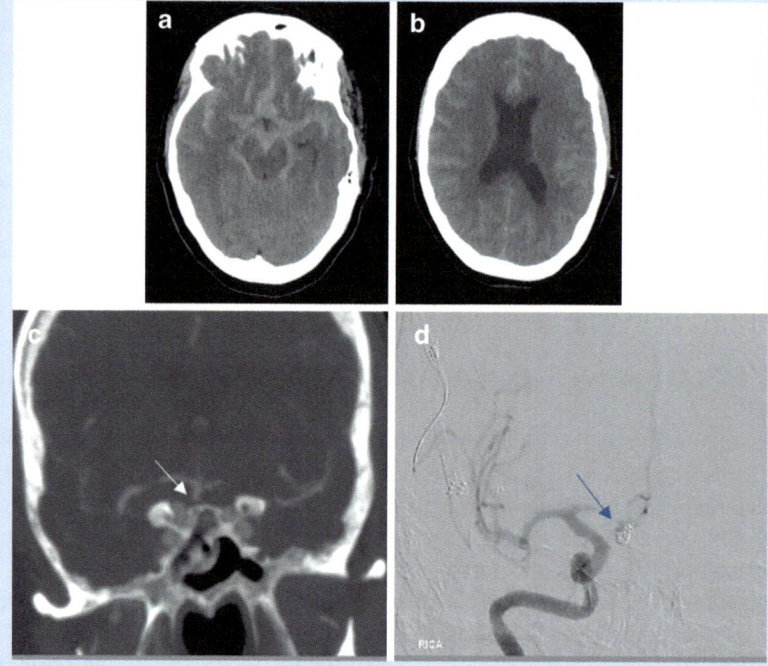

Diffuse subarachnoid blood (SAH) in the basal cisterns and bilateral hemispheres (a, b). Inferiorly directed anterior communicating artery aneurysm (c), and conventional angiogram following aneurysm coiling (d)

Classification/Scales

Grading scales for SAH help identify high-risk patients and guide management. While no scale is perfect, they can help standardize communication between providers.

The Glasgow Coma Scale (GCS) is a universally accepted bedside scale for grading consciousness levels. The GCS incorporates eye-opening, verbal, and motor responses to evaluate the level of consciousness in neurologic patients (Table 29.2). Higher numbers mean intact functions. A lower score is associated with a worse outcome [14].

The Hunt and Hess Scale (Table 29.3) was developed to determine the severity of the SAH and predict survival based on the patient's clinical condition (Table 29.3) [8, 14].

The Modified Fisher Scale (Table 29.4) predicts the likelihood of cerebral vasospasm based on the amount and pattern of blood identified on the initial CT [14, 15].

Table 29.2 Glasgow Coma Scale. Scores range from 15 (best response) to 3 (totally unresponsive)

Assessment	Score
Eye opening	4 = Spontaneous
	3 = To sound
	2 = To pressure
	1 = None
Verbal response	5 = Oriented
	4 = Confused
	3 = Words, but not coherent
	2 = Sounds, but no words
	1 = None
Best motor response	6 = Obeys commands
	5 = Localizing
	4 = Normal flexion
	3 = Abnormal flexion
	2 = Extension
	1 = None
Total score	**3–15**

Table 29.3 Hunt and Hess

Grade	Findings	Mortality risk (%)
1	Asymptomatic or minimal headache; slight nuchal rigidity	30
2	Moderate to severe headache; nuchal rigidity; no focal neurologic deficit except cranial nerve palsy	40
3	Drowsy; confusion, lethargy, or mild focal neurologic deficit except cranial nerve palsy	50
4	Stuporous; moderate to severe hemiparesis; early decerebrate rigidity; vegetative disturbances	80
5	Deep coma; decerebrate posturing; moribund	90

Table 29.4 Modified Fisher Scale

Grade	Modified Fisher Scale	Risk of vasospasm (%)
0	No SAH or IVH	0
1	Minimum, focal, or diffuse thin SAH, no IVH in either ventricle	24
2	Minimum, focal, or diffuse thin SAH with IVH in both ventricles	15–33
3	Thick, focal, or diffuse SAH, no IVH	33–35
4	Thick, focal, or diffuse SAH with IVH present	40

Table 29.5 World Federation of Neurological Surgeons Scale

Grade	Glasgow Coma Scale	Motor deficit
1 (good)	15	No motor deficit
2 (good)	13–14	No motor deficit
3 (good)	13–14	Motor deficit
4 (poor)	7–12	With or without deficit
5 (poor)	3–6	With or without deficit

The scale is often used with the Hunt and Hess scale to communicate the severity of illness among clinicians and within research [10].

The World Federation of Neurological Surgeons Scale (Table 29.5) predicts outcomes using GCS and motor deficits. A higher grade is associated with worse outcomes [8, 14].

Preoperative Management

If a patient survives the initial SAH, a feared complication of a ruptured aneurysm is rebleeding. Rebleeding can occur in 8–23% of patients within 72 h of the initial SAH and carries a high mortality rate. Treating an aneurysm through coiling or clipping significantly reduces the risk of rebleeding. Institutions generally follow an ultra-early (within the first 24 h) aneurysm repair protocol since most rebleeding events occur within this timeframe. Preoperative management before securing the aneurysm focuses on patient stabilization, minimizing complications, and decreasing the risk of rebleeding (Fig. 29.4) [16].

Blood Pressure Control

Elevated blood pressure increases the risk of rebleeding and is associated with worse outcomes [8]. It is reasonable to consider a goal of <160 mmHg or mean arterial pressure (MAP) <110 mmHg for unsecured aneurysms using short-acting agents that allow titration, such as nicardipine, labetalol, or clevidipine [8, 9]. Hydralazine may be appropriate if the patient is bradycardic. Nitroprusside and nitroglycerin should be avoided because of the increased vasodilatory effect and

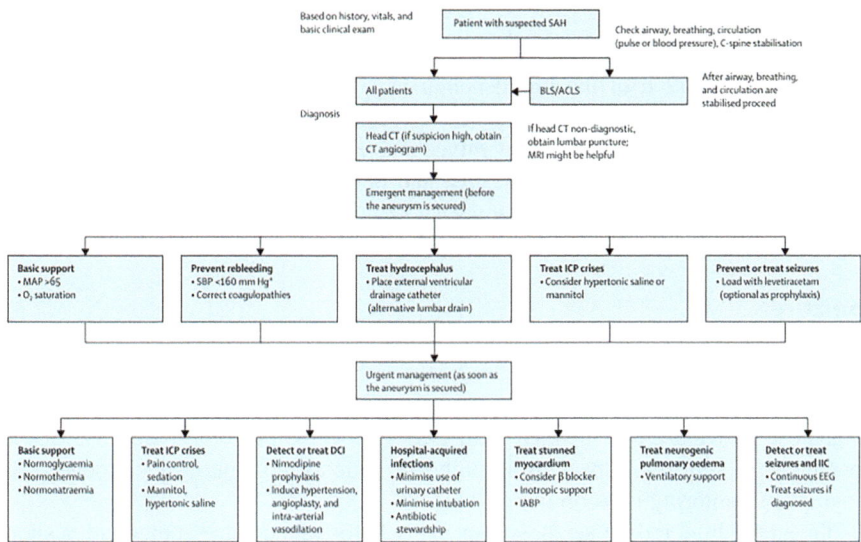

Fig. 29.4 aSAH management. (Reprinted with permission from Claassen J and S Park, Lancet, 2022 [17])

increase in ICP [4]. Overaggressive BP reduction can lead to hypotension and should be avoided to avoid complications [8, 9, 18].

Antifibrinolytic Therapy

Some ruptured aneurysms may not require urgent intervention. In such cases, delayed aneurysm treatment may require an antifibrinolytic agent like tranexamic acid to reduce the risk of rebleeding [3]. Avoid prolonged use (>72 h) of antifibrinolytics due to the risk of increased deep-vein thrombosis, stroke, and myocardial infarction.

Temperature

Fever is one of the most common complications associated with aSAH, occurring in approximately 41–72% of patients, and is associated with worse outcomes [11, 19]. During the first 72 h, fevers are primarily associated with the release of inflammatory cytokines in response to blood in the subarachnoid space, but other infections should still be ruled out. Fevers should be treated aggressively with acetaminophen and surface cooling devices. Shivering should be avoided since it decreases brain tissue oxygenation with institutional shivering protocols [19].

Hyperglycemia

Within the first 72 h of the initial hemorrhage, 75% of patients will experience hyperglycemia [20]. SAH triggers inflammation, increasing glucose production and insulin resistance, leading to hyperglycemia. Hyperglycemia is associated with increased ICU length of stay, mortality, and poor outcomes. Therefore, treatment with target serum glucose levels between 130 and 180 mg/dL is critical [21].

Seizure

In aSAH, seizure development is associated with higher SAH grade, lower GCS at presentation, rebleeding, and vasospasm [22]. Nonconvulsive seizures occurring in comatose patients are associated with DCI and worse outcomes. Because of the potential for seizures, especially in high-risk patients, continuous electroencephalography monitoring is recommended [1].

Given the high risk of seizures, especially before aneurysm securement, a short course (3–7 days) of anti-seizure medication is common. Phenytoin is not recommended due to unpredictable pharmacokinetics, requiring monitoring of levels, poor effects on cognition, and worse outcomes [1, 9, 22]. Levetiracetam is often the drug of choice due to lower drug-drug interactions and adverse effects. Treatment should be tapered after aneurysm securement unless the patient continues to have seizures [1].

Cardiac and Pulmonary Complications

Aneurysmal SAH impacts cardiac and pulmonary function, often within minutes of aneurysmal rupture, but should not delay urgent surgery. While the pathophysiological changes are complex, the associated cardiac complications are most likely related to catecholamine release/toxicity and sympathetic hyperactivity [3, 23, 24]. The increase in ICP leads to reduced cerebral perfusion and oxygenation of the brain tissue. The sympathetic nervous system responds by increasing systemic blood pressure. Increased blood pressure stimulates the parasympathetic system, leading to bradycardia [23]. Further increases in ICP lead to brainstem compression, causing irregular respirations and apnea. This combination of findings is known as Cushing's triad.

Electrocardiograph (ECG) abnormalities occur in 80–100% of patients with aSAH. ECG changes include ST-segment depression or elevation, T-wave inversion, increased U-waves, prolonged QTc intervals, atrial fibrillation, ventricular tachycardia, and fibrillation. In addition, elevated serum troponin levels occur in approximately 30% of patients [1, 3, 16, 25]. An echocardiogram may reveal reversible wall motion abnormalities, apical ballooning, and Takotsubo cardiomyopathy [3]. These cardiac-specific changes occur more often in patients with higher Hunt and Hess scores (>2) and are associated with an increased risk of DCI and mortality [5, 25].

Pulmonary complications, including neurogenic pulmonary edema (NPE), acute respiratory distress syndrome, pulmonary embolism, and pneumonia, occur in 20–30% of patients with aSAH independently of cardiac function or cardiac abnormalities [3, 5, 16]. NPE is associated with catecholamine and sympathetic release and occurs more often in patients with ruptured posterior aneurysms [16]. An observational study found lung injury associated with higher Hunt and Hess and lower GCS scores [26].

Acute Pain Management

Controlling pain from headaches and craniotomy is challenging. Research shows that 50% of patients experience ongoing headaches for the first year, decreasing to 28% at 10 years [27]. The cause of headache pain is complicated and multifactorial, associated with inflammation of cerebral arteries, meningeal irritation due to blood in the subarachnoid space, and increased ICP. Headaches cause significant suffering and require individualized treatment plans, including analgesic agents (Table 29.6) [28]. Acetaminophen is the most commonly used analgesic during the acute phase. Yet, it has limited pain relief and associated hepatic injury with doses over 3–4 g/day. Opioids are the second-line treatment even though they remain inadequate and obscure the neurological exam due to sleepiness. A combination of opioids and

Table 29.6 Current pharmaceutical treatment options for headache following subarachnoid hemorrhage [29]

Drug class	Examples	Efficacy	Drawbacks	Route of administration
Miscellaneous analgesic	Acetaminophen	– Limited based on current evidence, but offset by benign side effect profile	– Limit to 4 g/day due to concern for hepatotoxicity	Oral/ intravenous
Opioid	Morphine, codeine, tramadol, oxycodone, fentanyl	– Mixed evidence – Multiple studies show limited to no pain relief for these patients, one study found benefit in only patients treated with clipping	– Negative side effect profile – One study suggested possible vasospasm	Oral/ intravenous

(continued)

Table 29.6 (continued)

Drug class	Examples	Efficacy	Drawbacks	Route of administration
NSAID	Aspirin, ibuprofen, ketorolac	– Limited evidence	– Possible vasospasm with ketorolac – Risk of bleeding in unsecured aneurysms	Oral/intravenous
Anesthetics	Bupivacaine, Ropivacaine + dexamethasone	– Effective in acute alleviation of refractory post-SAH headache	– Invasive – Data lacking on long-term pain control	Local injection
Corticosteroid	Dexamethasone	– Likely ineffective (difficult to assess as these agents are typically given for other indications, not pain)	– Hyperglycemia	Intravenous
Electrolyte solution	Magnesium sulfate	– May be effective as an adjunct for refractory pain	– Risk of magnesium toxicity	Intravenous
Gabapentinoids	Pregabalin, gabapentin	– Likely effective as an adjunct for perioperative pain control and headache at 24 h	– Pregabalin was not assessed for persistent headache, and gabapentin data from observational study only	Oral

acetaminophen is superior to opioids alone. NSAIDs should be avoided, if possible, before aneurysm surgery because of the increased risk of bleeding. Intravenous magnesium may decrease the severity of headaches [19, 29, 30].

Anemia

Oxygen delivery and uptake to brain tissue relies on cerebral blood flow, arterial oxygen content, and extraction. Anemia reduces the amount of oxygen delivered to the brain, which can lead to ischemic complications. Anemia (hemoglobin <11 g/dL) occurs in 80% of patients, typically within the first 4 days, and is associated with poor outcomes and increased mortality [25, 31, 32]. Risk factors for anemia requiring blood transfusion are older age, female gender, higher grade, and numerous comorbidities [33].

The hemoglobin threshold for transfusion is not clear. However, data and most clinicians support transfusion if hemoglobin falls below 10 g/dL [33].

Aneurysm Treatment

Surgical options include either clip ligation (requiring craniotomy or an opening in the skull) or catheter-based neuroendovascular coiling. Several clinical trials have demonstrated that the endovascular approach has better recovery rates at 2 months and 1 year post-rupture, and patients are more likely to be independent. Clipping was shown to be associated with a higher risk of seizure development. Not all ruptured aneurysms are amenable to endovascular treatment, however. Some ruptured aneurysms present with an intracerebral hematoma causing mass effect requiring emergent decompression. In some instances, the hematoma can be evacuated after endovascular intervention. In others, craniotomy to evacuate the blood is needed before aneurysm treatment.

Post-Discharge Management

Outcomes following aSAH have greatly improved due to the advancements in surgical procedures and early intervention, with most patients discharged home [18]. Nevertheless, many survivors continue to confront cognitive, emotional, and physical complications. Post-discharge recovery requires a minimum of 6–8 weeks. However, survivors generally require at least 3–6 months to return to premorbid function [34]. Poor outcomes were associated with older age, poor admission neurological status (GCS <8), need for external ventricular drainage, and vasospasm [35]. Assessing functional and psychological impairments during follow-up guides individualized treatment plans and rehabilitation for improved outcomes and independence.

Fatigue, Cognitive, and Mood disorders

Post-aSAH fatigue is common (up to 69.7% of patients in one study) and can remain steady over 1–7 years [36]. Fatigue is likely associated with the severity of hemorrhage, dopamine imbalance, depression, anxiety, sleep disturbances, and motor weakness [37]. Identifying fatigue may be challenging. Treatable conditions like mood disorders, sleep disturbances, vitamin deficiency, hypothyroidism, adrenal insufficiency, or anemia should be ruled out [38]. Validated questionnaires can assist in identifying mood and cognitive disorders, as well as chronic symptoms of fatigue [37].

Memory impairment ranges from mild to severe, often presenting within 3 months of aneurysmal rupture. Deficits include difficulty remembering names, written or spoken information, processing speed, face recognition, response inhibition,

Table 29.7 Assessment tools [10, 39]

Disorder	Assessment tool
Depression	Patient Health Questionnaire-9 (PHQ-9)
	Beck Depression Inventory (BDI)
	Center for Epidemiologic Studies Depression (CES-D)
	Geriatric Depression Scale (GDS)
	Hospital Anxiety and Depression (HADS)
Anxiety and post-traumatic stress disorder	State-Trait Anxiety Inventory
	Structured Clinical Interview for Axis-1 Disorders
	Wimbledon Self-Report Scale
Cognitive impairment	Montreal Cognitive Assessment (MoCA)
	Mini-Mental State Examination (MMSE)
	Telephone Interview for Cognitive Status (TICS)
Quality of life	Health-Related Quality Of Life (HRQoL)
	EuroQoL-5 Dimensions (EQ-5D)
Sexual dysfunction	Female Sexual Function Index
	International Index of Erectile Function

impaired attention, poor working memory, or remembering directions [39]. These patients require a memory specialist for optimal management.

Mood disorders like depression, anxiety, and post-traumatic stress disorder are common in patients during the first year after aSAH. They are more frequent in patients with a history of psychiatric illness. Symptoms can be related to fear of SAH recurrence (a form of post-traumatic stress), financial stress, long-term disability, heightened sense of mortality, hypervigilance and anxiety over new symptoms, and having intercourse (especially if the aneurysmal rupture occurred during sex) [34].

These impairments negatively impact the quality of life and the ability to return to work, with over 50% of survivors unable to resume previous work and social activities [39]. Post-discharge follow-up should include screening patients for cognitive and mood disorders utilizing validated assessment tools (Table 29.7) and, if indicated, referring patients for additional neuropsychological testing to aid management [10]. Treatment may include pharmacological, psychotherapy, and rehabilitation.

Anosmia

At least 25–33% of patients will experience anosmia (loss of smell) after aSAH. Anosmia is linked to loss of appetite, decreased nutritional intake, decreased weight, reduced QOL, and decreased libido. Safety issues, such as the inability to detect smoke, gas, or spoiled food, may be life-threatening [34]. There is no specific proven treatment for anosmia. Unfortunately, recovery is rare in surgical patients, but occurs frequently in those treated endovascularly. Safety education, such as using smoke and propane gas detectors, is essential [40].

Seizures

The incidence of seizures post-aSAH ranges between 8 and 15%. Seizures may occur years after the initial SAH and can be associated with rebleeding [9, 41]. Seizure onset and late epilepsy risk factors include aneurysm location in the MCA territory, higher Hunt and Hess and Fisher grade scores, surgical clipping, and intracerebral hemorrhage. For SAH patients who experience seizures, ASM should be continued post-discharge to prevent recurrent seizures within 2 years. Seizures that occur during the first week or later may require prolonged treatment and should be managed postoperatively by an epileptologist [9].

Chronic Headache

SAH is associated with a high risk of persistent headaches compared to other stroke subtypes. Patients often describe the post-SAH headache as pressing, stabbing, pulling, dull, or throbbing [42]. Treatment of chronic headaches includes analgesic medications (listed in the acute section), with commonly used analgesics being opioids and the combination of acetaminophen, butalbital, and caffeine (A/B/C). Gabapentin has success in decreasing pain and reducing the need for opioids, as well as providing anxiolytic, antiemetic, and anti-seizure benefits. NSAIDs may increase the risk of aneurysm rebleeding. Nerve blocks have shown promise in studies completed during hospitalization, but have not been studied in the post-discharge chronic SAH headache population. Additional treatments include cognitive-behavioral therapy, relaxation techniques, and acupuncture [42].

Hyponatremia

Defined as serum sodium <135 meq/L, hyponatremia following aSAH is commonly associated with cerebral salt wasting (CSW) or syndrome of inappropriate antidiuretic hormone (SIADH) and may require continued treatment and monitoring post-discharge. CSW requires sodium and water replacement, while SIADH is often treated with fluid restriction [43]. Patients discharged on treatment for hyponatremia or SIADH should have their serum sodium level checked approximately 1 week after discharge. Regardless of the cause, if the serum sodium level drops below 120 mEq/L, the patient should be sent to the local ED for treatment, close monitoring, and possible hospitalization [44].

Fluid restrictions are difficult to follow, often leading to poor compliance [45]. If recommended at discharge, a negative fluid balance goal of >500 mL/day effectively increases plasma sodium levels [46]. Sodium chloride tablets will increase water excretion and sodium levels and are relatively inexpensive [47].

Modifiable Risk Factors

The most common modifiable risk factors for aneurysm formation, growth, and rupture are hypertension and cigarette smoking, followed by alcohol intake and substance use, such as cocaine [34]. Hypertension contributes to aneurysm development, growth, and rupture through disturbances in vascular resistance and arterial wall damage. Adding cigarette smoking leads to a 15-fold increase in subarachnoid hemorrhage risk, and that risk is proportional to the number of cigarettes smoked daily [48].

About 4.5% of aSAH occur during sexual activity and 30% at rest [49]. Home care post-clipping, the provider should instruct the patient to avoid strenuous activity, such as lifting anything >5 pounds, yard or housework, and sexual activity for 2 weeks or as per the neurosurgeon's recommendation. Encourage daily leisure physical activity, such as walking, gradually increasing the distance. (Recommendations regarding driving, air travel, and returning to work will be individualized based on patient outcome at discharge).

Intracranial Aneurysm Imaging Follow-Up and Screening

Post-EVT aneurysm imaging follow-up includes serial imaging and clinic follow-up. Follow-ups should be at 3–6 months, 12–24 months, and 3–5 years after the procedure and are arranged by the neurosurgery clinic. Approximately 5–10% of patients will develop new aneurysms over time [50]. Magnetic resonance angiography (MRA) is the preferred method for follow-up imaging. Computed tomography angiography (CTA) is not helpful for coiled aneurysms because the platinum coils lead to CT artifact and obscure the actual aneurysm [50].

> **Clinical Pearls**
> - Rebleeding after aSAH increases mortality and poor outcomes. Prompt identification and treatment of ruptured aneurysm is recommended to prevent rebleeding.
> - Aneurysm treatment depends on patient and aneurysm characteristics and is determined by neurosurgeons or neuro-interventionalists. Grading scales aid shared decision-making.
> - Hemodynamic monitoring, blood pressure management, and maintaining euvolemia are critical in decreasing complications.
> - Prophylactic antiepileptic drugs are often used until an aneurysm is secured; new-onset seizures should be treated for a longer duration.
> - Clinical deterioration may be a sign of cerebral vasospasm and delayed cerebral ischemia.
> - Early nimodipine administration decreases DCI risk and improves functional outcomes.

Clinical Trials

ULTRA Trial evaluated if ultra-early and short-term use of tranexamic acid after subarachnoid hemorrhage improved clinical outcomes at 6 months. The trial enrolled 955 patients with aneurysm subarachnoid hemorrhage, with 480 assigned to tranexamic acid and 475 assigned to the control group (usual care). There was no significant difference in outcomes between groups [51].

BRAT Trial compared the safety and efficacy of surgical clipping versus endovascular coil embolization for ruptured aneurysms. Patients were followed for 6 years. Of the 471 patients enrolled, 362 (77%) had a saccular aneurysm, with 181 each assigned to the clipping and coiling groups. 95% of the clipped aneurysms were obliterated entirely, compared to 40% of the coiled aneurysms at the 6-year follow-up. There was no difference in morbidity, but retreatment rates and complete obliteration favored clipping [52].

References

1. Tawk R, Hasan T, D'Souza C, Peel J, Freeman W. Diagnosis and treatment of unruptured intracranial aneurysms and aneurysmal subarachnoid hemorrhage. Mayo Clin Proc. 2021;96(7):1970–2000. https://doi.org/10.1016/j.mayocp.2021.01.005.
2. Renowden S, Nelson R. Management of incidental unruptured intracranial aneurysms. Pract Neurol. 2020;20(5):347–55. https://doi.org/10.1136/practneurol-2020-002521.
3. Osgood M. Aneurysmal subarachnoid hemorrhage: review of the pathophysiology and management strategies. Curr Neurol Neurosci Rep. 2021;21(9):50–61. https://doi.org/10.1007/s11910-021-01136-9.
4. Marcolini E, Hine J. Approach to the diagnosis and management of subarachnoid hemorrhage. West J Emerg Med. 2019;20(2):203–11. https://doi.org/10.5811/westjem.2019.1.37352.
5. Rouanet C, Silva S. Aneurysmal subarachnoid hemorrhage: current concepts and updates. Archivos De Neuro-Psiquiatria. 2019;77(11):806–14. https://doi.org/10.1590/0004-282X20190112.
6. Xia C, Hoffman H, Anikpezie N, Philip K, Wee C, Choudhry R, Otite O. Trends in the incidence of spontaneous subarachnoid hemorrhage in the United States, 2007–2017. Neurology. 2023;10(100):e123–32. https://doi.org/10.1212/WNL.0000000000201340.
7. Eisinger R, Sorrentino Z, Lucke-Wold B, Zhou S, Barlow B, Hoh B, Maciel C, Busl K. Severe headache trajectory following aneurysmal subarachnoid hemorrhage: the association with lower sodium levels. Brain Inj. 2022;36(4):579–85. https://doi.org/10.1080/02699052.2022.2055146.
8. Patel S, Parikh A, Okorie O. Subarachnoid hemorrhage in the emergency department. Int J Emerg Med. 2021;14(1):31–9. https://doi.org/10.1186/s12245-021-00353-w.
9. Hoh B, Ko N, Amin-Hanjani S, Chou S, Cruz-Flores S, Dangayach N, Derdeyn C, Du R, Hänggi D, Hetts S, Lfejika N, Johnson R, Keigher K, Leslie-Mazwi T, Luck-Wold B, Rabinstein A, Robicsek S, Stapleton C, Suarez J, Tjoumakaris S, Welch B. 2023 Guideline for the management of patients with aneurysmal subarachnoid hemorrhage: a guideline from the American Heart Association/American Stroke Association. Stroke. 2023;54:e1–e57. https://doi.org/10.1161/STR.0000000000000436.
10. Wilson SE, Ashcraft S, Troiani L. Aneurysmal subarachnoid hemorrhage: management by the advanced practice provider. J Nurse Pract. 2019;15:553–8. https://doi.org/10.1016/j.nurpra.2019.05.017.

11. Schatlo B, Fathi A, Fandino J. Management of aneurysmal subarachnoid haemorrhage. Swiss Med Wkly. 2014;144:1–9. https://doi.org/10.4414/smw.2014.13934.
12. Yoon N, McNally S, Taussky P, Park M. Imaging of cerebral aneurysms: a clinical perspective. Neurovasc Imaging. 2016;2(6):1–7. https://doi.org/10.1186/s40809-016-0016-3.
13. Thompson BG, Brown RD, Amin-Hanjani S, Broderick J, Cockroft K, Connolly S, Duckwiler G, Harris C, Howard V, Johnston C, Meyers P, Molyneux A, Ogilvy C, Ringer A, Torner J. Guidelines for the management of patients with unruptured intracranial aneurysms. A guideline for healthcare professionals from the American Heart Association/American Stroke Association. Stroke. 2015;46:2368–400. https://doi.org/10.1161/STR.0000000000000070.
14. Rosen D, Macdonald L. Subarachnoid hemorrhage grading scales: a systematic review. Neurocrit Care. 2005;2:110–8. https://doi.org/10.1385/NCC:2:2:110.
15. Frontera J, Claassen J, Schmidt JM, Wartenberg K, Temes R, Connolly ES, Macdonald RL, Mayer S. Prediction of symptomatic vasospasm after subarachnoid hemorrhage the modified fisher scale. Neurosurgery. 2006;59(1):21–7. https://doi.org/10.1227/01.neu.0000243277.86222.6c.
16. Sharma D. Perioperative management of aneurysmal subarachnoid hemorrhage. Anesthesiology. 2020;133:1283–305. https://doi.org/10.1097/ALN.0000000000003558.
17. Claassen J, Park S. Spontaneous subarachnoid haemorrhage. Lancet. 2022;400(10355):846–62. https://doi.org/10.1016/S0140-6736(22)00938-2. Epub 2022 Aug 16. PMID: 35985353; PMCID: PMC9987649.
18. D'Souza S. Aneurysmal subarachnoid hemorrhage. J Neurosurg Anesthesiol. 2015;27(3):222–40. https://doi.org/10.1097/ANA.0000000000000130.
19. Boling B, Groves T. Management of subarachnoid hemorrhage. Crit Care Nurse. 2019;39(5):58–67. https://doi.org/10.4037/ccn2019882.
20. Santana D, Mosteiro A, Pedrosa L, Llull L, Torné R, Amaro S. Clinical relevance of glucose metrics during the early brain injury period after aneurysmal subarachnoid hemorrhage: an opportunity for continuous glucose monitoring. Front Neurol. 2022;13:1–9. https://doi.org/10.3389/fneur.2022.977307.
21. Onur O, Fink G, Karamatsu J, Schwab S. Aneurysmatic subarachnoid hemorrhage. Neurol Res Pract. 2019;1(15):1–6. https://doi.org/10.1186/s42466-019-0015-3.
22. Panczykowski D, Pease M, Zhao Y, Weiner G, Ares W, Crago E, Jankowitz B, Ducruet A. Prophylactic antiepileptics and seizure incidence following subarachnoid hemorrhage: a propensity score-matched analysis. Stroke. 2016;47:1754–60. https://doi.org/10.1161/STOKEAHA.116.013766.
23. Wybraniec M, Mizia-Stec K, Kryzyxh L. Neurocardiogenic injury in subarachnoid hemorrhage: a wide spectrum of catecholamine-mediated brain–heart interactions. Cardiol J. 2014;21(3):220–8. https://doi.org/10.5603/CJ.a2014.0019.
24. Green D, Burns J, DeFusco C. ICU management of aneurysmal subarachnoid hemorrhage. J Intensive Care Med. 2013;28(6):341–54. https://doi.org/10.1177/0885066611434100.
25. Garg R, Bar B. Systemic complications following aneurysmal subarachnoid hemorrhage. Curr Neurol Neurosci Rep. 2017;17:1–7. https://doi.org/10.1007/s11910-017-0716-3.
26. Towner J, Rahmani R, Zammit C, Khan I, Paul D, Bhalla T, Roberts D. Mechanical ventilation in aneurysmal subarachnoid hemorrhage: systematic review and recommendations. Crit Care. 2020;24(575):1–8. https://doi.org/10.1186/s13054-020-03269-8.
27. Gaastra B, Carmichael H, Galea I, Bulters D. Duration and characteristics of persistent headache following aneurysmal subarachnoid hemorrhage. Headache. 2022;62(10):1376–82. https://doi.org/10.1111/head.14418.
28. Glisic E, Gardiner L, Josti L, Dermanelian E, Ridel S, Dziodzio J, McCrum B, Enos B, Lerwick P, Fraser G, Muscat P, Riker R, Ecker R, Florman J, Seder D. Inadequacy of headache management after subarachnoid hemorrhage. Am J Crit Care. 2018;25(2):136–43. https://doi.org/10.4037/ajcc2016486.
29. Sorrentino ZA, Laurent D, Hernandez J, Davidson C, Small C, Dodd W, Lucke-Wold B. Headache persisting after aneurysmal subarachnoid hemorrhage: a narrative review of

pathophysiology and therapeutic strategies. Headache. 2022;62(9):1120–32. https://doi.org/10.1111/head.14394. Epub 2022 Sep 16.

30. Hile G, Cook A. Treatment of headache in aneurysmal subarachnoid hemorrhage: multimodal approach. Interdiscip Neurosurg. 2020;22:100857. https://doi.org/10.1016/j.inat.2020.100857.

31. Ayling O, Ibrahim G, Alotaibi N, Gooderham P, Macdonald L. Anemia after aneurysmal subarachnoid hemorrhage is associated with poor outcome and death. Stroke. 2018;49:1859–65. https://doi.org/10.1161/STROKEAHA.117.020260.

32. Maher M, Schweizer T, Macdonald L. Treatment of spontaneous subarachnoid hemorrhage guidelines and gaps. Stroke. 2020;51:1326–32. https://doi.org/10.1161/STROKEAHA.119.025997.

33. Mofor P, Oduguwa E, Tao J, Barrie U, Kenfack Y, Montgomery E, Edukugho D, Rail B, Hicks W, Pernik M, Adeyemo E, Caruso J, Ahmadieh T, Bagley C, Sillero R, Aoun S. Postoperative transfusion guidelines in aneurysmal cerebral subarachnoid hemorrhage: a systematic review and critical summary of available evidence. World Neurosurg. 2022;158:234–43. https://doi.org/10.1016/jwneu.2021.12.007.

34. Rinkel G, Greebe P. Subarachnoid hemorrhage in clinical practice. Cham: Springer International Publishing; 2015. p. 12–5. https://doi.org/10.1007/978-3-319-17840-0.

35. Cinotti R, Putegnat JB, Lakhal K, Desal H, Chenet A, Buffenoir K, Frasca D, Allaouchiche B, Asehnoune K, Rozec B. Evolution of neurological recovery during the first year after subarachnoid haemorrhage in a French University Centre. Anaesth Crit Care Pain Med. 2019;38:251–7. https://doi.org/10.1016/j.accpm.2018.10.002.

36. Western E, Sorteberg A, Brunborg C, Nordenmark T. Prevalence and predictors of fatigue after aneurysmal subarachnoid hemorrhage. Acta Neurochir. 2020;162:3107–16. https://doi.org/10.1007/s00701-020-04538-9.

37. Western E, Nordenmark T, Sorteberg W, Karic T, Sorteberg A. Fatigue after aneurysmal subarachnoid hemorrhage: clinical characteristics and associated factors in patients with good outcome. Front Behav Neurosci. 2021;15:1–15. https://doi.org/10.3389/fnbeh.2021.633616.

38. Kutlubaev M, Mead G. Chapter 29: Fatigue after stroke. In: Godefroy O, editor. The behavioral and cognitive neurology of stroke. 2nd ed. Cambridge: Cambridge University Press; 2013. p. 375–86. https://doi.org/10.1017/CB09781139058988.

39. Nussbaum ES, Mikoff N, Paranjape GS. Cognitive deficits among patients surviving aneurysmal subarachnoid hemorrhage. A contemporary systematic review. Br J Neurosurg. 2021;35(4):384–401. https://doi.org/10.1080/02688697.2020.1859462.

40. Holbrook EH, Leopold D. Disorders of taste and smell. Medscape. 2022;2:2022. https://emedicine.medscape.com/article/861242-overview.

41. Ramos M, Teixeira M, Figueiredo E. Seizures and epilepsy following subarachnoid hemorrhage: a review on incidence, risk factors, outcome, and treatment. Arquivos Brasileiros de Neurocirurgia. 2018;37(3):206–12. https://doi.org/10.1055/s-0038-1672202.

42. Huckhagel T, Klinger R, Schmidt N, Regelsberger J, Westphal M, Czorlich P. The burden of headache following aneurysmal subarachnoid hemorrhage: a prospective single-center cross-sectional analysis. Acta Neurochir. 2020;16:893–903. https://doi.org/10.1007/s00701-020-04235-7.

43. Shah K, Turgeon R, Gooderham P, Ensom M. Prevention and treatment of hyponatremia in patients with subarachnoid hemorrhage: a systematic review. World Neurosurg. 2021;109:222–9. https://doi.org/10.1016/j.wneu.2017.09.182.

44. Adrogué H, Tucker B, Madias N. Diagnosis and management of hyponatremia a review. JAMA. 2022;380(3):280–91. https://doi.org/10.1001/jama.2022.1176.

45. Peri A, Groché C, Berardi R, Runkle I. SIADH: differential diagnosis and clinical management. Endocrine. 2017;55:311–9. https://doi.org/10.1007/s12020-016-0936-3.

46. Martin-Grace J, Tomkins M, O'Reilly M, Thompson C, Sherlock M. Approach to the patient: hyponatremia and the syndrome of inappropriate antidiuresis (SIAD). J Clin Endocrinol Metabol. 2022;107:2362–76. https://doi.org/10.1210/clinem/dgac245.

47. Buffington M, Abreo K. Hyponatremia: a review. J Intensive Care Med. 2016;31(4):223–36. https://doi.org/10.1177/0885066614566794.

48. Toth G, Cerejo R. Intracranial aneurysms: review of current science and management. Vasc Med. 2018;23(3):276–88. https://doi.org/10.1177/1358863X18754693.
49. Mallereau C, Todeschi J, Lefevre E, Chibbaro S, Proust F, Cebula H. Is physical activity a trigger factor for subarachnoid hemorrhage? Neurochirurgie. 2022;68(3):315–9. https://doi.org/10.1016/j.neuchi.2021.06.011.
50. Soize S, Gawlitza M, Raoult H, Pierot L. Imaging follow-up of intracranial aneurysms treated by endovascular means. Why, when, and how? Stroke. 2016;47:1407–12. https://doi.org/10.1161/STROKEAHA.115.011414.
51. Post R, Germans M, Tjerkstra M, Vergouwen M, Jellema K, Koot R, Kruyt N, Willems P, Wolfs J, de Beer F, Verbaan D. Ultra-early tranexamic acid after subarachnoid haemorrhage (ULTRA): a randomized controlled trial. Lancet. 2021;397(10269):112–8. https://doi.org/10.1016/S0140-6736(20)32518-6.
52. Spetzler R, Zabramski J, McDougall C, Albuquerque F, Hills N, Wallace R, Nakaji P. Analysis of saccular aneurysms in the barrow ruptured aneurysm trial. J Neurosurg. 2018;128(1):120–5. https://doi.org/10.3171/2016.9.JNS161301.

Poststroke Complications

30

Jeremy Bingham and Deborah Kerrigan

Introduction

Neurological worsening is a feared event for any admitted stroke patient. A multitude of complications following a stroke can lead to a worsening of clinical status (Table 30.1). It is important to develop a rapid differential when patients decline to order appropriate tests and perhaps even reverse the symptoms.

Hemorrhagic transformation (HT) or hemorrhagic conversion of ischemic tissue is a very common sequelae of ischemic stroke. In ischemic stroke, both the brain tissue and the walls of the blood vessels in that region are injured. Injury to the blood-brain barrier leads to extravasation of blood into the stroke "bed," a.k.a. hemorrhagic transformation. HT is often clinically insignificant and only detected on imaging (Fig. 30.1), but if severe, it can cause clinical deterioration by compressing surrounding brain structures or causing seizures. Clinically significant HT is measured by a worsening of the patient's National Institutes of Health Stroke Scale score (NIHSS) of four or more [1–3]. Asymptomatic HT warrants follow-up imaging to monitor for expansion, but patients with clinical deterioration warrant transfer to an intensive care unit.

The risk of developing spontaneous HT is highest within the first 2 weeks following a severe stroke. Risk factors for HT include advanced patient age, hyperglycemia, thrombocytopenia, larger infarct size, embolic strokes (not lacunes), elevated blood pressure, and thrombolytic therapy. If HT occurs after thrombolytics or with anticoagulation, follow reversal protocols (discussed in another chapter). Antiplatelet agents are generally safe in small volume of HT, but anticoagulation (if urgently needed) may increase the risk of expansion and should be carefully considered. For patients with atrial fibrillation, it is prudent to wait until HT is stable before initiating anticoagulation.

J. Bingham · D. Kerrigan (✉)
Vanderbilt University Medical Center, Nashville, TN, USA
e-mail: Jeremy.Bingham@va.gov; Deborah.L.Kerrigan@vumc.org

© The Author(s), under exclusive license to Springer Nature Switzerland AG 2024
H. P. Amin (ed.), *Stroke for the Advanced Practice Clinician*,
https://doi.org/10.1007/978-3-031-66289-8_30

Table 30.1 Causes of neurological worsening

Recurrent stroke	Neurological complications	Systemic complications
– Thromboembolism	– Seizures	– Infection
– Failure of collateral flow	– Edema	– Dehydration
– Hemorrhagic conversion of ischemic stroke	– Hydrocephalus	– Malnutrition
– Hematoma growth	– Delirium	– Deep vein thrombosis/pulmonary embolism
		– Sedating medications
		– Cardiac complications

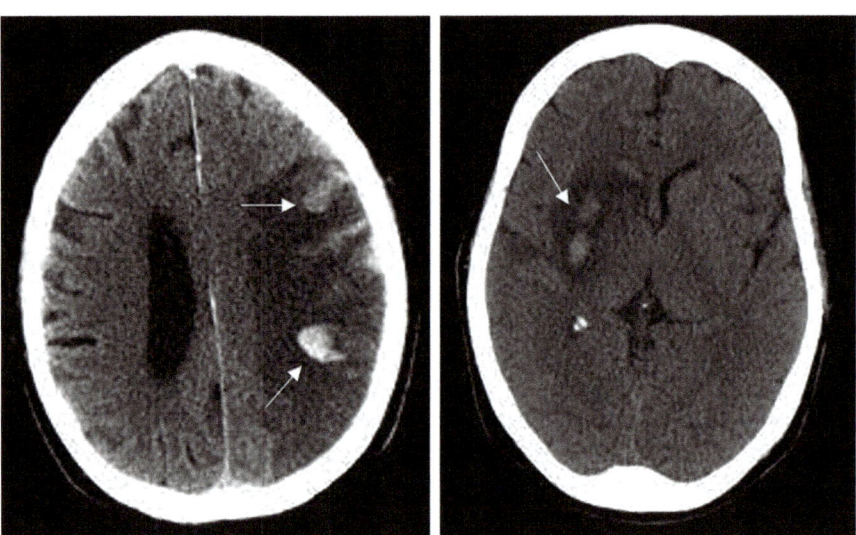

Fig. 30.1 Hemorrhagic transformation/conversion following ischemic stroke. Note the patchy hyperdense blood (white arrows) within a large hypodense area of ischemia

Blood pressure deviations can result in neurological worsening. Many stroke patients will be hypertensive early in their course and will autoregulate down on their own. The concept of permissive hypertension for ischemic stroke encapsulates this phenomenon, as overaggressive BP reduction can lead to hypotension and worsening ischemia. Avoiding hypotension by establishing a clear *lower limit* is particularly important for patients with severe stenosis in the carotid or intracranial vessels. Conversely, untreated hypertension for hemorrhage patients can lead to expansion and clinical worsening. Communicating clear blood pressure parameters to nursing and during signout to the next provider can reduce these deviations.

Dysphagia is impaired swallowing due to weakness of the swallowing mechanism. It occurs with strokes in the cortex, cerebellum, or brainstem. Difficulty forming a food bolus, delayed swallow reflex, disrupted cough reflex, and impaired coordination of chewing and swallowing musculature can occur. Dysphagia leads to aspiration (food or mucus particles entering the airway), which leads to pneumonia, increased length of stay, malnutrition, fever, and delirium.

Stroke patients should be screened for dysphagia early in the hospital stay (ideally in the emergency room) and educated on aspiration signs and symptoms. The initial screen assesses a patient's level of consciousness, ability to maintain a safe swallowing position, and facial motor functions using the 3 oz. swallow evaluation from the Yale Swallow Protocol. Swallowing is assessed by asking the patient to drink 3 oz. of water from a cup or straw with sequential swallows (slow and steady) but without stopping. The screen fails if the patient stops, coughs, or has excessive throat clearing while drinking. Other signs of dysphagia and indicators of aspiration risk include slowed speech, dysarthria, coughing or "wet" quality of speech after oral intake, retained food in the mouth after swallowing, nasal regurgitation, or respiratory distress.

When a patient shows signs or symptoms of dysphagia or fails a bedside 3-ounce water challenge, a more comprehensive screening by a speech-language pathologist (SLP) is necessary. Fiberoptic Endoscopic Evaluation of Swallowing (FEES) is a bedside procedure using a transnasal endoscope to visualize the patient's larynx and pharynx (Fig. 30.2). The test assesses for aspiration and the degree of dysphagia. The SLP may recommend no oral intake (nil per os, NPO) if the patient fails, a diet consistency based on their swallowing ability, and prognosticate swallowing

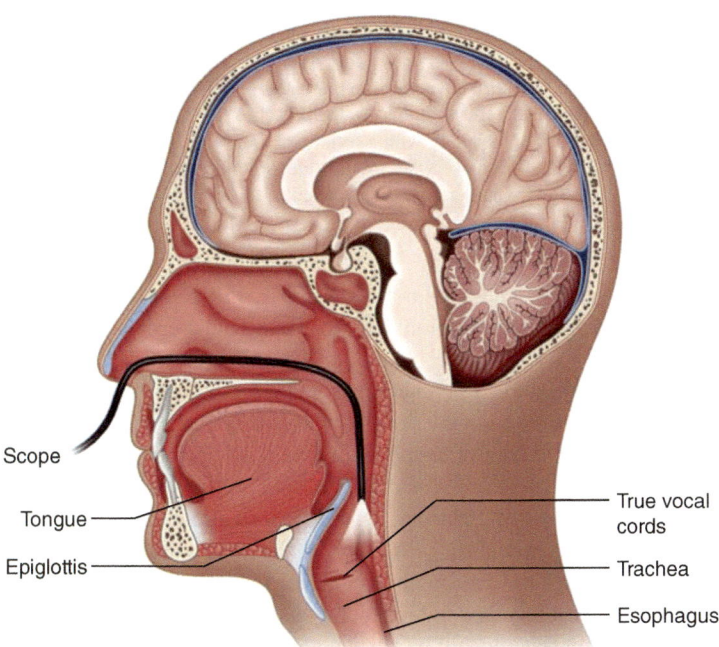

Fig. 30.2 Fiberoptic endoscopic evaluation of swallowing (FEES)

Table 30.2 Pros and cons of fiberoptic endoscopic evaluation of swallowing (FEES)

Pros	Cons
– Visualizes the anatomy of the nasopharynx, supraglottis, and vocal cords	– Does not visualize all phases of the swallowing process
– No radiation exposure for the patient or clinician	– Can miss trace aspiration
– Allows for multiple different food consistencies to be tested	– Can be uncomfortable due to a nasopharyngoscope
– Can be performed outpatient or at the bedside	– Contraindicated with facial trauma
– Can assess patients in isolation or in those too medically unstable to leave the intensive care unit	
– Can be performed on morbidly obese patients	

Table 30.3 Examples of dietary consistencies and modifications

Thin liquids	Water. There is no special consistency. It can easily flow through cups and straws
Moderately thick liquids/liquidized foods	Can be drunk from a cup but require some effort to pass through a straw. It will pass through the tongs of a fork easily. Examples include honey and honey-like consistency.
Extremely thick liquids/pureed foods	Usually eaten with a spoon and can fall off a spoon easily if tilted. If held on a fork, it will not drip through the tongs easily. It cannot pass through a straw or be drunk from a cup. They do not require chewing. Examples include mashed potatoes and applesauce.
Minced and moist foods	These can be eaten with a spoon or fork. Small lumps may be in the food, but they should be easily squashed with the tongue. Examples include finely minced fruits and vegetables or meats chopped to 4 mm width and 15 mm length.
Soft and bite-sized foods	These can be eaten with a fork or spoon. They do not require a knife and do not require the patient to bite and tear off any food, but they are required to chew. Examples include cooked and soft meat that can be broken apart easily with a fork or spoon.
Easy to chew foods/normal diet	This includes everyday foods with soft and tender textures to unrestricted textures. There are no size restrictions.

Source: IDDSI Framework, 2019 [4]

recovery (weeks versus months or not at all). While incredibly helpful, the test is somewhat invasive and has limitations (Table 30.2). Diet consistencies are reviewed in Table 30.3.

For many stroke patients, a percutaneous endoscopic gastrostomy (PEG) tube, a temporary tube inserted through the skin into the stomach, allows patients to continue getting nutrition in the setting of dysphagia while leaving the hospital to begin rehabilitation. It can be removed after several months when patients regain their swallowing ability. Delaying PEG tube placement for repeat swallow evaluations in the hopes of minor improvements extends hospital stays and increases the risk of complications. Even if a patient "passes" a FEES with a pureed or thick liquid diet, consider whether they can consistently, safely, and independently eat enough daily to meet their caloric needs. If not, PEG tube should still be considered. Discussion of PEG tube placement with the patient or their surrogate decision-makers should involve careful contemplation and assessment of their wishes, predicted quality of life, and what the patient would consider acceptable. Not surprisingly, stroke patients who require PEG tubes generally have higher mortality within 1 year of their initial stroke, often due to the severity of the stroke itself combined with other comorbid conditions. A stroke team should guide the patient and family about the overall prognosis and likelihood of PEG tube removal down the road. Declining PEG tube placement may be appropriate in older or neurologically devastated patients who are unlikely to make meaningful neurological recovery and would not want artificial means of nutrition. At that point, the patient would effectively transition to end-of-life care.

Deep vein thrombosis (DVT), a blood clot forming inside the deep veins, is a common and feared complication for all hospitalized patients, particularly hemiparetic stroke patients. Stroke patients have a high risk for DVT and venous thromboembolism (VTE), with over 10% experiencing VTE within 3 months due to immobility and increased clotting factors [6–8]. Sometimes, DVT can also be the cause of a stroke. VTE occurs when a thrombus breaks off the DVT and travels into the systemic circulation. For example, a VTE can travel to the pulmonary artery causing a pulmonary embolism (PE), which can be fatal.

For the ischemic stroke patient, VTE prophylaxis will likely include compression therapy to enhance venous return and pharmacologic measures, including low-molecular-weight heparin (LMWH) such as enoxaparin, dalteparin, or low-dose unfractionated heparin. LMWH may be more beneficial than unfractionated heparin. Some studies suggest lower rates of VTE, PE, major bleeding, and heparin-induced thrombocytopenia with LMWH [9, 10]. Pharmacologic therapy is superior to non-pharmacological devices such as compression devices alone [11–13]. Patients treated with intravenous thrombolysis should not start pharmacologic VTE prophylaxis for at least 24 h to reduce the risk of hemorrhagic transformation.

For hemorrhagic stroke patients, mechanical compression therapy should be initiated within the first 24 h [14]. After the hemorrhage has stabilized, pharmacologic prophylaxis should be added within 1–4 days and continue throughout the hospitalization and rehabilitation. VTE prophylaxis after discharge is less clear and should be considered on a case-by-case basis, such as for those with severe lower extremity weakness or prolonged immobility [15].

Early poststroke seizures (EPSS), occurring within 7–14 days of the index stroke, can cause decreased levels of consciousness, abnormal movements, sensory changes, respiratory distress, and other complications. Recent stroke is the most common cause of seizures in adults and affects up to 20% of stroke patients. Poststroke seizures are due to the release of intracellular contents from damaged neurons, blood products from hemorrhage, or irritation of the parenchyma in the setting of ischemia [16–21].

EPSS may not continue and should be distinguished from poststroke epilepsy, which is likely a lifelong condition. The management of poststroke epilepsy is discussed in a separate chapter. EPSS are more common with intracerebral hemorrhage (ICH) or larger ischemic strokes [16, 17, 20]. The 2018 Guidelines for the Early Management of Patients with Acute Ischemic Stroke and the 2015 Guidelines for the Management of Spontaneous Intracerebral Hemorrhage suggest using antiseizure medication (ASM) only for clinical seizures or concerning EEG, but not for seizure prophylaxis for all stroke patients [5, 14]. The choice of ASM should be individualized based on the patient's renal function, liver function, other medications, comorbidities, and seizure type [22].

Incontinence, a lack of voluntary control of urination or defecation, occurs in approximately half of all stroke patients in the acute stroke period and 25% at hospital discharge. The normal micturition reflex (the act of urination) involves inhibitory signals from the brain that suppress the urge to void. An interruption in this pathway results in detrusor hyperreflexia (bladder overactivity), the most common cause of urinary incontinence (UI) (Table 30.4). This uninhibited contraction of the bladder increases urinary urgency and frequency, resulting in incontinence. Detrusor *hypo*reflexia, the inability of the bladder to contract and empty, can be caused by diabetes, neuropathy, immobility, and some medications. Impaired voiding is a significant risk for urinary tract infections (UTI). Overflow incontinence occurs when the bladder is unable to empty properly, leading to urine leakage. This can be caused by weak detrusor muscles, which prevent the bladder from fully emptying [23, 24].

Other causes of bowel and bladder issues in stroke patients include impaired ability to communicate the need to eliminate, impaired mobility, disrupted sensory pathways, or decreased cognition [24–26]. Identifying which patients may have these difficulties can avoid complications later.

There aren't many validated interventions to treat incontinence. A thorough assessment for non-stroke-related causes of impaired elimination, such as symptom chronicity, medications, or prostate enlargement, is important. Urology consult for urodynamic studies and the measurement of post-void residuals can help to determine the type of incontinence, which is important as each is treated differently. An elimination routine should be scheduled, including regularly using a bedpan, commode, or urinal. The routine use of an indwelling urinary catheter for incontinence is discouraged due to the risk of catheter-associated UTI and other complications, which are reported care quality markers and are not reimbursable by Medicare in the United States.

Poststroke fever occurs in about half of all stroke patients during their hospitalization, typically within the first 2 days of their index stroke. Fever is associated with worse outcomes and increased mortality [14, 28]. A typical fever workup

Table 30.4 Types of poststroke urinary incontinence, derived from Mehdi et al. [27]

Detrusor hyperreflexia and urge incontinence	• Due to direct damage to the neuro-micturition pathways • Involuntary leakage of urine accompanied or preceded by urgency
Detrusor hyporeflexia and overflow incontinence	• Due to initial loss of bladder tone and non-stroke factors • Dribbling and/or continuous leakage of urine associated with incomplete bladder emptying and urinary retention
Impaired awareness urinary incontinence	• Reduced ability to be aware of bladder signals before leakage, to take notice of eventual leakage, or both
Functional incontinence	• Communicative, cognitive, and mobility difficulties leading to urinary incontinence despite normal bladder function
Stress incontinence	• Not directly caused by stroke but a preexisting problem that may be exacerbated
Transient causes of urinary incontinence	• Reversible causes such as medications, urinary tract infections, fecal impaction, and delirium

should include blood cultures, urinalysis, chest X-ray, and evaluation of all lines, tubes, and catheters the patient may have in place. A skin exam may reveal a pressure wound. DVT can also be a source of fever. Central fever due to a brain injury and hypothalamic temperature dysregulation should only be considered after ruling out more common causes, and is often a diagnosis of exclusion. Prophylactic antibiotics are not recommended for fever without evidence of infection. Patients should be kept normothermic, defined as a temperature of <38 °C [5]. To treat a fever is to treat its underlying cause. However, pharmacologic treatments such as acetaminophen or bromocriptine (in the setting of a central fever) or physical cooling with cooling blankets, ice packs, and fans can also be considered.

Poststroke delirium is an acute onset (with onset over hours to days), fluctuating disturbance in the level of consciousness characterized by inattention and disorganized thinking. It is further categorized as hyperactive, hypoactive, and mixed delirium based on the patient's behavior pattern (Table 30.5). Delirium occurs in 10–30% of stroke patients and is associated with increased mortality at 1 year. Patients who experience delirium have a hospital stay averaging more than a week or longer than those who do not [29, 30]. Predictors of delirium include right hemisphere or anterior circulation strokes, increased stroke severity with an NIHSS of ≥8, the presence of brain atrophy on imaging, prior cognitive or sensory impairment, prolonged hospital stays, and ICU admissions [31].

The pathophysiology of delirium is poorly understood, though it is likely multifactorial. Etiologies include disrupted sleep/wake cycles, medication side effects, infection, seizures, and metabolic derangements. The development of delirium, therefore, mandates a thorough workup and evaluation for any treatable complications that arise during hospitalization.

Treatment for delirium is based on the underlying etiology. At a minimum, frequently reorienting confused patients, providing home hearing aids or glasses, reducing overstimulation, encouraging a regular sleep-wake cycle, early mobilization, and appropriate nutrition are all helpful. Removing overnight neurologic examinations might be helpful in select stable patients so the patient can sleep uninterrupted. Pharmacologic treatment is used for agitated patients who do not respond to non-pharmacologic measures. No FDA-approved drugs exist for treating delirium in the US. While antipsychotics are typically used as an off-label treatment for

Table 30.5 Poststroke delirium

Features: Abrupt onset, impaired attention, fluctuating level of consciousness, disorganized speech

Hypoactive	Hyperactive
Inattentive	Hypervigilant
Slow speech	Restless
Lethargic	Labile emotions
Staring	Loud or fast speech
Apathetic	Motor agitation

severe agitation in delirious patients, there is not enough evidence to recommend any particular agent, with typical and atypical antipsychotics demonstrating similar efficacy in controlling symptoms. Benzodiazepines, however, should be avoided in delirium-related agitation, as they are associated with paradoxical worsening of long-term delirium (unless alcohol withdrawal is suspected, in which case they are preferred) [25].

Poststroke pain is a debilitating complication in an estimated 30% of stroke patients. Multiple types of pain occur poststroke, including musculoskeletal pain, thalamic pain syndrome, also known as central poststroke pain (CPSP), headache, and peripheral nerve pain. Disruptions in the sensory systems lead to CPSP, affecting pain, temperature, touch, position, and vibration sensations received by the skin's sensory receptors. CPSP is typically seen after a thalamic stroke and can manifest as contralateral pain from stimuli that usually are not painful (allodynia), pain felt to be worse than usual for a given stimulus (hyperalgesia), and abnormal or unpleasant sensations like burning, tingling, or aching (dysesthesias). CPSP is most common in the subacute and chronic periods after a stroke, beginning around day 15 and continuing indefinitely, and often changes in severity throughout the day [32, 33].

Treatment of CPSP is challenging and individualized, requiring trials of different agents at different doses before finding a regimen that works. Numbness following a stroke is not treatable, however. Treatment of CPSP includes antidepressants, ASM, electrical or magnetic stimulation, and acupuncture. Tricyclic antidepressants such as amitriptyline and nortriptyline are commonly used, as are the serotonin and norepinephrine reuptake inhibitors (SNRI) duloxetine and venlafaxine. ASMs such as pregabalin and gabapentin are also widely used. Other helpful ASMs include carbamazepine, lamotrigine, zonisamide, and oxcarbazepine [32, 34].

Clinical Pearls
- Hemorrhagic transformation may not always require treatment, but careful evaluation is critical for recognizing when it does.
- All patients should be screened for dysphagia. Prolonged dysphagia may require PEG tube placement to allow the patient to continue rehabilitation outside the acute hospital setting while safely getting nutrition.
- All ischemic and hemorrhagic stroke patients require DVT protection.
- ASM is only indicated after a poststroke seizure or abnormal EEG.
- Incontinence in stroke patients may be exacerbated by aphasia, hemiparesis, or cognitive impairments. Awareness of these factors can help treatment and prevent complications.
- Management of delirium involves ruling out treatable causes, maintaining regular sleep-wake cycles, and ensuring proper hearing and sight for older patients. Medications can improve sleep and prevent injury.

References

1. Hong JM, Kim DS, Kim M. Hemorrhagic transformation after ischemic stroke: mechanisms and management. Front Neurol. 2021;12:703258. https://doi.org/10.3389/fneur.2021.703258.
2. Spronk E, Sykes G, Falcione S, Munsterman D, Joy T, Kamtchum-Tatuene J, Jickling GC. Hemorrhagic transformation in ischemic stroke and the role of inflammation. Front Neurol. 2021;12:1–15. https://doi.org/10.3389/fneur.2021.661955.
3. Thomas SE, Plumber N, Venkatapathappa P, Gorantla V. A review of risk factors and predictors for hemorrhagic transformation in patients with acute ischemic stroke. Int J Vasc Med. 2021;2021:4244267. https://doi.org/10.1155/2021/4244267.
4. International Dysphagia Diet Standardization Initiative. "IDDSI—IDDSI Framework." 2019. Iddsiorg. iddsi.org/Framework. Accessed 7 Mar 2024.
5. Powers WJ, Rabinstein AA, Ackerson T, Adeoye OM, American Heart Association Stroke Council. 2018 Guidelines for the early management of patients with acute ischemic stroke: a guideline for healthcare professionals from the American Heart Association/American Stroke Association. Stroke. 2018;49(3):e46. https://doi.org/10.1161/STR.0000000000000158.
6. Amin AM, Lin J, Thompson S, Wiederkehr D. Rate of deep-vein thrombosis and pulmonary embolism during the care continuum in patients with acute ischemic stroke in the United States. BMC Neurol. 2013;13:17. https://doi.org/10.1186/1471-2377-13-17.
7. Dennis M, Mordi N, Graham C, Sandercock P. The timing, extent, progression and regression of deep vein thrombosis in immobile stroke patients: observational data from the CLOTS multicenter randomized trials. J Thromb Haemost. 2011;9(11):2193–200. https://doi.org/10.1111/j.1538-7836.2011.04486.x.
8. Kelly J, Rudd A, Lewis R, Hunt BJ. Venous thromboembolism after acute stroke. Stroke. 2001;32(1):262–7. https://doi.org/10.1161/01.str.32.1.262.
9. Junqueira DR, Perini E, Penholati RR, Carvalho MG. Unfractionated heparin versus low molecular weight heparin for avoiding heparin-induced thrombocytopenia in postoperative patients. Cochrane Database Syst Rev. 2012;12(9):CD007557. https://doi.org/10.1002/14651858.CD007557.pub2.
10. Kamphuisen PW, Agnelli G. What is the optimal pharmacological prophylaxis for the prevention of deep-vein thrombosis and pulmonary embolism in patients with acute ischemic stroke? Thromb Res. 2007;119(3):265–74. https://doi.org/10.1016/j.thromres.2006.03.010.
11. Lansberg MG, O'Donnell MJ, Khatri P, Lang ES, Nguyen-Huynh MN. Antithrombotic and thrombolytic therapy for ischemic stroke: antithrombotic therapy and prevention of thrombosis, 9th ed: American College of Chest Physicians Evidence-Based Clinical Practice Guidelines. Chest. 2012;141(2 Supp):e601S–36S. https://doi.org/10.1378/chest.11-2302.
12. Samama MM, Cohen AT, Cohen JY, Desjardins L. A comparison of enoxaparin with placebo for the prevention of venous thromboembolism in acutely ill medical patients. Prophylaxis in Medical Patients with Enoxaparin Study Group. N Engl J Med. 1999;341(11):793–800. https://doi.org/10.1056/NEJM199909093411103.
13. Tapson VF, Decousus H, Pini M, Chong BH, Froehlich JB, IMPROVE Investigators. Venous thromboembolism prophylaxis in acutely ill hospitalized medical patients: findings from the International Medical Prevention Registry on Venous Thromboembolism. Chest. 2007;132(3):936–45. https://doi.org/10.1378/chest.06-2993.
14. Hemphill JC III, Greenberg SM, Anderson CS, Becker K, Bendok BR, American Heart Association Stroke Council; Council on Cardiovascular and Stroke Nursing; Council on Clinical Cardiology. Guidelines for the management of spontaneous intracerebral hemorrhage: a guideline for healthcare professionals from the American Heart Association/American Stroke Association. Stroke. 2015;46(7):2032–60. https://doi.org/10.1161/STR.0000000000000069.
15. Amin A, Neuman WR, Lingohr-Smith M, Menges B, Lin J. Venous thromboembolism prophylaxis and risk in the inpatient and outpatient continuum of care among hospitalized acutely ill patients in the US: a retrospective analysis. Adv Ther. 2019;36(1):59–71. https://doi.org/10.1007/s12325-018-0846-2.

16. Doria JW, Forgacs PB. Incidence, implications, and management of seizures following ischemic and hemorrhagic stroke. Curr Neurol Neurosci Rep. 2019;19(7):37. https://doi.org/10.1007/s11910-019-0957-4.

17. Graham NS, Crichton S, Koutroumanidis M, Wolfe CD, Rudd AG. Incidence and associations of poststroke epilepsy: the prospective South London stroke register. Stroke. 2013;44(3):605. https://doi.org/10.1161/STROKEAHA.111.000220.

18. Hauser WA, Annegers JF, Kurland LT. Incidence of epilepsy and unprovoked seizures in Rochester, Minnesota: 1935–1984. Epilepsia. 1993;34(3):453–68. https://doi.org/10.1111/j.1528-1157.1993.tb02586.

19. Kilpatrick CJ, Davis SM, Tress BM, Rossiter SC, Hopper JL, Vandendriesen ML. Epileptic seizures in acute stroke. Arch Neurol. 1990;47(2):157–60. https://doi.org/10.1001/archneur.1990.00530020053014.

20. Myint PK, Staufenberg EF, Sabanathan K. Post-stroke seizure and post-stroke epilepsy. Postgrad Med J. 2006;82(971):568–72. https://doi.org/10.1136/pgmj.2005.041426.

21. Zelano J, Holtkamp M, Agarwal N, Lattanzi S, Trinka E, Brigo F. How to diagnose and treat post-stroke seizures and epilepsy. Epileptic Disord. 2020;22:252–63. https://doi.org/10.1684/epd.2020.1159.

22. Wang JZ, Vyas MV, Saposnik G, Burneo JG. Incidence and management of seizures after ischemic stroke: systematic review and meta-analysis. Neurology. 2017;89(12):1220. https://doi.org/10.1212/WNL.0000000000004407.

23. Hebjorn S, Andersen JT, Walter S, Dam AM. Detrusor hyperreflexia. A survey on its etiology and treatment. Scand J Urol Nephrol. 1976;10(2):103. https://doi.org/10.3109/00365597609179667.

24. Winstein CJ, Stein J, Arena R, Bates B, American Heart Association Stroke Council, Council on Cardiovascular and Stroke Nursing, Council on Clinical Cardiology, and Council on Quality of Care and Outcomes Research. Guidelines for adult stroke rehabilitation and recovery: a guideline for healthcare professionals from the American Heart Association/American Stroke Association. Stroke. 2016;47(6):98. https://doi.org/10.1161/STR.0000000000000098.

25. Ross JJ, Dressler DD, McKean SC, Scheurer D, editors. Principles and practice of hospital medicine. 2nd ed. McGraw-Hill Education; 2016.

26. Gelber DA, Good DC, Laven LJ, Verhulst SJ. Causes of urinary incontinence after acute hemispheric stroke. Stroke. 1993;24(3):378. https://doi.org/10.1161/01.str.24.3.378.

27. Mehdi Z, Birns J, Bhalla A. Post-stroke urinary incontinence. Int J Clin Pract. 2013;67(11):1128–37. https://doi.org/10.1111/ijcp.12183.

28. Wrotek SE, Kozak WE, Hess DC, Fagan SC. Treatment of fever after stroke: conflicting evidence. Pharmacotherapy. 2011;31(11):1085–91. https://doi.org/10.1592/phco.31.11.1085.

29. Shaw RC, Walker G, Elliott E, Quinn TJ. Occurrence rate of delirium in acute stroke settings: systematic review and meta-analysis. Stroke. 2019;50(11):3028. https://doi.org/10.1161/STROKEAHA.119.025015.

30. Shi Q, Presutti R, Selchen D, Saposnik G. Delirium in acute stroke: a systematic review and meta-analysis. Stroke. 2012;43(3):645–9. https://doi.org/10.1161/STROKEAHA.111.643726.

31. Oldenbeuving AW, de Kort PL, Jansen BP, Algra A. Delirium in the acute phase after stroke: incidence, risk factors, and outcome. Neurology. 2011;76(11):993. https://doi.org/10.1212/WNL.0b013e318210411f.

32. Dydyk AM, Munakomi S. Thalamic pain syndrome. StatPearls—NCBI bookshelf. NCBI. 2022. https://www.ncbi.nlm.nih.gov/books/NBK554490/#article-30011.s6. Accessed 11 Dec 2022.

33. Paolucci S, Iosa M, Toni D, Barbanti P, Bovi P, Neuropathic Pain Special Interest Group of the Italian Neurological Society. Prevalence and time course of post-stroke pain: a multicenter prospective hospital-based study. Pain Med. 2016;17(5):19. https://doi.org/10.1093/pm/pnv019.

34. Treister AK, Hatch MN, Cramer SC, Chang EY. Demystifying poststroke pain: from etiology to treatment. PM R. 2017;9(1):63. https://doi.org/10.1016/j.pmrj.2016.05.015.

Goals of Care Discussions

31

Emily Alston and Lee Chung

> *"Cure sometimes, comfort always"*
>
> —*Hank Dunn*

Goals of Care Discussions

Despite improved treatment capabilities for acute stroke patients, a significant portion of stroke survivors will have significant disabilities and die due to stroke-related issues. In 2020, stroke was associated with over 160,000 deaths in the United States. Approximately 64% of those deaths occurred outside the acute hospital phase [1]. This means that many stroke survivors leave the acute hospital with a poor prognosis. Identifying those patients and having empathetic and thoughtful conversations with patients and their families are a challenge every clinician faces.

With modern-day medicine, patients and families face difficult choices about potentially life-prolonging medical treatments. Surgical procedures such as tracheostomies and feeding tubes have improved the odds of patients' survival from devastating strokes. Cardiopulmonary resuscitation (CPR) can help regain cardiac function in the event of a cardiac arrest. However, increasing the *length* of life does not always mean improving the *quality* of life. Discussing goals of care (GOC) helps identify acceptable treatment options based on patient wishes and circumstances. Aggressive interventions would be reasonable for patients who prioritize

E. Alston · L. Chung (✉)
University of Utah, Salt Lake City, UT, USA
e-mail: Emily.Alston@hsc.utah.edu; lee.chung@hsc.utah.edu

© The Author(s), under exclusive license to Springer Nature Switzerland AG 2024
H. P. Amin (ed.), *Stroke for the Advanced Practice Clinician*,
https://doi.org/10.1007/978-3-031-66289-8_31

living despite reliance on others for care and artificial means of nutrition and breathing. Other patients may prefer focusing on comfort and hospice care if losing independence would not meet their standard for life.

GOC discussions can be one of the biggest challenges for healthcare providers to navigate. These discussions should establish trust, educate, and align goals to promote patient and family-centered care. Providers should recognize that each patient and family has unique experiences, expectations, and beliefs that frame their perspectives in GOC conversations. Providers should acknowledge limitations in risk scores, personal views, or biases based on their own experiences and might consider asking for a second opinion from experienced colleagues in complex cases [2].

Before initiating GOC discussion with the patient and their family, it is crucial to gather all necessary information. There are many studies and prediction models to help estimate prognosis, such as mortality and disability, in stroke. The iScore and ICH score can help predict mortality following ischemic and hemorrhagic stroke, respectively. However, these scores should be an aid, not the primary means of predicting a patient's outcome. Prognosticating for patients with stroke should be individualized using the clinician's estimates based on their experience and the best available evidence from the literature, including model-based outcome predictions from well-validated studies. However, it is important to note that these scales are not perfect. Errors in prognostication can have significant consequences, including premature withdrawal of treatment or overtreatment, causing excessive suffering, burden, and costs. Therefore, providers should work with patients and surrogate decision-makers to incorporate prognostic models, *patient preferences*, and clinician experience to guide decision-making.

If multiple providers participate in a meeting, it is helpful to identify who will "lead." At the start of the meeting, all participants should introduce themselves, and the team lead should explain the purpose of the meeting. In most stroke cases, the patient will unlikely be able to participate in a GOC discussion. There may be a point person for the family, but addressing every family member's concerns equally is important. Some relatives may be less informed or have differing views than others, and family dynamics may become quickly apparent. Being present, honest, listening to concerns, and answering all questions are essential to building trust.

Tips for Conducting a GOC Meeting

We will now review the components of the meeting, which may or may not follow the sequence we provide. Ask what the patient and family know about the diagnosis, treatments given, and the patient's current state. This is a great time to clarify misunderstandings, define terminology, fill any gaps, and get everyone on the same page. Next, ask what the patient was like before their stroke, what they would define as an acceptable quality of life, and what the most important aspects of recovery might be to them.

At that point, the family will likely turn to the treatment team for their prognosis and recommendations. The medical provider's objective is to give enough information to help the patient and family make informed medical decisions. That typically comes in the form of a "best case scenario" question or the likelihood of a meaningful recovery.

Let us take a moment to discuss the burden of decision-making. It is a common phenomenon that is rarely discussed. It is a silent pressure that a provider or family may feel about making the best decision for their patient or loved one. If a patient cannot communicate, the family serves as their voice to convey their wishes in the current circumstances. Emphasize to family that they are not "making the decision" but instead conveying what their loved one would want in their current situation. Treatment choices are up to the patient. The healthcare team and the family come together to honor and respect the patient's wishes. Below, we give some examples of questions to learn more about the patient's perspective.

If [Mary] was sitting next to us, what would she decide?
Or
What would align with [John's] wishes?

These questions help start a conversation about what the patient would want. Even if the family and patient never had a direct conversation about how they would define acceptable quality of life, they have powerful insight into how the patient lived their daily life and what they value. If the likelihood of a meaningful neurological recovery is low, but the patient would still want to proceed with a percutaneous endoscopic gastrostomy (PEG) tube for feeding or tracheostomy for breathing support, it would be reasonable to move forward. If the patient does not want to live in a dependent state with artificial means of support, then the care priorities "shift" to what the patient would prioritize: comfort. In many institutions, this involves palliative care or hospice teams.

The Disability Paradox and Cognitive Biases

Deciding what a "good" outcome for a patient is an additional challenge, particularly for patients who cannot speak for themselves. The "disability paradox" is a phenomenon where individuals with serious disabilities actually rate their quality of life much higher than others might predict, possibly due to disabled individuals adapting to new conditions and reinterpreting their lives and social roles [3]. These patients can take control of their lives by learning what *is* possible, setting new goals and values, and remaining connected in social networks.

Cognitive biases can result in the disability paradox. Over-estimating the emotional impact that a disability may have on an individual is called forecasting bias, and focusing effects occur when patients anchor on what function is "gone" rather than appreciating the functions that remain [2]. Self-awareness of one's own potential biases is an important step to overcoming them when establishing GOC. Once goals are established, the medical care team can discuss specific interventions outlined below.

Surgical Discussions

Tracheostomy

Mechanical ventilation is required when patients cannot breathe safely on their own. After weeks of requiring mechanical ventilation, patients may require the placement of a tracheostomy tube. A tracheostomy is a surgical procedure that creates an opening in the neck, allowing a tube to be inserted into the trachea for ventilation, bypassing the nose and mouth. Common reasons for tracheostomy placement include upper airway obstruction or insufficient airway protection from stroke, neuromuscular disease, or traumatic brain injury.

Here is an example of an approach to the possibility of tracheostomy. "Due to the severity of 'stroke' [name the disease process], we are entering a phase where we need to discuss possible long-term treatment options. We have been monitoring [patient's name] respiratory status closely for the last few days, and at this time, we cannot extubate. Our goal is to align with [patient's name] wishes. Let us review the medical options available and answer any questions."

Long-term care decisions are made based on the disease process, not because the team is choosing to ask difficult questions. Stress that decisions must be made when a disease process has "entered into a new phase," and the provider is a guide to help answer questions.

Percutaneous Endoscopic Gastrostomy (PEG) tube

Patients with dysphagia (inability to safely swallow) will initially get nutrition via a nasogastric tube (NGT). However, feeding via NGT is temporary, since prolonged use beyond 2–3 weeks can lead to nasal pressure ulcers, tissue necrosis, or gastric bleeding. If a patient requires long-term assistance with feeding, then a PEG tube is the next step. Dysphagia can improve over months to the point where a patient can return to eating and drinking by mouth. Like tracheostomy, a PEG can be removed if a patient recovers their ability to swallow.

A challenge for the provider is prognosticating whether a patient will require a tracheostomy or PEG tube indefinitely, and this is based on the provider's clinical assessment and experience. Some patients have clear advanced directives that they would not want long-term artificial nutrition or mechanical ventilation. However, these procedures might still be warranted in a patient with a reasonable chance of recovery.

DNR/DNI Status

Do Not Resuscitate (DNR) and Do Not Intubate (DNI) are designations made by the patient or family in the event of severe or catastrophic illnesses. Patients may arrive at the hospital with these designations already in place, but many times not. When is the best time to bring up DNR/DNI status? When the patient is admitted to the hospital with a significant condition (stroke), a change in clinical status, or a request from the patient/family to discuss would all be appropriate times.

When discussing code status, review the prognosis and data of survival post-CPR. Survival to discharge after in-hospital CPR is 6–15%, and CPR will not improve function or restore health to prior levels. Careful wording and language are crucial when discussing this topic, as it can be a sensitive subject. Establish that the conversation is happening now to address possible emergency healthcare decisions in the future. Like GOC discussions, DNR/DNI discussions require clear patient and family understanding to be successful. For stroke patients, it is essential to separate possible cardiac and respiratory events from the neurological sequelae of the stroke. This helps set expectations that even after CPR or intubation, the patient will still have stroke deficits. While this seems intuitive, it helps frame whether the patient may want aggressive measures that do not alter their neurological prognosis. Clear language like, "If your heart stops, you will die. Do you want us to use heroic measures to attempt to bring you back?" If the GOC are comfort, then intubation and CPR would not be appropriate.

Hospice Care: Inpatient vs Outpatient Hospice

Many services are available to patients who wish to focus on comfort and quality of life. Palliative care and hospice services are available nationwide for anyone with a severe illness in inpatient and outpatient settings. It is appropriate at any age and any stage in a severe illness. The goal is to optimize the quality of life for both the patient and the family. Hospice care is used for those with a life-limiting progressive or terminal illness with 6 months or less to live if the disease runs its normal course.

Though hospice and palliative care are widely available, some communities may not yet have programs in place. Even so, a patient can still receive comfort measures. Comfort care seeks to make the patient more comfortable despite serious illness while also addressing the family's needs.

Comfort Care Measures: What It Means for the Provider

When a patient comes under our care, the focus is on curing the underlying disease process. Sadly, sometimes, a cure is not possible. Other times, the burden of treatment or disease severity is not acceptable to the patient. When this happens, clinicians should shift away from the goal of curing to the goal of preparing for a comfortable and dignified death. In most cases, this decision comes gradually over time. When a family decides to transition to comfort care, assure them that choosing comfort measures does not mean care stops, but the focus of care has shifted to what their loved one would prioritize at this moment in their life. The medical team will continue the best nursing care, focusing on comfort, easing pain, and breathing.

Table 31.1 Difficult questions

"God is going to bring me a miracle":	How much time do I have left?	Are you saying there is nothing more you can do?

– I hope that for you too. Remember, no "buts"! (Supporting)
– I really admire and respect your faith (Respecting)
– Having faith is very important (Respecting)
– Can you share with me what a miracle might be like for you? (Exploring)
	(This question may mean many things. The patient may be scared; they want to know so they can plan; they are suffering). Exploring what they want to know can be very helpful.)
	– That is a great question. I am going to answer it the best that I can. Can you tell me what you are worried about? (Exploring)
		– I cannot even imagine how (NAME EMOTION) this must be
		– It sounds like you might be feeling (NAMING/ EXPLORING)
		  – Alone
		  – Scared
		  – Frustrated
		– I wish we had a treatment that would cure (make your illness go away). Our team is here to help you through this. (Supporting)

Are you telling me my dad is dying? These responses will affirm the question empathetically so do not use them if the patient is not dying – I wish I had better news – This must be such a shock for you. (NAMING) – I can't even imagine how difficult this can be. (Understanding)	Are you giving up on me? – No, never give up on anyone! I want to ensure we get you the best care possible to address what is happening now – I wish we had more curative treatments to offer. Our team is committed to helping you in every way we can. (Supporting) – We will get through this together. (Supporting) It sounds like you might be feeling Alone Scared – We will work hard to get you the resources and support that you need (supporting)	My dad is a fighter! – He is. He is such a strong person and has been through so much. (Respecting) – I really admire how much you care about your dad. (Respecting) – Seeing him so sick must be so (Name Emotion). (Naming) Tell me more about your dad and what matters most to him. (Exploring)

Special Consideration: In a study of attitudes of palliative care nurses, the majority felt that the "death rattle" was the most distressing symptom for families. Educate families to normalize the disease process for the family. This helps put their mind at rest that their loved one is not suffering [4].

Documentation Tips: There is no standard documentation for medical charts. It is important to document patients' values, goals, and preferences, as well as the specific content of the GOC discussed. Table 31.1 lists common or challenging scenarios and possible responses.

Clinical Pearls
- Understanding that your personal biases and beliefs may not be the same as a patient's or their families, and asking for a colleague's assistance in complex cases is helpful.
- GOC conversations should be conducted for all stroke patients.
- Comfort care/palliative/hospice care shifts the focus of care to what the patient would prioritize at that point in their life.
- In a study of attitudes of palliative care nurses, 100% felt "death rattle" was the most distressing symptom for families. Educate families to normalize the disease process for the family. This helps put their mind at rest that their loved one is not suffering.

References

1. Tsao CW, Aday AW, Almarzooq ZI, Alonso A, Beaton AZ, Bittencourt MS, Boehme AK, Buxton AE, Carson AP, Commodore-Mensah Y, Elkind MSV, Evenson KR, Eze-Nliam C, Ferguson JF, Generoso G, Ho JE, Kalani R, Khan SS, Kissela BM, Knutson KL, Levine DA, Lewis TT, Liu J, Loop MS, Ma J, Mussolino ME, Navaneethan SD, Perak AM, Poudel R, Rezk-Hanna M, Roth GA, Schroeder EB, Shah SH, Thacker EL, VanWagner LB, Virani SS, Voecks JH, Wang NY, Yaffe K, Martin SS. Heart Disease and Stroke Statistics-2022 update: a report from the American Heart Association. Circulation. 2022;145(8):e153–639. https://doi.org/10.1161/CIR.0000000000001052.
2. Holloway RG, Arnold RM, Creutzfeldt CJ, Lewis EF, Lutz BJ, McCann RM, Rabinstein AA, Saposnik G, Sheth KN, Zahuranec DB, Zipfel GJ, Zorowitz RD. American Heart Association Stroke Council, Council on Cardiovascular and Stroke Nursing, and Council on Clinical Cardiology. Palliative and end-of-life care in stroke: a statement for healthcare professionals from the American Heart Association/American Stroke Association. Stroke. 2014;45(6):1887–916. https://doi.org/10.1161/STR.0000000000000015. Epub 2014 Mar 27.
3. Albrecht GL, Devlieger PJ. The disability paradox: high quality of life against all odds. Soc Sci Med. 1999;48(8):977–88. https://doi.org/10.1016/s0277-9536(98)00411-0.
4. Dunn H. Hard choices for loving people. Quality of life. 6th ed. A&A; 2016. p. 15–41.

Discharge Planning

Julia Gray and Michael Lyerly

Introduction

Discharge planning should begin as early as possible during a patient's hospitalization. The goal is to work with the patient, their family, and the interdisciplinary team to decide the most appropriate and safest plan for the transition of care. By identifying barriers early, a thoughtful care plan will decrease hospital readmissions, increase patient safety and satisfaction, and reduce the overall length of stay. As patient advocates, healthcare providers need transparency and input from our entire frontline team to accomplish this goal.

Discharge Planning Team

Everyone needs to be on the same page regarding disposition planning. Best practice involves daily interdisciplinary discussions, or rounds, regarding the patient's wants and needs well before discharge. These discussions can be in the form of sit-down table rounds to discuss each patient on the team, a video conference call, an easily accessible group document or log where opinions or concerns can be noted, or daily phone conference calls. In-person meetings are preferred, since they decrease confusion or misinformation, promote engagement, create a cohesive atmosphere where everyone feels heard, and ensure increased privacy around sensitive medical or social information. These discussions should happen away from patient care areas to ensure patient confidentiality but should also be in a central location to allow ease of access for the team. Depending on complexity, each patient should typically take 2–5 min to discuss.

J. Gray · M. Lyerly (✉)
University of Alabama, Birmingham, AL, USA
e-mail: jngray@uabmc.edu; mlyerly@uabmc.edu

© The Author(s), under exclusive license to Springer Nature Switzerland AG 2024
H. P. Amin (ed.), *Stroke for the Advanced Practice Clinician*,
https://doi.org/10.1007/978-3-031-66289-8_32

- *Healthcare Providers* (MDs, PAs, and APRNs) can update the patient's medical progress and communicate anticipated medical needs after discharge.
- *Nursing* has the closest pulse on the day-to-day progress and needs of the patient. They spend the most time with the patient and bring vital medical and social information to the group. They help initiate discussions on removing certain lines, catheters, or restraints and bring any new concerns to the group. Nurses can also aid in discussions about readiness for transitioning the patient to a different level of care (e.g., ICU, step-down, and acute care floor).
- *Therapists* will help determine appropriate discharge rehab recommendations. Physical and occupational therapists should discuss the patient's mobility, independence level, and safety awareness. Speech therapists will aid with cognition, language deficits, and swallowing evaluations. Therapy needs may change from day to day or remain static, but assessments should remain current.
- *Case Management/Care Coordination* can help identify barriers such as social issues, insurance status, and outside resource needs (financial assistance, transportation, medical equipment, and support groups). Case Management, usually composed of a licensed social worker or RN case manager, will consider therapy recommendations, medical needs, and insurance coverage to present disposition options. They also guide discussion on ethical situations, including next of kin or designated medical decision-makers. They should work very closely with the patients and families to educate them on options and obtain preferences.
- *Pharmacists* can help with discussions on Joint Commission recommendations/requirements regarding DVT prophylaxis, antiplatelet agents, and statins, simplify medication regimens, and identify prescription co-pay concerns. They can also help educate the patient on new medications, assist with transitioning between IV and oral medications, and create an appropriate medication schedule before discharge. At some institutions, pharmacists may be able to deliver some medications to the bedside before discharge.

Stroke Nurse Navigator

Having a stroke nurse navigator within the multidisciplinary discharge planning team is helpful. The stroke navigator serves as a primary resource for patients during treatment and coordinates care transitions for stroke patients and their families (Table 32.1). They can follow up on discharge barriers and assist with arranging services to transition patients out of the hospital and bridge them before their first post-hospital follow-up visit. A best practice is to embed the nurse navigator in the care team, so that they can be involved in daily conversations on rounds. In this manner, the navigator knows all facets of the patient's discharge planning.

Finally, involving the patient, family, and caregivers is crucial in discharge planning. Patients and their families would not be involved in the daily interdisciplinary team rounds but should be updated regularly about these discussions. To allow for realistic planning, the team should be transparent about how much help or supervision the patient will require after discharge. Caregivers may need to take extended

Table 32.1 Role of stroke nurse navigators

Practice domains	Patient and family experience	Best practice
EMS emergency care	• Introduction to the stroke code evaluation • Neurological assessments • Patient/family/staff bedside teaching and support	• Stroke team member • ED/RN liaison • Targeting target treatment times
Critical care (endovascular therapy, and intensive care)	• Patient/family/staff bedside teaching • Facilitating family/provider communication	• SBAR hand-offs to IR, PACU, and NICU • Treatment times • Documentation of care
Recovery care	• Stroke service rounding • Patient and family teaching • RN consultation • Transitions of care rounding	• Care plan update • Metrics review • Patient/staff education • Discharge coordination • Follow-up appointments
Discharge follow-up	• Coordination of medical appointments, outpatient diagnostic testing, home care services, rehabilitation therapies	• 7-day follow-up phone calls • Medication adherence • Extended cardiac services • 90-day outcome metrics
Community outreach	• Provider follow-up • Support groups, community resources, transportation • VNA liaison	• Community hospital support • Stamp-out-stroke programs • Stroke awareness month

EMS emergency medical services, *ED* emergency department, *RN* registered nurse, *SBAR* Situation–Background–Assessment–Recommendation, *PACU* post-anesthesia care unit, *NICU* neurological intensive care unit, *VNA* Visiting Nurse Association
Courtesy of Kaile Neuschatz, RN* and Karin Nystrom, APRN*
*Yale-New Haven Hospital

leave from work, arrange patient sitters or other caregivers, prepare their home, oversee finances and assets, arrange care for dependent children or pets, and provide support and care in rehab facilities.

Disposition Options for Stroke Patients

Once the interdisciplinary team is established, it is crucial to understand all discharge options. While some patients may be able to be discharged directly to home without further rehabilitation needs, many will have ongoing rehabilitation or long-term care needs that will require coordination from their care team. Different rehabilitation levels depend on the patient's therapy requirements, medical needs, and caregiver support. The insurance status of the patient is a significant factor in determining disposition. Many patients cannot afford out-of-pocket rehabilitation services, and Case Management may be able to help identify other outside resources. In addition, some insurance plans only cover certain therapy benefits, making it essential to consider this information early on in disposition planning. A challenging situation is when the patient has no insurance coverage and minimal or no family support yet will require either inpatient rehabilitation or long-term care. The process for filing for Medicaid or institutional Medicare (public insurance options) is lengthy. The process should be started as soon as possible for patients without insurance and with a high likelihood of acute rehab or long-term care needs. We will briefly requirements for different levels of rehab here:

- *Acute Care Inpatient Rehabilitation*: Patients must tolerate at least 3 hours of rehabilitation daily. To qualify, they must have needs in at least two therapy disciplines (Physical, occupational, and speech). The patient will stay in a facility similar to a hospital where they will be assigned therapists, a nurse, and a medical team. An important factor to consider when discussing inpatient rehabilitation is that most facilities will want the hospital team to identify the support plan for the patient after they have met their rehabilitation goals. This ensures that the patient will have a safe disposition with the appropriate level of supervision or aid.
- *Subacute Rehabilitation*: Patients receive approximately 1 hour of therapy daily between all three disciplines. This option is more appropriate than acute rehab for patients who are not able to tolerate aggressive rehab due to frailty, fatigue, alertness, large neurologic deficits, or long-term disposition needs. Patients have access to therapists, nursing care, and medical provider oversight.
- *Outpatient Therapy*: These patients can be discharged home safely and go to an outpatient rehab facility for about an hour, three-to-five times per week. Patients must be capable of transferring in and out of the car and have access to transportation to and from the appointment.
- *Home Health Therapy*: This is an excellent option for patients with minimal deficits or who cannot access outpatient therapy. Therapists can visit the patient's residence one-to-four times weekly for about 30 min to an hour.
- *Long-Term Acute Care Hospitals*: Some patients may have ongoing medical needs that a skilled nursing facility or acute inpatient rehab hospital cannot manage. The most common example is a patient who cannot be weaned from ventilator support. A long-term acute care hospital allows patients to stay for several months to gradually wean ventilator support and work toward getting the patient medically ready to discharge to therapy or home.
- *Nursing Home Care*: Patients with large stroke deficits sometimes are unable to participate in therapy and are unable to care for themselves. If they do not have 24/7 supervision by their family or caretakers who can meet their healthcare needs, then a nursing home will be a good option. They will receive 24/7 nursing care, including clinical assessments, assistance with bathing, feeding, and turning, and medical attention for any issues.

Unique Situations and Challenges

Unfortunately, not all patients have support or financial means for housing or basic needs, so knowledge about local group homes or shelters will be beneficial. The case management team is aware of these facilities and their admission requirements. These facilities typically require patients to ambulate independently (or with an assistive device), self-administer all medications, be self-reliant for eating and drinking, and communicate their needs. These programs have resources to aid with permanent or temporary housing and job opportunities.

Patients at the end of life can be discharged to a skilled nursing facility, palliative care hospital unit, or even home with hospice. Giving families realistic predictions of life expectancy and caregiver burden helps them decide between home care or facilities. It is important to have an honest discussion about whether the caregiver has the physical ability and support to provide around-the-clock care for the patient. The team should also ask the family about the patient's preferences for end-of-life care and location and incorporate that information into disposition discussions. Hospice is a service that focuses on patient comfort with a nurse, case manager, and medical provider team, and can give specialized support and education to the family on what to expect during end-of-life care.

Regardless of the type of facility, families and patients may have unrealistic expectations or will refuse specific centers based on anecdotes from others or limited online reviews. Encourage the patient's family or support team to call or tour the facility choices before discharge. Sharing the medical team's broader experience with a particular facility can be helpful. Remind the family that stays in rehab are temporary, and explain that prolonging hospital stays to wait for specific centers to have open beds increases the risk of medical complications and negatively affects long-term recovery. It can be challenging to explain to a family why their loved ones may not be eligible for a particular rehab or disposition choice, so knowing the differences in these levels of care can help the healthcare team members explain. Educating the family and asking them to consider all options early is essential. The finalized disposition plan should have buy-in from all parties to be safe, ensure patient and family satisfaction, and, above all, get patients the appropriate care they need.

Clinical Pearls
- Establish a multidisciplinary team of healthcare providers, nurses, therapists, social workers, and case management to hold daily discussions on discharge planning.
- Discharge planning should start early during the patient's hospitalization, and regular meetings should update the patient's progress and ongoing needs.
- Patients have various discharge options. It is important to familiarize oneself with available community resources and their admission requirements.
- Involve the patient and their family in disposition discussions. Provide realistic and honest expectations to help plan for the next steps in the patient's care.

Further Reading

American Stroke Association. Choosing the right stroke rehab facility. 2022. www.stroke.org. https://www.stroke.org/en/life-after-stroke/stroke-rehab/choosing-the-right-stroke-rehab-facility. Accessed 31 Dec 2022.

Stroke Rehab

33

Divya Viswanathan and Carolin Dohle

Introduction

Stroke is the number one cause of disability in the United States today [1]. With so many more people surviving their initial stroke, the role of rehabilitation becomes increasingly important. Rehabilitation starts in the acute care setting. Assessments by physical therapy (PT), occupational therapy (OT), and speech therapy (SLP) are part of the Get With the Guidelines recommendations for acute stroke care.

Physical Therapists focus on walking, lower extremity mobility, and endurance. They are experts in prescribing appropriate lower extremity bracing for support during standing and ambulation. In the acute care setting, PTs evaluate the appropriate level of mobility for a patient, distance that a patient can ambulate as well as the level of assistance required for mobility, and recommend the appropriate post-acute setting.

Occupational Therapists focus on upper extremity strength and range of motion (ROM), transfers to and from bed, toileting, dressing, grooming, and overall activities of daily living. OTs also assess the patient for visual deficits such as hemineglect or visual field cut and assess cognition as part of their evaluation.

Speech Language Pathologists assess speech production, comprehension, articulation, cognition, and swallowing. They also assess a patient's ability to swallow and recommend appropriate consistencies of solids and liquids.

All disciplines are essential when deciding on the right post-acute patient setting. During interdisciplinary team rounds, the therapists share the level of assistance a patient needs. Table 33.1 describes common terms used during rounds to describe a patient's level of dependence.

Scores like the GG Score and Activity Measure for Post-Acute Care (AM-PAC) help measure ability following a stroke and predict the level of assistance required

D. Viswanathan · C. Dohle (✉)
Westchester Medical Center, Valhalla, NY, USA
e-mail: divya.viswanathan@wmchealth.org; carolin.dohle@wmchealth.org

Table 33.1 Common levels of assistance patients may require

Level of assistance	Description
Total assistance	Patient is completely unable to care for themselves and cannot help at all with any mobility efforts
Maximal assistance	Patient can perform about 25% of the mobility tasks, and depends on their caregivers for the other 75%
Moderate assistance	Patient can perform about 50% of the mobility tasks, and depends on their caregivers for the other 50%
Minimal assistance	Patient can perform about 75% of the mobility tasks, and depends on their caregivers for the other 25%
Contact guard assistance	The caregiver has one or two hands on the patients' body, but the patient can complete 100% of the mobility tasks
Stand-by assistance	The patient does not require hands-on help, but the caregiver should be close by in cases of loss of balance or safety needs
Independent	The patient can perform the task and does not require anyone to be close to them for safety purposes

upon hospital discharge [2, 3]. The AM-PAC asks how much help the patient needs with the following activities: Bed mobility, sit-to-stand and stand-to-sit, supine-to-sit, seated transfers, ambulation, stair climbing, bathing, clothing, grooming, eating, and toileting. These scores can be translated into daily mobility goals for the patient.

What are the Options for Rehab?

When discharging patients, one might feel overwhelmed by the number of available options—it is almost like alphabet soup! Let's dive into the options.

Inpatient Rehab Facilities (IRFs) are entities regulated by CMS [4]. Patients receive at least 3 h of therapy per day, 5 days a week, or 15 h over a 7-day period, whichever works better for the patient/therapy team. IRFs have all therapeutic modalities, such as PT, OT, and SLP, on staff and available to patients and are staffed by physicians who see patients daily. To qualify for an IRF, the patient must tolerate 3 h of therapy per day. Therapy can include pre-gait activities, such as transfers, standing, and toileting. However, the patient has to be able to participate in therapy and has a reasonable potential for improvement in some way. Patients should also have a chance of eventually returning home; a patient who requires long-term custodial care will likely not be a good IRF candidate. IRF frequently have certified rehabilitation RNs for patient care, neuropsychologists who can perform in-depth cognitive assessments, and therapeutic recreation therapists who reintegrate patients into society by providing therapeutic leisure activities designed to further the rehabilitation process [5].

Skilled Nursing Facilities (SNFs) that provide rehabilitation services are sometimes called subacute rehabilitation facilities. They provide skilled nursing to stroke survivors and a varying amount of rehabilitation but may not have all therapy modalities available [6]. Patients get varying degrees of therapy and may get more group sessions instead of individualized therapy. Nursing is skilled but usually not specialized. SNFs are required to have skilled nursing for at least 8 h/day on site. Physician supervision is also less frequent than IRF, with CMS requiring the patients to be seen by a physician once in 30 days for the first 90 days and once every 60 days after that. SNFs are appropriate for patients who cannot tolerate a more intense level of rehabilitation or are unlikely to go home. Medicare covers SNF stays for up to 100 days. Long-term care is usually not paid for by Medicare and is either paid for out of pocket or covered by Medicaid.

Studies have shown that stroke patients have a higher level of motor recovery and independence following therapy at an IRF versus an SNF [7, 8]. The Guidelines for Adult Stroke Rehabilitation and Recovery reiterate that "stroke patients who are candidates for post-acute rehabilitation receive organized, coordinated, interprofessional care" and recommend that "stroke survivors who qualify for and have access to IRF care receive treatment in an IRF in preference to a SNF" [9].

Long-Term Acute Care Hospitals (LTACH) can provide ongoing intensive medical care and rehabilitation services for patients [10]. Patients who are ventilator-dependent for a prolonged period or have complex wound or pain management needs may qualify for an LTACH. The length of stay in an LTACH has to be at least 25 days, reflecting that these patients are usually among the most medically complex.

Home Health Agencies (HHA) can provide care in outpatient settings if a patient is deemed safe for discharge home after their acute care hospitalization. To qualify for HHA visits, the patient must be homebound, and providers must complete a face-to-face encounter certifying they have met with the patient and that they are, in fact, homebound.

Recovery After Stroke

The rate of recovery following a stroke varies depending on the severity of the stroke, age, and overall health of the patient [11]. While most stroke survivors can experience some level of recovery in the first few weeks or months after the stroke, the most rapid improvement occurs in the first few days or weeks [12]. However, motor and speech recovery can continue for many months or even years after the stroke for some individuals. The modified Rankin Scale (mRS) can be used to assess the patient's functional status after the stroke [13]. A lower mRS score at 90 days may indicate that the patient has made good progress in their recovery and has a higher level of functional independence (Table 33.2).

True recovery after a stroke with improvement in strength or dexterity (rather than the patient simply adapting to their disability) is likely due to neuroplasticity. Neuroplasticity refers to the ability of the brain to change and adapt in response to certain experiences, learning, and injury involving the reorganization of neural connections and the formation of new neurons and synapses [14, 15]. Research has shown that learning new skills, socializing, PT, and exercise can stimulate neuroplasticity and improve brain function [16–18].

Table 33.2 Modified Rankin Scale

Score	Description
0	No symptoms
1	No significant disability, despite symptoms; able to perform all usual duties and activities
2	Slight disability; unable to perform all previous activities but able to look after own affairs without assistance
3	Moderate disability; requires some help, but able to walk without assistance
4	Moderate to severe disability; unable to walk without assistance and unable to attend to own bodily needs without assistance
5	Severe disability: bedridden, incontinent, and requires constant nursing care and attention
6	Dead

Common Issues in Stroke Rehabilitation

Spasticity

Spasticity is a motor disorder characterized by a "velocity-dependent" increase in the tonic stretch reflex (muscle tone) [19]. In other words, the faster one tries to bend or straighten a spastic arm, the tighter it will feel. It is frequently described as a "catch and release" phenomenon, where rapid flexion or extension of the affected joint results in an initial "catch" (the resistance), followed by a slower "release" (movement but slower with increased resistance) through the remainder of the movement [20, 21]. Spasticity is a common phenomenon after stroke, affecting 17–46% of stroke survivors within their first year of recovery, and can become chronic [22, 23].

Spasticity is graded on the Modified Ashworth Scale (MAS) [24]. An MAS of 1 indicates a mostly intact ROM, and an MAS of 4 indicates that the joint is nearly impossible to move. Spasticity that is allowed to continue unchecked and is not addressed by regular stretching and potential treatment can lead to contractures. Contractures indicate that the joint is stuck in a specific position and cannot be moved. Tendons and muscle tissue become fibrotic, limiting the potential of rehabilitating and using a contracted limb in daily activities [25]. One should pay special attention to the palm and evaluate whether there is any evidence of fingernails digging into the palm and causing skin injury. If the patient has difficulty opening their hand, ask for OT evaluation for solinting and consider rolling up a small towel and placing it in their palm to keep the hand open and dry. A spastic plantarflexed ankle (pointing down) can make it difficult for the patient to put their heel on the ground during walking, resulting in circumduction at the hip joint and impairing balance during ambulation [26]. Bracing a plantarflexed ankle with a specialized Multi-Podus boot can help keep the ankle in a more natural position. Proper ankle position is critical to avoid injury when standing and ambulating.

Unchecked spasticity can lead to bone and joint issues in the long term, such as adhesive capsulitis, subluxation of joints, and complex regional pain syndrome [27].

To test for arm spasticity, hold the patient's elbow with one hand and the forearm with another hand and passively flex and extend. Cupping the underside of the knee with both hands and lifting the leg is helpful to test for leg spasticity. If the leg has normal or flaccid tone, the heel of that foot should drag along the bed. If the leg has increased tone, the heel may lift as the leg is lifted.

Spasticity in the upper extremity is often disabling. However, spasticity in the leg can be helpful for weight-bearing purposes. Medications are often used as a first-line treatment of spasticity, such as Lioresal (Baclofen®), but can affect a patient's level of alertness and cognition and increase the risk of falls, especially at higher dosages [28]. As such, patients may benefit from a more targeted approach. Physiatrists (MDs trained in rehabilitation medicine) and neurologists can adminis-ter intramuscular botulinum toxin (Botox® or Xeomin®) to "loosen" the spastic muscles and improve the ROM, avoiding systemic side effects of oral agents [29, 30]. Botox treatment every 3 months should be in conjunction with physical and OT, providing additional stretching, strengthening, and mobility exercises. Nerve blocks and chemoneurolysis with phenol injections are further treatment options, albeit less commonly used than botulinum toxin injections [31, 32]. For patients with significant spasticity that is not responsive to oral antispasmodics and who have generalized spasticity that is not amenable to Botox injections, an intrathecal pump that delivers Baclofen directly into the spinal fluid may be an option [33, 34]. These pumps are usually implanted by a neurosurgeon and managed by a physiatrist.

Hemiplegic Shoulder and Central Pain

A hemiplegic arm can misalign the shoulder joint, where the humeral head is par-tially dislocated from the glenohumeral joint. This phenomenon is called "sublux-ation" and can lead to pain and impaired shoulder mobility. Shoulder pain is relatively common after a stroke, affecting up to 22% of stroke survivors [35]. Shoulder joint ultrasounds can show bicep tendon effusions, tendinopathy, or rota-tor cuff injuries [36]. Prevention of hemiplegic shoulder pain starts in the acute care setting, with avoidance of pulling on the affected shoulder joint, correct positioning in bed, support of the affected arm with a pillow or lab tray sitting upright in a chair or wheelchair, using a sliding board for transfers and considering the use of a sling during transfer and mobility exercises [37]. Treatment options for shoulder pain include electrical stimulation such as transcutaneous electrical stimulation or neuro-muscular electrical stimulation (NMES), corticosteroid injections into the shoulder joint, and botulinum toxin injections into the muscles of the rotator cuff to help alleviate spasticity [38, 39].

Central pain is a burning sensation caused by a lesion in the central nervous sys-tem anywhere along the somatosensory pathways (like a thalamic stroke) [40, 41]. Central post-stroke pain affects approximately 5–7% of stroke survivors and can begin, while the patients are still in acute care [42, 43]. Central pain is challenging to treat and, in many cases, requires trials of several different agents and doses.

Pharmaceutical treatment options exist, with Amitriptyline and Lamotrigine being the most well-studied drugs [44, 45]. However, Gabapentin is frequently used in the clinical setting and may be a reasonable alternative when the other medications are contraindicated or ineffective [46].

Hemispatial Neglect

Hemispatial neglect is often called a "cortical sign," leading to a lack of awareness of the contralateral side, and is most commonly associated with right hemispheric strokes [47, 48]. Hemispatial neglect can be a significant barrier to rehabilitation and recovery but, fortunately, tends to improve in most patients within 3 months [49, 50]. Multiple strategies exist to treat patients with neglect. One strategy is visual scanning training, where the patient is presented with various stimuli (like letters and symbols) and asked to point out specific ones [51, 52]. This strategy can be combined with sensory stimulation for added benefit [53, 54]. Having the patient visually scan to the left helps retrain the brain to improve spatial awareness. Prism adaptation is another strategy that uses prism glasses that contain special lenses to pull items from the left into the central visual space. Newer studies using brain stimulation and virtual reality have also shown encouraging results [55, 56].

Motor Impairment

Constraint-Induced Movement Therapy (CIMT)

Despite having some movement and function in the affected extremity, stroke survivors often rely on the unaffected side, because it is easier to grab something quickly with the "normal" hand, even if it is the "non-dominant" side. Avoiding the affected side is called "learned non-use," which limits recovery and ultimately leads to atrophy and spasticity. To combat learned non-use, therapists sometimes employ CIMT. In this technique, the use of the unaffected hand is limited by placing it in a mitt, forcing the use of the affected hand in everyday life [57, 58]. CIMT, coupled with purposeful movement therapy, has been shown to improve hand function if done for several hours per day and several days per week. A similar concept can be applied to SLP, called constraint-induced aphasia therapy (CIAT) [59]. With CIAT, two stroke survivors are paired up and must describe pictures to each other, all without using gestures or other non-verbal communication. For obvious reasons, for both CIMT and CIAT, patients must have some degree of baseline ability to participate. Completely paralyzed or mute patients would not be suitable candidates for this therapy.

Neuromuscular Electrical Stimulation (NMES)

NMES uses electrical stimulation to achieve muscle contraction by stimulating motor units through electrical stimulation of the corresponding motor nerve [60, 61]. When paired with functional training, this therapy is called functional electrical stimulation. Multiple studies have shown the benefit of NMES on motor relearning in both the upper and lower extremities after stroke [62, 63]. The benefit of NMES is its low cost and relative portability. A trained OT or PT is required to place electrodes correctly. However, certain devices are available that incorporate the electrodes into a brace, making it more user-friendly. These systems exist for the upper and lower extremities [64].

Novel Rehabilitation Strategies

Rehabilitation robotics is a hot topic in stroke rehabilitation. For upper extremity robotic devices, the affected extremity is affixed to the machine (Fig. 33.1). The patient is then encouraged to move their affected extremity through a pre-determined set of exercises aided by a target that moves on a screen based on the patient's movements. Most robots allow the patient to start the movement, complete it as much as possible, and then guide the affected extremity through the rest of the ROM [65]. Lower extremity robotic devices also exist where the patient's body weight is supported in a harness, and the legs are guided through the walking movement. The

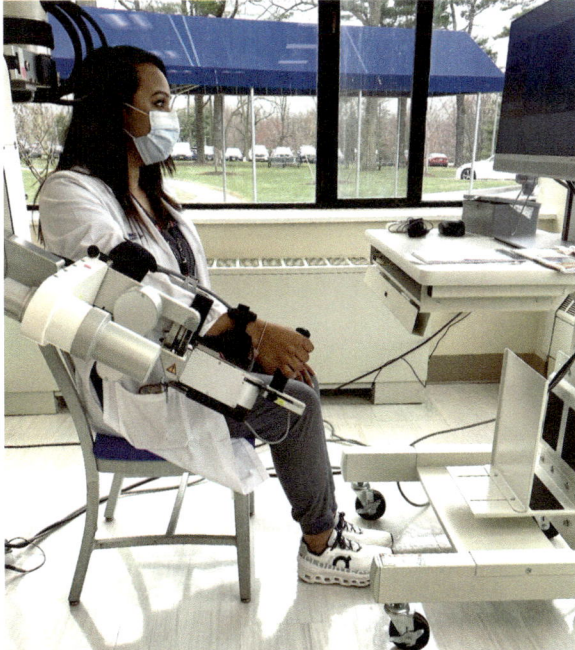

Fig. 33.1 Upper extremity rehabilitation robotics

advantage of rehabilitation robotics is that they can deliver hundreds of repetitions in one session versus only 30–50 repetitions in a standard PT or OT session [66]. Rehabilitation robots can also help measure the patient's progress. Visualizing data can be rewarding to patients, who often fail to appreciate smaller improvements. The "gaming" aspect of the robots can be engaging and entertaining for patients. However, these devices are still quite costly, and current evidence has not demonstrated that robotic rehabilitation is superior to intensive, hands-on training by a PT or OT [67, 68]. Therefore, these devices are not widely used at this time.

Noninvasive Brain Stimulation

Two methods of noninvasive brain stimulation are repetitive transcranial magnetic stimulation (rTMS) and transcranial direct current or electrical stimulation (tDCS or TES) [69]. rTMS employs repetitive, highly focused magnetic pulses that create electrical fields in the cortex [70]. If performed occurs over the motor cortex, a contraction in the corresponding muscle can be seen. In rTMS, the magnetic pulse is discharged so frequently that, depending on the interval between pulses, it either results in cortical excitability or depression. According to the Hebbian principle of "neurons that fire together wire together," rTMS increases neuroplasticity [71].

Conversely, TES uses a low-intensity constant current that flows between an anode and cathode placed over the skull (Fig. 33.2) [72]. Both techniques are

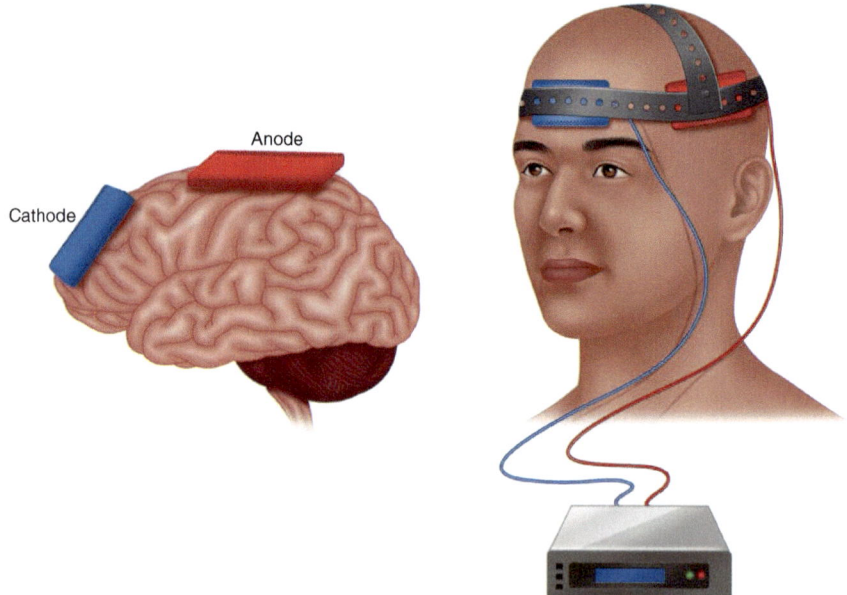

Fig. 33.2 Transcranial electrical stimulation stimulates the cortex through a continuous low-voltage current

painless and can change cortical excitability after stimulation, usually for minutes to hours [73]. The benefit of TES over TDCS is that it is portable and of lower cost. rTMS has been shown to improve arm function, lower extremity mobility, and balance after stroke [74]. Newer studies have also found an effect of both rTMS and TES on dysphagia [75, 76]. Both modalities have been used to reduce the burden of neglect, and rTMS can improve communication in patients with aphasia [77, 78].

Virtual Reality

Game systems such as the Nintendo Wii® or Microsoft Xbox Kinect® have been explored in rehabilitation [79]. Systems in which the patient uses a virtual reality headset and moves their arm in a virtual environment have been developed. While interactive environments are engaging and motivating for the patient, and patients reported high enjoyment with these systems, the EVREST trial did not demonstrate the superiority of gaming systems for motor recovery compared to simple recreational activities (playing cards, bingo, or ball games) [80].

Assistive Devices

As patients progress through their recovery, they often require different types of assistive devices to help them with their mobility. Some commonly prescribed devices are described here.

Bracing: Splints and Braces can help stabilize a limb for mobility and help counteract the adverse effects of spasticity.

Boots: Boots preventing foot-drop and plantarflexion can be used when the patient is lying in bed. These boots help align the foot in a neutral position. Many boots have a kickstand that can prevent the foot from falling into an abducted position, which leads to a pathological and painful external rotation in the hip joint.

AFO and AAFO: An ankle–foot orthosis (AFO, fixed ankle joint) or articulated AFO (AAFO and mobile ankle joint) helps clear the foot over the floor during ambulation. Some braces have a knee strap, which can help prevent knee buckling. AAFOs can have springs and pins that limit movement in one direction (such as pins that limit plantarflexion) but help with movement in the other direction (such as springs helping with dorsiflexion). This feature can help counteract knee buckling and hyperextension and help with foot clearance while allowing the patient to move the ankle joint within a specific range.

Walkers: The most common type of walker is a rolling walker (RW), which has wheels in the front and rubber tips in the back. RWs give stability, while the patient is ambulating. Hemi-walkers exist for patients who are paretic on one side and can only navigate the walker with one side of their bodies. Platform walkers are for patients who need additional help stabilizing the upper extremity.

Canes: Instead of a single-point cane, stroke patients with hemiparesis often use a cane with a four-pronged tip, a so-called quad cane. Quad canes give additional stability on the unaffected side, so the patient can maneuver the paretic side.

References

1. Ma VY, Chan L, Carruthers KJ. Incidence, prevalence, costs, and impact on disability of common conditions requiring rehabilitation in the United States: stroke, spinal cord injury, traumatic brain injury, multiple sclerosis, osteoarthritis, rheumatoid arthritis, limb loss, and back pain. Arch Phys Med Rehabil. 2014;95(5):986–95.
2. Warren M, Knecht J, Verheijde J, Tompkins J. Association of AM-PAC "6-Clicks" basic mobility and daily activity scores with discharge destination. Phys Ther. 2021;101(4):pzab043.
3. Li CY, Kuo YF, Ottenbacher K. Using GG items to characterize self-care and mobility performance in stroke. Am J Occup Ther. 2021;75(Supplement_2):7512510224p1.
4. Miller EL, Murray L, Richards L, Zorowitz RD, Bakas T, Clark P, Billinger SA. Comprehensive overview of nursing and interdisciplinary rehabilitation care of the stroke patient: a scientific statement from the American Heart Association. Stroke. 2010;41(10):2402–48.
5. Long AF, Kneafsey R, Ryan J, Berry J. The role of the nurse within the multi-professional rehabilitation team. J Adv Nurs. 2002;37(1):70–8.
6. Leon J, Cheng M, Dunbar J. Trends in special care: the 1995 National Nursing Census of Sub-Acute Units. ASPE; 1997.
7. Deutsch A, Granger CV, Heinemann AW, Fiedler RC, DeJong G, Kane RL, Trevisan M. Poststroke rehabilitation: outcomes and reimbursement of inpatient rehabilitation facilities and subacute rehabilitation programs. Stroke. 2006;37(6):1477–82.
8. Kane RL, Chen Q, Blewett LA, Sangl J. Do rehabilitative nursing homes improve the outcomes of care? J Am Geriatr Soc. 1996;44(5):545–54.
9. Winstein CJ, Stein J, Arena R, Bates B, Cherney LR, Cramer SC, Zorowitz RD. Guidelines for adult stroke rehabilitation and recovery: a guideline for healthcare professionals from the American Heart Association/American Stroke Association. Stroke. 2016;47(6):e98–e169.
10. Liu K, Baseggio C, Wissoker D, Maxwell S, Haley J, Long S. Long-term care hospitals under Medicare: facility-level characteristics. Health Care Financ Rev. 2001;23(2):1.
11. Hachinski V, Iadecola C, Petersen RC, Breteler MM, Nyenhuis DL, Black SE, Leblanc GG. National Institute of Neurological Disorders and Stroke–Canadian stroke network vascular cognitive impairment harmonization standards. Stroke. 2006;37(9):2220–41.
12. Prabhakaran S, Zarahn E, Riley C, Speizer A, Chong JY, Lazar RM, Krakauer JW. Interindividual variability in the capacity for motor recovery after ischemic stroke. Neurorehabil Neural Repair. 2008;22(1):64–71.
13. Chye A, Hackett ML, Hankey GJ, Lundström E, Almeida OP, Gommans J, Lung T. Repeated measures of modified Rankin scale scores to assess functional recovery from stroke: AFFINITY study findings. J Am Heart Assoc. 2022;11(16):e025425.
14. Nudo RJ. Recovery after brain injury: mechanisms and principles. Front Hum Neurosci. 2013;7:887.
15. Nudo RJ, Milliken GW, Jenkins WM, Merzenich MM. Use-dependent alterations of movement representations in primary motor cortex of adult squirrel monkeys. J Neurosci. 1996;16(2):785.
16. Davidson RJ, McEwen BS. Social influences on neuroplasticity: stress and interventions to promote well-being. Nat Neurosci. 2012;15(5):689.
17. Pin-Barre C, Laurin J. Physical exercise as a diagnostic, rehabilitation, and preventive tool: influence on neuroplasticity and motor recovery after stroke. Neural Plast. 2015;2015:1.
18. Teixeira-Machado L, Arida RM, de Jesus Mari J. Dance for neuroplasticity: a descriptive systematic review. Neurosci Biobehav Rev. 2019;96:232–40.

19. Lance JW. Pathophysiology of spasticity and clinical experience with baclofen. In: Spasticity: disordered motor control. Year Book; 1980. p. 185–204.
20. Urban PP, Wolf T, Uebele M, Marx JJ, Vogt T, Stoeter P, Wissel J. Occurrence and clinical predictors of spasticity after ischemic stroke. Stroke. 2010;41(9):2016–20.
21. Trompetto C, Marinelli L, Mori L, Pelosin E, Currà A, Molfetta L, Abbruzzese G. Pathophysiology of spasticity: implications for neurorehabilitation. Biomed Res Int. 2014;2014:354906.
22. Wissel J, Manack A, Brainin M. Toward an epidemiology of poststroke spasticity. Neurology. 2013;80(3 Supplement 2):S13–9.
23. Katoozian L, Tahan N, Zoghi M, Bakhshayesh B. The onset and frequency of spasticity after first ever stroke. J Natl Med Assoc. 2018;110(6):547–52.
24. Bohannon RW, Smith MB. Interrater reliability of a modified Ashworth scale of muscle spasticity. Phys Ther. 1987;67(2):206–7.
25. McDonald CM. Limb contractures in progressive neuromuscular disease and the role of stretching, orthotics, and surgery. Phys Med Rehabil Clin N Am. 1998;9(1):187–211.
26. Rodda J, Graham HK. Classification of gait patterns in spastic hemiplegia and spastic diplegia: a basis for a management algorithm. Eur J Neurol. 2001;8:98–108.
27. Zorowitz RD, Gillard PJ, Brainin M. Poststroke spasticity: sequelae and burden on stroke survivors and caregivers. Neurology. 2013;80(3 Supplement 2):S45–52.
28. Hudgson P, Weightman D. Baclofen in the treatment of spasticity. Br Med J. 1971;4(5778):15–7.
29. Rosales RL, Chua-Yap AS. Evidence-based systematic review on the efficacy and safety of botulinum toxin-A therapy in post-stroke spasticity. J Neural Transm. 2008;115:617–23.
30. Kaji R, Osako Y, Suyama K, Maeda T, Uechi Y, Iwasaki M, GSK1358820 Spasticity Study Group. Botulinum toxin type A in post-stroke upper limb spasticity. Curr Med Res Opin. 2010;26(8):1983–92.
31. Elovic EP, Esquenazi A, Alter KE, Lin JL, Alfaro A, Kaelin DL. Chemodenervation and nerve blocks in the diagnosis and management of spasticity and muscle overactivity. PM&R. 2009;1(9):842–51.
32. Botte MJ, Abrams RA, Bodine-Fowler SC. Treatment of acquired muscle spasticity using phenol peripheral nerve blocks. Orthopedics. 1995;18(2):151–9.
33. Dvorak EM, Ketchum NC, McGuire JR. The underutilization of intrathecal baclofen in post-stroke spasticity. Top Stroke Rehabil. 2011;18(3):195–202.
34. Meythaler JM, Guin-Renfroe S, Brunner RC, Hadley MN. Intrathecal baclofen for spastic hypertonia from stroke. Stroke. 2001;32(9):2099–109.
35. Lindgren I, Jonsson AC, Norrving B, Lindgren A. Shoulder pain after stroke: a prospective population-based study. Stroke. 2007;38(2):343–8.
36. Huang YC, Liang PJ, Pong YP, Leong CP, Tseng CH. Physical findings and sonography of hemiplegic shoulder in patients after acute stroke during rehabilitation. J Rehabil Med. 2010;42(1):21–6.
37. McKenna LBK. Hemiplegic shoulder pain: defining the problem and its management. Disabil Rehabil. 2001;23(16):698–705.
38. Koog YH, Jin SS, Yoon K, Min BI. Interventions for hemiplegic shoulder pain: systematic review of randomised controlled trials. Disabil Rehabil. 2010;32(4):282–91.
39. Xie HM, Guo TT, Sun X, Ge HX, Chen XD, Zhao KJ, Zhang LN. Effectiveness of botulinum toxin a in treatment of hemiplegic shoulder pain: a systematic review and meta-analysis. Arch Phys Med Rehabil. 2021;102(9):1775–87.
40. Roosink M, Buitenweg JR, Renzenbrink GJ, Geurts AC, IJzerman MJ. Altered cortical somatosensory processing in chronic stroke: a relationship with post-stroke shoulder pain. NeuroRehabilitation. 2011;28(4):331–44.
41. Klit H, Finnerup NB, Jensen TS. Central post-stroke pain: clinical characteristics, pathophysiology, and management. Lancet Neurol. 2009;8(9):857–68.
42. Bashir AH, Abdullahi A, Abba MA, Mukhtar NB. Central poststroke pain: its profile among stroke survivors in Kano, Nigeria. Behav Neurol. 2017;2017:9318597.

43. Tang A, Thickbroom G, Rodger J. Repetitive transcranial magnetic stimulation of the brain: mechanisms from animal and experimental models. Neuroscientist. 2017;23(1):82–94.
44. Leijon G, Boivie J. Central post-stroke pain—a controlled trial of amitriptyline and carbamazepine. Pain. 1989;36(1):27–36.
45. Vestergaard K, Andersen G, Gottrup H, Kristensen BT, Jensen TS. Lamotrigine for central poststroke pain: a randomized controlled trial. Neurology. 2001;56(2):184–90.
46. Kim JS. Post-stroke pain. Expert Rev Neurother. 2009;9(5):711–21.
47. Coslett HB. Apraxia, neglect, and agnosia. Continuum (Minneap Minn). 2018;24(3):768–82.
48. Esposito E, Shekhtman G, Chen P. Prevalence of spatial neglect post-stroke: a systematic review. Ann Phys Rehabil Med. 2021;64(5):101459.
49. Ramsey LE, Siegel JS, Baldassarre A, Metcalf NV, Zinn K, Shulman GL, Corbetta M. Normalization of network connectivity in hemispatial neglect recovery. Ann Neurol. 2016;80(1):127–41.
50. Wee JY, Hopman WM. Comparing consequences of right and left unilateral neglect in a stroke rehabilitation population. Am J Phys Med Rehabil. 2008;87(11):910–20.
51. Luukkainen-Markkula R, Tarkka IM, Pitkänen K, Sivenius J, Hämäläinen H. Rehabilitation of hemispatial neglect: a randomized study using either arm activation or visual scanning training. Restor Neurol Neurosci. 2009;27(6):665–74.
52. Pereira Ferreira H, Lopes ALM, Raggio Luiz R, Cardoso L, André C. Is visual scanning better than mental practice in hemispatial neglect? Results from a pilot study. Top Stroke Rehabil. 2011;18(2):155–61.
53. Saevarsson S, Kristjánsson Á, Halsband U. Strength in numbers: combining neck vibration and prism adaptation produces additive therapeutic effects in unilateral neglect. Neuropsychol Rehabil. 2010;20(5):704–24.
54. Polanowska K, Seniów J, Paprot E, Leśniak M, Członkowska A. Left-hand somatosensory stimulation combined with visual scanning training in rehabilitation for post-stroke hemineglect: a randomised, double-blind study. Neuropsychol Rehabil. 2009;19(3):364–82.
55. Salazar APS, Vaz PG, Marchese RR, Stein C, Pinto C, Pagnussat AS. Noninvasive brain stimulation improves hemispatial neglect after stroke: a systematic review and meta-analysis. Arch Phys Med Rehabil. 2018;99(2):355–66.
56. Kim YM, Chun MH, Yun GJ, Song YJ, Young HE. The effect of virtual reality training on unilateral spatial neglect in stroke patients. Ann Rehabil Med. 2011;35(3):309–15.
57. Grotta JC, Noser EA, Ro T, Boake C, Levin H, Aronowski J, Schallert T. Constraint-induced movement therapy. Stroke. 2004;35(11_suppl_1):2699–701.
58. Kwakkel G, Veerbeek JM, van Wegen EE, Wolf SL. Constraint-induced movement therapy after stroke. Lancet Neurol. 2015;14(2):224–34.
59. Szaflarski JP, Ball AL, Grether S, Al-Fwaress F, Griffith NM, Neils-Strunjas J, Reichhardt R. Constraint-induced aphasia therapy stimulates language recovery in patients with chronic aphasia after ischemic stroke. Med Sci Monit. 2008;14(5):CR243.
60. Reed B. The physiology of neuromuscular electrical stimulation. Pediatr Phys Ther. 1997;9(3):96–102.
61. Sheffler LR, Chae J. Neuromuscular electrical stimulation in neurorehabilitation. Muscle Nerve. 2007;35(5):562–90.
62. Chae J, Sheffler L, Knutson J. Neuromuscular electrical stimulation for motor restoration in hemiplegia. Top Stroke Rehabil. 2008;15(5):412–26.
63. Hong Z, Sui M, Zhuang Z, Liu H, Zheng X, Cai C, Jin D. Effectiveness of neuromuscular electrical stimulation on lower limbs of patients with hemiplegia after chronic stroke: a systematic review. Arch Phys Med Rehabil. 2018;99(5):1011–22.
64. Everaert DG, Stein RB, Abrams GM, Dromerick AW, Francisco GE, Hafner BJ, Kufta CV. Effect of a foot-drop stimulator and ankle–foot orthosis on walking performance after stroke: a multicenter randomized controlled trial. Neurorehabil Neural Repair. 2013;27(7):579–91.
65. Volpe BT, Krebs HI, Hogan N, Edelstein L, Diels C, Aisen M. A novel approach to stroke rehabilitation: robot-aided sensorimotor stimulation. Neurology. 2000;54(10):1938–44.

66. Lum PS, Godfrey SB, Brokaw EB, Holley RJ, Nichols D. Robotic approaches for rehabilitation of hand function after stroke. Am J Phys Med Rehabil. 2012;91(11):S242–54.
67. Lo AC, Guarino PD, Richards LG, Haselkorn JK, Wittenberg GF, Federman DG, Peduzzi P. Robot-assisted therapy for long-term upper-limb impairment after stroke. N Engl J Med. 2010;362(19):1772–83.
68. Lohse KR, Lang CE, Boyd LA. Is more better? Using metadata to explore dose–response relationships in stroke rehabilitation. Stroke. 2014;45(7):2053–8.
69. Webster BR, Celnik PA, Cohen LG. Noninvasive brain stimulation in stroke rehabilitation. NeuroRx. 2006;3(4):474–81.
70. Xing Y, Zhang Y, Li C, Luo L, Hua Y, Hu J, Bai Y. Repetitive transcranial magnetic stimulation of the brain after ischemic stroke: mechanisms from animal models. Cell Mol Neurobiol. 2022;43:1487–97.
71. Yoon KJ, Lee YT, Han TR. Mechanism of functional recovery after repetitive transcranial magnetic stimulation (rTMS) in the subacute cerebral ischemic rat model: neural plasticity or anti-apoptosis? Exp Brain Res. 2011;214:549–56.
72. Korai SA, Ranieri F, Di Lazzaro V, Papa M, Cirillo G. Neurobiological after-effects of low intensity transcranial electric stimulation of the human nervous system: from basic mechanisms to metaplasticity. Front Neurol. 2021;12:587771.
73. Bao SC, Khan A, Song R, Tong RKY. Rewiring the lesioned brain: electrical stimulation for post-stroke motor restoration. J Stroke. 2020;22(1):47.
74. Etoh S, Noma T, Ikeda K, Jonoshita Y, Ogata A, Matsumoto S, Kawahira K. Effects of repetitive transcranial magnetic stimulation on repetitive facilitation exercises of the hemiplegic hand in chronic stroke patients. J Rehabil Med. 2013;45(9):843–7.
75. Simons A, Hamdy S. The use of brain stimulation in dysphagia management. Dysphagia. 2017;32(2):209–15.
76. Liao X, Xing G, Guo Z, Jin Y, Tang Q, He B, Mu Q. Repetitive transcranial magnetic stimulation as an alternative therapy for dysphagia after stroke: a systematic review and meta-analysis. Clin Rehabil. 2017;31(3):289–98.
77. Fierro B, Brighina F, Bisiach E. Improving neglect by TMS. Behav Neurol. 2006;17(3–4):169–76.
78. Naeser MA, Martin PI, Treglia E, Ho M, Kaplan E, Bashir S, Pascual-Leone A. Research with rTMS in the treatment of aphasia. Restor Neurol Neurosci. 2010;28(4):511–29.
79. Deutsch JE, Brettler A, Smith C, Welsh J, John R, Guarrera-Bowlby P, Kafri M. Nintendo wii sports and wii fit game analysis, validation, and application to stroke rehabilitation. Top Stroke Rehabil. 2011;18(6):701–19.
80. Saposnik G, Cohen LG, Mamdani M, Pooyania S, Ploughman M, Cheung D, Bayley M. Efficacy and safety of non-immersive virtual reality exercising in stroke rehabilitation (EVREST): a randomised, multicentre, single-blind, controlled trial. Lancet Neurol. 2016;15(10):1019–27.

Pharmacology

34

Abdalla A. Ammar and Kent A. Owusu

Introduction

Medical management of stroke involves using pharmacological agents that target different aspects of stroke pathophysiology. For example, antithrombotics prevent clotting for acute stroke treatment and primary and secondary stroke prevention. Risk factor management with blood pressure, lipid, and glucose management all help in future stroke prevention. For providers, the key is knowing when a medication may or may not be appropriate for patients based on its pharmacology and patient factors. This chapter provides an overview of the pharmacologic options for managing stroke patients, their mechanisms of action, and recommended administration protocols, which are supplemented by tables for easy reference.

Before we dive into the medications, let us review some pharmacology terms that will be used in this chapter:

1. **Agonist**: A drug that binds to a receptor to enhance its function.
2. **Antagonist**: A drug that binds to a receptor to block its function.
3. **Efficacy**: Maximum response a drug can achieve.
4. **Half-life**: The time it takes for a drug concentration in the body to be reduced by one-half of the original amount. Typically, after 4–5 half-lives, the drug's plasma concentration in the body should be negligible.
5. **Mechanism of action**: How the drug works.
6. **Onset**: Time between the administration of a drug and first noticeable effects.
7. **Parenteral**: Any route of drug administration other than oral (through the digestive tract).

A. A. Ammar (✉)
New York Presbyterian Hospital, New York, NY, USA
e-mail: svf9004@nyp.org

K. A. Owusu
Yale New Haven Hospital, New Haven, CT, USA
e-mail: Kowusu@sturdyhealth.org

8. **Peak effect**: Maximum effect of a medication.
9. **Pharmacodynamics**: Interactions of a drug and target receptors.
10. **Pharmacokinetics**: How a drug is absorbed, distributed, metabolized, and eliminated by the body.
11. **Placebo**: A form of treatment with no effect, also known as a "sugar pill" or "dummy."
12. **Prodrug**: A drug that requires activation once in the body to exert its effects.

Fibrinolytic Therapy

Intrinsic fibrinolysis occurs through the activation of plasminogen into plasmin, which in turn breaks down fibrin clots. The most commonly used tissue–plasminogen activators for managing acute ischemic stroke are alteplase (t-PA) and tenecteplase (TNK) (Refer to the table 8.1 in Chap. 8 for a comparison). Alteplase is similar to endogenous t-PA made by the body and is made using recombinant DNA. TNK is a novel fibrinolytic similar to alteplase but has specific mutations at three sites, resulting in a 15-fold higher fibrin specificity (meaning that it is more specific for clots) [1, 2]. TNK is also more resistant than t-PA to Plasminogen Activator Inhibitor, the enzyme that inhibits the activity of plasminogen activators, giving the drug a much longer half-life than alteplase. That difference allows for more convenient administration with TNK with a single bolus push, whereas t-PA requires a bolus followed by an hour-long infusion. Both thrombolytics share the same efficacy [1, 2].

Early pharmacologic reperfusion with intravenous thrombolytics improves functional outcomes post-ischemic stroke [3, 4]. Multiple studies have compared TNK to t-PA and found a lower risk of systemic bleeding, similar risk of intracerebral hemorrhage (ICH), and efficacy for treating stroke, with a trend toward higher spontaneous recanalization rates for LVO with TNK [5–9]. Although TNK did not demonstrate superiority over alteplase in these studies, tenecteplase is recommended as an alternative to t-PA [10].

Antithrombotics: Antiplatelets vs. Anticoagulants

The terms antithrombotics, anticoagulants, and antiplatelets are often misused. Antithrombotics, also known as blood thinners, include all antiplatelets and anticoagulants. More specifically, antiplatelet agents affect platelet activity and are used in patients with arterial disease and small vessel strokes (Table 34.1). Anticoagulants are more potent blood thinners that affect the coagulation cascade and prevent clot formation in slower-flow areas like the venous system or cardiac chambers. Knowing when to use these agents requires understanding the stroke mechanism. Warfarin is the oldest oral anticoagulant (but still widely used), and direct oral anticoagulants (DOACs) are newer with multiple important advantages (Table 34.2).

Table 34.1 Common antiplatelets in stroke setting [11–24]

	Mechanism of action	Dosing	Pharmacokinetics	Patient care considerations
Salicylate				
Aspirin	Irreversibly inhibits cyclooxygenase, prostaglandin derivative formation, and thromboxane A2, thus inhibiting platelet aggregation	Ischemic stroke/ transient ischemic attack: 81 mg	Onset of action: 1–4 h Duration: 5–7 days (reminder life span of the platelets) It is metabolized through hydrolyzation into active metabolite salicylate Half-life: parent 15–20 min; active metabolite salicylate 3 h Elimination: Urine	Allergy symptoms include hives, itching, or wheezing within an hour of taking tablet Use with caution in platelets with thrombocytopenia
P2Y12 antagonist; thienopyridine				
Clopidogrel	Prodrug that biotransforms to an active metabolite that, in turn, is an irreversible inhibitor of P2Y12	Ischemic stroke/ transient ischemic attack: 75 mg once daily	Onset of action: 2 h post-loading dose Peak effect: 6 h post-loading dose Duration: 5–7 days (reminder life span of the platelets) Hepatically metabolized via CYP2C19 to an active metabolite Half-life: 6 h (parent drug); 30 min Elimination: urine (50%); feces (46%)	Metabolic activation of clopidogrel is affected by polymorphisms in CYP2C19 High risk for bleeding when combined with aspirin, other anticoagulants, nonsteroidal anti-inflammatory drugs, and antidepressant drugs (e.g., selective serotonin reuptake inhibitors) CYP2C19 is inhibited by proton pump inhibitors, decreasing clopidogrel efficacy
P2Y12 antagonist; non-thienopyridine				

(continued)

Table 34.1 (continued)

	Mechanism of action	Dosing	Pharmacokinetics	Patient care considerations
Ticagrelor	Reversible inhibitor of P2Y12	Minor ischemic stroke or high-risk transient ischemic attack: loading dose 80 mg once orally Maintenance 90 mg twice daily orally	Onset of action: 30 min post-loading dose Peak effect: 2 h post-loading dose Duration: 2–8 h Hepatically metabolized via CYP3A4/5 to an active metabolite Half-life: 7 h (parent drug); 9 h (active metabolite)	High risk for bleeding when combined with aspirin, other anticoagulants, nonsteroidal anti-inflammatory drugs, and antidepressant drugs (e.g., selective serotonin reuptake inhibitors) Drug interactions with potent inhibitors of CYP3A (e.g., ketoconazole, itraconazole, voriconazole, and ritonavir) and potent inducers of CYP3A (e.g., rifampin, phenytoin, carbamazepine, and phenobarbital)
Glycoprotein IIb/IIIa inhibitors				
Eptifibatide	Glycoprotein IIb/IIIa inhibitors	Loading dose: 90–180 µg/kg followed by 0.5–2 µg/kg/min for 24 h	Onset of action: 5 min post-loading dose Peak effect: 1 h Duration: 4–8 h post-infusion discontinuation Half-life: 2.5 h Elimination: 50% renal	Thrombocytopenia occurs in 0.5–1% of patients
Tirofiban		Loading dose: 25 µg/kg over 5 min followed by 0.15 µg/kg/min	Onset of action: 10 min post-loading dose Duration: 4–8 h post-infusion discontinuation Half-life: 2 h Elimination: 65% renal	Is reduced in patients with creatinine clearance of less than 60 mL/min Thrombocytopenia occurs in 0.5–1% of patients

CYP cytochrome P450, *h* hours, *IV* intravenous, *min* minutes, *PO* per os

Table 34.2 Common anticoagulants in stroke patients

Drug class	Agents	Dosing	Pharmacokinetics	Dose adjustments consideration	Special considerations
Direct thrombin inhibitors	Argatroban	IV: 2–10 µg/kg/min Titrate to aPTT goals	Onset of action: immediate Half-life: ~45 min Metabolism: hepatic Elimination: biliary excretion	Hepatic failure: 0.5 mg/kg/min. Avoid use in severe hepatic impairment	PT/INR will falsely increase with administration
	Bivalirudin	IV bolus dose of 0.75 mg/kg, followed by a continuous infusion of 1.75 mg/kg/h Titrate to aPTT goal	Onset of action: immediate Half-life: ~25 min Metabolism: hepatic and proteolysis Elimination: 20% of the dose is renally eliminated	CrCl 15–60 mL/min: 15–50% dose reduction CrCl < 15 mL/min: avoid the use	PT/INR will falsely increase with administration
	Dabigatran	Non-valvular AF and VTE: 150 mg PO twice daily Hip DVT prophylaxis: 110 mg PO on day 1, then 220 mg PO once daily × 35 days	Onset of action: 1 h Half-life: 12–17 h Metabolism: hepatocytes and enterocytes Elimination: biliary 20%; renally 80%	NVAF: CrCl 15–30 mL/min: 75 mg twice daily VTE treatment and hip DVT prophylaxis: CrCl 15–30 mL/min: avoid the use CrCl < 15 mL/min: avoid the use	Delayed absorption with food Avoid opening, crushing, or chewing the capsule as it increases its bioavailability Significant drug–drug interaction with verapamil, amiodarone, rifampin, and potent P-glycoprotein inhibitors

(continued)

Table 34.2 (continued)

Drug class	Agents	Dosing	Pharmacokinetics	Dose adjustments consideration	Special considerations
Factor-Xa inhibitors	Apixaban	2.5–10 mg q12h (based on indication)	Onset of action: 3–4 h Half-life: ~12 h Elim: renally (~27%) Feces	NVAF: If a patient meets 2 of the 3 criteria: SCr ≥ 1.5 mg/dL, weight ≤60 kg, age ≥80 years, decrease dose to 2.5 mg BID VTE treatment: dose adjustment not recommended	Least renally cleared oral factor-Xa inhibitor Significant drug–drug interaction with CYP inhibitors (such as ketoconazole and ritonavir) and CYP inducers (such as phenytoin, carbamazepine, and rifampin)
	Edoxaban	30–60 mg daily	Onset of action: 1–2 h Half-life: 10–14 h Elim: hepatic and renally	NVAF: CrCl > 95 mL/min: not recommended CrCl 15–50 mL/min: 30 mg daily CrCl < 15 mL/min: not recommend VTE treatment: CrCl ≥ 51 mL/min: none CrCl 15–50 mL/min: 30 mg daily CrCl < 15 mL/min: not recommend	Least drug–drug interactions of oral factor-Xa inhibitors Significant drug–drug interaction with rifampin and potent P-gp inhibitors
	Enoxaparin	Prophylaxis: 30–40 mg daily or q12h Treatment: 1 mg/kg q12h or 1.5 mg/kg daily (based on indication)	Onset of action: 3–5 h Half-life 4.5–7 h Elim: renally	VTE prophylaxis: CrCl < 30 mL/min: 30 mg daily VTE treatment: CrCl < 30 mL/min: 1 mg/kg daily	–
	Fondaparinux	2.5–10 mg daily (weight based)	Onset of action: 2–3 h Half-life 17–21 h Elim: renally	No specific recommendations provided VTE prophylaxis: CrCl 20–50 mL/min: Consider 1.5 mg daily	–
	Rivaroxaban	10–30 mg daily (based on indication)	Onset of action: 2–4 h Half-life: 5–9 h Elim: renally (66%)	NVAF: CrCl 15–50 mL/min: 15 mg daily CrCl < 15 mL/min: not recommend VTE treatment: CrCl ≥ 51 mL/min: none CrCl 15–50 mL/min: 30 mg daily CrCl < 15 mL/min: not recommend	Significant drug–drug interaction with CYP inhibitors (such as ketoconazole, itraconazole, and ritonavir) and CYP inducers (such as phenytoin, carbamazepine, and rifampin)

Thrombin inhibitor	Unfractionated heparin	Varies depending on the therapeutic indication and targeted aPTT	Onset of action: IV: immediate SQ: 3 h Half-life: depending on dose (30–150 min) Elim: renally	–	Often used to "challenge" stroke patients with high bleeding risk who also require anticoagulation
Vitamin K antagonist	Warfarin	Dose varies depending on the therapeutic indication and targeted INR	Onset of action: variable Half-life: 20–60 h Hepatic metabolism Renally (92%)	Consider dose adjustment in renal and hepatic impairment	Genetic variations in the 2C9 isoenzymes and VKOR1 have been associated with differences in dose requirements Significant food–drug interaction with vitamin K rich food (kale, spinach, collards, chard, broccoli, cabbage, and Brussel sprouts) Significant drug–drug interaction interactions with drugs that inhibit or induce CYP 2C9, 1A2, and 3A4 isoenzymes

Adapted from H. Prabhakar et al. *Anticoagulants in Use*. Singapore: Springer Nature; 2022. https://doi.org/10.1007/978-981-19-0954-2_32

aPTT activated partial thromboplastin time, *BID* twice daily, *CrCl* creatinine clearance, *CYP* cytochrome, *DVT* deep vein thrombosis, *h* hours, *INR* international normalized ratio, *IV* intravenous, *NVAF* non-valvular atrial fibrillation, *PT* prothrombin time, *PO* oral, *VTE* venous thromboembolism

Antiplatelet Agents

Platelets have a crucial role in controlling bleeding (hemostasis) by aggregating at a site of vascular injury and forming a "platelet plug." Platelet aggregation can lead to the formation of a thrombus, which can cause vascular stenosis or occlusion, leading to stroke or myocardial infarction, primarily when it occurs on an atherosclerotic lesion.

Aspirin is the most common antiplatelet agent and exerts its activity by irreversibly inhibiting both cyclooxygenase and prostacyclin activity, preventing platelet aggregation [25, 26]. Aspirin has an onset of action of 60 min, and platelets stay inhibited for their entire lifespan (5–7 days). Common side effects of aspirin are dose-related upper gastrointestinal discomfort and bleeding [25, 26].

Aspirin is a cornerstone for the secondary prevention of ischemic stroke. The AHA recommends administering aspirin to patients with acute ischemic stroke within 24–48 h after symptom onset and delaying administering aspirin until 24 h in those patients who received thrombolytics [27]. In patients with minor non-cardioembolic ischemic stroke (defined as NIHSS score ≤3) and did not receive thrombolytics, starting dual antiplatelet therapy with two agents within 24 h of symptom onset for 21–90 days has been shown to reduce recurrent ischemic stroke [27].

Dipyridamole inhibits platelet activity and acts as a mild vasodilator to increase blood flow. Combined with aspirin, it makes the twice-daily drug Aggrenox. Dipyridamole interferes with platelet function by augmenting prostacyclin-related platelet aggregation inhibition and vasodilation through inhibiting phosphodiesterase enzyme. Aggrenox is approved for secondary prevention of ischemic stroke; however, it may cause severe headaches due to vasodilation [28]. Initiating Aggrenox at once-daily dosing for 1–2 weeks and then increasing it to twice daily may reduce the risk of developing headaches.

Clopidogrel is a P2Y12 antagonist. Activation of the P2Y12 receptor on platelet membranes stimulates platelet aggregation. A potent group of antiplatelet agents includes P2Y12 receptor antagonists. Clopidogrel (brand name is Plavix) is a pro-drug, meaning that it needs to be activated (in this case by the liver) to its active metabolite. This metabolite binds to and irreversibly inhibits the P2Y12 receptor, blocking its activity. Clopidogrel can be used for patients with aspirin allergy, but it can also cause rash and GI upset. Ticagrelor is another oral P2Y12 inhibitor administered twice daily with a more rapid onset and offset of action than clopidogrel [29, 30]. Cangrelor is a reversible P2Y12 inhibitor that can be administered parenterally as a bolus followed by an infusion. Cangrelor effect on platelet aggregation is within minutes and it has a very short half-life [11, 31].

Glycoprotein IIb/IIIa Receptor Inhibitors are antiplatelet agents that bind to and inhibit their receptors, preventing platelet aggregation. Eptifibatide and tirofiban are the only two available glycoproteins IIb/IIIa Inhibitors, with abciximab discontinued in 2019 [12, 13]. Table 34.2 summarizes some data for the use of glycoprotein IIb/IIIa Inhibitors l for the management of stroke patients.

Anticoagulants

Warfarin has been around for quite some time. In the 1920s, cattle were dying from internal bleeding after eating moldy sweet clover hay. The Wisconsin Alumni Research Foundation funded a study in 1940 that identified coumarin as the active compound causing the bleeding. Coumarin was then sold as rat poison in 1948, named Warfarin after the funding agency, and approved for use in humans in 1954 as an anticoagulant! Warfarin inhibits the activation of vitamin K-dependent coagulation proteins: factors II (prothrombin), VII, IX, and X, endogenous anticoagulants, and proteins C and S [32]. Warfarin has a peak effect of 4 h and a variable half-life of 20–60 h [32].

Warfarin is absorbed quickly, but it can take 48 h or longer to become therapeutic. The International Normalized Ratio (INR) measures warfarin efficacy, with a typical therapeutic range between 2 and 3 for atrial fibrillation [33, 34]. The dosing regimen and time to therapeutic INR are different for every patient, and a lot of dose tinkering is needed on initiation. Warfarin has clinically significant drug–food and drug–drug interactions with vitamin K-containing foods, which can decrease Warfarin's anticoagulation effect [35]. Warfarin is hepatically metabolized mainly through cytochrome P450 (CYP) 2C9, and medications inhibit that this enzyme can also result in significant drug–drug interactions with Warfarin [36]. It is crucial to check for interactions with any new medication for patients taking warfarin. Table 34.2 reviews pharmacokinetics in more detail, and Tables 34.3 and 34.4 review reversal options for all anticoagulants.

Unfractionated Heparin (UFH) and Low-Molecular-Weight Heparin (LMWH) are intravenous and subcutaneous options for anticoagulation. They inhibit free thrombin by binding to both antithrombin and thrombin, ultimately preventing the conversion of fibrinogen to fibrin, a major ingredient in clots [41, 42]. Intravenous UFH has an immediate onset of action, while subcutaneous LMWH has an onset of action of 20–30 min. UFH half-life depends on the route of

Table 34.3 Common reversal strategies of anticoagulants [37–40]

Agents	Dialyzable	Reversal agent (intravenous)
Direct thrombin inhibitors		
Argatroban	20% over 4 h	• aPCC (50 units/kg) OR
Bivalirudin	25% over 4 h	• 4-Factor PCC (50 units/kg) OR
		• FFP 15–20 mL/kg OR
		• rFVIIa 20 μg/kg and may repeat
		• Monitor aPTT to confirm reversal
Dabigatran	57–68% over 4 h	• If a patient presents within 2–3 h from ingestion, administer enteral activated charcoal 50 g (caution—aspiration risk)
		• Idarucizumab 5 g (2.5 g × 2 doses)
Factor-Xa inhibitors		
Apixaban	Minimal	• If a patient presents within 2–3 h from ingestion, administer enteral activated charcoal 50 g (caution—aspiration risk)
Rivaroxaban	No	
		• Andexanet alpha (refer to Table 34.4 for recommended dosing) OR
		• 4-Factor PCC 25–50 units/kg OR
		• rFVIIa 40 μg/kg OR
		• aPCC 50 units/kg
Edoxaban	No	• If a patient presents within 2–3 h from ingestion, administer enteral activated charcoal 50 g (caution—high aspiration risk)
		• 4-Factor PCC 25–50 units/kg OR
		• rFVIIa 40 μg/kg OR
		• aPCC 50 units/kg
Enoxaparin	No	• Protamine partially reverses the anticoagulant effect of LMWHs (~60%)
		• If <8 h since the last dose: 1 mg protamine:1 mg enoxaparin OR 100 units dalteparin (max: 50 mg)
		• If 8–12 h since the last dose: 0.5 mg protamine: 1 mg enoxaparin OR 100 units dalteparin (max: 25 mg)
		• If >12 h since the last dose: unlikely to be of benefit; may consider in patients with renal dysfunction (max: 25 mg)
		• Monitor factor Xa activity to confirm reversal
Fondaparinux	Yes, 20%	• Weak data for reversal effect with the following but may consider:
		– 4-Factor-PCC 50 units/kg OR
		– rFVIIa 20 μg/kg and may repeat ×1
		• Protamine not effective
Thrombin inhibitor		
Unfractionated heparin	No	• Protamine neutralizes heparin
		• 1 mg per 100 units of heparin administered if stopped immediately
		• 0.5 mg per 100 units of heparin administered if stopped 30 min ago
		• 0.25 mg per 100 units of heparin administered if stopped >2 h ago
Vitamin K antagonist		

(continued)

Table 34.3 (continued)

Agents	Dialyzable	Reversal agent (intravenous)
Warfarin	No	• Vitamin K 2.5–10 mg IV (onset 4–12 h) or 1–5 mg PO (onset 12–24 h) • 4-Factor PCC (in addition to vitamin K) – INR 2–3.9: 25 units/kg (max 2500 units) – INR 4–6: 35 units/kg (max 3500 units) – INR >6: 50 units/kg (max 5000 units) Recheck INR 30 min after 4-Factor PCC administered • Additional 500 units may be given for clinically significant bleeding, repeat INR ≥1.4 OR • FFP 20–30 mL/kg (in addition to vitamin K)

Adapted from *Crit Care Clin.* 2023 Jan;39(1):171–213, Copyright Elsevier (2023)
aPCC activated prothrombin complex concentrate, *aPTT* activated partial thromboplastin time, *FXa* factor Xa, *FFP* fresh frozen plasma, *IV* intravenous, *PO* per os, *PCC* prothrombin complex concentrate, *rFVIIa* recombinant factor VIIa, *INR* International Normalized Ratio

Table 34.4 Andexanet-alpha dosing recommendation [37–40]

Factor Xa inhibitor	Factor Xa inhibitor last dose	Time since the last dose of FXa inhibitor		Low-dose regimen	High dose regimen
		<8 h or unknown	≥8 h		
Rivaroxaban	≤10 mg	Low dose	Low dose	*Bolus*: 400 mg over 15 min	*Bolus*: 800 mg over 30 min
	>10 mg/unknown	High dose		*Infusion*: 480 mg over 2 h (4 mg/min)	*Infusion*: 960 mg over 2 h (8 mg/min)
Apixaban	≤5 mg	Low dose			
	>5 mg/unknown	High dose			

administration and the dose administered, with a mean half-life of 90 min. Due to UFH's short half-life, it is administered as a continuous intravenous infusion to achieve therapeutic efficacy. UFH efficacy can be measured by activated partial thromboplastin time (aPTT) and anti-factor Xa (anti-Xa) analysis. Even though anti-Xa measures direct heparin activity, aPTT is more widely used due to its availability and lower cost than anti-Xa analysis.

UFH can be used in stroke patients who require more urgent anticoagulation and are at risk of hemorrhagic conversion. The benefit of UFH is that if hemorrhage is detected, it can be stopped and reversed quickly with protamine sulfate. Heparin-induced thrombocytopenia (HIT) is a known complication of heparin, whereby an immune-mediated response leads to platelet activation and a drop in platelet count.

Direct Thrombin Inhibitors bind thrombin directly to inhibit its activity. Thrombin is a key enzyme responsible for forming clots.

- **Bivalirudin and Argatroban** are intravenous and commonly used in patients with HIT [43]. Bivalirudin is hepatically metabolized, with 20% of the dose being renally eliminated; thus, dose adjustment is warranted in patients with poor renal function [44]. Both agents can increase the INR [45, 46].
- **Dabigatran** etexilate, used to treat atrial fibrillation, is an oral prodrug that is converted to the active drug dabigatran (a DOAC). Dabigatran directly and reversibly inhibits both free and clot-bound thrombin [47, 48]. Capsules should not be crushed or opened, as the oral bioavailability of dabigatran will increase by 75% if opened [49]. Dabigatran is renally cleared and thus requires renal dose adjustment in patients with renal impairment [50].

Factor Xa Inhibitors work by binding directly to factor Xa, inhibiting thrombin generation. Multiple landmark trials have shown a significant reduction in the rates of intracranial hemorrhage compared to Warfarin for the management of non-valvular atrial fibrillation [51–53]. All three are considered DOACs, and you will notice that they conveniently have "Xa" in their names.

- **Apixaban** is absorbed rapidly from the gastrointestinal tract, with a peak effect in 3–4 h, and a half-life of 12 h [54]. Notice that the half-life is much shorter than Warfarin, just like all the DOACs. Recommended dose adjustments for apixaban differ based on the indication: 5 mg twice daily for atrial fibrillation or 2.5 mg twice daily if the patient has two of the following criteria: a serum creatinine ≥ 1.5 mg/dL, weight ≤ 60 kg, or age ≥ 80 years [54].
- **Edoxaban** is absorbed rapidly from the gastrointestinal tract, with a peak effect of 1–2 h and a half-life of 10–14 h. Edoxaban is primarily renally eliminated and is not recommended in patients with CrCl <15 mL/min [55]. It is not used as often as the other DOACs for the treatment of AF.
- **Rivaroxaban** has a peak effect of 2–4 h and a 5–9 h half-life. It is recommended to administer rivaroxaban with the largest meal of the day for doses above 15 mg to maximize absorption. For the indication of atrial fibrillation, in patients with CrCl, between 15 and 50 mL/min, the rivaroxaban dose should be reduced to 15 mg once daily. Rivaroxaban should be avoided in patients with CrCl less than 15 mL/min due to an increased risk of bleeding compared to Warfarin [56].

Concomitant administration of rivaroxaban and potent P-gp and CYP3A inhibitors or inducers should be avoided [57].

Parenteral Factor Xa Inhibitors
- **Fondaparinux** is a subcutaneous drug that exhibits its anticoagulant effect through the inhibition of factor Xa. Fondaparinux is the preferred agent in patients with HIT due to its negligible cross-reactivity with HIT antibodies [58, 59]. Fondaparinux has a peak effect of 2–3 h and a long half-life of 17–21 h [60]. Anticoagulant effects last 2–4 days after the discontinuation of therapy in patients with normal renal function. Fondaparinux is renally eliminated, and its use is contraindicated in patients with CrCl less than 30 mL/min [60].
- **Enoxaparin** is a subcutaneous drug that exerts its anticoagulant effect through inhibiting factor Xa with little impact on thrombin (approximately 14:1). After the subcutaneous administration of 40 mg, enoxaparin has an anti-factor Xa peak effect of 3–5 h and a terminal half-life between 4.5 and 7 h. Routine monitoring of anti-factor Xa concentrations is not necessary for all patients; however, for obese, underweight, renally impaired, or pregnant patients, anti-factor Xa monitoring is warranted. In mechanical heart valve bridging, the recommended anti-factor Xa goals are 0.5–1 units/mL in non-pregnant patients and 0.8–1.2 units/mL in pregnant patients [61]. For VTE prophylaxis, the recommended anti-factor Xa level is 0.2–0.6 units/mL in pregnant patients and 0.2–0.4 units/mL in trauma patients [61, 62].

Antihypertensive Drugs

AHA guidelines recommend that patients who present with elevated blood pressure and are eligible for thrombolytic treatment should have a systolic blood pressure (SBP) goal of less than 185 mmHg and a diastolic blood pressure goal of <110 mmHg before IV fibrinolytic administration. Blood pressure should be less than 180/105 mmHg for the first 24 h post-thrombolytic treatment [10, 27]. For patients with acute ICH, AHA guidelines recommend an SBP goal of 140 mmHg in patients who present with SBP between 150 and 220 mmHg and <220 mmHg (to a target range of 140–160 mmHg) in patients who present with SBP >220 mmHg [63]. For aneurysmal subarachnoid hemorrhage, the optimal blood pressure goal is not clear. The guidelines recommend maintaining <160 mmHg or mean arterial pressure <110 mmHg in the acute SAH setting [64, 65]. Given the acute nature of these conditions, parenteral medications are the most effective. Table 34.5 highlights the most common antihypertensive drugs used in the acute setting.

Table 34.5 Common parenteral antihypertensive agents [39, 66, 67]

	Mechanism of action	Dosing	Pharmacokinetics	Patient care considerations
Vasodilators				
Hydralazine	Potent arterial vasodilator decreasing afterload	IV bolus 10–20 mg every 30 min as needed IM: 10–40 mg every 30 min as needed	Onset: IV: 10 min, IM: 20 min Duration: IV: 1–4 h, IM: 2–6 h Half-life: 2–8 h	It can cause reflex tachycardia, headache, flushing
Calcium channel blockers				
Nicardipine	Dihydropyridine; peripherally selective to L-type calcium channel blockers. Inhibit calcium influx through calcium channels along the vascular smooth muscle, leading to vasodilation	IV 5–15 mg/h Increase rate by 2.5 mg/h every 5–15 min	Onset: 5–15 min Duration: 0.5–2 h Half-life: 2 h	It can cause reflex tachycardia, headache, nausea, flushing Contraindicated in patients with severe aortic stenosis
Clevidipine		IV 1–2 mg/h Increase rate by 1–2 mg/h every 90 s to a maximum dose of 21 mg/24 h (for more aggressive dosing, may double rate every 90 s up to a dose of 16 mg/h, then increase by 2 mg/h once within 10 mmHg of goal blood pressure to a typical max of 24 mg/h)	Onset: 1–4 min Duration: 90 s Half-life: 1 min	Contraindication in patients with soy or egg product allergy (as it is formulated in a lipid compound) and severe aortic stenosis Provides 2 kcal/mL—adjust nutritional support as needed Monitor triglycerides, lipase, and amylase Discard vials within 12 h due to the risk of bacterial growth It can cause reflex tachycardia
Nimodipine		Enteral: 60 mg every 4 h or 30 mg q 2 h for 21 consecutive days	Onset: 0.25–1 h Half-life: 1–2 h	Indicated for use in aneurysmal subarachnoid hemorrhage to decrease delayed cerebral ischemia (no indication for hypertension)
Beta-blockers				

(continued)

Table 34.5 (continued)

	Mechanism of action	Dosing	Pharmacokinetics	Patient care considerations
Esmolol	Beta selective antagonist	IV 25–300 µg/kg/min Increase rate by 25 µg/kg/min every 3–5 min	Onset: 1–2 min Duration: 10–20 min Half-life: 9 min	Avoid in a patient with systolic heart failure
Labetalol	Combined alpha and beta antagonist	IV bolus: 10–20 mg; may repeat escalating doses by 20–80 mg every 5–10 min as needed IV 0.5–10 mg/min. Increase dose by 1–2 mg/min every 2 h	Onset: 2–5 min Peak effect: 5–15 min Duration: 2–18 h Half-life: 4–8 h	Avoid in a patient with systolic heart failure
Metoprolol	Beta selective antagonist	IV bolus: 5–15 mg every 5–15 min as needed	Onset: 5–20 min Duration 2–6 h Half-life: 3–4 h	Avoid in a patient with systolic heart failure Due to the long duration of the activity, it is less titratable and can cause extended, unintentional correction of blood pressure
Angiotensin-converting enzyme inhibitor				
Enalaprilat	Inhibits ACE preventing the conversion of angiotensin I to angiotensin II, a potent vasoconstrictor	IV bolus: 1.25 mg over 5 min every 6 h. maximum dose: 5 mg/dose every 6 h	Onset: 15 min Duration: 6 h Half-life: 35 h	It can cause angioedema, cough, hyperkalemia Due to the long duration of the activity, it is less titratable and can cause extended, unintentional correction of blood pressure Use in pregnancy is contraindicated

Adapted from *Crit Care Clin*. 2023 Jan;39(1):171–213, Copyright Elsevier (2023)
ACE angiotensin-converting enzyme, *IV* intravenous, *IM* intramuscular

Table 34-5. Statin Dose Equivalents and Intensities					
Statin					
Atorvastatin		5	10	20	40	80
Rosuvastatin			5	10	20	40
Simvastatin	5	10	20	40	80	
Pravastatin	10	20	40	80		
Lovastatin	10	20	40	80		
Fluvastatin	20	40	80			
Yellow: Low intensity (expected 30% LDL reduction), Orange: Moderate intensity (< 50% LDL reduction), Red: High intensity (≥ 50% LDL reduction)						

Fig. 34.1 Statin dose equivalents and intensities. Yellow: low intensity (expected 30% LDL reduction), Orange: moderate intensity (<50% LDL reduction), Red: high intensity (≥50% LDL reduction)

Dyslipidemia

Targeted therapies for dyslipidemia, including 3-hydroxy-3-methylglutaryl coenzyme A reductase inhibitors (statins), have been shown to reduce the risk of cardiovascular disease and stroke among patients with coronary heart disease and those at increased risk for cardiovascular disease [68]. Figure 34.1 reviews statin options and dose equivalencies. In addition, statins have been shown to decrease the risk of stroke among patients with a history of stroke or TIA [69]. Beyond statins, ezetimibe, and proprotein convertase subtilisin/kexin type 9 (PCSK9), inhibitors reduce the risk of stroke and cardiovascular events in patients at cardiovascular risk [70]. Most recently, Icosapent ethyl (Vazkepa) was shown to reduce the risk of cardiovascular events, including myocardial infarctions and strokes, in people with controlled LDL-C and elevated triglycerides [71].

There is some evidence to suggest that having extremely low cholesterol levels may increase the risk of ICH. However, the benefit of lipid-lowering therapy outweighs the risk [71–73]. The most common side effect related to statin therapy impacting patient adherence is related to statin-associated muscle symptoms (myalgias) [74]. Different statins have different degrees of lipophilicity, which influences the distribution of statins in muscle tissue. Simvastatin is the most lipophilic and commonly associated with myalgias, whereas rosuvastatin and pravastatin are the least [74]. While most statin-related muscle symptoms have been reported with simvastatin and lovastatin, all currently available statins have been associated with some muscle side effects, including rhabdomyolysis [74].

References

1. Coutts SB, Dubuc V, Mandzia J, et al. Tenecteplase-tissue-type plasminogen activator evaluation for minor ischemic stroke with proven occlusion. Stroke. 2015;46:769–74.
2. Tanswell P, Modi N, Combs D, Danays T. Pharmacokinetics and pharmacodynamics of tenecteplase in fibrinolytic therapy of acute myocardial infarction. Clin Pharmacokinet. 2002;41:1229–45.

3. National Institute of Neurological Disorders and Stroke. Tissue plasminogen activator for acute ischemic stroke. N Engl J Med. 1995;333:1581–7.
4. Hacke W, Kaste M, Bluhmki E, et al. Thrombolysis with alteplase 3 to 4.5 hours after acute ischemic stroke. N Engl J Med. 2008;359:1317–29.
5. Parsons M, Spratt N, Bivard A, et al. A randomized trial of tenecteplase versus alteplase for acute ischemic stroke. N Engl J Med. 2012;366:1099–107.
6. Huang X, Cheripelli BK, Lloyd SM, et al. Alteplase versus tenecteplase for thrombolysis after ischaemic stroke (ATTEST): a phase 2, randomised, open-label, blinded endpoint study. Lancet Neurol. 2015;14:368–76.
7. Logallo N, Novotny V, Assmus J, et al. Tenecteplase versus alteplase for management of acute ischaemic stroke (NOR-TEST): a phase 3, randomised, open-label, blinded endpoint trial. Lancet Neurol. 2017;16:781–8.
8. Campbell BC, Mitchell PJ, Churilov L, et al. Tenecteplase versus alteplase before endovascular thrombectomy (EXTEND-IA TNK): a multicenter, randomized, controlled study. Int J Stroke. 2018;13:328–34.
9. Campbell BCV, Mitchell PJ, Churilov L, et al. Effect of intravenous tenecteplase dose on cerebral reperfusion before thrombectomy in patients with large vessel occlusion ischemic stroke: the EXTEND-IA TNK part 2 randomized clinical trial. JAMA. 2020;323:1257–65.
10. Powers WJ, Rabinstein AA, Ackerson T, et al. Guidelines for the early management of patients with acute ischemic stroke: 2019 update to the 2018 guidelines for the early management of acute ischemic stroke: a guideline for healthcare professionals from the American Heart Association/American Stroke Association. Stroke. 2019;50:e344–418.
11. Kengreal [package insert]. Cary, NC: Chiesi USA, Inc.; 2022.
12. Tirofiban [package insert]. Greenville, NC: Amdipharm Limited; 2022.
13. Eptifibatide [package insert]. Bridgewater, NJ: Amneal Pharmaceuticals LLC; 2021.
14. Eikelboom JW, Hirsh J, Spencer FA, Baglin TP, Weitz JI. Antiplatelet drugs: antithrombotic therapy and prevention of thrombosis, 9th ed: American College of Chest Physicians Evidence-Based Clinical Practice Guidelines. Chest. 2012;141:e89S–e119S.
15. Gilchrist IC, O'Shea JC, Kosoglou T, et al. Pharmacodynamics and pharmacokinetics of higher-dose, double-bolus eptifibatide in percutaneous coronary intervention. Circulation. 2001;104:406–11.
16. Cheema AA, Teklinski AH, Maria V, Chilukuri K, Frank JJ, Gosselin MO. Recurrent acute profound thrombocytopenia related to readministration of eptifibatide. J Interv Cardiol. 2006;19:99–103.
17. Coons JC, Barcelona RA, Freedy T, Hagerty MF. Eptifibatide-associated acute, profound thrombocytopenia. Ann Pharmacother. 2005;39:368–72.
18. Tardiff BE, Jennings LK, Harrington RA, et al. Pharmacodynamics and pharmacokinetics of eptifibatide in patients with acute coronary syndromes: prospective analysis from PURSUIT. Circulation. 2001;104:399–405.
19. Van Tuyl JS, Newsome AS, Hollis IB. Perioperative bridging with glycoprotein IIb/IIIa inhibitors versus cangrelor: balancing efficacy and safety. Ann Pharmacother. 2019;53:726–37.
20. Huxtable LM, Tafreshi MJ, Rakkar AN. Frequency and management of thrombocytopenia with the glycoprotein IIb/IIIa receptor antagonists. Am J Cardiol. 2006;97:426–9.
21. Llevadot J, Coulter SA, Giugliano RP. A practical approach to the diagnosis and management of thrombocytopenia associated with glycoprotein IIb/IIIa receptor inhibitors. J Thromb Thrombolysis. 2000;9:175–80.
22. Brilinta [package insert]. Wilmington, DE: AstraZeneca Pharmaceuticals LP.; 2021.
23. Prasugrel [package insert]. Durham, NC: Accord Healthcare, Inc.; 2019.
24. Clopidogrel [package insert]. Wilmington, DE: Graviti Pharmaceuticals Inc.; 2022.
25. Awtry EH, Loscalzo J. Aspirin. Circulation. 2000;101:1206–18.
26. Pillinger MH, Capodici C, Rosenthal P, et al. Modes of action of aspirin-like drugs: salicylates inhibit erk activation and integrin-dependent neutrophil adhesion. Proc Natl Acad Sci USA. 1998;95:14540–5.
27. Whelton PK, Carey RM, Aronow WS, et al. 2017 ACC/AHA/AAPA/ABC/ACPM/AGS/APhA/ASH/ASPC/NMA/PCNA Guideline for the prevention, detection, evaluation, and

management of high blood pressure in adults: a report of the American College of Cardiology/ American Heart Association Task Force on Clinical Practice Guidelines. Hypertension. 2018;71:e13–e115.

28. Aspirin and extended-release dipyridamole [package insert]. Princeton, NJ: Dr. Reddy's Laboratories Inc.; 2021.

29. Wang D, Yang XH, Zhang JD, Li RB, Jia M, Cui XR. Compared efficacy of clopidogrel and ticagrelor in treating acute coronary syndrome: a meta-analysis. BMC Cardiovasc Disord. 2018;18:217.

30. Guerra DR, Tcheng JE. Prasugrel: clinical development and therapeutic application. Adv Ther. 2009;26:999–1011.

31. Cortez GM, Monteiro A, Sourour N, et al. The use of cangrelor in neurovascular interventions: a multicenter experience. Neuroradiology. 2021;63:925–34.

32. Product Information: COUMADIN(R) oral tablets, intravenous injection, warfarin sodium oral tablets, intravenous injection. Princeton, NJ: Bristol-Myers Squibb Company; 2010.

33. Nutescu EA, Burnett A, Fanikos J, Spinler S, Wittkowsky A. Erratum to: Pharmacology of anticoagulants used in the treatment of venous thromboembolism. J Thromb Thrombolysis. 2016;42:296–311.

34. Pengo V, Biasiolo A, Pegoraro C. A simple scheme to initiate oral anticoagulant treatment in outpatients with nonrheumatic atrial fibrillation. Am J Cardiol. 2001;88:1214–6.

35. O'Reilly RA, Rytand DA. "Resistance" to warfarin due to unrecognized vitamin K supplementation. N Engl J Med. 1980;303:160–1.

36. Weser JK, Sellers E. Drug interactions with coumarin anticoagulants. 2. N Engl J Med. 1971;285:547–58.

37. Frontera JA, Lewin JJ III, Rabinstein AA, et al. Guideline for reversal of antithrombotics in intracranial hemorrhage: a statement for healthcare professionals from the Neurocritical Care Society and Society of Critical Care Medicine. Neurocrit Care. 2016;24:6–46.

38. Bower MM, Sweidan AJ, Shafie M, Atallah S, Groysman LI, Yu W. Contemporary reversal of oral anticoagulation in intracerebral hemorrhage. Stroke. 2019;50:529–36.

39. Brophy GM, Human T, Shutter L. Emergency neurological life support: pharmacotherapy. Neurocrit Care. 2015;23(Suppl 2):S48–68.

40. January CT, Wann LS, et al. 2019 AHA/ACC/HRS focused update of the 2014 AHA/ACC/ HRS guideline for the management of patients with atrial fibrillation: a report of the American College of Cardiology/American Heart Association Task Force on Clinical Practice Guidelines and the Heart Rhythm Society. Heart Rhythm. 2019;16:e66–93.

41. Tulinsky A. Molecular interactions of thrombin. Semin Thromb Hemost. 1996;22:117–24.

42. Product Information: heparin sodium injection, USP, heparin sodium injection, USP. Kalamazoo, MI: Pharmacia and Upjohn Company; 2000.

43. Alban S. Pharmacological strategies for inhibition of thrombin activity. Curr Pharm Des. 2008;14:1152–75.

44. Robson R, White H, Aylward P, Frampton C. Bivalirudin pharmacokinetics and pharmacodynamics: effect of renal function, dose, and gender. Clin Pharmacol Ther. 2002;71:433–9.

45. Gosselin RC, Dager WE, King JH, et al. Effect of direct thrombin inhibitors, bivalirudin, lepirudin, and argatroban, on prothrombin time and INR values. Am J Clin Pathol. 2004;121:593–9.

46. Garcia DA, Baglin TP, Weitz JI, Samama MM. Parenteral anticoagulants: antithrombotic therapy and prevention of thrombosis, 9th ed: American College of Chest Physicians Evidence-Based Clinical Practice Guidelines. Chest. 2012;141:e24S–43S.

47. Blech S, Ebner T, Ludwig-Schwellinger E, Stangier J, Roth W. The metabolism and disposition of the oral direct thrombin inhibitor, dabigatran, in humans. Drug Metab Dispos. 2008;36:386–99.

48. Stangier J. Clinical pharmacokinetics and pharmacodynamics of the oral direct thrombin inhibitor dabigatran etexilate. Clin Pharmacokinet. 2008;47:285–95.

49. Stangier J, Stahle H, Rathgen K, Fuhr R. Pharmacokinetics and pharmacodynamics of the direct oral thrombin inhibitor dabigatran in healthy elderly subjects. Clin Pharmacokinet. 2008;47:47–59.

50. Eriksson BI, Quinlan DJ, Weitz JI. Comparative pharmacodynamics and pharmacokinetics of oral direct thrombin and factor xa inhibitors in development. Clin Pharmacokinet. 2009;48:1–22.
51. Giugliano RP, Ruff CT, Braunwald E, et al. Edoxaban versus warfarin in patients with atrial fibrillation. N Engl J Med. 2013;369:2093–104.
52. Granger CB, Alexander JH, McMurray JJ, et al. Apixaban versus warfarin in patients with atrial fibrillation. N Engl J Med. 2011;365:981–92.
53. Patel MR, Mahaffey KW, Garg J, et al. Rivaroxaban versus warfarin in nonvalvular atrial fibrillation. N Engl J Med. 2011;365:883–91.
54. Apixaban [package insert]. Princeton, NJ: Bristol-Myers Squibb; 2019.
55. Edoxaban [package insert]. Basking Ridge, NJ: Daiichi Sankyo Co., LTD.; 2021.
56. Chan KE, Edelman ER, Wenger JB, Thadhani RI, Maddux FW. Dabigatran and rivaroxaban use in atrial fibrillation patients on hemodialysis. Circulation. 2015;131:972–9.
57. Rivaroxaban [package insert]. Titusville, NH: Janssen Pharmaceuticals; 2020.
58. Cuker A, Arepally GM, Chong BH, et al. American Society of Hematology 2018 guidelines for management of venous thromboembolism: heparin-induced thrombocytopenia. Blood Adv. 2018;2:3360–92.
59. Schindewolf M, Steindl J, Beyer-Westendorf J, et al. Use of fondaparinux off-label or approved anticoagulants for management of heparin-induced thrombocytopenia. J Am Coll Cardiol. 2017;70:2636–48.
60. Fondaparinux [package insert]. Research Triangle Park, NC: GlaxoSmithKline; 2009.
61. Bates SM, Greer IA, Middeldorp S, Veenstra DL, Prabulos AM, Vandvik PO. VTE, thrombophilia, antithrombotic therapy, and pregnancy: antithrombotic therapy and prevention of thrombosis, 9th ed: American College of Chest Physicians Evidence-Based Clinical Practice Guidelines. Chest. 2012;141:e691S–736S.
62. Nyquist P, Bautista C, Jichici D, et al. Prophylaxis of venous thrombosis in neurocritical care patients: an evidence-based guideline: a statement for healthcare professionals from the Neurocritical Care Society. Neurocrit Care. 2016;24:47–60.
63. Greenberg SM, Ziai WC, Cordonnier C, et al. 2022 Guideline for the management of patients with spontaneous intracerebral hemorrhage: A guideline from the American Heart Association/American Stroke Association. Stroke. 2022;53:e282–361.
64. Connolly ES Jr, Rabinstein AA, Carhuapoma JR, et al. Guidelines for the management of aneurysmal subarachnoid hemorrhage: a guideline for healthcare professionals from the American Heart Association/American Stroke Association. Stroke. 2012;43:1711–37.
65. Diringer MN, Bleck TP, Claude Hemphill J III, et al. Critical care management of patients following aneurysmal subarachnoid hemorrhage: recommendations from the Neurocritical Care Society's Multidisciplinary Consensus Conference. Neurocrit Care. 2011;15:211–40.
66. Rhoney D, Peacock WF. Intravenous therapy for hypertensive emergencies, Part 2. Am J Health Syst Pharm. 2009;66:1448–57.
67. Aggarwal M, Khan IA. Hypertensive crisis: hypertensive emergencies and urgencies. Cardiol Clin. 2006;24:135–46.
68. Sacco RL, Adams R, Albers G, et al. Guidelines for prevention of stroke in patients with ischemic stroke or transient ischemic attach: a statement for healthcare professionals from the American Heart Association/American Stroke Association Council on Stroke: co-sponsored by the Council on Cardiovascular Radiology and Intervention: the American Academy of Neurology affirms the value of this guideline. Stroke. 2006;37:577–617.
69. Amarenco P, Bogousslavsky J, Callahan A III, et al., Stroke Prevention by Aggressive Reduction in Cholesterol Levels (SPARCL) Investigators. High-dose atorvastatin after stroke or transient ischemic attack. N Engl J Med. 2006;355(6):549–59.
70. Sohn SI. Dyslipidemia and hemorrhagic stroke. In: Lee SH, Kang MK, editors. Stroke revisited: dyslipidemia in stroke. Stroke revisited. Singapore: Springer; 2021. https://doi.org/10.1007/978-981-16-3923-4_4.
71. Peterson BE, Bhatt DL, Steg PG, et al., REDUCE-IT Investigators. Treatment with icosapent ethyl to reduce ischemic events in patients with prior percutaneous coronary intervention: insights from REDUCE-IT PCI. J Am Heart Assoc. 2022;11(6):e022937.

72. Yaghi S, Elkind MS. Lipids and cerebrovascular disease: research and practice. Stroke. 2015;46(11):3322–8.
73. Tsankof A, Tziomalos K. The role of lipid-lowering treatment in the secondary prevention of ischemic stroke. Diseases. 2021;10(1):3.
74. Wiggins BS, Backes JM, Hilleman D. Statin-associated muscle symptoms—a review: individualizing the approach to optimize care. Pharmacotherapy. 2022;42(5):428–38.

The Interdisciplinary Stroke Team

35

Sharon Bottomley and Jason Sico

Introduction

Ischemic stroke, transient ischemic attacks (TIAs), and intracerebral hemorrhages are often attributed to underlying, sometimes long-standing, chronic conditions such as hypertension, diabetes, hyperlipidemia, atrial fibrillation, carotid artery disease, and obstructive sleep apnea (OSA) [1, 2]. Some conditions are not yet known and require further investigation. Based on findings from such testing as arrhythmia monitoring, echocardiography, carotid ultrasound, and polysomnography/home sleep testing, care needs for stroke and TIA survivors may be complex and multifaceted. Post-stroke/TIA patients may also have additional rehabilitation and support needs based on stroke severity and residual deficits. Cognitive, mood, and pain disorders are common and need to be considered after a cerebrovascular event, and not evaluating and managing such conditions may profoundly interfere with delivering effective secondary preventive strategies and patient participation in rehabilitation [1, 3, 4]. Adding to the complexities of post-stroke/TIA care includes multiple transitions between settings (e.g., hospital to rehab or an extended care facility and hospital/rehab center to home) [5] and handoffs between healthcare providers (e.g., inpatient ICU/neurology/stroke/hospitalist medicine teams to outpatient primary care or neurology). Every transition point is fraught with opportunities for mistakes and gaps in care. Finally, care needs for stroke patients may evolve over time, and providers should be prepared to address those needs [2, 6, 7].

S. Bottomley
Veterans Affairs Medical Center, West Haven, CT, USA
e-mail: sharon.bottomley@va.gov

J. Sico (✉)
Yale School of Medicine, New Haven, CT, USA
e-mail: Jason.Sico@va.gov

A single provider cannot deliver all the high-quality, high-value, individually tailored, and evidence-based post-stroke/TIA care required for stroke patients. Thus, post-stroke/TIA care coordinated across various disciplines can improve post-cerebrovascular event outcomes, including improvements in vascular risk factor management, functional recovery, and pain. It can also be more cost-effective than similar patients who did not receive comparable care [2]. In the literature and clinical care, "multidisciplinary" care and "interdisciplinary" care are often used synonymously. Multidisciplinary care is "a group of individuals from various disciplines involved in a project but working independently." In contrast, interdisciplinary care is "groups of professionals who work together to develop collaborative processes and plans for patients" [8–10]. We will use "interdisciplinary care" throughout this chapter. We will discuss the specific roles of important team members in providing interdisciplinary cerebrovascular care teams. Finally, we will provide case studies to illustrate advanced practice clinicians (APCs) working across disciplines and within interdisciplinary care teams. The tables provides an overview of subspecialty referrals and services that these practitioners may offer.

Evaluation and Management of Cerebrovascular Risk Factors

The 2021 Guidelines for the Prevention of Stroke in Patients with Stroke and TIA highlighted the importance of interdisciplinary care in the management of cerebrovascular risk factors in two of its "Top 10 Take-Home Messages for the Secondary Stroke Prevention Guideline" [3], noting the importance of a team-based approach in post-cerebrovascular event risk factor care in both intensive medical management and patient behavior change related to medication compliance, diet, and exercise. Guiding principles for post-stroke and TIA care include a patient-centric focus promoting functional recovery, identifying barriers, providing evidence-based treatment to cerebrovascular risk factor management, and evaluating and addressing new needs that have resulted from a cerebrovascular event across the continuum of post-stroke/TIA care while leaning on the expertise from each team member.

Primary care is primarily the home of longitudinal, evidence-based management of post-ischemic stroke/TIA cerebrovascular risk factor evaluation and management [4]. APCs have a long and rich tradition of practicing within primary care settings and are very likely to see stroke patients in follow-up. When delivering interdisciplinary post-stroke/TIA care, APCs may find themselves as the "quarterback" working with a multitude of healthcare providers, the combination of which would primarily be driven by the needs of comorbidities of individual patients (Fig. 35.1) [4].

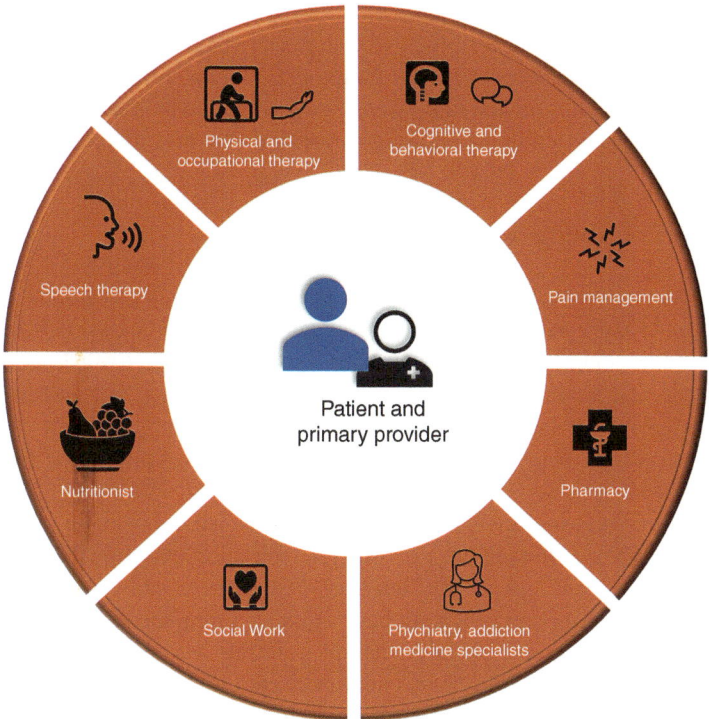

Fig. 35.1   Interdisciplinary stroke team

Stroke Evaluations

Various risk factors cause stroke, sometimes known and sometimes unknown. Defining stroke etiology (i.e., small vessel, large vessel, and cardioembolic) helps focus the discussion on specific conditions. Studies have shown that treating multiple risk factors—combining antithrombotic agents with antihypertensive, statin, and diabetes therapy—with exercise, dietary modifications, and lifestyle counseling can lead to an 80% reduction in recurrent cerebrovascular events [5].

Often, a stroke etiology is unknown and needs further workup. A comprehensive secondary prevention plan requires knowing what vascular risk factors are known and contributed to a stroke and what unknown risk factors may still need to be ruled out. For example, older stroke patients may need cardiac monitoring to rule out atrial fibrillation. Stroke clinics may be able to perform monitoring, but a cardiology referral is required in many cases. Close collaboration with a cardiology clinic for timely initiation of monitoring *and* review of results is important to reduce future stroke risk effectively. Young patients often need broad hematological or genetic evaluations to rule out hereditary or acquired genetic conditions. Having a network of specialized doctors and knowing which patients require their services ensure that patients receive appropriate and thorough evaluations to prevent recurrent strokes.

Utilizing Rehabilitation Specialists

According to the AHA/ASA Primary Care of Adult Patients After Stroke Scientific Statement, "Unmet needs for physical rehabilitation, activities of daily living, mobility, pain control, and communication remain prevalent" [6]. Rehabilitation should focus on maximizing function, improving quality of life, and journeying with patients as they strive to regain as much independence as possible. All stroke patients require physical and occupational therapy evaluations in the hospital to determine rehab needs.

A rehabilitation assessment can help identify deficiencies in cognition, comprehension, speech, swallowing, vision, strength, sensation, balance, and performing complex, coordinated, purposeful activities [7]. Patients can benefit from more speech and language therapy if they have ongoing communication or swallowing difficulties [8]. Outpatient physical therapy referrals are warranted to regain or improve gross motor skills, improve endurance, increase range of motion, and treat pain. Occupational therapists attend to fine motor skills, focusing on how patients perform activities and the role of these activities during their daily lives and delivering therapies that address deficits in cognition, sensation, and behavior. Physical Medicine and Rehabilitation (PM&R) providers, also known as physiatrists, are medical doctors who work closely with therapists to coordinate rehabilitation care across different disciplines and are particularly helpful for complex disabilities. They use a range of treatment options, including more invasive procedures and pharmacotherapies, to manage spasticity. They also help select additional therapies, such as functional electrical stimulation, transcutaneous electrical nerve stimulation, and other adjunctive therapies to improve upper and lower extremity motor recovery [7].

Patients often get referred to physical, occupational, and speech therapy after a stroke, but many times, for a variety of reasons, may not follow through. Barriers include lack of access to transportation, severe language impairment or non-English speaking patients, elderly or isolated patients with no support system, or a history of mood disorders limiting motivation to participate. To identify patients who might benefit from rehabilitation but are not receiving it, it is important to determine the status of active therapy referrals and inquire about issues with ambulation or daily activities, recent falls, and unmet long-term goals (i.e., returning to work or driving). This is especially important for patients who may have been overlooked or not received adequate care in the past.

A real-world limiting factor to therapies is insurance coverage. Uninsured patients are often unable to get beds at rehab facilities, leading to extended hospital stays. In the outpatient setting, some insurances will only cover a certain number of sessions, and getting more may require an appeal from the provider.

Pain

Pain after a stroke can limit functional recovery and occur in about 10–30% of stroke patients. Pain can be attributed to various causes, including musculoskeletal pain caused by spasticity and contractures, fractures, arthritis, adhesive capsulitis, and shoulder subluxation. Patients with hemiparesis are at risk of shoulder subluxation during transfers. Patients may also place more weight on joints on the unaffected side, potentially increasing the risk of injury or joint deterioration. This kind of pain is aching and throbbing and may require joint imaging and referral to physical therapy or orthopedics in addition to pain control. Complex regional pain syndrome or central post-stroke pain can occur after thalamic and parietal ischemic strokes affecting the sensory cortex [9, 10]. This pain manifests as burning, tingling, pins and needles, or hypersensitivity to normal sensations like touch. Treating central neuropathic pain is complex and often involves trying different neuropathic pain medications and adjusting doses while monitoring for side effects. This is best done by a neurologist or pain specialist. The most used medications for central pain include gabapentin, lamotrigine, pregabalin, and amitriptyline.

Mood and Cognitive Specialists

Having cognitive and mental health specialists as part of an interdisciplinary clinic is incredibly valuable. Patients reporting cognitive symptoms after a stroke may benefit from a referral to a neuropsychologist, whereas psychologists are more trained to focus on emotions. Neuropsychologists can conduct validated screening of cognition in the context of affective disorders such as depression, anxiety, and post-traumatic stress disorder, stress, pain, social isolation, as well as screen for alcohol or polysubstance use and inquire about diet and exercise [2].

A behavioral psychologist may be more appropriate for patients suffering from anxiety, stress, and depression after a traumatic medical event like a stroke, without cognitive symptoms. Clinical psychologists embrace the biopsychosocial model of health, recognizing the interconnectedness of biological and psychosocial components of health and illness [11, 12].

For many patients, short-term memory loss is the first sign of a cognitive problem. It can be difficult for a primary care provider to separate normal, age-related cognitive symptoms from a more concerning picture. It is important to determine whether cognitive difficutlies affect a patient's day-today functioning, including manging finances and ability to navigate. Predictors of developing post-stroke cognitive impairment include older age, premorbid cognitive and functional decline, history of prior stroke, and lower socioeconomic status [13]. Cognitive symptoms may be primarily due to a stroke but can also be exacerbated by mood disorders, medications, or medical conditions like sleep apnea, anemia, nutritional deficiencies, or hypothyroidism. Therefore, in addition to cognitive screening, ruling out other conditions is also important for patients complaining of memory difficulty. Cognitive screening tools that are less reliant on language-based tasks, such as the Montreal Cognitive Assessment test (MoCA), are preferred and can be administered in the primary care clinic. Referrals to neuropsychology and geriatric or memory clinics may be helpful based on the results or patient complaints of cognitive symptoms.

Patients, who live alone, are frequent no-shows to the clinic or have significant impairments, should be screened for depression. Post-stroke depression, post-traumatic stress, and anxiety are common affective disorders experienced by stroke survivors, with a frequency of 33–41% reported within the first 6 months and a slight reduction to 25% by 12 month post-cerebrovascular event [1, 14, 15]. Post-stroke depression leads to lower medication compliance, less engagement with medical providers and rehabilitation, and a lower quality of life. It also increases hospitalization rates within 12 months following a stroke and prolongs hospital stays [1]. In addition to treating emotional disorders, psychologists can also provide techniques to improve medication compliance, promote smoking cessation [16], and spearhead continuous positive airway pressure (CPAP) desensitization clinics [17, 18].

Social workers provide a wide range of services for stroke patients, including emotional support for patients and caregivers adjusting to a new reality, assistance accessing healthcare resources, insurance coverage, and financial assistance programs. They also ensure medication access and know community resources such as support groups and social assistance programs. Social workers are particularly helpful for vulnerable populations such as those without insurance, those with cognitive issues, those who struggle with substance use, or those who have limited resources or access to healthcare.

In the inpatient setting, social workers engage the family and patient, coordinating meetings if necessary, insurance coverage, and discharge planning. In the outpatient setting, social workers may be available through a home care agency or accountable care organization. The outpatient social worker helps to follow through on discharge goals, identifies any barriers to success, such as issues with prescriptions or prescribed services, and provides ongoing social support.

Lifestyle Concerns

Many lifestyle choices increase the risk of stroke, such as diet and substance use. Poor diet quality is an independent risk factor for mortality in stroke. Unfortunately, many medical providers do not get sufficient training to counsel patients on diet. Knowledge of the Mediterranean and DASH diets might be sufficient for providers counseling patients without advanced medical or socioeconomic problems (Table 35.1). However, a referral to a nutritionist can be helpful for patients with advanced diabetes, obesity or malnutrition, hypertension or renal disease, or limited resources to develop an individual nutrition assessment and diet plans. Patients struggling with substance abuse, including alcohol and drugs, can benefit from the expertise of addiction medicine specialists. These specialists can provide counseling and develop inpatient or outpatient detox and treatment plans. Consulting addiction medicine teams early is also linked with shorter hospital stays for this patient population.

Clinical Pearls
- Outpatient cerebrovascular care for stroke or TIA survivors is complex and requires interdisciplinary attention.
- An APC is central to delivering cerebrovascular care, ensuring proper diagnostic testing, managing vascular risk factors, and addressing comorbidities impacting rehabilitation potential, quality of life, and overall health.
- Knowing roles and referral processes for specialists can make caring for complex stroke patients more efficient and comprehensive (Table 35.2).

Table 35.1 Brief comparison of DASH and Mediterranean diets

Dash diet	Mediterranean diet
The goal is to reduce blood pressure	The goal is to promote overall cardiovascular health
Key emphasis is on limiting sodium intake (<1500–2300 mg daily)	Focuses more on moderation, derived from Mediterranean cuisine
Prioritizes potassium, magnesium, and calcium intake plus sodium restriction	Emphasizes whole foods like fruits, vegetables, whole grains, healthy fats, and lean proteins
Data have shown significant reductions in BP within 8 weeks	Lower cardiovascular events in this diet supplemented with extra-virgin olive oil or nuts

Table 35.2 Roles and responsibilities of interdisciplinary stroke/TIA team members in the provision of outpatient care

Clinical practitioner	Roles and responsibilities
APP and primary care physician	Long-term management of vascular risk factors
	Oversees necessary referrals and care coordination initiatives
	Ensures that necessary post-discharge care is in place and provides clinical services within the month following discharge, especially when time-dependent therapies may have been recommended (e.g., discontinuation of dual antiplatelet therapy after 21 days, resuming home antihypertensive regimen and carotid revascularization)
	Assess for acute and chronic pain, including musculoskeletal pain and central pain syndromes
	Screen for commonly encountered post-stroke cognitive and mental health conditions, including depression, anxiety, and post-traumatic stress disorder
	Manage complex mental health conditions

(continued)

Table 35.2 (continued)

Clinical practitioner	Roles and responsibilities
Neurologist	Guides completeness of evaluation for stroke/TIA etiologies and the need for additional testing or follow-up central nervous system imaging
	Treats pain, specifically post-stroke central pain syndromes
	Manages both early and late post-stroke epilepsy
	Performs neurotoxin injection(s) for spasticity [19]
	Coordinates with APP/Primary Care Physician and other specialists, especially when interventions (e.g., PFO closure and carotid revascularization) are proposed
Clinical pharmacist	Monitoring for effectiveness, tolerability, and effectiveness of pharmacotherapies, including following vital signs and laboratory values
	Up-titrating and tapering pharmacotherapies, especially antihypertensive, hyperlipidemia, and diabetes medication as needed
	Managing anticoagulation
	Assessing medication adherence with standardized assessments (e.g., Morisky Medication Adherence Scale-8) [20]
	Understanding whether physical limitations impair medication use (e.g., difficulty swallowing larger pills and impaired dexterity affecting self-administration of insulin)
	Patient counseling and education about diagnosed health conditions, pharmacotherapies, and stroke signs and symptoms
	Medication reconciliation, especially at key transition points
Dietician/nutritionist	Dietary counseling, with a focus on low-sodium and diets that incorporate elements of the Mediterranean and DASH diets [3, 4]
	Monitor weight and adequacy of protein intake, especially among more frail patients and those with dysphagia
	Work collaboratively to develop and promote weight loss strategies among obese patients
	Provides guidance specific to vascular risk factors, specifically hypertension, diabetes, hyperlipidemia, and obesity [21]

(continued)

Table 35.2 (continued)

Clinical practitioner	Roles and responsibilities
Rehabilitation medicine (physical medicine and rehabilitation physician, physical and occupational therapist)	The focus is on maximizing rehabilitation and recovery while understanding the impact of a cerebrovascular event on independent activities of daily living (ADLs) and ADLs
	Assess functional status (e.g., through functional independence measure), mobility, and balance
	Assess fall risk (e.g., through Morse Fall Scale) [2, 22]
	Discern the presence of hand and limb spasticity (e.g., through Ashworth/modified Ashworth Scale) [23, 24] and adhesive capsulitis [25]
	Considers interventions and pharmacotherapies for the management of motor deficits and extremity spasticity
	Evaluate for equipment needs
	Advise on exercise (with a focus on aerobic exercise, neuromuscular, and resistance training)
	Evaluates for agnosias, other visual–spatial impairments, constructional skill impairments, apraxia, and alcalculia [26]
	Leads home assessments
	Conducts cognitive assessments [e.g., Montreal Cognitive Assessment (MOCA)] [27]
	Performs neurotoxin injection(s) for spasticity [19]
Psychologist (including health psychology, neuropsychology, and rehabilitation psychology)	Conducts cognitive assessments (e.g., MOCA) and formal neuropsychiatric testing
	Screens for affective disorders [e.g., post-stroke depression with Patient Health Questionnaire-2 (PHQ-2)] [1]
	Addresses diet, exercise, smoking cessation, alcohol, and polysubstance use [11]
	Assesses for self-efficacy [28] and social isolation
	Deliver therapies designed to promote coping with a new diagnosis or diagnoses
	Teaches continuous positive airway pressure (CPAP) desensitization techniques [17]
	Evaluate for and, when necessary, augment medication compliance
	Deliver psychological intervention to promote smoking cessation [16, 18]
Speech language pathologist	Assesses for the presence, degree, and type of dysphagia
	Diagnoses and manages communication disorders, including cognitive–communication disorders, aphasia, and motor-speech disorders [8]
	Oversees swallowing rehabilitation and neuromuscular re-education of voice and swallowing muscles, especially among patients with dysphagia, dysarthria, and dyspraxia
Sleep medicine provider	Diagnose and manage obstructive sleep apnea (OSA), insomnia, and other sleep-disordered breathing [29, 30]

(continued)

Table 35.2 (continued)

Clinical practitioner	Roles and responsibilities
Cardiologist	Interpretation of Holter monitor and other extended arrhythmia, and implantation of loop recorders
	Perform and interpret transthoracic/transesophageal echocardiography
	Advise and, when appropriate, perform patent foramen ovale closure and carotid revascularization
	Long-term management of congestive heart disease and valvular heart disease
	Provide recommendations on long-term vascular risk reduction strategies, especially among those with comorbid cardiac disease [31]
Vascular surgeon	Advise and, when appropriate, perform carotid revascularization
Nephrologist	Interprets ambulatory blood pressure monitoring studies [32]
	Evaluate and manage refractory hypertension [33]
Social worker and case manager	Assessing for social isolation and determining the needs of the individual patient and their family/caregivers [34]
	Understanding caregiver tasks and discerning if caregiver burnout is present
	Determine if language, cultural, and health literacy barriers may exist in accessing healthcare
	Assist the patient and family in the adjustment process
	Aid in continuity and coordination of interdisciplinary care and liaise between patient/caregivers/family and APP/other healthcare providers [7]

Case Studies

Case #1: Management of Treatment-Resistant Hypertension Ischemic Stroke

History: A 72-year-old right-handed Black male with a past medical history significant for hypertension, hyperlipidemia, diabetes, and prior cigarette smoking (50-pack year history and stopped smoking 5 years prior) is seen in your clinic 6 weeks after being discharged with a right middle cerebral artery stroke. He was discharged to short-term rehabilitation and returned home 2 weeks ago. His wife accompanied him to his clinic appointment. The patient and his wife report taking his stroke preventive medications as prescribed, including HCTZ 25 mg once daily, lisinopril 40 mg daily, amlodipine 10 mg daily, atorvastatin 80 mg daily, and ASA 81 mg daily. A home blood pressure log review indicates readings ranging between 150–190 and 90–110 mmHg. His wife lays out his medications daily and confirms adherence.

Physical Examination: 170/100 mmHg and pulse of 80 beats/min. The cardiac exam showed a regular rate and no murmurs, rubs, or gallops. NIHSS of 5 (mild left lower facial droop, some effort against gravity in the left upper extremity with evidence of spasticity, decreased sensation over left upper extremity, and mild dysarthria).

Interventions: You have reviewed that he appropriately takes his medications and has not had difficulty swallowing his pills. They have brought in the automated blood pressure monitor that they use at home. You have confirmed that the cuff is an adequate fit and that blood pressure readings are not being taken in the spastic upper extremity, as this may affect accuracy [32]. A screen for OSA with the STOP-Bang (snoring, tiredness, observed apnea, blood pressure, Body Mass Index, age, neck size, and gender) [35] reveals a score of 5 (high risk for OSA) [35]. A referral for home sleep testing is made. You have the patient start taking his ACE inhibitor in the evening, recognizing that many stroke survivors have a 'non-dipping' blood pressure response and that two ways to correct this are to treat OSA when diagnosed and to have patients take an ACE inhibitor in the evening [32]. You also give them literature on the DASH diet to educate them on lowering sodium intake to further lower blood pressure.

Follow-Up: Four weeks later, his pressure improved to 158/90 mmHg, and his sleep study showed an apnea/hypopnea index of 32 events/h, consistent with severe OSA. He has a referral to sleep medicine for positive airway pressure treatment. They use less salt in their cooking and are eating less packaged food. You coordinate discussions with his primary care provider regarding starting another hypertensive agent, waiting to see how his blood pressure improves with treatment of his OSA or referral for other etiologies of uncontrolled hypertension.

Case #2: Post-stroke Depression and Impairing Participation in Rehabilitation
History: A 58-year-old primarily Spanish-speaking woman is seen in a follow-up for a left internal capsule ischemic stroke 4 months prior. During her hospitalization, she was diagnosed with hyperlipidemia and diabetes (with a hemoglobin A1c of 12.3%). At this time of her discharge, her NIHSS was 12 (partial paralysis of the right lower face and no movement of either the right upper or lower extremity and severe dysarthria). She was discharged to an extended care facility. With an interpreter, you learn that she was functionally independent and working full-time before her stroke. She was started on aspirin daily, atorvastatin 80 mg daily, and metformin 500 mg twice a day. The aide accompanying her today notes that the patient has shown reduced effort with physical and occupational therapy over the last 3 months.

Physical Examination: BP: 110/60, HR 82. Her NIHSS is now 7. She is fluent in Spanish with mild dysarthria. She has upper and lower extremity spasticity, with a modified Ashworth Scale of 3 [36] (i.e., a considerable increase in tone with difficult passive movement) in both affected extremities. She appears withdrawn and occasionally tearful, but no uncontrollable outbursts of crying or laughing (pseudobulbar affect) [37]. Her STOP–BANG score is 2 (low risk for OSA). Her Patient Health Questionnaire (PHQ)-2 score was 6 (with a score of 3 or more suggesting that a depressive disorder is likely), and PHQ-9 was 17 (moderately severe depression). She has suicidal ideations, not suicidal intent. Your suicide assessment is low acute risk and low chronic risk. You also complete a PTSD checklist, and her score is <33 (consistent with her being less likely to have PTSD) [38].

Interventions: You diagnose her with post-stroke depression, responsible for her being less engaged with rehabilitation, appearing withdrawn, and her PHQ-2 scores. Post-stroke PTSD or pseudobulbar affect are unlikely. The psychologist discusses the diagnosis of post-stroke depression and pharmacological and non-pharmacological therapies. She agrees to start escitalopram 10 mg daily and for a referral to health psychology for cognitive behavioral therapy [39, 40]. She is given information about the Suicide and Crisis Lifeline. While her STOP–BANG score is low, you recognize that OSA screening instruments have poorer sensitivity in the ischemic stroke population [41]. She agrees to a sleep study. She agrees to referrals to Rehabilitation Medicine for neurotoxin injection for post-stroke spasticity, combined with physical and occupational therapy [42].

Follow-Up: Four months later, she has completed 20 sessions of CBT and has been compliant with her escitalopram. She reports an improved mood and her aide reports she has been more engaged with PT and OT. She has had one round of botulinum injections in her right upper and lower extremity. Her dysarthria has improved, though she has had minimal improvement in her strength and spasticity. Her sleep study showed an apnea/hypopnea index of 22 events/h, consistent with moderate OSA. She was started on auto-PAP.

References

1. Towfighi A, Ovbiagele B, Husseini NE, Hackett ML, Jorge RE, Kissela BM, Mitchell PH, Skolarus LE, Whooley MA, Williams LS. Poststroke depression: a scientific statement for healthcare professionals from the American Heart Association/American Stroke Association. Stroke. 2017;48:e30–43. https://doi.org/10.1161/STR.0000000000000113.
2. Schmid AA, Kapoor JR, Miech EJ, Kuehn D, Dallas MI, Kerns RD, Lo AC, Concato J, Phipps MS, Couch CD, et al. A multidisciplinary stroke clinic for outpatient care of veterans with cerebrovascular disease. J Multidiscip Healthc. 2011;4:111–8. https://doi.org/10.2147/jmdh.S17154.
3. Kleindorfer DO, Towfighi A, Chaturvedi S, Cockroft KM, Gutierrez J, Lombardi-Hill D, Kamel H, Kernan WN, Kittner SJ, Leira EC, et al. 2021 Guideline for the prevention of stroke in patients with stroke and transient ischemic attack: a guideline from the American Heart Association/American Stroke Association. Stroke. 2021;52:e364–467. https://doi.org/10.1161/STR.0000000000000375.
4. Kernan WN, Viera AJ, Billinger SA, Bravata DM, Stark SL, Kasner SE, Kuritzky L, Towfighi A. Primary care of adult patients after stroke: a scientific statement from the American Heart Association/American Stroke Association. Stroke. 2021;52:e558–71. https://doi.org/10.1161/str.0000000000000382.
5. Hackam DG, Spence JD. Combining multiple approaches for the secondary prevention of vascular events after stroke. Stroke. 2007;38:1881–5. https://doi.org/10.1161/STROKEAHA.106.475525.
6. Heron N, Kee F, Mant J, Cupples ME, Donnelly M. Rehabilitation of patients after a transient ischaemic attack or minor stroke: pilot feasibility randomised trial of a home-based prevention programme. Br J Gen Pract. 2019;69:e706–14. https://doi.org/10.3399/bjgp19X705509.

7. U.S. Department of Veterans Affairs. VA/DOD clinical practice guideline for the management of stroke rehabilitation. J Rehabil Res Dev. 2010;47:1–43.
8. Dilworth C. The role of the speech-language pathologist in acute stroke. Ann Indian Acad Neurol. 2008;11:S108–s118.
9. Treister AK, Hatch MN, Cramer SC, Chang EY. Demystifying poststroke pain: from etiology to treatment. PM R. 2017;9:63–75. https://doi.org/10.1016/j.pmrj.2016.05.015.
10. Flaster M, Meresh E, Rao M, Biller J. Central poststroke pain: current diagnosis and treatment. Top Stroke Rehabil. 2013;20:116–23. https://doi.org/10.1310/tsr2002-116.
11. Wahass SH. The role of psychologists in health care delivery. J Family Community Med. 2005;12:63–70.
12. Kusnanto H, Agustian D, Hilmanto D. Biopsychosocial model of illnesses in primary care: a hermeneutic literature review. J Family Med Prim Care. 2018;7:497–500. https://doi.org/10.4103/jfmpc.jfmpc_145_17.
13. Rost NS, Brodtmann A, Pase MP, van Veluw SJ, Biffi A, Duering M, Hinman JD, Dichgans M. Post-stroke cognitive impairment and dementia. Circ Res. 2022;130:1252–71. https://doi.org/10.1161/CIRCRESAHA.122.319951.
14. Shi Y, Yang D, Zeng Y, Wu W. Risk factors for post-stroke depression: a meta-analysis. Front Aging Neurosci. 2017;9:218. https://doi.org/10.3389/fnagi.2017.00218.
15. Garton ALA, Sisti JA, Gupta VP, Christophe BR, Connolly ES. Poststroke post-traumatic stress disorder. Stroke. 2017;48:507–12. https://doi.org/10.1161/STROKEAHA.116.015234.
16. Akpanudo SM, Price JH, Jordan T, Khuder S, Price JA. Clinical psychologists and smoking cessation: treatment practices and perceptions. J Community Health. 2009;34:461–71. https://doi.org/10.1007/s10900-009-9178-0.
17. Chernyak Y. Improving CPAP adherence for obstructive sleep apnea: a practical application primer on CPAP desensitization. MedEdPORTAL. 2020;16:10963. https://doi.org/10.15766/mep_2374-8265.10963.
18. Lightfoot K, Panagiotaki G, Nobes G. Effectiveness of psychological interventions for smoking cessation in adults with mental health problems: a systematic review. Br J Health Psychol. 2020;25:615–38. https://doi.org/10.1111/bjhp.12431.
19. Ozcakir S, Sivrioglu K. Botulinum toxin in poststroke spasticity. Clin Med Res. 2007;5:132–8. https://doi.org/10.3121/cmr.2007.716.
20. Moon SJ, Lee W-Y, Hwang JS, Hong YP, Morisky DE. Accuracy of a screening tool for medication adherence: a systematic review and meta-analysis of the Morisky Medication Adherence Scale-8. PLoS One. 2017;12:e0187139. https://doi.org/10.1371/journal.pone.0187139.
21. Riegel GR, Ribeiro PAB, Rodrigues MP, Zuchinali P, Moreira LB. Efficacy of nutritional recommendations given by registered dietitians compared to other healthcare providers in reducing arterial blood pressure: systematic review and meta-analysis. Clin Nutr. 2018;37:522–31. https://doi.org/10.1016/j.clnu.2016.12.019.
22. Perell KL, Nelson A, Goldman RL, Luther SL, Prieto-Lewis N, Rubenstein LZ. Fall risk assessment measures: an analytic review. J Gerontol A. 2001;56:M761–6. https://doi.org/10.1093/gerona/56.12.M761.
23. Plantin J, Pennati GV, Roca P, Baron JC, Laurencikas E, Weber K, Godbolt AK, Borg J, Lindberg PG. Quantitative assessment of hand spasticity after stroke: imaging correlates and impact on motor recovery. Front Neurol. 2019;10:836. https://doi.org/10.3389/fneur.2019.00836.
24. Hugos CL, Cameron MH. Assessment and measurement of spasticity in MS: state of the evidence. Curr Neurol Neurosci Rep. 2019;19:79. https://doi.org/10.1007/s11910-019-0991-2.
25. Hsu JE, Anakwenze OA, Warrender WJ, Abboud JA. Current review of adhesive capsulitis. J Shoulder Elb Surg. 2011;20:502–14. https://doi.org/10.1016/j.jse.2010.08.023.
26. Rowland TJ, Cooke DM, Gustafsson LA. Role of occupational therapy after stroke. Ann Indian Acad Neurol. 2008;11:S99–s107.
27. Chiti G, Pantoni L. Use of Montreal cognitive assessment in patients with stroke. Stroke. 2014;45:3135–40. https://doi.org/10.1161/STROKEAHA.114.004590.
28. Torrisi M, De Cola MC, Buda A, Carioti L, Scaltrito MV, Bramanti P, Manuli A, De Luca R, Calabrò RS. Self-efficacy, poststroke depression, and rehabilitation outcomes: is there

a correlation? J Stroke Cerebrovasc Dis. 2018;27:3208–11. https://doi.org/10.1016/j.jstrokecerebrovasdis.2018.07.021.

29. Hepburn M, Bollu PC, French B, Sahota P. Sleep medicine: stroke and sleep. Mo Med. 2018;115:527–32.
30. Koo DL, Nam H, Thomas RJ, Yun CH. Sleep disturbances as a risk factor for stroke. J Stroke. 2018;20:12–32. https://doi.org/10.5853/jos.2017.02887.
31. Doehner W, Leistner DM, Audebert HJ, Scheitz JF. The role of cardiologists on the stroke unit. Eur Heart J Suppl. 2020;22:M3–M12. https://doi.org/10.1093/eurheartj/suaa160.
32. Sico JJ, Phipps MS, Klar Yaggi H, Burrus N, Ferguson J, McClain V, Austin C, Li X, Bravata DM. Ambulatory blood pressure monitoring among patients with cerebrovascular disease. Blood Press Monit. 2011;16:211–7. https://doi.org/10.1097/MBP.0b013e32834b4d6c.
33. Howard VJ, Tanner RM, Anderson A, Irvin MR, Calhoun DA, Lackland DT, Oparil S, Muntner P. Apparent treatment-resistant hypertension among individuals with history of stroke or transient ischemic attack. Am J Med. 2015;128:707–714.e702. https://doi.org/10.1016/j.amjmed.2015.02.008.
34. Ue B. Social work and the stroke patient. Clin Orthop Relat Res. 1978;(131):101–3.
35. Pivetta B, Chen L, Nagappa M, Saripella A, Waseem R, Englesakis M, Chung F. Use and performance of the STOP-Bang Questionnaire for obstructive sleep apnea screening across geographic regions: a systematic review and meta-analysis. JAMA Netw Open. 2021;4:e211009. https://doi.org/10.1001/jamanetworkopen.2021.1009.
36. Harb A, Kishner S. Modified Ashworth Scale. In: StatPearls. Treasure Island, FL: StatPearls Publishing LLC; 2023.
37. Goldin DS. Pseudobulbar affect: an overview. J Psychosoc Nurs Ment Health Serv. 2020;58:19–24. https://doi.org/10.3928/02793695-20200624-08.
38. Ashbaugh AR, Houle-Johnson S, Herbert C, El-Hage W, Brunet A. Psychometric validation of the English and French versions of the post-traumatic stress disorder checklist for DSM-5 (PCL-5). PLoS One. 2016;11:e0161645. https://doi.org/10.1371/journal.pone.0161645.
39. Starkstein SE, Hayhow BD. Treatment of post-stroke depression. Curr Treat Options Neurol. 2019;21:31. https://doi.org/10.1007/s11940-019-0570-5.
40. Wang S-B, Wang Y-Y, Zhang Q-E, Wu S-L, Ng CH, Ungvari GS, Chen L, Wang C-X, Jia F-J, Xiang Y-T. Cognitive behavioral therapy for post-stroke depression: a meta-analysis. J Affect Disord. 2018;235:589–96. https://doi.org/10.1016/j.jad.2018.04.011.
41. Sico JJ, Yaggi HK, Ofner S, Concato J, Austin C, Ferguson J, Qin L, Tobias L, Taylor S, Vaz Fragoso CA, et al. Development, validation, and assessment of an ischemic stroke or transient ischemic attack-specific prediction tool for obstructive sleep apnea. J Stroke Cerebrovasc Dis. 2017;26:1745–54. https://doi.org/10.1016/j.jstrokecerebrovasdis.2017.03.042.
42. Francisco GE, McGuire JR. Poststroke spasticity management. Stroke. 2012;43:3132–6. https://doi.org/10.1161/STROKEAHA.111.639831.

Primary Prevention of Stroke: Identifying High-Risk Patients

Jessica Kaslow and Walter N. Kernan

Introduction

Stroke is the most important preventable threat to brain health, which the American Heart Association defines as "an optimal capacity to function adaptively in the environment." Even the loss of a small amount of brain tissue to ischemic or hemorrhagic injury, depending on anatomic location, can affect a person's adaptive function by changing how they think, communicate, move, or feel [1].

Over 600,000 US residents have a first stroke each year, among whom 60,000 will die acutely and 300,000 will survive with permanent physical or cognitive impairment, including vascular dementia. The 600,000 clinical events are in addition to a far greater number of so-called subclinical or "silent" events (e.g., clinically unrecognized infarctions and white matter injury) that contribute to cognitive impairment, dementia, and impaired mobility. As a cause of death, stroke ranks fifth in the US and second worldwide.

Primary prevention of stroke is highly effective. By one estimate, the risk of stroke in persons over 65 years of age fell 40% in the US between 1988 and 2008 [2]. This remarkable trend has been attributed to progress in reducing cigarette smoking and improving treatment for hypertension, hyperlipidemia, and atrial fibrillation.

This progress is impressive, but there is more that can be done. Even with modern care, over 50% of stroke events could be prevented by reaching more patients who are not currently at goal for hypertension, tobacco exposure, dyslipidemia, diet quality, atrial fibrillation, excessive alcohol use, and other stroke risk factors [3, 4]. This chapter highlights the risk factors for cerebrovascular disease and provides strategies to help patients control them. Preventive measures for stroke should also be part of an intentional effort to prevent other conditions caused by

J. Kaslow · W. N. Kernan (✉)

Yale School of Medicine, New Haven, CT, USA

e-mail: Jessica.kaslow@yale.edu; walter.kernan@yale.edu

shared risk factors such as inactivity, overweight, hypertension, dyslipidemia, coronary artery disease, peripheral vascular disease, chronic kidney disease, and diabetes. Delivering preventive care to more eligible persons, improving its quality, and investing in research for new approaches to maintaining health can lead to further progress.

Individual Risk Factors for Stroke

Stroke risk factors can be modifiable or nonmodifiable. The most common modifiable risk factors for both stroke and coronary artery disease are listed in Table 36.1 according to population prevalence, and nonmodifiable risk factors are listed in Table 36.2. Most risk factors have a dose-dependent association, such that the risk of stroke or heart disease increases as the severity of the risk factor increases (e.g., less physical activity, higher body mass index, and higher usual blood pressure).

Table 36.1 Selected modifiable risk factors for stroke and acute myocardial infarction in US adults according to population prevalence [5–12]

Risk factor	Adult prevalence (%)	Approximate strength of association with risk	
		Stroke	AMI
Physical inactivity	75	+	+
Poor quality diet	46	++	+
Obesity	43	++	++
Hypertension	32	++	+
Inadequate sleep[a]	30	+	+
Serum lipids	29	+	++
Cigarette smoking	15	++	++
Diabetes	12	+++	+++
Atrial fibrillation	1	+++	Not applicable

AMI acute myocardial infarction

List does not include the social determinants of health that are discussed separately in the text. List includes well-documented risk factors with prevalence >10% or very high relative risk (i.e., ≥2.0). For some (inactivity, poor diet quality, obesity, hypertension, lipids), risk of stroke or MI increases directly with the magnitude of the factor

[a] Association of short or long sleep duration with risk for ischemic stroke is uncertain. Hemorrhagic stroke may be associated with short sleep duration. Obstructive sleep apnea is associated with stroke and heart disease risk

Table 36.2 Selected nonmodifiable risk factors for stroke

- Age
- Sex (men > women)
- Family history of young stroke (<60 years of age)

Physical Inactivity Epidemiologic research shows a near-linear relationship between more physical activity and lower risk for stroke, heart disease, and all-cause mortality [13–16]. Benefits for the prevention of cardiovascular mortality begin with as few as 2700 steps/day and increase up to about 9000 steps/day. In general, for an equivalent amount of time, more intensive activity (e.g., jogging vs. walking at a normal pace) confers greater benefit [17]. Physical inactivity can be recognized by the absence of recreational exercise in a person with a sedentary occupation.

Poor Quality Diet Healthier diets are associated with reduced risk for cardiovascular disease, including stroke [18]. Healthy diets include a total energy intake that achieves or maintains a healthy weight, plenty of fruits and vegetables, whole grains, healthy sources of protein (primarily plants and fish, lean cuts of meat), healthy oils, and nuts/legumes [19]. Healthy diets are low in animal fats, salt, and concentrated sweets. The Mediterranean, DASH, and plant-based diet patterns are healthy diets. Reducing sodium intake (a key feature of the DASH diet) is particularly important for reducing blood pressure; compared with usual sodium intake, a daily intake of 500 mg sodium is associated with a 6 mmHg drop in systolic blood pressure [20].

Obesity As weight increases above normal (i.e., BMI 18.5–24.9 in non-Asian persons and 18.5–22.9 in Asian persons), the risk increases for cardiovascular disease, diabetes, and several other chronic conditions [21–24]. However, BMI itself is an imperfect measure of risk because it fails to account precisely for variations in fat distribution and total body fat that explain most of the adverse effects of adiposity [25]. The ratio of waist-to-hip helps with this problem and may be considered a risk modifier to accompany BMI.

Hypertension Throughout middle and older age, there is a linear association between usual blood pressure and increased risk for cardiovascular disease, including stroke [26–29]. Risk appears to increase starting with systolic blood pressure of 115 mmHg and diastolic blood pressure of 75 mmHg [26]. There are no available clear estimates of the age-specific absolute increment in risk for stroke for a defined time interval and defined baseline or sustained SBP. However, during approximately 4 years of therapy, a 5 mmHg reduction in SBP is associated with a 13% reduction in risk for stroke [30].

Inadequate Sleep Very little sleep, too much sleep, and specific sleep disorders (e.g., obstructive sleep apnea) may increase the risk for stroke and heart disease [31–33]. The optimal sleep duration is 7–9 h for most adults. Sleep was recently added to the AHA's "Life Essential 8" elements of cardiovascular preventive health [34].

Dyslipidemia Cholesterol and triglycerides are transported in lipoproteins, including LDL, VLDL, and HDL. Of these, LDL is the most atherogenic [35]. Observational research demonstrates that higher total cholesterol and LDL are associated with increased risk for coronary heart disease. Although the association with risk for ischemic stroke is weaker [34–36] than other risk factors, clinical trials of cholesterol-lowering therapy show similar reductions in rates of coronary heart disease and ischemic stroke [33]. However, LDL-C is the main lipoprotein target for primary prevention of atherosclerotic cardiovascular disease (ASCVD), including stroke. Other lipoproteins, including Lp(a) and apoB (both related to LDL-C), are considered risk-enhancing factors and may be appropriate to measure in selected patients [35]. Of note, total cholesterol, and LDL-C are each inversely related to risk for hemorrhagic stroke; in other words, aggressive over-reduction in LDL to very low levels (generally <30–40 mg/dL) has been shown to increase the risk of hemorrhage. However, this effect on public health is much smaller than the association [35–37] between higher serum cholesterol levels and death from ischemic stroke and overall cardiovascular disease [34].

Cigarette Smoking Current cigarette smoking is a significant risk factor for all forms of ASCVD, including coronary heart disease, ischemic stroke, and peripheral arterial disease. It is also probably a risk factor for hemorrhagic stroke, particularly in the young, but this topic is controversial [38, 39]. Smoking cessation results in a reduction in risk toward that of nonsmokers [40, 41].

Diabetes Diabetes increases the risk for stroke through several mechanisms (e.g., hypertension, dyslipidemia, inflammation, and hyperglycemia) that lead to atherosclerosis [42, 43].

Atrial Fibrillation Atrial fibrillation can cause clots to form in the left atrial appendage that subsequently embolize to the brain. On average, atrial fibrillation is associated with a four- to fivefold increase in the risk of stroke. However, not every person with atrial fibrillation is at equal risk. The CHAD2DS2VASc score can stratify patients into low, moderate, or high risk to help guide decisions on medical management [44]. It is recommended that anticoagulation be considered for patients with a score of ≥ 1 for men or ≥ 2 for women. The benefit of routine screening for AF is unclear [45]. Most professional groups recommend monitoring for symptoms such as palpitations, syncope, shortness of breath, and chest pain during routine patient encounters to warrant monitoring.

Asymptomatic Carotid Stenosis Usually detected incidentally or after an auscultated bruit on exam, asymptomatic carotid stenosis refers to narrowing (usually from plaque) without a history of attributable TIA or stroke. Randomized clinical trials have demonstrated a reduced risk for ipsilateral ischemic stroke and perioperative morbidity with carotid endarterectomy, compared with medical management, in patients with 60–99% stenosis. In these trials, the annual risk for stroke in medically treated patients was about 3%. More recent observational studies show a lower risk for stroke in medically treated patients to less than 1% [46]. Asymptomatic carotid stenosis may still increase the risk for stroke, but with modern medical therapy (e.g., antiplatelet, statin, and BP reduction), it is not clear that surgery provides additional benefit. Chapter 20 has a more detailed discussion of this complex topic.

Among the nonmodifiable risk factors, age is the most important factor. Between ages 20–44 and 75–84, the average risk increases more than 20-fold [47]. Data suggest that race is also associated with stroke risk. Like age, race is commonly described as a nonmodifiable risk factor. However, this classification does not recognize the modifiable social and economic factors that confound the associations between race and stroke risk. These include suboptimal access to medical care, poverty, adverse living environments (e.g., food deserts or lack of outdoor recreation space), and difficulty accessing higher education. Ethnicity is also associated with stroke risk, and the same modifiable social and economic factors likely explain this association.

Three additional factors classified as nonmodifiable are low birth weight, menopause, hypertensive disorders of pregnancy, and family history. Of these, a family history of ASCVD has the clearest diagnostic and therapeutic implications as it is considered a risk-enhancing factor in selecting persons for treatment of stage 1 hypertension and for cholesterol-lowering therapy.

Multivariable Instruments for Risk Estimation

The Pooled Cohort Equation is a helpful tool that estimates the combined 10-year risk for nonfatal myocardial infarction, coronary heart disease death, or fatal or nonfatal stroke [48]. This approach recognizes the shared risk factors for stroke and coronary artery disease. The Pooled Cohort Equation has recently been replaced by the updated PREVENT tool [49].

The Framingham Stroke Risk Score (created in 1991 and revised in 2018 for improved performance) combines several stroke risk factors (age, SBP, hypertension therapy, cardiovascular disease, diabetes, active cigarette smoking, and atrial fibrillation) to estimate 10-year risk [50]. Adding coronary artery calcification modestly improves the discriminant ability of the revised Framingham Score [51].

Risk Reduction

It is helpful to recognize that stroke prevention is already in the workflow for adult preventive care. The standard medical history, family history, review of systems, physical exam, and laboratory testing (i.e., lipid profile, basic metabolic profile, and A1c) include all the information needed to estimate and manage stroke risk. Putting the brain front and center (where it should be), however, may require added time to call a patient's attention to the brain and the added benefit for the brain in achieving overall cardiovascular risk reduction. This section summarizes the key steps in achieving optimal preventive brain care in adult primary care. These tasks can be done, of course, over multiple visits. Key points are summarized in the text box.

Approach Prevention with Patient-Centered Care Skills

Most adults in primary care will have cardiovascular risk factors; some will not be aware, and others may not be ready to take medications or change their behaviors. They may have misperceptions or other barriers to self-care. We recommend taking a long view of risk management and using skills in patient-centered care to help each patient achieve personal goals in a supportive, consistent environment. Patient-centered care includes respect for patients' values, preferences, and expressed needs; coordination of care among providers, specialists, and ancillary services; clear communication, including information about long-term implications of risk factors; physical comfort; and emotional support [52].

Many patients are not familiar with stroke in the same way they know heart health or cancer prevention. When education is needed, we often turn to online material from the US CDC, the American Heart Association, or the JAMA Patient Page [53], but there are other sources, including YouTube videos such as the British Heart Association's "What is a stroke?." These materials can be displayed during a clinic visit. Despite advances in acute stroke treatment, many patients do not present to medical care in a timely way to be eligible. Educating patients on identifying stroke symptoms and the need for prompt medical attention can mean the difference between preserving independence versus living with a significant disability. Most electronic medical record systems also include printable educational material.

Discover Risk Factors and Estimate ASCVD Risk

Most risk factors for stroke will be discovered during the routine health maintenance exam. This is not to underestimate the effort to ask about and chart these risk factors. Diet, sleep, and physical activity require conversation to understand a patient's current practices. The American Heart Association has developed *Life's Essential 8* to help clinicians in this conversation. In line with Table 36.1, Life's Essential 8 are diet, physical activity, nicotine exposure, sleep health, body mass index, blood lipids, blood glucose, and blood pressure [34].

When reviewing family history, ask about coronary heart disease and stroke, specifically. A history of a first-degree relative with heart disease or stroke at a young age should prompt further discussion for details of the diagnosis and risk factors in the family member. A first degree relative with premature atherosclerotic heart or brain disease may identify a patient who is themselves at high risk and for whom early initiation of risk reducing therapy (e.g., cholesterol or blood pressure lowering therapy) may be warranted [54].

For many adults (e.g., stage 1 hypertension, moderately elevated LDL without ASCVD), calculating their 10-year risk for ASCVD using the AHA pooled cohort equation (or the more recent PREVENT tool) will be necessary to guide the management of blood pressure and lipids.

Manage Specific Risk Factors

Table 36.3 lists the basic management for the major stroke risk factors (which include all major risk factors for coronary heart disease). Here, we provide additional details.

Table 36.3 Treatment goals for selected modifiable risk factors for stroke in adults

Risk factor	When to start treatment	Goal[a]
Physical inactivity	All patients	150 min/week moderate intensity or 75 min/week vigorous intensity exercise[b]
Poor quality diet	All patients	Adherence to healthy diet
Overweight/ obesity	BMI ≥25 kg/m²[a]	BMI 18.5 –24.9 kg/m²[a]
Hypertension	• ≥130/≥80 with clinical CVD or 10-year ASCVD risk ≥10% • ≥140/≥90 most others	<130/80 (<130 systolic blood pressure age ≥ 65, diastolic blood pressure not considered)
Inadequate sleep	All patients	7 to <9 h/night
Dyslipidemia	• Severe primary hypercholesterolemia (LDL-C ≥190 mg/dL) • LDL-C ≥70 mg/dL, age 40–75 and diabetes • LDL-C ≥70 mg/dL without diabetes based on risk for ASCVD	• In persons with known ASCVD, lower LDL-C ≥50%; in general, lower LDL-C is better • In persons at high risk for ASCVD, reduce LDL-C to <70 mg/dL
Cigarette smoking	Current smokers	Abstinence
Diabetes	At diagnosis	A1c <7.0%, optimal medical Rx
Atrial fibrillation	Based on risk	On anticoagulation if indicated

BMI body mass index, *CVD* cardiovascular disease, *ASCVD* atherosclerotic cardiovascular disease, *LDL-C* low density lipoprotein-cholesterol, *A1c* hemoglobin A1C

Goals in this table are based on professional guidelines [34, 35, 38, 55, 56], which readers are encouraged to consult for further detail; those for diabetes [56], hypertension [55], and dyslipidemia [35] are particularly important

[a] Normal BMI for Asian persons by WHO criteria is 18.5–22.9 kg/m², overweight 23–27.5 g/m², and ≥27.5 kg/m² obese. Weight assessment and management should be modified by consideration of waist-hip circumference, which modifies risk for obesity-related conditions [57]

[b] Moderate exercise includes walking briskly, slow bicycling, gardening, and golf. Vigorous includes race-walking, jogging, running, swimming laps, more than slow bicycling [58]

Physical Activity Prescription For patients who say they do not exercise, review the benefits of meeting professional guidelines for 150 min/week of moderate exercise (e.g., walking, slow bicycling, slow stationary cycling, and gardening) or 75 min a week of vigorous exercise (e.g., fast walking, jogging, faster stationary cycling, and swimming) [59]. If sedentary, encourage patients to start with a low level of an activity they enjoy. Walking 7–10,000 steps a day is often an excellent way to start.

Nutrition Counseling For patients with a poor-quality diet, explore reasons, including knowledge, customs, financial barriers, or access. When knowledge or customs are at play and patients have internet access, recommend the USDA website and the MyPlate campaign (www.myplate.gov). Recommend eating fruits, vegetables, whole grains, low-fat dairy, healthy oils such as olive, avocado, sesame or safflower, fish, or lean meat, and avoiding sugary and fatty foods. Refer to a nutritionist if available.

Weight Management Professional guidelines for weight management recommend early use of medication therapy, particularly GLP-1 receptor agonist therapy if intensive counseling is unavailable or fails [60]. GLP-1 receptor agonists are indicated for most patients with DMII and obesity. Metabolic surgery is an option for patients with T2D and BMI ≥ 40 kg/m^2 (≥ 37.5 in Asian American persons) or BMI 35–39.9 kg/m^2 (32.5–37.4 kg/m^2 in Asian American persons) who do not achieve adequate weight loss and improvement in comorbidities with nonsurgical methods [61]. Because weight management is more successful with newer therapies and because there are more options, consider referral early to a provider with certification or an endocrinologist with experience.

Blood Pressure Management For diagnosis and management of hypertension, we recommend consulting the current guidelines from the AHA [55]. All patients should be advised to monitor their blood pressure at home and use the results to take specific action.

Sleep Testing and Counseling Patients with suspected OSA (i.e., excessive daytime sleepiness and at least two of the following three criteria: habitual snoring, witnessed apnea or gasping or choking, or hypertension) should undergo polysomnography [62]. All others should be asked about sleep duration, reminded of AHA duration guidelines (7–9 h/night), and offered help with sleep as needed.

Lipid Management The US Centers for Disease Control and Prevention recommends that most adults be screened for high cholesterol every 4–6 years. To manage results, we recommend consulting the current AHA guidelines, which recommend statin therapy for primary prevention in selected adults depending on

LDL-C level, comorbidity, and calculated 10-year ASCVD risk [35]. Target LDL-C reduction for patients on treatment for primary prevention depends on estimated risk for ASCVD. For "high risk" patients ($\geq$20% 10 years risk), the goal recommended by the AHA is to reduce LDL-C by $\geq$50% [35].

Smoking Cessation Most people who smoke wants to quit. The most effective approach to helping them includes combined counseling (which can be brief) and pharmacotherapy, often with a combination of agents with different mechanisms of action (e.g., nicotine plus varenicline) [63]. Close follow-up by clinicians to support quit efforts is essential. Many current smokers will be eligible for lung cancer screening.

Diabetes Care For diagnosis and management of diabetes, we recommend consulting the recommendations published annually in January by the American Diabetes Association [56]. A1c should be checked at least every 6 months for most patients.

Avoid Therapeutic Inertia

A common reason that patients do not achieve therapeutic goals for chronic conditions, including hypertension and diabetes, is the failure of healthcare providers to titrate treatment when opportunities arise. This is termed therapeutic inertia. To avoid inertia, try these actions: (1) call the patient's attention to each risk factor that is not controlled as soon as it is identified, (2) unless there is evidence of ongoing progress toward the therapeutic goal, titrate treatment, change treatment, or create a plan for one or the other, and (3) if the patient is not at goal for a risk factor, schedule early follow-up.

Clinical Pearls
- Stroke prevention is already part of the typical workflow for adult preventive health in primary care.
- Good stroke prevention is a crucial part of preventing all cardiovascular diseases due to shared risk factors.
- Be explicit with patients that brain health is a goal for preventive care.
- Be intentional in identifying stroke risk and using patient-centered skills to help patients address any risk factors that are not controlled.
- Check patient knowledge about stroke and fill in gaps.
- Identify and remediate barriers to self-care for risk reduction.
- Plan to modify risk factors according to guidelines.
- Schedule timely follow-ups to monitor progress.
- To avoid therapeutic inertia, name the risk factor and make a plan to get it under control, mindful of the patient's preferences, values, goals, and individual barriers.

References

1. Gorelick PB, Furie K, Iadecola C, Smith EE, Waddy SP, Lloyd-Jones DM, Bae H-J, Bauman MA, Dichgans M, Duncan PW, et al. Defining optimal brain health in adults. A presidential advisory from the American Heart Association/American Stroke Association. Stroke. 2017;48:e284–303.
2. Fang MC, Perraillon MC, Ghosh K, Cutler DM, Rosen AB. Trends in stroke rates, risk, and outcomes in the United States, 1988–2008. Am J Med. 2014;127:608–15.
3. Hankey GJ. Population impact of potentially modifiable risk factors for stroke. Stroke. 2020;51:719–28.
4. Yusuf S, Hawken S, Ounpuu S, Dans T, Avezum A, Lanai F, McQueen M, Budaj A, Pais P, Varigos J, et al. Effect of potentially modifiable risk factors associated with myocardial infarction in 52 countries (the INTEREART study): case-control study. Lancet. 2004;364:937–52.
5. Zhang Y, Moran AE. Trends in the prevalence, awarensss, treatment, and control of hypertension among young adults in the United States 1999–2014. Hypertension. 2017;70:736–42.
6. Flegal KM, Kruszon-Moran D, Carroll MD, Fryar CD, Ogden CL. Trends in obesity among adults in the United States. JAMA. 2016;315:2284–91.
7. Jamal A, King BA, Neff LL, Whitmill J, Babb SD, Graffunder CM. Current cigarette smoking among adults—Unites States 2005–2015. MMWR Morb Mortal Wkly Rep. 2016;65:1205–11.
8. Whitfield GP, Carlson SA, Ussery EN, Fulton JE, Galuska DA, Petersen R. Trends in meeting physical activity guidelines among urban and rural dwelling adults—United States 2008–2015. MMWR Morb Mortal Wkly Rep. 2019;68:513–8. https://doi.org/10.1136/bmj.m4573.
9. Rehm CD, Penalvo JL, Afshin A, Mozaffarian D. Dietary intake among US adults, 1999–2012. JAMA. 2016;315:2542–53.
10. Goff DC, Bertoni AG, Kramer HC, Bonds D, Blumenthal RS, Tsai MT, Psaty BM. Dylipidemia prevalence, treatment, and control in the multi-ethnic study of atherosclerosis (MESA). Circulation. 2006;113:647–56.
11. Mercado C, DeSimone AK, Odome E, Gillespie C, Ayala C, Loustalot F. Prevalence of cholesterol treatment eligibility and medication use among adults—United States, 2005–2012. MMWR Morb Mortal Wkly Rep. 2015;64:1305–11.
12. Go AS, Hylek EM, Phillips KA, Chang Y, Henault LE, Selby JV, Singer DE. Prevalence of diagnosed atrial fibrillation in adults: national implications for rhythm management and stroke prevention: the AnTicoagulation and Risk Factors in Atrial Fibrillation (ATRIA) Study. JAMA. 2001;285:2370–5. https://doi.org/10.1001/jama.285.18.2370.
13. Wendel-Vos GCW, Schuit AJ, Feskens EJM, Boschuizen WMM, Saris WHM, Kromhout D. Physical activity and stroke. A meta-analysis of observational data. Int J Epidemiol. 2004;33:787–98.
14. Lee CD, Folsom AR, Blair SN. Physical activity and stroke risk. A meta-analysis. Stroke. 2003;34:2475–82.
15. Shigdel R, Dalen H, Sui X, Lavie CJ, Wisloff U, Ernsten L. Cardiorespiratory fitness and the risk of first acute myocardial infarction: the HUNT Study. J Am Heart Assoc. 2019;8:e010293. https://doi.org/10.1161/JAHA.118.010293.
16. Sattelmair J, Pertman J, Ding EL, Kohl HW, Haskell WL, Lee I-M. Dose response between physical activity and risk of coronary heart disease: a meta-analysis. Circulation (New York, NY). 2011;124:789–95. https://doi.org/10.1161/CIRCULATIONAHA.110.010710.
17. Stens NA, Bakker EA, Manas A, Buffart LM, Ortega FB, Lee D, Thompson PD, Thijssen DHJ, Eijsvogels TMH. Relationship of daily step counts to all-cause mortality and cardiovascular events. J Am Coll Cardiol. 2023;82:1483–94.
18. Fung TT, Pan A, Hou T, Mozaffarian D, Rexrode KM, Willett WC, Hu FB. Food quality score and the risk of coronary artery disease: a prospective analysis in 3 cohorts. Am J Clin Nutr. 2016;104:65–72.
19. Lichtenstein AH, Appel LJ, Vadiveloo M, Hu FB, Kris-Etherton PM, Rebholz CM, Sacks FM, Thornkide AN, Van Horn L, Wylie-Rosett J, et al. Dietary guidance to improve

cardiovascular health: a scientific statement from the American Heart Association. Circulation. 2021;144:e472. https://doi.org/10.1161/CIR.0000000000001031.

20. Gupta DK, Lewis CE, Varady KA, Su YR, Madjur MS, Lackland DT, Reis JP, Wang TJ, Lloyd-Jones DM, Allen NB. Effect of dietary sodium on blood pressure. A crossover trial. JAMA. 2023;330:2258–66.

21. Kroll ME, Green J, Beral V, Sudlow CLM, Brown A, Kirichek O, Price A, Yang TO, Reeves GK, for the Million Women Study Collaboration. Adiposity and ischemic and hemorrhagic stroke. Prospective study in women and meta-analysis. Neurology. 2016;87:1473–81.

22. Kurth T, Gaziano JM, Berger K, Kase CS, Rexrode KM, Cook NR, Buring JE, Manson JE. Body mass index and the risk of stroke in men. Arch Intern Med. 2002;162:2557–62.

23. Kurth T, Gaziano JM, Rexrode KM, Kase CS, Cook NR, Manson JE, Buring JE. Prospective study of body mass index and risk of stroke in apparently healthy women. Circulation. 2005;111:1992–8.

24. Khan SS, Ning H, Wilkins JT, Allen N, Marnethon M, Berry JD, Sweis RN, Lloyd-Jones DM. Association of body mass index with lifetime risk of cardiovascular disease and compression of morbidity. JAMA Cardiol. 2018;3:280–7.

25. Liu B, Du Y, Snetselaar LG, Wallace RB, Bao W. Trends in obesity and adiposity measures by race or ethnicity among adults in the United States 2011–18: populations based study. BMJ. 2021;372:n365.

26. Prospective Studies Collaboration. Age-specific relevance of usual blood pressure to vascular mortality; a meta-analysis of individual data for one million adults in 61 prospective studies. Lancet. 2002;360:1903–13.

27. Rapsomaniki E, Timmis A, George J, Pujadas-Rodriguez M, Shah AD, Denazas S, White IR, Caulfield MJ, Deanfield JE, Smeeth L, et al. Blood pressure and incidence of twelve cardiovascular diseases: lifetime risk, healthy life-years lost, and age-specific associations in 1.25 million people. Lancet. 2014;383:1899–911.

28. Willey JZ, Moon YP, Khahn E, Rodriguez CJ, Rundek T, Cheung K, Sacco RL, Elkind MS. Population attributable risks of hypertension and diabetes for cardiovascular disease and stroke in the Northern Manhattan Study. J Am Heart Assoc. 2014;3:e001106.

29. Clark D, Colantonio LD, Min Y-I, Hall ME, Zhao H, Mentz RJ, Shimbo D, Ogedegbe G, Howard G, Levitan EB, et al. Population attributable risk for cardiovascular disease associated with hypertension in black adults. JAMA Cardiol. 2019;4:1194–202.

30. The Blood Pressure Lowering Treatment Trialists' Collaboration. Pharmacological blood pressure lowering for primary and secondary prevention of cardiovascular disease across different levels of blood pressure: an individual participant-level data meta-analysis. Lancet. 2021;397:1625–36.

31. Yaggi HK, Concato J, Kernan WN, Lichtman JH, Brass LM, Mohsenin V. Obstructive sleep apnea as a risk factor for stroke and death. N Engl J Med. 2005;353:2034–41.

32. Yang X, Chen H, Li S, Pan L, Jia C. Association of sleep duration with the morbidity and mortality of coronary artery disease: a meta-analysis of prospective studies. Heart Lung Circ. 2015;24:1180–90. https://doi.org/10.1016/j.hlc.2015.08.005.

33. Titova OE, Michaelsson K, Larsson SC. Sleep duration and stroke: prospective cohort study and Mendelian randomization analysis. Stroke. 2020;51:3279–85. https://doi.org/10.1161/STROKEAHA.120.029902.

34. Lloyd-Jones DM, Allen NB, Anderson CAM, Black T, Brewer LC, Foraker RE, Grandner MA, Lavretsky H, Perak MA, Sharma G, et al. Life's essential 8: updating and enhancing the American Heart Association's Construct of Cardiovascular Health: a presidential advisory from the American Heart Association. Circulation. 2022;146:e18–43.

35. Grundy SM, Stone NJ, Bailey AL, Beam C, Birtcher KK, Blumenthal RS, Braun LT, de Ferranti S, Faiella-Tommasino J, Forman DE, et al. 2018 AHA/ACC/AACVPR/AAPA/ABC/ACPM/ADA/AGS/AphA/ASPC/NLA/PCNA guideline on the management of blood cholesterol. A report of the American College of Cardiology/American Heart Association Task Force on Clinical Practice Guidelines. J Am Acad Coll Cardiol. 2019;73(24):e285–350.

36. Sun L, Clarke R, Bennett D, Guo Y, Walters RG, Hill M, Parish S, Millwood IY, Bian Z, Chen Y, et al. Causal associations of blood lipids with risk of ischemic stroke and intracerebral hemorrhage in Chinese adults. Nat Med. 2019;25:569–74.
37. Iso H, Jacobs DR, Wentworth D, Neaton JD, Cohen J, Group ftMR. Serum cholesterol levels and six-year mortality from stroke in 350,977 men screened for the multiple risk factor intervention trial. N Engl J Med. 1989;320:904–10.
38. Meschia JF, Bushnell C, Boden-Albala B, Braun LT, Bravata DM, Chaturvedi S, Creager MA, Eckel RH, Elkind MSV, Fornage M, et al. Guidelines for the primary prevention of stroke. A statement for healthcare professionals from the American Heart Association/American Stroke Association. Stroke. 2014;45:3754–832.
39. Feldmann E, Broderick JP, Kernan WN, Viscoli CM, Brass LM, Brott T, Morgenstern LB, Wilterdink JL, Horwitz RI. Major risk factors for intracerebral hemorrhage in the young are modifiable. Stroke. 2005;36:1881–5.
40. Critchley JA, Capewell S. Mortality risk reduction associated with smoking cessation in patients with coronary heart disease. JAMA. 2003;290:86–97.
41. Wannamethee SG, Shaper AG, Whincup PH, Walker M. Smoking cessation and the risk of stroke in middle-aged men. JAMA J Am Med Assoc. 1995;274:155–60.
42. Kernan WN, Forman R, Inzucchi SE. Caring for patients with diabetes in stroke neurology. Stroke. 2022;54:894. https://doi.org/10.1161/STROKEAHA.122.038163.
43. The Emerging Risk Factors Collaboration. Diabetes mellitus, fasting blood glucose concentration, and risk of vascular disease: a collaborative meta-analysis of 102 prospective studies. Lancet. 2010;375:2215–22.
44. Beaser AD, Cifu AS. Management of patients with atrial fibrillation. JAMA. 2019;321:1100–1.
45. US Preventive Services Task Force. Screening for atrial fibrillation. US Preventive Services Task Force Recommendation Statement. JAMA. 2022;327:360–7.
46. Chang RW, Tucker L-Y, Rothenberg KA, Lancaster E, Faruqu RM, Kuang HC, Flint AC, Avins AL, Nguyen-Huynh MN. Incidence of ischemic stroke in patients with asymptomatic severe carotid stenosis without surgical intervention. JAMA. 2022;327:1974–82.
47. Madsen TE, Khoury JC, Leppert M, Alwell K, Moomaw CJ, Sucharew H, Woo D, Ferioli S, Martini S, Adeoye O, et al. Temporal trends in stroke incidence over time by sex and age in the GCNKSS. Stroke. 2020;51:1070–6.
48. Goff DC, Lloyd-Jones DM, Bennet G, Coady S, D'Agostino RB, Gibbons R, Greenland P, Lackland DT, Levy D, O'Donnell CJ, et al. 2013 ACC/AHA guideline on the assessment of cardiovascular risk. A report of the American College of Cardiology/American Heart Association Task Force on Practice Guidelines. J Am Coll Cardiol. 2014;63:2935–59.
49. SS Khan, et al. Circulation. 2024;149:430–49.
50. Dufouil C, Beiser A, McLure LA, Wolf PA, Tzourio C, Howard VJ, Westwood AJ, Himali JJ, Sullivan L, Aparicio HJ, et al. Revised Framingham Stroke Risk Profile to reflect temporal trends. Circulation. 2017;135:1145–59.
51. Flueckiger P, Longstreth W, Herrington D, Yeboah J. Revised Framingham Stroke Risk Score, nontraditional risk markers, and incident stroke in a multiethnic cohort. Stroke. 2018;49:363–9.
52. Delbanco T, Gerteis M. A patient-centered view of the clinician-patient relationship. Waltham, MA: UpToDate; 2022.
53. Hwang MY. Prevent a first stroke. JAMA. 1999;281:1146.
54. Arnett DK, Blumental RS, Albert MA, Buroker AB, Goldberger ZD, Al E. 2019 ACC/AHA guideline on the primary prevention of cardiovascular disease. Circulation. 2019;4:1043.
55. Whelton PK, Al E. 2017 ACC/AHA/AAPA/ABC/ACPM/AGS/AphA/ASH/ASPC/NMA/PCNA guideline for the prevention, detection, evaluation, and management of high blood pressure in adults. J Am Acad Coll Cardiol. 2017.
56. ElSayed NA, Aleppo G, Aroda VR, Bannuru RR, Brown FM, Bruemmer D, Collins BS, Hilliard ME, Isaacs D, Johnson EL, et al. Pharmacologic approaches to glycemic treatment: Standards of Care in Diabetes—2023. Diabetes Care. 2023;46(Suppl 1):S140–57.

57. Garvey WT, Mechanick JI, Brett EM, Garber AJ, Hurley DL, Jastreboff AM, Nadolsky K, Pessah-Pollack R, Plodkowski R, Reviewers of the AACE/ACE Obesity Clinical Practice Guidelines. American Association of Clinical Endocrinologists and American College of Endocrinology comprehensive clinical practice guidelines for medical care of patients with obesity. Endocr Pract. 2016;22:842–84.

58. Piepoli MF, Hoes AW, Agewall S, Albus C, Brotons C, Catapano AL, Cooney MT, Corrà U, Cosyns B, Deaton C, Graham I, Hall MS, Hobbs FDR, Løchen ML, Löllgen H, Marques-Vidal P, Perk J, Prescott E, Redon J, Richter DJ, Sattar N, Smulders Y, Tiberi M, van der Worp HB, van Dis I, Verschuren WMM, Binno S, ESC Scientific Document Group. 2016 European guideline on cardiovascular disease prevention in clinical practice. Eur Heart J. 2016;37:2315–81.

59. Piercy KL, Troiano RP, Ballard RM, Carlson SA, Fulton JE, Galuska DA, George SM, Olson RD. The physical activity guidelines for Americans. JAMA. 2018;320:2020–8.

60. Grunvald E, Shah R, Hernaez R, Chandar AK, Pickett-Blakely O, Teigen LM, Harindhanavudhi T, Sultan S, Singh S, Davitkov P, et al. AGA clinical practice guideline on pharmacological interventions for adults with obesity. Gastroenterology. 2022;163:1198–225. https://doi.org/10.1053/j.gastro.2022.08.045.

61. American Diabetes Association. Obesity and weight management for the prevention and treatment of type 2 diabetes: Standards of Care in Diabetes—2023. Diabetes Care. 2023;46(Suppl 1):s128–39.

62. Kapur VK, Auckley DH, Chowdhuri S, Kuhlmann DC, Mehra R, Ramar K, Harrod CG. Clinical practice guideline for diagnostic testing for adult obstructive sleep apnea: an American Academy of Sleep Medicine Clinical Practice Guideline. J Clin Sleep Med. 2017;13:479–504.

63. Rigotti NA, Kruse GR, Livingstone-Banks J, Hartmann-Boyce J. Treatment of tobacco smoking: a review. JAMA. 2022;327:566–77. https://doi.org/10.1001/jama.2022.0395.

After the Stroke (Secondary Prevention) 37

Sharon Bottomley, Jennifer Picagli, and Jason Sico

After an ischemic stroke or transient ischemic attack (TIA), delivering high-quality, evidence-based secondary prevention is of paramount importance. This includes addressing known vascular risk factors through pharmacological and nonpharmacological approaches, additional workup for unknown risk factors, and treating newly identified risk factors targeting "goals" or targets put forward by the American Heart Association/American Stroke Association (AHA/ASA) and other professional organizations [1]. Understanding the plan for blood thinners is also essential. Patients with atrial fibrillation will need lifelong anticoagulation, whereas patients with stroke due to atherosclerosis may get placed on a short course of dual antiplatelet therapy followed by monotherapy [1–3]. Multiple interventions may be needed to achieve health targets. For example, a patient may be on multiple blood pressure (BP) agents and later be found to have a poor diet and severe obstructive sleep apnea (OSA). Treatment of OSA and diet counseling with a nutritionist may help patients finally reach their target BP [4, 5]. This chapter will highlight the important recommendations for secondary prevention, refer readers to other sections of this book for more in-depth discussions on evaluating and managing other risk factors, and provide an outpatient "checklist" that can be used in the clinic.

A stroke clinic follow-up includes briefly reviewing the hospital course, reviewing pertinent workup results, discussing stroke mechanism and secondary prevention plan, rehab and recovery status, and answering patient questions and concerns.

S. Bottomley
Veterans Affairs Medical Center, West Haven, CT, USA
e-mail: sharon.bottomley@va.gov

J. Picagli
Yale New Haven Hospital, New Haven, CT, USA
e-mail: jennifer.picagli@yale.edu

J. Sico (✉)
Yale School of Medicine, New Haven, CT, USA
e-mail: Jason.Sico@va.gov

© The Author(s), under exclusive license to Springer Nature Switzerland AG 2024
H. P. Amin (ed.), *Stroke for the Advanced Practice Clinician*,
https://doi.org/10.1007/978-3-031-66289-8_37

This task becomes even more challenging when considering that stroke patients may have impaired language processing and memory difficulty, and benefit from using simple terminology and repetition of key pieces of information. Patients may need multiple visits to cover everything. A written after-visit summary helps improve understanding and recall of the information discussed during the visit.

Hypertension, Hyperlipidemia, Diabetes and the Role of Pharmacotherapies, Regular Exercise and Diet

Hypertension

Blood pressure (BP) reduction can have a significant impact on stroke recurrence. Permissive hypertension in the acute poststroke inpatient setting must be followed by gradual BP reduction with close follow-up to ensure the patient eventually reaches the target. Normal BP is now <120/80 mmHg [1]. As with primary prevention, lifestyle modification and nonpharmacologic therapy, including a healthy diet, weight management, and physical activity, should be considered part of a secondary prevention plan.

Current guidance is to start antihypertension pharmacotherapy for high-risk individuals, such as those age 65 or older, with known cardiovascular disease, diabetes, or chronic kidney disease, when the BP is ≥130/80 mmHg. As hypertension is such a common risk factor, appropriately aggressive treatment is warranted. Telehealth visits and home self-monitoring of BP can encourage patients to actively participate in care, be more closely monitored, and promote titration without risking side effects like hypotension, dizziness, and fatigue. Home BP telemonitoring and pharmacist case management successfully lowered BP by at least 10 mmHg and were found to be a cost-saving treatment method [6]. Antihypertensive treatment reduced the risk of recurrent stroke and disabling or fatal stroke in a linear pattern [7].

Gradual reduction over weeks is important to avoid overcorrection. One study using real-world data noted a higher risk of death in the 12 months after discharge from an ischemic stroke or TIA when a systolic BP of ≤105 mmHg was obtained 90 days after hospitalization. An optimal range of systolic BP of 115–124 mmHg has been suggested [8].

Hyperlipidemia

For lipid-lowering treatment in very high-risk individuals (patients with a history of stroke and multiple high-risk conditions), treatment with a high-intensity statin, either atorvastatin 80 mg daily or rosuvastatin 20 mg daily, is recommended. If LDL-C remains >70 mg/dL, or nonhigh-density lipoprotein is >100 mg/dL, ezetimibe or PSCK9 inhibitors (evolocumab or alirocumab) can be added (Fig. 37.1). Guidelines recommend ezetimibe, a generic drug with proven efficacy and safety [1]. Given the cost of PSCK9 inhibitors, their use may be more determined by

Fig. 37.1 Proposed algorithm for lipid management based on AHA guidelines [2]. *Fasting lipids should be checked 4–12 weeks after statin initiation, and if needed, dose adjustments every 3–12 months thereafter

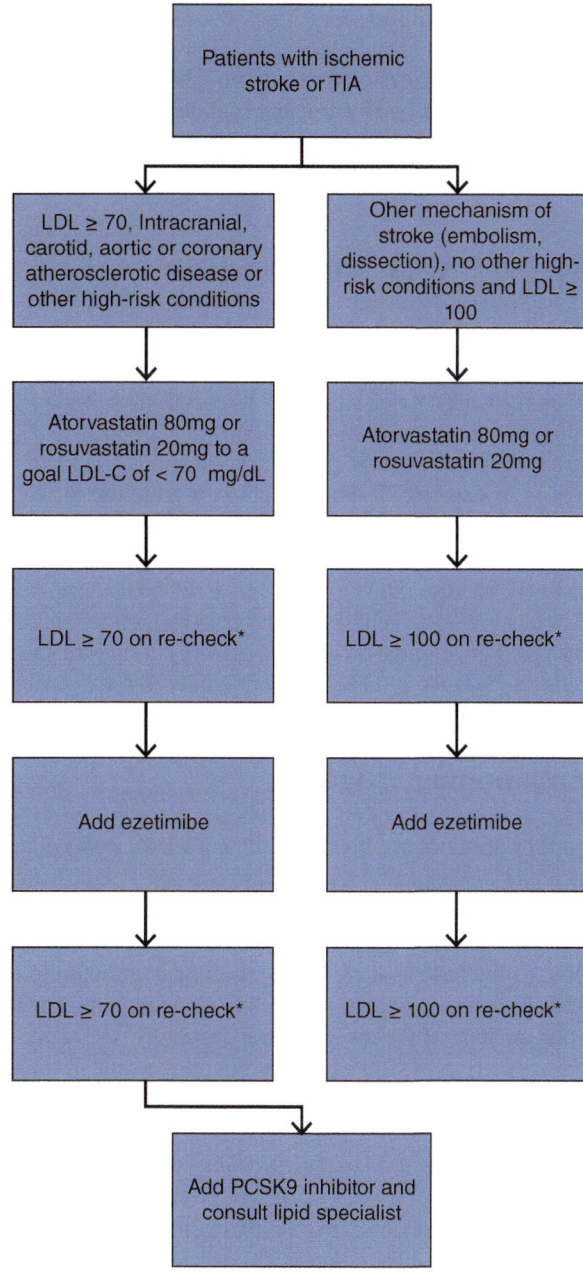

economics and payers to document justification for therapy [9]. Fasting is not routinely needed for lipid testing, as fasting and nonfasting numbers are relatively similar, except in those with nonfasting triglycerides >440 mg/dL, in which fasting levels should be assessed [10].

Diabetes

Lifestyle and disease-modifying nonpharmacologic treatment should continue. As per AHA/ASA [1], all the patients should be screened for diabetes poststroke, with the goal hemoglobin A1c of ≥7%. Goals, however, can be liberalized in older adults, those with comorbidities or limited life expectancy.

Regular Physical Activity and Diet

Regular physical activity reduces cerebrovascular risk and aids recovery when patients with residual neurological deficits are discharged. Able patients should engage in at least moderate-intensity aerobic activity for a minimum of 10 min four times per week or vigorous activity for a minimum of 20 min twice a week. Referring to a supervised exercise program is helpful for patients with deficits that impair their ability to exercise. It is reasonable for patients to follow a diet low in sodium and rich in fruits, vegetables, whole grains, fish, low-fat dairy, and legumes and nuts. The DASH (Dietary Approaches to Stop Hypertension) diet is a helpful framework to lower sodium intake for patients with hypertension. Likewise, the Mediterranean diet has lowered the risk of cerebrovascular and cardiovascular events. There is an overlap between the two diets regarding food, but the DASH diet also focuses on reducing sodium to about 1500 mg daily to lower BP.

Antithrombotic Agents

Antithrombotics are pivotal in the long-term management of patients with cerebro-vascular disease and include anticoagulants (which inhibit the coagulation cascade and fibrin formation) and antiplatelets (which inhibit activation and aggregation of platelets through various mechanisms) [2, 11]. Antiplatelets commonly used in practice include aspirin, clopidogrel, the combination of dipyridamole and aspirin, and, to a lesser extent, ticagrelor. Anticoagulation routinely includes Vitamin K antagonists and Direct Oral Anticoagulants (DOACs). The general guiding principles related to the use of antithrombotic agents after an ischemic stroke or TIA are given as follows:

1. Some antithrombotic agent is universally recommended for patients after cerebrovascular disease, barring the presence of contraindications.
2. Dual antiplatelet (DAPT) regimens (aspirin, Plavix, ticagrelor) are recommended for short courses (weeks to months) for specific scenarios, including high-risk TIA and mild ischemic stroke [2, 3], ischemic stroke secondary to severe intracranial atherosclerosis, and recent coronary or carotid artery stent. *In the clinic, identify the duration of DAPT recommended on hospital discharge and ensure the patient is aware.*

3. Long-term dual antiplatelet therapy is not recommended as it increases bleeding risk.
4. Antiplatelets are recommended for managing embolic stroke of uncertain source unless an indication for anticoagulation is discovered.
5. Anticoagulation is preferred over antiplatelet for cerebrovascular events related to atrial fibrillation.

Atrial Fibrillation

Monitoring for Suspected Atrial Fibrillation

Longer-term monitoring is recommended for patients with a suspected embolic stroke of unknown etiology. Current AHA/ASA guidelines recommend at least a 30-day monitoring period. However, with implantable devices, the detection of AF increased with a longer duration of monitoring, up to 3 years, leading to more patients being treated with anticoagulation [12]. The duration or frequency of atrial fibrillation events does not change the need for anticoagulation in patients who have had a stroke [13].

Treatment of Diagnosed Atrial Fibrillation

Anticoagulation is recommended for patients diagnosed with atrial fibrillation, as oral anticoagulation reduces the risk of stroke by 60–80%. DOACs (apixaban, dabigatran, edoxaban, or rivaroxaban) are preferred over warfarin, as DOACS are equivalent or superior to warfarin for stroke prevention and have lower rates of intracerebral hemorrhage [14]. DOACs, in addition, do not interact with food and do not require the routine monitoring that warfarin does.

In clinic, make sure to tell patients on DOACs that after only a few missed doses, these medications are out of the system, and the patient is unprotected from another stroke. The message is to reinforce adherence.

Vitamin K antagonists are recommended for patients with mechanical valves and valvular atrial fibrillation due to a moderately to severely stenosed mitral valve [15].

Contraindications and Alternatives/Special Circumstances Related to Anticoagulation of Atrial Fibrillation

Absolute contraindications to anticoagulation include spontaneous intracranial hemorrhage (not traumatic or secondary to a lesion that was treated), an intracranial neoplasm, recurrent life-threatening gastrointestinal or other bleeding events, and severe bleeding disorders, including severe thrombocytopenia [16].

Aspirin plus clopidogrel may be used for patients who refuse anticoagulation; however, the combination is inferior to anticoagulation, and the benefit of aspirin monotherapy may be offset by increased bleeding risk [17].

A thrombus in the LAA (left atrial appendage) can occur in the setting of atrial fibrillation and is best visualized by transesophageal echocardiography (TEE). In a literature review, the recommended treatment is a 4-week course of warfarin. However, resolution rates on repeat TEE are 63–89%. Results with DOACs were variable and have shown lower rates of resolution. Individuals with AF at high risk of bleeding with anticoagulation can be referred for consideration for left atrial appendage closure, which then removes the need for anticoagulation. However, patients require a short course of anticoagulation following the procedure [18].

Restarting Anticoagulation After Traumatic Intracranial Hemorrhage

When to restart anticoagulation after a traumatic intracranial hemorrhage should be decided in consultation with neurosurgery due to variable patient factors and data. A single institutional study at a level 1 trauma center revealed that patients with atrial fibrillation and traumatic intracranial hemorrhage (ICH) were restarted on anticoagulation 30 days after the ICH [19]. While off anticoagulation, patients are at higher risk of thrombosis and cardiac embolism. Other studies have confirmed safety with earlier reinitiation, including restarts at 7–13 days [20–23].

These results are in contrast to studies involving warfarin-associated intracranial hemorrhage (without trauma) when the optimal timing for resumption of warfarin therapy appeared to be between 7 and 8 weeks after intracranial hemorrhage [24]. If there are microbleeds on MRI, however, CAA may be a contributing factor, in which case that patient may be at high risk of recurrent hemorrhage. In most cases, a head CT should be performed to confirm that the hematoma has resolved before resuming anticoagulation [25].

Carotid Artery Disease

Assessing extracranial and intracranial vasculature is standard of care in the acute evaluation of a new cerebrovascular event [2]. Patients with older age, male sex, and such vascular risk factors as a history of hypertension, diabetes, hyperlipidemia, chronic kidney disease, cigarette smoking, and lower levels of physical activity are at greater risk for developing extracranial carotid artery stenosis [26, 27]. Extracranial carotid artery imaging can be accomplished via CTA, MRA, or carotid ultrasound. Medical management, with particular attention to atherosclerotic vascular risk factors, is a mainstay for patients found to have either asymptomatic or symptomatic carotid artery disease. Decisions related to carotid artery intervention are typically addressed during hospitalization for stroke and incorporate whether carotid artery stenosis is ipsilateral to the stroke, the severity of stenosis, and the degree of post-cerebrovascular disability. Patients who undergo endarterectomy are typically managed on single-agent monotherapy, whereas patients who receive stents will be on a short course of dual antiplatelet therapy. All the patients who undergo carotid intervention will get serial follow-up imaging that the surgery team should direct. Monitoring asymptomatic carotid stenosis may be done more frequently (every 3–6 months) initially, then spaced further out after demonstrating stability.

Smoking Cessation

For smokers, tobacco use should be assessed at each healthcare visit, and individuals who use tobacco should be strongly advised to quit. Counseling in combination with drug therapy is recommended. Nicotine replacement therapy, bupropion hydrochloride sustained release, and varenicline all improve tobacco cessation rates. If nicotine replacement is used, the combination of short- and long-acting forms of replacement is recommended. The simplified "AAR" model, which encourages clinicians to ask patients about tobacco use, advises them to quit and refers them to telephone quitlines or other evidence-based cessation interventions, may be more feasible in a busy clinic (Fig. 37.2). This brief counseling is effective, and a combination of behavioral approaches and medication management increases the chances of success. Telephone support and individual or group therapy may also be used [12].

Counselling Regarding Alcohol and Drug Abuse Disorders

Alcohol consumption should be limited to ≤2 drinks per day for men and ≤1 drink per day for nonpregnant women in individuals who choose to drink alcohol. Abstinence from alcohol or reduction in consumption for heavy drinkers is recommended through appropriate counseling and referral to treatment programs. Referral to an appropriate treatment program for patients who abuse drugs that have been associated with stroke, such as cocaine and amphetamines, is recommended [13].

Obstructive Sleep Apnea

Obstructive sleep apnea (OSA) is underdiagnosed and undertreated. It is an independent risk factor for recurrent cerebrovascular events [28–30]. Treatment of OSA may also improve how well other vascular risk factors may be controlled. OSA has been independently associated with hypertension, with greater OSA severity being correlated with the presence of hypertension [4, 5, 28]. OSA is also associated with glucose metabolism, and a higher apnea-hypopnea index (AHI) is associated with poorer glycemic control among those with diabetes mellitus [28].

All stroke patients should be screened for OSA, but current guidelines do not highlight which patients should receive sleep study testing. While several tools developed and validated in the general population predict the presence of OSA on formal sleep testing (e.g., snoring, tiredness, observed apnea, high BP, body mass index, age, neck circumference, and gender [STOP-BANG]), these instruments perform poor when used to screen patients with cerebrovascular disease for OSA [29]. All the patients who are overweight, have large neck circumference, snore, or report

Tobacco Cessation in the Stroke Patient

Providers should be familiar with the basics of nicotine replacement tlierapy (NRT), options for pharmacologic assistance, and at least one local or otherwise accessible resource to the patient. Clinicians seeing many stroke or vascular patients may benefit from taking part in formal tobacco cessation training programs.

The Council for Tobacco Treatment Training Programs maintains a list of accredited programs in the United States and a few abroad at https://ctttp.org/accredited-programs/. The CDC also maintains a list of resources for providers at https://www.cdc.gov/tobacco/patient-care/education-training/index.html. Many programs offer Continuing education, including those directed toward public health, pulmonology, cardiovascular providers, pharmacists, dentists, respiratory therapists, and social workers. Some states require substance abuse or addiction continuing education and may have additional resources developed locally.

States offer tobacco cessation programs, but counseling should supplement local resources.

Principles of Tobacco Cessation Counseling

Basic models for substance cessation counseling include

'AAR'	"The Five As":
•Ask about tobacco use	• Ask about tobacco use
• Advise quitting	• Advise quitting
• Refer to resources	• Assess readiness to quit
	• Assist smokers who are ready to quit
	• Arrange follow-up

Engaging with the patient about their tobacco use and contextualizing it can help gauge their readiness, perceived barriers, and other potential health concerns. It may be helpful to not only discuss the effect of tobacco use on the patient's stroke but to bring in a holistic health model. For example, a patient who has only been taught (perhaps exhaustively, in their estimation) about the influence of smoking on lung health may respond more actively to a discussion about stroke, claudication, impaired wound healing, or oral health.

Motivational interviewing is a common technique taught in substance cessation programs, in which the patient is assisted in finding her or his reasons for making a positive change in their health. While these may not overtly align with tlie medical rationale for tlie same - for example, many patients report financial reasons to stop smoking (online smoking cost calculators can be eye-opening)–they align with the patient's values and lead to the same desired outcome: a tobacco-free lifestyle.

Document cessation discussions and communicate efforts with other providers. Social work and psychological counseling can help stroke patients cope and address substance use.

Fig. 37.2 Smoking cessation counseling

daytime drowsiness or headaches should consider a sleep study. Polysomnography is a zero-risk evaluation with a high potential benefit. Many centers offer home testing, which removes a barrier for patients who do not want to sleep at a clinic.

Continuous positive airway pressure (CPAP) is the gold standard for OSA treatment; however, non-PAP alternatives are available and are increasingly being used in clinical practice. In addition to improving AHI, treating OSA can improve the control of other comorbid vascular risk factors, promote neurological recovery, and reduce the risk of future vascular events [5]. Patients may be more motivated to use the therapy as prescribed if they are educated that regular CPAP use can result in improvement in neurological recovery, especially when started soon after a cerebrovascular event [5]. Like other treatments, adherence should be monitored, given that at least 4 h per night of use is recommended to improve outcomes [30].

Assessing Fall Risk

Falls are common after an ischemic stroke, ranging from 7% to 73% in the days to the first year after a cerebrovascular event [31]. Risk factors for falls include severity and type of poststroke neurological disability, psychomotor slowness, cognitive impairment, alterations in mental status, depression, anxiety, insomnia, impaired postural control with standing and walking, urinary tract infections, and male gender [31, 32]. Falls can be a significant source of morbidity and mortality, with complications including impaired quality of life and mental health, hematomas (including intracranial), and closed and open bone fractures.

Fall Risk and Anticoagulation

A history of falls or a high risk of falling is associated with intracranial hemorrhage. However, the risk does not appear to differ between patients treated with warfarin, aspirin, or no anticoagulant therapy. Patients with a CHADS2 score or higher benefited from anticoagulation, whether or not they were deemed a fall risk [33]. Elderly patients, in particular, derive the greatest benefit from anticoagulation [34]. In addition, it has been estimated that an individual would have to fall 295 times in 1 year for the risk of a fall-related major bleed to outweigh the benefit of warfarin in reducing the risk of stroke [35].

In patients with frequent falls, even injurious falls, the benefits of anticoagulation usually outweigh the bleeding risks. Management should include interventions designed to mitigate fall risk, including but not limited to safety assessments, referral to physical therapy, and visual testing. However, discussing the care plan with the patient and relevant caregivers and respecting patient autonomy is necessary. Patients at the end of life, for whom anticoagulation may be burdensome and of less perceived benefit, may also be considered for discontinuation of therapy [16].

Fall Risk and Blood Pressure Management

BP management postcerebrovascular events can be complicated, given that these patients may have dysautonomia following cerebrovascular events and yet require BP medications to treat hypertension [36]. Approximately one-third of stroke patients will have orthostatic hypotension, with most also having concomitant hypertension [37]. Orthostasis may be more common when the a patient is more hypertensive [38]. Orthostasis is also a risk factor for falls [39], especially among more frail individuals [40].

In clinic, inquiring about symptoms consistent with orthostasis (e.g., lightheadedness, generalized weakness) and measuring BP and pulse in multiple positions (e.g., lying down to sitting, sitting to standing). Spacing out antihypertensive may be helpful when patients report symptoms of orthostasis a few hours after taking multiple medications simultaneously.

Structured Approach to First Poststroke/TIA Visit

A checklist of items to review at the first poststroke visit can assist with the organization of care (Fig. 37.3). A list of discharge medications and appropriate rehabilitation and home care services referrals should be confirmed. Arrangements for

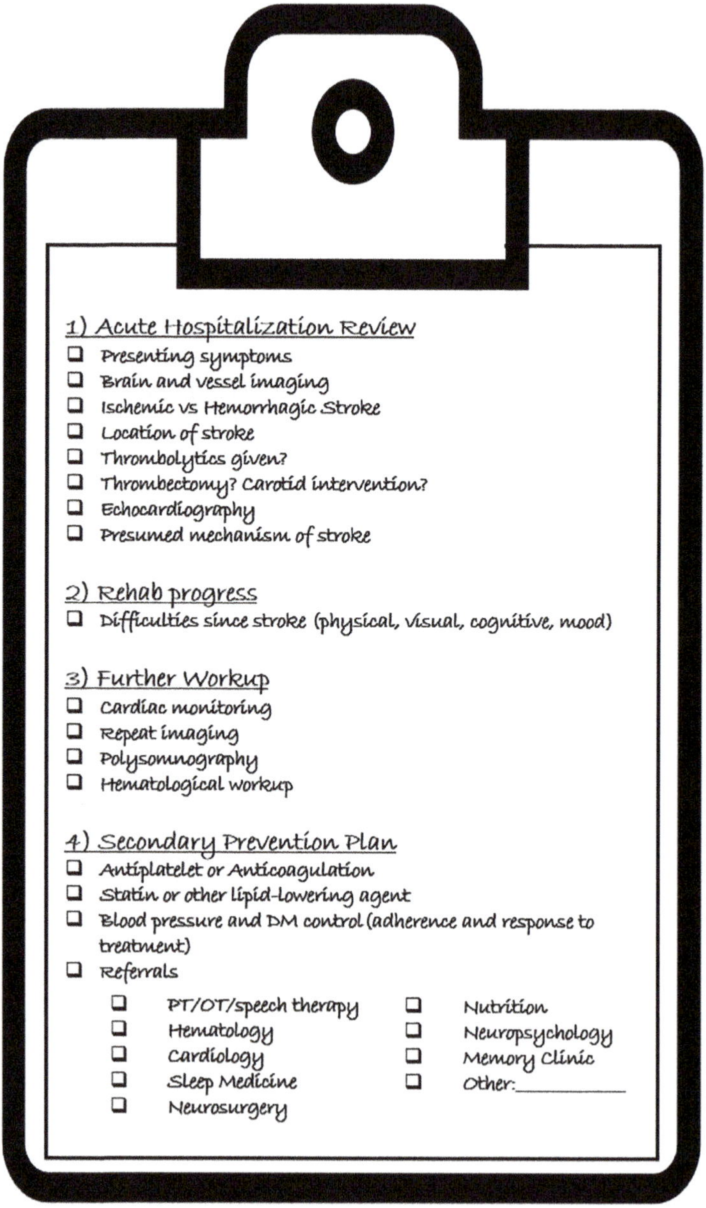

Fig. 37.3 Poststroke follow-up checklist

extended cardiac monitoring and polysomnography may need to be initiated at the outpatient visit.

Follow-Up

The frequency of follow-up visits is determined by patient needs and ongoing workup. Telehealth became a popular method of seeing patients during the COVID-19 pandemic, and some institutions continue to offer this option for follow-up appointments. Choosing which patients are appropriate for this method is challenging. Keep in mind that neurological examinations are drastically limited during virtual visits, and discussions may not be as comprehensive as in face-to-face meetings. Face-to-face visits should still be considered the gold standard, especially for high-risk patients where a detailed exam may pick up new deficits and should still be the first option. Telehealth may be reasonable, however, for patients with great difficulty with transportation due to disability or resources or for patients who would otherwise have to travel great distances, and a conversation via telehealth would suffice. If used appropriately, telehealth allows the provider to maintain regular contact with patients who may otherwise be lost to follow-up.

> **Clinical Pearls**
> - A comprehensive stroke follow-up includes reviewing the hospitalization, results, stroke mechanism, secondary prevention, rehab status, and answering questions and concerns. This may require multiple visits to cover.
> - Using simple terms and repeating essential pieces of information is very helpful to stroke patients in understanding why their stroke occurred and the plan to prevent future strokes.
> - Telehealth may be appropriate for certain patients, but face-to-face visits should be the first option.

References

1. Del Brutto VJ, et al. Antithrombotic therapy to prevent recurrent strokes in ischemic cerebrovascular disease: JACC Scientific Expert Panel. J Am Coll Cardiol. 2019;74(6):786–803.
2. Kleindorfer DO, et al. 2021 Guidelines for the prevention of stroke in patients with stroke and transient ischemic attack: a guideline for the American Heart Association/American Stroke Association. Stroke. 2021;52(7):e364–467.
3. Brown DL, et al. Benefits and risks of dual versus single antiplatelet therapy for secondary stroke prevention: a systematic review for the 2021 guideline for the prevention of stroke in patients with stroke and transient ischemic attack. Stroke. 2021;52(7):e468–79.
4. Ou YH, Tan A, Lee CH. Management of hypertension in obstructive sleep apnea. Am J Prev Cardiol. 2023;13:100475.
5. Bravata DM, et al. Diagnosing and treating sleep apnea in patients with acute cerebrovascular disease. J Am Heart Assoc. 2018;7(16):e008841.

6. Padwal RS, et al. Cost effectiveness of home blood pressure monitoring and case management in the secondary prevention of cerebrovascular disease in Canada. J Clin Hypertens. 2019;22(2):159–68.
7. Katsanos AH, et al. Blood pressure reduction and secondary stroke prevention: a systematic review and meta-regression analysis of randomized clinical trials. Hypertension. 2017;69:171–9.
8. Sico JJ, et al. Real-world analysis of two ischaemic stroke and TIA systolic blood pressure goals on 12-month mortality and recurrent vascular events. Stroke Vasc Neurol. 2024; https://doi.org/10.1136/svn-2023-002759.
9. Lepor NE, Kereiakes DJ. The PSCK9 inhibitors: a novel therapeutic target enters clinical practice. Am Health Drug Benefits. 2015;8(9):483–9.
10. Nordestgaard BG. A test in context: lipid profile, fasting versus non-fasting. J Am Coll Cardiol. 2017;70(13):1637–46.
11. Tsoumani ME, Tselepis AD. Antiplatelet agents and anticoagulants: from pharmacology to clinical practice. Curr Pharm Des. 2017;23(9):1279–93.
12. Sanna T, et al. Cryptogrenic stroke and underlying atrial fibrillation. N Engl J Med. 2014;370(26):2478–86.
13. Bridge F, Thijs V. How and when to screen for atrial fibrillation after stroke: insights from insertable cardiac monitoring devices. Stroke. 2016;18(2):121–8.
14. Ruff CT, et al. Comparison and of the efficacy and safety of new oral anticoagulants with warfarin in patients with atrial fibrillation: a meta-analysis of randomized trials. Lancet. 2014;383(9921):955–62.
15. Wigle P, et al. Anticoagulation: updated guidelines for outpatient management. Am Fam Physician. 2019;100(7):426–34.
16. Hagerty T, Rich MW. Fall risk and atrial fibrillation in the elderly: a delicate balance. Cleve Clin J Med. 2017;84(1):35–40.
17. Connolly SJ, et al. Dabigatran versus warfarin in patients with atrial fibrillation. N Engl J Med. 2009;361(12):1139–51.
18. Patel M, et al. Diagnosis and treatment of intracardiac thrombus. J Cardiovasc Pharmacol. 2021;78(3):361–73.
19. Naylor RM, et al. Timing of restarting anticoagulation and antiplatelet therapies after traumatic subdural hematoma—a single institution experience. World Neurosurg. 2021;150:e203–8.
20. Chipman AM, et al. Therapeutic anticoagulation inpatients with traumatic brain injuries and pulmonary emboli. J Trauma Acute Care Surg. 2020;89:592–5355.
21. Byrnes MC, et al. Therapeutic anticoagulation can be safely accomplished in selected patients with traumatic intracranial hemorrhage. World J Emerg Surg. 2012;7:25.
22. Puckett Y, et al. Safest time to resume oral anticoagulation in patients with traumatic brain injury. Cureus. 2018;10(7):e2920.
23. Matsushima K, et al. Anticoagulation therapy in patients with traumatic brain injury: an Eastern Association for the Surgery of Trauma Multicenter Prospective Study. Surgery. 2021;169(2):470–6.
24. Penlert J, Overholser R, Asplund K, et al. Optimal timing of anticoagulant treatment after intracerebral hemorrhage in patients with atrial fibrillation. Stroke. 2017;48(2):314–20.
25. Jung IH, Yun JH, Kim SJ, Chung J, Lee SK. Anticoagulation and antiplatelet agent resumption timing following traumatic brain injury. Korean J Neurotrauma. 2023;19(3):298–306.
26. Ismail A, et al. Carotid artery stenosis: a look into the diagnostic and management strategies, and related complications. Cureus. 2023;15(5):e38794.
27. Paraskevas KI, et al. Cholesterol, carotid artery disease and stroke: what the vascular specialist needs to know. Ann Transl Med. 2020;8(19):1265.
28. Kapa S, Kuniyoshi FHS, Somers VK. Sleep apnea and hypertension: interactions and implications for management. Hypertension. 2008;51(3):605–8.
29. Sico JJ, et al. Development, validation, and assessment of an ischemic stroke or transient ischemic attack-specific prediction tool for obstructive sleep apnea. J Stroke Cerebrovasc Dis. 2017;26(8):1745–54.

30. Dissanayake HU, et al. Obstructive sleep apnea therapy for cardiovascular risk reduction— time for a rethink? Clin Cardiol. 2021;44(12):1729–38.
31. Denissen S, et al. Interventions for preventing falls in people after stroke. Cochrane Database Syst Rev. 2019;10(10):CD008728.
32. Persson CU, Hansson P-O. Determinants of falls after stroke based on data on 5065 patients from the Swedish Väststroke and Riksstroke Registers. Sci Rep. 2021;11(1):24035.
33. Gage BF, et al. Incidents of intracranial hemorrhage in patients with atrial fibrillation who are prone to fall. Am J Med. 2005;118:612–7.
34. Lip GY, et al. Stroke and major bleeding risk in elderly patients aged greater than or equal to 75 years with atrial fibrillation: the Loire Valley atrial fibrillation project. Stroke. 2015;46:143–50.
35. Man-son-Hing M, et al. Choosing antithrombotic therapy for elderly patients with atrial fibrillation who are at risk for falls. Arch Intern Med. 1999;159:677–85.
36. Rodriguez J, et al. Poststroke alterations in heart rate variability during orthostatic challenge. Medicine. 2017;96(14):e5989.
37. Phipps MS, et al. Orthostatic hypotension among outpatients with ischemic stroke. J Neurol Sci. 2012;314(1–2):62–5.
38. Raber I, et al. Orthostatic hypotension in hypertensive adults: Harry Goldblatt Award for Early Career Investigators 2021. Hypertension. 2022;79(11):2388–96.
39. Hohtari-Kivimäki U, et al. Orthostatic hypotension is a risk factor for falls among older adults: 3-year follow-up. J Am Med Dir Assoc. 2021;22(11):2325–30.
40. Shaw BH, et al. Relationships between orthostatic hypotension, frailty, falling and mortality in elderly care home residents. BMC Geriatr. 2019;19(1):80.

Social Determinants of Health

38

Gino Paolucci and Rebecca Karb

Introduction

Stroke is a leading cause of death and disability in the United States [1–5]. While preventative efforts to reduce cardiovascular risk factors and advances in acute stroke care have decreased overall stroke incidence and mortality over the past decade, disparities rooted in the social determinants of health (SDOH) have persisted. Healthy People 2030 defines SDOH as "the conditions in the environments where people are born, live, learn, work, play, worship, and age that affect a wide range of health, functioning, and quality-of-life outcomes and risks" [6]. SDOH include factors such as socioeconomic status and wealth, education and employment opportunities, safe housing, neighborhood environments, social support networks, and access to healthcare. The differential distribution of these social and economic resources is, in turn, influenced by structural factors such as racism and discrimination, sexism, and ableism. Inequities have been identified along every aspect of the stroke continuum, from stroke recognition to acute treatment to post-stroke care (Fig. 38.1). In this chapter, we will outline documented disparities in stroke care and opportunities for reducing inequities in clinical practice.

G. Paolucci
Rhode Island Hospital, Providence, RI, USA
e-mail: gpaolucci@lifespan.org

R. Karb (✉)
Warren Alpert School of Medicine, Providence, RI, USA
e-mail: rebecca.karb@brownphysicians.org

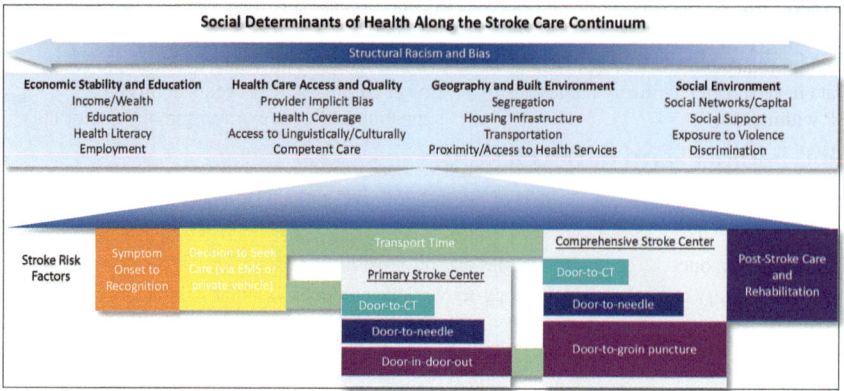

Fig. 38.1 Social determinants of health along the stroke care continuum

Disparities in Stroke Incidence

The risk of first-time stroke is almost twice as high for Blacks compared to Whites in the United States [2–7]. Moreover, despite overall declines in the death rates from stroke, Latinos have actually seen increases in stroke mortality over the past decade [1]. Excess stroke risk among racial/ethnic minorities can be attributed in part to disparities in well-established stroke risk factors such as hypertension, diabetes, atrial fibrillation, heart disease, and smoking, which should be best understood as mediating the relationship between SDOH and stroke risk.

Sex and gender are also important contributors to differences in stroke risk factors and incidence. In the United States in 2019, stroke was the third leading cause of death in women, compared with fifth in men (resulting in 55,000 more fatal strokes among women) [8]. This gender-associated risk is recognized and reflected in stroke risk assessment tools, most notably the CHADS-VAS2 score, which incorporates the female sex as a moderate risk enhancer for stroke due to atrial fibrillation. Results from the Women's Health Initiative showed an almost 50% higher risk of stroke for Black women compared to White women, mediated in part by differences in risk factors and socioeconomic status [8]. Women are also more likely than men to present with atypical stroke symptoms (e.g., mental status and behavioral changes, generalized weakness, and fatigue) [9].

While race/ethnicity and gender disparities have been well documented, research on LGBTQI+ stroke disparities is still emerging, with most attention on the transpopulation [10, 11]. In a recent prospective study of approximately 5000 trans women matched to cisgender men and women, trans women had a significantly elevated stroke risk compared with ciswomen [10]. While this association was particularly strong for trans women on estrogen hormone therapy, the disparity holds even amongst those not on hormonal treatment. This increased risk potentially speaks to sociocultural effects (e.g., experiences of discrimination) on cardiovascular health.

Stroke Recognition and Prehospital Care

The treatment of acute stroke is time-sensitive. Therefore, prompt awareness of stroke symptoms and presentation to a Stroke Center is crucial for morbidity and mortality outcomes. In studies on stroke awareness and recognition, lower education levels, non-White race, and immigrant status are all associated with both decreased knowledge of stroke symptoms and delayed presentation to the Emergency Department [12]. Small-scale, targeted efforts to improve stroke awareness in these communities have shown promising results [7].

Using Emergency Medical Services (EMS) for transportation to the hospital for stroke care results in shorter transportation times and faster medical evaluation [3, 4]. Yet, the usage of EMS differs across demographic groups and geographic space. Low socioeconomic status has been associated with a lower likelihood of contacting EMS for stroke symptoms [3]. In a review of studies that detected racial disparities in emergency services, EMS usage was lower by as much as 40% in Latino patients, 20% in Asian patients, and 21% in African American patients compared with White patients [13].

Delays in stroke recognition and decision delay (the time from recognition to the decision to seek medical evaluation) determine the time from last known well (LKW) upon presentation to the Emergency Department, which ultimately determines the eligibility for interventions such as tPA and mechanical thrombectomy. A greater proportion of White patients arrive within 3 h from the onset of stroke symptoms compared to Black and Latino patients—a result of both delayed recognition of stroke symptoms and decision delays in presentation [12, 13].

Social isolation is a major barrier to stroke recognition and timely presentation. In a systematic review, social isolation and poor social relationships were associated with a 32% increase in stroke risk [14]. Individuals living in rural areas are also more likely to be socially isolated. Older women are more likely than men to live alone and be socially isolated, which sometimes results in significant delays in treatment [15]. A retrospective cohort analysis of stroke patients in New York found that women are significantly more likely than men to be found by others in their homes after a severe stroke (the commonly used phrase "found down") [16].

Geography also plays an important role in stroke care; options for acute treatment depend on proximity and access to certified stroke centers. A study of all the certified primary and comprehensive stroke centers in the United States found that rural census tracts with greater representation of elderly, American Indian, uninsured people, or low median income are generally more distant from stroke care [17, 18].

Emergency Department Stroke Care

Door-to-computed tomography time (DTCT) measures the time elapsed between a patient's arrival to the ED and a non-contrast CT of the brain; a DTCT time of ≤25 min is the established AHA/ASA target goal for patients with suspected strokes.

Delays in obtaining a CT can result in longer door-to-needle (DTN) times, delayed therapeutic interventions, and worse stroke outcomes. A Florida-based study found that overall DTCT times have been steadily improving over the past decade, yet race and gender disparities have been constant. Women and Black patients are less likely to achieve a DTCT ≤25 min, which may reflect differences in the mode of arrival to the ED (as EMS often prenotifies the ED of stroke arrivals, thus expediting care) as well as differences in provider evaluation [19].

Door to tPA and tPA Declination

Currently, alteplase (tPA) is the only FDA-approved medical treatment for acute ischemic stroke. Patients treated with tPA within 3 h of symptom onset are more likely to have minimal or no disability in the months following a stroke. In a recent review, White patients receive tPA treatment at the highest rates, followed by Black, Latino, Asian, and Native American patients [2]. Among the subset of patients that do receive tPA, White patients and men are more likely to receive it in under 45 min from arrival to the ED [20]. Rural and nonteaching hospitals are also less likely to give tPA and less likely to achieve the target door-to-needle (DTN) times [3]. This may be due to low tPA usage in small hospitals where neurologists are not always available.

The low rate of tPA administration for Black patients may be partly due to a higher tPA refusal rate [21]. The consent process for tPA involves a detailed but very time-sensitive discussion of the risks and benefits and can seem rushed to many patients. The long history of systemic mistreatment of Black patients within the healthcare system has led to well-founded mistrust that may explain hesitation and refusal of tPA.

Large Vessel Occlusion and Thrombectomy

The 2015 landmark ischemic stroke trials showed efficacy and improved outcomes for patients with large vessel occlusion [22] treated with thrombectomy, paving the way for endovascular therapy (EVT) to become the standard of care. Despite an overall increase in EVT incidence since 2015, disparities exist based on race, socioeconomic status, age, and geography [2–4, 23]. The rise of EVT for stroke is multifactorial, including increased availability, better systems of care, and improved public awareness [3]. In comparing the rates of endovascular therapy in Black, Hispanic, and Native American patients versus White patients, administration of EVT is significantly higher in White patients [2, 3, 24].

Awareness of stroke symptoms, access to healthcare, income, insurance status, cultural, and language barriers all may factor into this disparity [3]. Uninsured patients also receive EVT at lower rates. In comparing the incidence of EVT across socioeconomic groups, those with lower income were less likely to undergo EVT [25]. This could be due to a lack of symptom recognition and the fact that those with

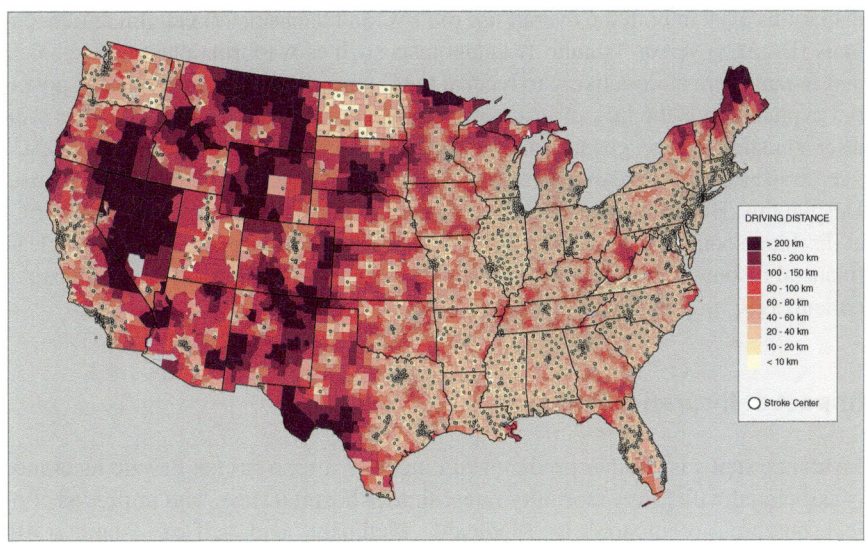

Fig. 38.2 A map of the United States indicating distances to the nearest stroke-ready hospital, with deeper colors indicating further distances. (Source: Yu et al. [17])

lower socioeconomic status were more distant from a certified stroke center [17]. In the same vein, patients across all races living in rural areas were less likely to receive EVT compared to those in metropolitan areas [3] and had higher stroke mortality [26]. Not surprisingly, some of these social determinants also factor into outcomes. Patients with lower socioeconomic status or who live in rural areas were less likely to be functionally independent at 90 days, had increased hospital mortality, and had longer times to stroke treatment due to distance to stroke-ready hospitals (Fig. 38.2). Interestingly, the difference is less significant when adjusting for factors such as stroke severity, perhaps suggesting that those with lower SES may not immediately recognize symptoms and present later in the course of their stroke [27]. While EVT may still be offered up to 24 h from symptom onset, the eligibility criteria are stricter in the extended windows, and some patients may no longer benefit. At last, disparity exists in the rates of EVT in patients aged 80 and older compared with those who are younger. Pre-stroke baseline function is an important consideration when considering EVT. Older patients also have less favorable functional outcomes with increased mortality and are more likely to be discharged to hospice care [23].

Inpatient Hospital Care of Acute Stroke

Anticoagulation

The use of oral anticoagulation (OAC) in eligible patients can dramatically reduce the risk of ischemic stroke caused by atrial fibrillation. However, racial and gender disparities exist in both the overall use of OAC and the use of direct oral anticoagulants (DOACs) versus Vitamin K antagonists such as warfarin. Blacks, Hispanics, and Asians were all less likely to receive OAC when compared to Whites. A potential explanation is the lack of insurance; however, usage rates were still lower even after adjusting for age, gender, income, and insurance status [28]. The use of DOACs over warfarin has increased over the recent years given safety and ease of use. Despite this, Blacks have a higher rate of warfarin prescription (rather than DOAC) at discharge compared to Whites. While the exact reasons may not be entirely clear, financial resources may be a factor due to high copays for DOACs, even for insured patients [29].

Impact of Insurance Status

Insurance status is another predictor of outcomes after a stroke. Private insurance is associated with lower mortality rates, shorter hospital stays, and improved clinical outcomes compared to Medicaid, Medicare, and self-pay status [30]. Uninsured patients have less control of risk factors, may wait longer to seek treatment, and have more advanced cerebrovascular disease [30, 31]. Difficulty obtaining inpatient rehabilitation beds for uninsured patients also contributes to longer hospital stays [31]. Longer hospital stays also increase the risk of hospital-acquired complications, such as delirium, infection, skin breakdown, and deconditioning.

Poststroke Care and Secondary Prevention

Poststroke Rehabilitation

Poststroke rehabilitation is crucial for improving the functional status and quality of life of individuals impacted by stroke. Options include inpatient acute rehabilitation, skilled nursing subacute rehabilitation, in-home rehabilitation, and outpatient rehabilitation services. A concerning disparity exists with the odds of receiving any type of rehabilitation service based on race. Whites receive significantly more rehabilitation than Blacks, especially in inpatient rehab and home settings [32]. White stroke survivors have a higher rate of supplemental insurance and higher income, which may be a reason for the higher use of inpatient and home services [32, 33]. Of patients admitted to inpatient rehabilitation, those of lower socioeconomic status may have difficulty completing the full course due to transportation difficulties, lack of social support, and financial limitations [27]. Interestingly, women are less likely to go to inpatient rehabilitation than men, and patients with lower incomes were more likely to go to skilled nursing rehabilitation versus inpatient services with more aggressive rehab [33]. There do not appear to be any significant differences in discharges to homes between Whites and Blacks.

Stroke Survival

Although there has been an impressive decline in overall stroke mortality over the past two decades, racial disparities in the burden of stroke mortality remain substantial [34]. This difference can be seen across the stroke care continuum, from incidence to morbidity/mortality [34]. There is also an association between socioeconomic status and stroke mortality; long-term mortality from stroke is significantly higher in low-income patients compared to high-income patients [35]. Higher poststroke mortality is seen in disadvantaged neighborhoods and the less educated as well, with neighborhoods with a higher percentage of White residents and those with higher education seeing lower mortality [36, 37]. Interestingly, although women may be more affected by stroke, gender is not thought to be an independent risk for long-term stroke mortality after controlling for comorbid diseases [38].

Mitigation of Disparities

Although it may seem daunting, individual providers can act both independently and in collaboration with others to address health inequities. The first important task is to acknowledge and respect the trauma and historically rooted distrust that some communities have experienced within the healthcare system and work to rebuild trust in patient encounters. Interpreters can be incredibly helpful, especially for conversations centered on procedural consent. Hospitals should have patient navigators available to aid with translation and serve as patient advocates. Another critical area for advancement is increasing the diversity and cultural competence of the healthcare workforce. A diverse workforce that reflects the patient populations it serves has been shown to improve the quality of care and patient outcomes [39]. Another area to target is the education of healthcare workers. Embedding cultural competency training into continuing medical education can keep the healthcare workforce aware of changing demographics in the local community and provide tools for improving care to underserved groups [40]. On a community level, providers can partner with public and private organizations to advocate for more supportive health environments and public health policies aimed at reducing health inequities [41].

Summary

The overwhelming impact of stroke and its sequelae is influenced by several social determinants such as socioeconomic status, income, education, patient's neighborhood of residence, social support, and access to healthcare. Alarming trends exist in disparities among race, gender, socioeconomic status, insurance status, and proximity to healthcare. Some degree of disparity can be seen in every aspect of stroke care and spans from stroke recognition to post-discharge morbidity and mortality. As overall stroke care continues to improve, care must be taken to monitor differential access to, and benefit from, these advances. In clinical practice, awareness of the social determinants of disparities in stroke incidence and treatment is a critical step in the effort to reduce these inequities.

Clinical Pearls
- Be aware of racial and cultural disparities in acute stroke care.
- Medical interpreters may improve patient's understanding of acute stroke treatment and post-stroke education in the case of a language barrier.
- Understand that mistrust in the medical system by marginalized populations may lead to delays in stroke presentation and treatment.
- Clear and concise conversations surrounding consent for thrombolytic or endovascular therapy may help mitigate distrust in the medical system.
- Be aware that some groups may experience disparities based on neighborhood of residence or geography from stroke centers.

References

1. https://www.cdc.gov/stroke/facts.htm. Accessed 28 Nov 2023.
2. Ikeme S, Kottenmeier E, Uzochukwu G, Brinjikji W. Evidence-based disparities in stroke care metrics and outcomes in the United States: a systematic review. Stroke. 2022;53:670–9.
3. de Havenon A, Sheth K, Johnston KC, et al. Acute ischemic stroke interventions in the United States and racial, socioeconomic, and geographic disparities. Neurology. 2021;97(23):e2292–303.
4. O'Carroll CB, Demaerschalk BM. Racial, socioeconomic, and geographic disparities in acute stroke care in the United States. Neurology. 2021;97:1059–60.
5. Reshetnyak E, Ntamatungiro M, Pinheiro LC, et al. Impact of multiple social determinants of health on incident stroke. Stroke. 2020;51:2445–53.
6. Office of Disease Prevention and Health Promotion. Diabetes. Healthy people 2030. U.S. Department of Health and Human Services; n.d. https://health.gov/healthypeople/priority-areas/social-determinants-health.
7. Levine DA, Duncan PW, Hguyen-Huynh MN, Ogedegbe OG. Interventions targeting racial/ethnic disparities in stroke prevention and treatment. Stroke. 2020;51:3425–32.
8. Rexrode KM, Madsen TE, Yu AYX, et al. The impact of sex and gender on stroke. Circ Res. 2022;130:512–28.
9. Bushnell C, Howard VJ, Lisabeth L, Caso V, Gall S, Kleindorfer D, et al. Sex differences in the evaluation and treatment of acute ischaemic stroke. Lancet Neurol. 2018;17:641–50. https://doi.org/10.1016/S1474-4422(18)30201-1.
10. Getahun D, Nash R, Flanders WD, Baird TC, Becerra-Culqui TA, Cromwell L, Hunkeler E, Lash TL, Millman A, Quinn VP, et al. Cross-sex hormones and acute cardiovascular events in transgender persons: a cohort study. Ann Intern Med. 2018;169:205–13.
11. Diaz M, Rosendale N. Diagnosis, treatment, and prevention of stroke in transgender adults. Curr Treat Options Neurol. 2022;24:409–28.
12. Mszar R, Mahajan S, Valero-Elizondo J, et al. Association between sociodemographic determinants and disparities in stroke symptoms awareness among US young adults. Stroke. 2020;51:3552–61.

13. Mochari-Greenberger H, Xian Y, Hellkamp AS, et al. Racial/ethnic and sex differences in emergency medical services transport among hospitalized US stroke patients: analysis of the national Get With The Guidelines—Stroke Registry. J Am Heart Assoc. 2015;4:e002099.

14. Valtorta NK, Kanaan M, Gilbody S, et al. Loneliness and social isolation as risk factors for coronary heart disease and stroke: systematic review and meta-analysis of longitudinal observational studies. Heart. 2016;102:1009–16.

15. Reeves MJ, Prager M, Fang J, et al. Impact of living alone on the care and outcomes of patients with acute stroke. Stroke. 2014;45:3083–5.

16. Springer MV, Labovitz DL. The effect of being found with stroke symptoms on predictors of hospital arrival. J Stroke Cerebrovasc Dis. 2018;27:1363–7. https://doi.org/10.1016/j.jstrokecerebrovasdis.2017.12.024.

17. Yu CY, Blaine T, Panagos PD, Kansagra AP. Demographic disparities in proximity to certified stroke care in the United States. Stroke. 2021;52(8):2571–9. https://doi.org/10.1161/STROKEAHA.121.034493.

18. Thompson SG, Barber PA, Gommans JH, et al. Geographic disparities in stroke outcomes and service access. Neurology. 2022;99(4):e414–22.

19. Polineni SP, Perez EJ, Wang K. Sex and race-ethnic disparities in door-to-CT time in acute ischemic stroke: the Florida Stroke Registry. J Am Heart Assoc. 2021;10:e017543.

20. Oluwole SA, Wang K, Dong C. Disparities and trends in door to needle time: Florida Puerto Rico Collaboration to Reduce Stroke Disparities Study. Stroke. 2017;48(8):2192–7.

21. Mendelson SJ, Zhang S, Matsouaka R, et al. Race-ethnic disparities in rates of declination of thrombolysis for stroke. Neurology. 2022;98:e1596–604.

22. Goyal M, Menon BK, van Zwam WH, et al. Endovascular thrombectomy after large-vessel ischaemic stroke: a meta-analysis of individual patient data from five randomised trials. Lancet. 2016;387(10029):1723–31. https://doi.org/10.1016/S0140-6736(16)00163-X.

23. Adcock AK, Schwamm LH, Smith EE, et al. Trends in use, outcomes, and disparities in endovascular thrombectomy in US patients with stroke aged 80 years and older compared with younger patients. JAMA Netw Open. 2022;5(6):e2215869. https://doi.org/10.1001/jamanetworkopen.2022.15869.

24. Aroor SR, Asif KS, Potter-Vig J, et al. Mechanical thrombectomy access for all? Challenges in increasing endovascular treatment for acute ischemic stroke in the United States. J Stroke. 2022;24(1):41–8. https://doi.org/10.5853/jos.2021.03909.

25. Attenello FJ, Adamczyk P, Wen G, et al. Racial and socioeconomic disparities in access to mechanical revascularization procedures for acute ischemic stroke. J Stroke Cerebrovasc Dis. 2014;23(2):327–34. https://doi.org/10.1016/j.jstrokecerebrovasdis.2013.03.036.

26. Hammond G, Luke AA, Elson L, Towfighi A, Joynt Maddox KE. Urban-rural inequities in acute stroke care and in-hospital mortality. Stroke. 2020;51(7):2131–8. https://doi.org/10.1161/STROKEAHA.120.029318.

27. Salwi S, Kelly KA, Patel PD, et al. Neighborhood socioeconomic status and mechanical thrombectomy outcomes. J Stroke Cerebrovasc Dis. 2021;30(2):105488. https://doi.org/10.1016/j.jstrokecerebrovasdis.2020.105488.

28. Tedla YG, Schwartz SM, Silberman P, Greenland P, Passman RS. Racial disparity in the prescription of anticoagulants and risk of stroke and bleeding in atrial fibrillation patients. J Stroke Cerebrovasc Dis. 2020;29(5):104718. https://doi.org/10.1016/j.jstrokecerebrovasdis.2020.104718.

29. Sur NB, Wang K, Di Tullio MR, et al. Disparities and temporal trends in the use of anticoagulation in patients with ischemic stroke and atrial fibrillation. Stroke. 2019;50(6):1452–9. https://doi.org/10.1161/STROKEAHA.118.023959.

30. Fargen KM, Neal D, Blackburn SL, Hoh BL, Rahman M. Health disparities and stroke: the influence of insurance status on the prevalence of patient safety indicators and hospital-acquired conditions. J Neurosurg. 2015;122(4):870–5. https://doi.org/10.3171/2014.12.JNS14646.

31. Gezmu T, Gizzi MS, Kirmani JF, Schneider D, Moussavi M. Disparities in acute stroke severity, outcomes, and care relative to health insurance status. J Stroke Cerebrovasc Dis. 2014;23(2):e93–8. https://doi.org/10.1016/j.jstrokecerebrovasdis.2013.08.027.

32. Keeney T, Jette AM, Freedman VA, Cabral H. Racial differences in patterns of use of rehabilitation services for adults aged 65 and older. J Am Geriatr Soc. 2017;65(12):2707–12. https://doi.org/10.1111/jgs.15136.
33. Sandel ME, Wang H, Terdiman J, et al. Disparities in stroke rehabilitation: results of a study in an integrated health system in northern California. PM R. 2009;1(1):29–40. https://doi.org/10.1016/j.pmrj.2008.10.012.
34. Elkind MSV, Lisabeth L, Howard VJ, Kleindorfer D, Howard G. Approaches to studying determinants of racial-ethnic disparities in stroke and its sequelae. Stroke. 2020;51(11):3406–16. https://doi.org/10.1161/STROKEAHA.120.030424.
35. Andersen KK, Olsen TS. Social inequality by income in short- and long-term cause-specific mortality after stroke. J Stroke Cerebrovasc Dis. 2019;28(6):1529–36. https://doi.org/10.1016/j.jstrokecerebrovasdis.2019.03.013.
36. Osypuk TL, Ehntholt A, Moon JR, Gilsanz P, Glymour MM. Neighborhood differences in post-stroke mortality. Circ Cardiovasc Qual Outcomes. 2017;10(2):e002547. https://doi.org/10.1161/CIRCOUTCOMES.116.002547.
37. Elfassy T, Grasset L, Glymour MM, et al. Sociodemographic disparities in long-term mortality among stroke survivors in the United States. Stroke. 2019;50(4):805–12. https://doi.org/10.1161/STROKEAHA.118.023782.
38. Lambert C, Chaudhary D, Olulana O, et al. Sex disparity in long-term stroke recurrence and mortality in a rural population in the United States. Ther Adv Neurol Disord. 2020;13:1756286420971895. https://doi.org/10.1177/1756286420971895.
39. Jackson CS, Gracia JN. Addressing health and health-care disparities: the role of a diverse workforce and the social determinants of health. Public Health Rep. 2014;129(Suppl 2):57–61. https://doi.org/10.1177/00333549141291S211.
40. Weiner SJ. Advancing health equity by avoiding judgmentalism and contextualizing care. AMA J Ethics. 2021;23(2):E91–6. https://doi.org/10.1001/amajethics.2021.91.
41. Andermann A, CLEAR Collaboration. Taking action on the social determinants of health in clinical practice: a framework for health professionals. CMAJ. 2016;188(17–18):E474–83. https://doi.org/10.1503/cmaj.160177.

Poststroke Mood Disorders

39

Mary Ann Harmon, Neeharika Thottempudi, and Teng Peng

Introduction

Depression is a common and largely underrecognized and undertreated condition that can occur in up to 33% of stroke survivors [1]. Patients with poststroke depression (PSD) have worse functional outcomes, recurrent vascular events, worse quality of life, and higher mortality rates. Suicidality is also increased after stroke [2]. Depression can manifest in various ways, such as sadness, lack of appetite, irritability, anxiety, lack of motivation, and abnormal sleeping patterns. The APC must be able to identify PSD and be familiar with different methods to treat this condition. This chapter focuses on the pathophysiology, risk factors, screening, diagnosis, and treatment of PSD.

Pathophysiology and Risk Factors

The pathophysiology of PSD is not well understood but is likely due to a combination of biological and psychosocial risk factors. Biologic risk factors of PSD include the severity of stroke-related physical disability, post-stroke cognitive decline, and reduced brain amine levels. Compared to patients with other stroke-related physical impairments, patients who suffer from executive and language dysfunction are at

M. A. Harmon
Yale New Haven Hospital, New Haven, CT, USA
e-mail: maryann.harmon@yale.edu

N. Thottempudi
Carson Tahoe Health, Carson City, NV, USA
e-mail: neeharika.thottempudi@yale.edu

T. Peng (✉)
University of Florida School of Medicine, Gainesville, FL, USA
e-mail: Teng.Peng@neurology.ufl.edu

© The Author(s), under exclusive license to Springer Nature Switzerland AG 2024
H. P. Amin (ed.), *Stroke for the Advanced Practice Clinician*,
https://doi.org/10.1007/978-3-031-66289-8_39

469

significantly higher risk for PSD. Psychosocial risk factors for PSD include the lack of family and social support and a prior history of depression. PSD is more common in patients with left-sided strokes due to the presence of aphasia. However, studies have shown no association between PSD and stroke location, age, or education level. Ischemic strokes are associated with reduced levels of biogenic amines involved in pleasure and happiness, such as dopamine and serotonin. However, these associations are not well established and not routinely tested in the clinical setting [3, 4].

There are two main subtypes of PSD, early and late-onset PSD. Early-onset PSD appears in the first 3 months after the stroke. This form of depression develops more abruptly with symptoms that include melancholy, somatic symptoms (i.e., fatigue and body aches), and significant social dysfunction. In contrast, late-onset PSD, occurring beyond the first few months following a stroke, is more insidious and associated with the realization of functional limitations that result from the stroke. Both PSD subtypes typically occur in the first year after stroke and are critical to recognize and treat [3].

Patients with brain injury, including ischemic stroke, may experience pseudobulbar affect (PBA), which is often misdiagnosed as depression. PBA is characterized by involuntary and unpredictable crying, laughter, and anger. PSD is an internal mood disorder experienced by the patient, congruent with known psychological triggers, occurring over weeks to months, with a preserved ability to modulate outward expressions, and often occurs alongside other symptoms of depression. In contrast, PBA is an outward expression (affect) of a feeling, unregulated by traditional inhibitory controls, manifesting as brief, uncontrollable, and often inappropriate displays of emotion. Patients with PBA do not understand why they are feeling certain emotions, which can be highly exaggerated. PBA is thought to occur from dysregulation of neurotransmitter pathways. It is essential to distinguish between PBA and PSD to ensure that the patient receives the appropriate treatment. The combination of quinidine and dextromethorphan, known as Nuedexta, is an effective treatment for PBA.

It is worth mentioning that PSD does not only occur in the patient. A metaanalysis of over 1700 caregivers revealed that 40% of caregivers of stroke survivors had depressive symptoms, and 21% had anxiety [5]. While the caregiver may not be your patient, identifying excess caregiver stress and burden might open a conversation about needing additional help at home.

Screening

Patients with PSD may appear sad and tearful, often exhibiting poor eye contact. Patients with PSD may also be less willing to participate in therapies. Other times, their symptoms may be more subtle.

The Joint Commission recommends early recognition and treatment of PSD by screening all stroke patients before hospital discharge. In addition, PSD screening should also be performed at follow-up visits for at least the first year after stroke, when patients are at the highest risk for PSD. Several screening tools are used in research and clinical practice. These include the Geriatric Depression Scale (either the full 30-question version or the shorter 15-question version), the Montgomery-Asberg Depression Rating Scale, the Patient Health Questionnaire (PHQ-2 and PHQ-9), and the single-item screen [6]. The PHQ-2 and PHQ-9 are the most widely used questionnaires and can be administered by nursing staff (Tables 39.1 and 39.2). The single-item screen (do you often feel sad or depressed?) is easy to use and has a sensitivity and specificity of greater than 80% [7].

The PHQ-2 asks about the *frequency* of depressive symptoms. When assessing the stroke patient using the PHQ-2, the patient is asked, "Over the past 2 weeks, how often have you been bothered by (a) little interest or pleasure in doing things, (b) feeling down, depressed, or hopeless." The response for each question is scored 0 for not at all, 1 for several days, 2 for more than half the days, and 3 for nearly every day. Patients with a score of 3 or greater have a high likelihood of depression. They should then be evaluated with the PHQ-9, which helps diagnose and measure

Table 39.1 PHQ-2 screening instrument for depression

Over the past 2 weeks, how often have you been bothered by any of the following problems?	Not at all	Several days	More than half the days	Nearly every day
Little interest or pleasure in doing things	0	1	2	3
Feeling down, depressed, or hopeless	0	1	2	3

Table was adapted from Kroenke et al.'s [8] original publication
Scoring: A total score of 0–2 is considered negative for depression. A score of 3–6 is considered positive for depression and warrants further evaluation for major depressive disorder

Table 39.2 PHQ-9 Screening instrument for depression

Over the past 2 weeks, how often have you been bothered by any of the following problems?	Not at all	Several days	More than half the days	Nearly every day
Little interest or pleasure in doing things	0	1	2	3
Feeling down, depressed, or hopeless	0	1	2	3
Trouble falling or staying asleep, or sleeping too much	0	1	2	3
Feeling tired or having little energy	0	1	2	3
Poor appetite or overeating	0	1	2	3
Feeling bad about yourself or that you are a failure or have let yourself or your family down	0	1	2	3
Trouble concentrating on things, such as reading the newspaper or watching television	0	1	2	3
Moving or speaking so slowly that other people could have noticed? Or are you so fidgety or restless that you have been moving a lot more than usual?	0	1	2	3
Thoughts that you would be better off dead, or of hurting yourself in some way	0	1	2	3

Table was adapted from Kroenke et al.'s [10] original publication
Scoring: A total score of 0–4 is considered no depression, 5–9 mild depression, 10–14 moderate depression, 15–19 moderately severe depression, and 20–27 severe depression.

the severity of depression or any other diagnostic instrument. The PHQ-9 has additional questions about sleep, fatigue, appetite, feeling bad about oneself, concentration, slow movement, and thoughts about death or self-harm, with points assigned to the frequency of symptoms. The total score then helps stratify patients into mild, moderate, moderately severe, and severe categories of depression. Patients screening positive for the PHQ-9 should be referred to a social worker, psychosocial nurse practitioner, or other mental healthcare provider [9].

A common symptom of PSD is poststroke fatigue, which is often described as a feeling of exhaustion and lack of physical or mental energy. Poststroke fatigue is estimated to be present in up to 51% of stroke patients and can occur alone or concurrently with PSD [11]. There is no consensus on screening or treatment for poststroke fatigue. However, it is vital to identify patients who may be experiencing fatigue and acknowledge that this can occur in isolation or as a symptom of depression. Fatigue may also be due to other treatable conditions, such as malnutrition, dehydration, sleep apnea, polypharmacy or medication side effects, anemia, or thyroid disorders. Many stroke patients experience fatigue that often resolves within months, but severe or persistent fatigue warrants consideration of these other causes.

Diagnosis

The clinical interview with the patient is the gold standard for diagnosing depression. During the interview, the provider must determine if the patient meets the criteria for depression set forth by the Diagnostic and Statistical Manual of Mental Disorders 5 (DSM-5) developed by the American Psychiatric Association. Symptoms of depression are included in the PHQ-9 screening tool and include persistent feelings of sadness or depressed mood, loss of interest, persistent feelings of worthlessness, excessive guilt, frequent thoughts of death or suicide, difficulty concentrating, and increased or decreased sleep, motor activity, or appetite. To meet formal DMS-5 diagnostic criteria, the patient must have five or more of the symptoms above during a 2-week period, and at least one of the symptoms should be loss of interest or depressed mood [12]. The diagnosis of PSD can be established in the stroke clinic by the advanced practice provider. Still, patients may be referred to other mental health providers for more precise diagnosis or treatment. Having a mental health provider in your network willing to see these patients quickly can be beneficial. Depression can limit stroke patients' participation in therapy and lead to malnutrition during their most critical recovery window. Urgent evaluation and treatment can, therefore, significantly impact long-term function.

Depression is also associated with cognitive symptoms. It can be challenging to separate mood-related cognitive symptoms from memory impairment due to brain injury from stroke. For patients where it is unclear if cognitive symptoms are due to stroke or depression, neuropsychological testing may be helpful. The neuropsychological evaluation, performed by a psychiatrist or psychologist, consists of tests evaluating memory, language, attention, cognitive, executive, visuospatial, motor, and personality. It takes several hours to complete, with family often included in the initial interview. Results of the neuropsychologic exam can help clarify cognitive symptoms following a stroke and distinguish a neurodegenerative condition such as dementia from a mood disorder [13]. To find a neuropsychologist nearby, go to https://theaaacn.org/directory/. Be aware that wait times might be long. Since each visit is long, a neuropsychologist may only see one or two patients a day! When referring to a neuropsychologist, be sure to clarify whether they review their findings and recommendations with the patient or send their report to the referring provider.

Treatment

A worthy discussion of the treatment of depression is beyond the scope of this chapter. No guidelines help choose a specific treatment or medication for PSD. The most effective therapy combines psychosocial, pharmacological, and stroke-focused treatments such as physical therapy, cognitive rehabilitation, and prevention of new vascular events.

Due to the high prevalence of PSD and its negative effect on outcomes, several randomized controlled trials (RCTs) were done to study the impact of *routine use of* selective serotonin reuptake inhibitors (SSRIs) on functional outcomes. These trials include FLAME, FOCUS, EFFECTS, and AFFINITY. FLAME is a randomized control trial performed in nine centers across France and enrolled 118 patients with ischemic stroke and unilateral weakness. This trial concluded that fluoxetine, a SSRI, started between days 5 and 10 after symptom onset, improved motor recovery, and increased the chances of functional independence after 3 months [14]. FOCUS was another randomized placebo-controlled trial performed in the UK across 103 hospitals and enrolled 3127 patients with either ischemic stroke or intracerebral hemorrhage. Unlike the FLAME trial, the FOCUS trial did not demonstrate any functional outcome benefit of fluoxetine compared with placebo at 6 months [15]. However, the FLAME trial specifically enrolled patients with hemiplegia or hemiparesis, whereas the FOCUS trial enrolled patients with any focal neurological deficit. In the FOCUS trial, fluoxetine did reduce the occurrence of depression, but it did not translate into promoting functional recovery after stroke. The findings of the FOCUS trial were reproduced in the recently done EFFECTS and AFFINITY trials, with no improvement in functional outcome with oral fluoxetine taken for 6 months after stroke.

It is important to note that all the trials mentioned above enrolled patients regardless of whether they exhibited depressive symptoms. The results, therefore, should be taken with caution. While their conclusions suggest that treating *all* stroke patients with SSRI has not been shown to improve outcomes, they do not say treating a patient with depression is ineffective. Considering the impact that depression can have on stroke patients, it is still worth strongly considering treatment. As with any medical intervention, the risks and benefits of starting SSRIs should be considered and discussed with the patient before initiation.

A 2020 systematic review identified 49 trials involving 3342 participants that evaluated prophylactic treatment to prevent PSD. The study found little evidence to support the effectiveness of pharmacological or psychological therapies in preventing the development of PSD [16]. Therefore, antidepressants are not formally recommended for the prevention of PSD but can be considered on an individual basis during follow-up clinic visits. Another important aspect to consider while initiating treatment with SSRIs includes their interaction with the antiplatelet clopidogrel, as some SSRIs inhibit CYP2C19 (i.e., fluoxetine and fluvoxamine) and can reduce the effectiveness of clopidogrel. Sertraline and citalopram do not inhibit CYP2C19 and may be used safely in conjunction with clopidogrel.

Psychosocial interventions for PSD include cognitive behavioral therapy, alone or combined with antidepressants. Other interventions include care management, psychoeducation, family support, and behavioral activation. Emerging therapies for treating PSD include neuromodulation techniques that involve stimulation, inhibition, or modification of the electrical activity in the brain. Among them, repetitive transcranial magnetic stimulation (rTMS) has shown promising results, but most studies with rTMS have small sample sizes and inconsistent methodological quality. Patients interested in rTMS treatment should be referred to an institution with adequate psychiatric facilities to perform this procedure.

Clinical Pearls
- PSD is common but underdiagnosed.
- Patients with stroke should be screened for depression before hospital discharge and during follow-up appointments in the stroke clinic.
- Screening can be done using the PHQ-2, with follow-up with PHQ-9 for comprehensive evaluation in case of positive screening results.
- Caregiver fatigue and depression are common. Identification of caregiver struggles should lead to consideration of additional resources where appropriate.
- PSD diagnosis can be done by advanced practice clinicians in clinic or referred to mental health providers for further diagnosis or treatment options.
- PSD can limit participation in therapy and lead to malnutrition during a critical recovery window. Optimal treatment of PSD should include cognitive behavioral therapy alone or in combination with antidepressant medications.

Referenced Trials

FLAME Trial (2011): Double-blind, placebo-controlled clinical trial evaluating whether fluoxetine enhances motor recovery in patients with ischemic stroke and hemiplegia or hemiparesis. The trial enrolled 118 patients randomized to fluoxetine 20 mg daily or placebo for 3 months starting 5–10 days after the onset of stroke. All patients had physiotherapy. The study results showed that patients with moderate to severe motor deficits prescribed with fluoxetine had better motor recovery after 3 months [14].

FOCUS Trial (2019): Double-blind, placebo-controlled clinical trial evaluating whether fluoxetine improves functional outcomes, even if they did not have depression. Patients enrolled in this trial needed a diagnosis of stroke or intracerebral hemorrhage and a functional neurological deficit (less focus on motor hemiplegia or hemiparesis compared to the FLAME trial). This trial enrolled 3127 patients randomized to fluoxetine 20 mg daily or placebo for 6 months starting at 2–15 days after stroke onset. The study results showed that fluoxetine decreased the occurrence of depression but increased the frequency of bone fractures and did not improve functional outcomes [15]. One can argue, however, that an intervention that reduces stroke-related depression is certainly important!

EFFECTS Trial (2020): Double-blind, placebo-controlled trial evaluating whether fluoxetine 20 mg once daily for 6 months improved functional outcomes. This trial enrolled 1500 patients and found that fluoxetine did not improve functional outcomes compared to placebo (although they did find a reduced occurrence of depression but an increased occurrence of fractures and hyponatremia). This study was extended to 12 months with similar results [17].

AFFINITY Trial (2021): Double-blind, placebo-controlled trial evaluating whether fluoxetine 20 mg once daily for 6 months improved functional outcomes. This trial enrolled 1280 patients and found that fluoxetine did not improve functional outcomes compared to placebo. There was also no difference in falls, bone fractures, or seizures between treatment and placebo groups. This study was extended to 12 months with similar results [18].

References

1. Robinson RG, Jorge RE. Post-stroke depression: a review. Am J Psychiatry. 2016;173:221–31.
2. Harnod T, Lin C-L, Kao C-H. Risk of suicide attempt in poststroke patients: a population-based cohort study. J Am Heart Assoc. 2018;7:e007830.
3. Facucho-Oliveira J, Esteves-Sousa D, Espada-Santos P, Moura N, Albuquerque M, Fraga AM, Sousa S, Cintra P, Mendonça L, Pita F. Depression after stroke. Pract Neurol. 2021;21:384–91.
4. Loubinoux I, Kronenberg G, Endres M, Schumann-Bard P, Freret T, Filipkowski RK, Kaczmarek L, Popa-Wagner A. Post-stroke depression: mechanisms, translation and therapy. J Cell Mol Med. 2012;16:1961–9.
5. Loh AZ, Tan JS, Zhang MW, Ho RC. The global prevalence of anxiety and depressive symptoms among caregivers of stroke survivors. J Am Med Dir Assoc. 2017;18:111–6.
6. Mitchell PH. Nursing assessment of depression in stroke survivors. Stroke. 2016;47:e1–3.
7. Watkins CL, Lightbody CE, Sutton CJ, Holcroft L, Jack CIA, Dickinson HA, van den Broek MD, Leathley MJ. Evaluation of a single-item screening tool for depression after stroke: a cohort study. Clin Rehabil. 2007;21:846–52.
8. Kroenke K, Spitzer RL, Williams JBW. The Patient Health Questionnaire-2: validity of a two-item depression screener. Med Care. 2003;41:1284–92.
9. Williams LS, Brizendine EJ, Plue L, Bakas T, Tu W, Hendrie H, Kroenke K. Performance of the PHQ-9 as a screening tool for depression after stroke. Stroke. 2005;36:635–8.

10. Kroenke K, Spitzer RL, Williams JB. The PHQ-9: validity of a brief depression severity measure. J Gen Intern Med. 2001;16:606–13.
11. Paciaroni M, Acciarresi M. Poststroke fatigue. Stroke. 2019;50:1927–33.
12. American Psychiatric Association. Diagnostic and statistical manual of mental disorders: DSM-5. 5th ed. Arlington, VA: American Psychiatric Association; 2013.
13. Zucchella C, Federico A, Martini A, Tinazzi M, Bartolo M, Tamburin S. Neuropsychological testing. Pract Neurol. 2018;18:227–37.
14. Chollet F, Tardy J, Albucher J-F, Thalamas C, Berard E, Lamy C, Bejot Y, Deltour S, Jaillard A, Niclot P, et al. Fluoxetine for motor recovery after acute ischaemic stroke (FLAME): a randomised placebo-controlled trial. Lancet Neurol. 2011;10:123–30.
15. FOCUS Trial Collaboration. Effects of fluoxetine on functional outcomes after acute stroke (FOCUS): a pragmatic, double-blind, randomised, controlled trial. Lancet. 2019;393:265–74.
16. Medeiros GC, Roy D, Kontos N, Beach SR. Post-stroke depression: a 2020 updated review. Gen Hosp Psychiatry. 2020;66:70–80.
17. Lundström E, Isaksson E, Greilert Norin N, Näsman P, Wester P, Mårtensson B, Norrving B, Wallén H, Borg J, Hankey GJ, et al. Effects of fluoxetine on outcomes at 12 months after acute stroke. Stroke. 2021;52:3082–7.
18. Hankey GJ, Hackett ML, Almeida OP, Flicker L, Mead GE, Dennis MS, Etherton-Beer C, Ford AH, Billot L, Jan S, et al. Twelve-month outcomes of the AFFINITY Trial of fluoxetine for functional recovery after acute stroke: AFFINITY Trial Steering Committee on behalf of the AFFINITY Trial Collaboration. Stroke. 2021;52:2502–9.

Poststroke Cognitive Disorders

40

Naomi Lowe and Darren Volpe

Introduction

Per the DSM-V, dementia is defined as an acquired cognitive impairment in at least one cognitive domain that is severe enough to impact a person's independence. Daily activities such as driving and managing finances become too complex for the patient to do safely and independently. Mild cognitive impairment (MCI) is an acquired cognitive impairment that is not severe enough to limit independent functioning. Some patients with MCI will eventually progress to dementia, and some can return to a state of normal cognition if the cause is reversible.

Epidemiology and Risk Factors

Approximately 20% of dementias in the Western world are classified as vascular dementias [1]. The prevalence is increased in countries with a high burden of vascular risk factors, such as hypertension, hyperlipidemia, type 2 diabetes, obstructive sleep apnea, and smoking. Globally, up to 30% of dementias are related to cerebrovascular disease [1]. As is the case with any dementia, an aging population is the primary, nonmodifiable risk factor.

Differential Diagnosis

Let us outline the four main subtypes of dementia, which are important to remember when evaluating cognitive changes. Alzheimer's dementia is the most common cause of dementia in people over the age of 65. The pathology involves the

N. Lowe · D. Volpe (✉)
Yale School of Medicine, New Haven, CT, USA
e-mail: naomi.lowe@yale.edu; Darren.volpe@yale.edu

© The Author(s), under exclusive license to Springer Nature Switzerland AG 2024
H. P. Amin (ed.), *Stroke for the Advanced Practice Clinician*,
https://doi.org/10.1007/978-3-031-66289-8_40

accumulation of amyloid plaques and tau tangles within the brain tissue. Classic neuroimaging findings include atrophy (shrinking) of the hippocampi. Clinically, patients present primarily with short-term memory deficits. Rapid forgetting is the most common symptom that leads to referral to cognitive neurology clinics, although other cognitive domains may also be impacted.

Depending on regional differences, both Lewy body dementia and vascular dementia have been regarded as the second most common type of dementia [2, 3]. Lewy body dementia is an alpha-synucleinopathy, in which patients present with cognitive impairment in addition to parkinsonism on exam. Patients may show severe fluctuations in cognition and awareness, in addition to complex visual hallucinations. Other defining features include REM sleep behavior disorder and sensitivity to antipsychotics. Vascular dementia is caused by cerebrovascular disease, which reduces blood supply to the brain due to cerebral infarction or intraparenchymal hemorrhage. Subtypes will be discussed in detail below.

The fourth dementia subtype is frontotemporal lobar degeneration, caused by the accumulation of pathologic proteins in the frontal and temporal lobes. This type of dementia classically presents with stark changes in personality and behavior. Memory is often not impaired in the early stages. Neuroimaging will show atrophy in the frontal and anterior temporal lobes. This diagnosis is usually made in younger patients and is one of the most common causes of dementia in patients younger than 65 years of age [3].

Clinical Presentations of Vascular Dementias

Vascular dementias can be further classified by specific patterns of cerebrovascular disease. There are three main types:

1. **Leukoaraiosis**: Diffuse small vessel white matter disease. Also called "Binswanger's Disease."
2. **Multi-infarct dementia**: Cognitive impairment due to multiple larger infarcts occurring over time.
3. **Strategic focal lesions**: A focal infarct or hemorrhage in an area specifically involved in memory and cognitive processing.

These abnormalities are best detected on brain MRI; they can also be seen on CT imaging but with less definition. However, it is critical to take a careful history and perform a thorough neurologic examination to evaluate for any concurrent causes of cognitive impairment.

The following are more detailed explanations of the above three subtypes of vascular cognitive impairment, each with illustrative case presentations with imaging.

Leukoaraiosis

The most common subtype of vascular cognitive impairment is leukoaraiosis from chronic, small vessel ischemia commonly seen in patients with advanced cardiovascular risk factors. Clinically, these patients have slowed processing speed, often concurrent with slowed motor function and postural/balance mechanisms. They report difficulty recalling information, though their recall improves with cues and reminders (thus, difficulty with retrieval with intact encoding). In contrast, patients with Alzheimer dementia often have difficulty with recall and do not improve with cues or reminders (thus, difficulty with encoding due to hippocampal degeneration). Patients with leukoaraiosis usually have executive dysfunction (including difficulty with multitasking, organizing, and strategizing), as well as attentional deficits. The volume of white matter affected usually accumulates very slowly in the periventricular and subcortical white matter. Therefore, the presentation is usually one in which there is a gradual onset of memory/cognitive impairment, similar to the gradual onset of late-onset Alzheimer dementia. On the physical exam, the motor slowing may manifest as parkinsonism as the motor pathways from the frontal lobes to/from the basal ganglia and thalamus may be affected. This "parkinsonism" would be of a different mechanism than idiopathic Parkinson disease, in which there is a loss of dopaminergic input from the brain stem.

Case 1: Leukoaraiosis

A 70-year-old man presented to the neurology clinic with his wife, reporting a slowly progressive worsening of short-term memory and ability to multitask, with onset at approximately age 67. He could no longer play cards with his family, which he previously enjoyed immensely. He needed assistance from his wife to set up and take his medications and to balance the checkbook. His medical history includes smoking (three packs per day), hypertension, hyperlipidemia, and alcohol use disorder (in remission since age 40). Neuropsychological testing showed impairments in executive function, processing speed, and ATTENTION. FIGURE 40.1 shows two axial FLAIR MR images:

In images a and b of Fig. 40.1, there is severe, diffuse T2 hyperintensity (seen as white signal), indicating chronic microinfarctions throughout the white matter of the brain. This occurs slowly over time and thus causes gradual cognitive and motor deficits. The rate of progression varies, but a more rapid decline is expected if stroke risk factors are not modified. The patient continued to smoke and has become more dependent on his family for instrumental activities of daily living as time has gone on. He also developed parkinsonism over that time due to the effects of white matter disease on motor pathways.

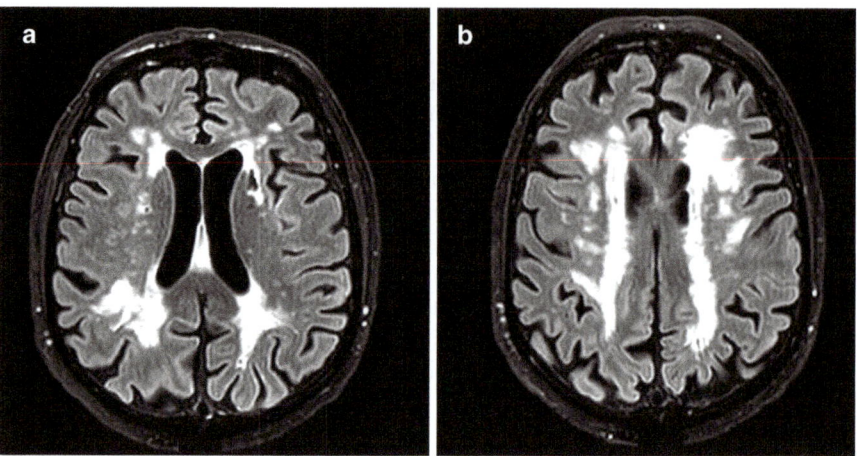

Fig. 40.1 Leukoaraiosis from chronic small vessel ischemia in a patient with a history of hypertension, hyperlipidemia, and heavy smoking

Multiinfarct Dementia

When learning about dementia subtypes, students are classically taught to identify vascular dementia as being of a stepwise cognitive decline. While this stepwise pattern is not seen with leukoaraiosis above (in which there is a gradual, progressive decline), it is indeed the pattern seen in multiinfarct dementia. In this syndrome, patients will show a sudden dropoff in cognitive function after a stroke, which will usually stabilize over months without further worsening until another stroke occurs.

Case 2: Multiinfarct Dementia
An 84-year-old woman presented to the emergency room with new, sudden-onset left-sided weakness. On exam, it was also noted that she was not looking toward the left. She previously had posterior circulation strokes causing visual field deficits with partial recovery, as well as a left thalamic stroke with right-sided numbness. These strokes had occurred over several years. After each stroke, there were combinations of visual, motor, sensory, and balance deficits, as well as initially mild but progressive levels of cognitive decline. The pattern was that after each stroke, there was a cognitive decline, which stabilized but then had a further decline after subsequent strokes. Ultimately, her cognitive function was severely impaired. Figure 40.2 shows two axial views on CT imaging performed several days after admission.

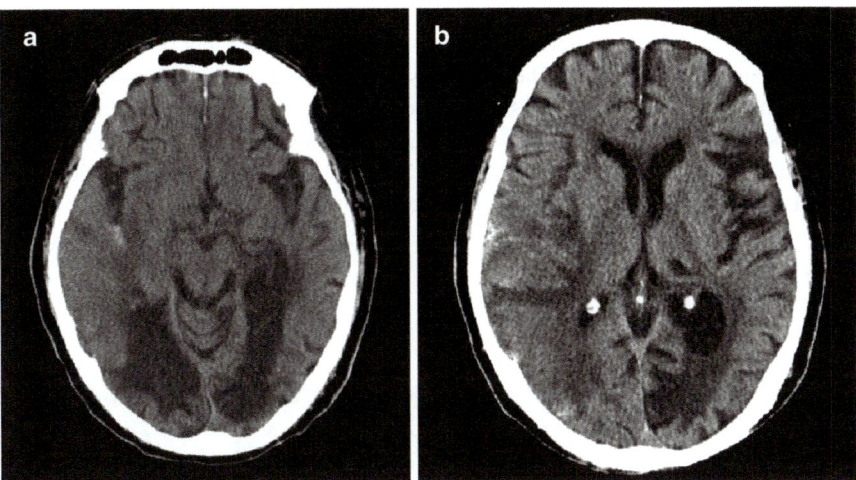

Fig. 40.2 Chronic bilateral posterior cerebral artery strokes (**a**), and bilateral middle cerebral artery and left thalamic strokes (**b**)

Case 3: Strategic Infarct

A 65-year-old man with a past medical history, including hypertension and hyperlipidemia, presented to the emergency room with a sudden onset of difficulty remembering conversations and names. Brain MRI revealed a focal infarction in the left anterior thalamus, part of the "circuit of Papez" subserving memory (Fig. 40.3). He had an initial decline immediately after the stroke, which remained stable over time with stable cognitive exams and abilities in instrumental activities of daily living.

Case 4: Strategic Infarct

A 70-year-old woman with a past medical history including diabetes, hypertension, hyperlipidemia, and smoking suddenly withdrew from conversation at the dinner table, not responding to others but still awake. She gradually appeared more drowsy, with occasional dysarthric utterances. She was taken to the emergency department, where she was following commands but with flat affect, without weakness or numbness in the extremities. She was able to speak in short phrases or sentences. Figure 40.4 shows the MRI of the brain (FLAIR sequences, axial views).

Over several years after these strokes, she did not have any further decline in behavior or memory. There were some improvements in the first few months, but she remained passive and only spoke when spoken to. She had occasional outbursts or impulsive behavior. Short-term memory was impaired, with rapid forgetting of conversations. She had poor attention and difficulty with executive function. Although these symptoms did not get progressively worse over several years, her cognitive behavioral status plateaued, and she never returned to her baseline.

Fig. 40.3 MRI FLAIR sequence with left anterior thalamic infarct (white arrow)

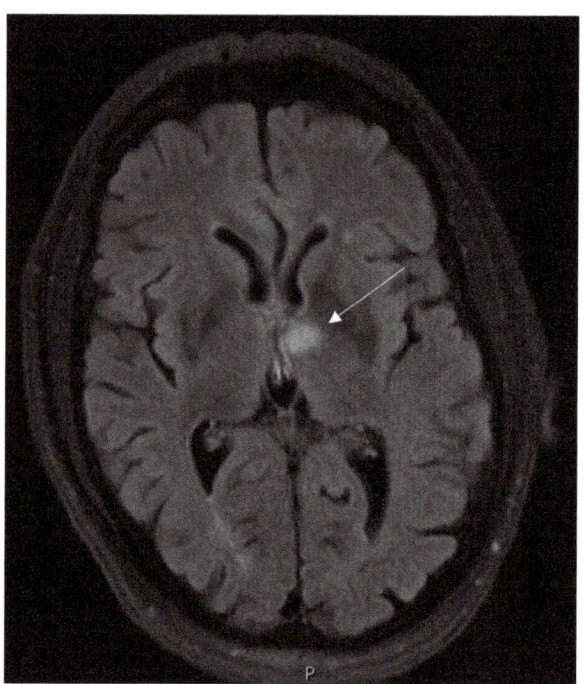

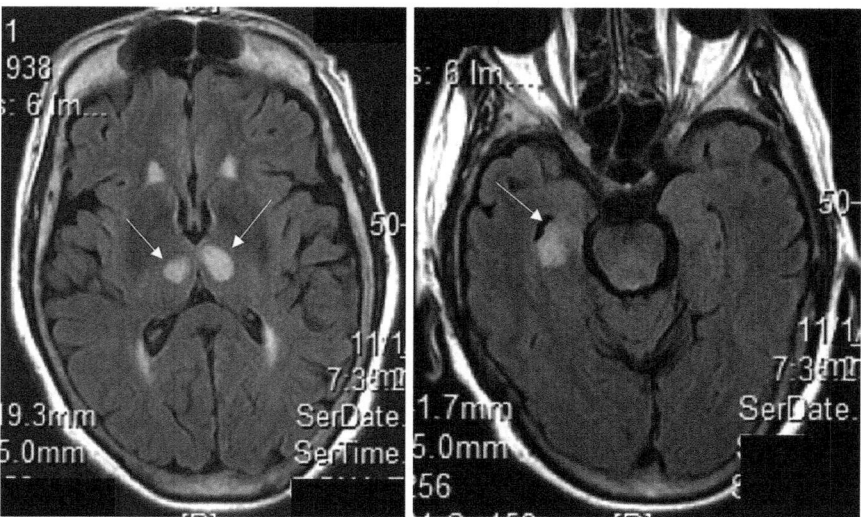

Fig. 40.4 Left: Bilateral thalamic infarcts involving dorsomedial nuclei, which have neurobehavioral functions related to motivation and impulse control. Right: Simultaneous infarct (via posterior circulation) in the right hippocampus, subserving episodic short-term memory

Strategic Infarct (or Hemorrhage)

A brain lesion caused by an infarct or hemorrhage, even of small size, can cause significant cognitive impairment if it occurs in a part of the brain involved in memory networks or other cognitive functions. Examples of these locations include the hippocampus or specific parts of the thalamus (there can be many other locations). Depending on the location, the patient may present with a sudden onset of short-term memory loss, cognitive slowing, or even behavioral changes. These infarcts can mimic other types of dementia, though the timeline and sudden onset would distinguish them from classic progressive, neurodegenerative disease.

Other Clinical Points

For individuals with multiple cerebrovascular/stroke risk factors, there may be more than one of the above subtypes of cognitive impairment occurring concurrently. For example, a single individual may have diffuse white matter disease, a strategically located lesion, or an accumulation of lacunar or larger-vessel infarctions. They may also demonstrate signs of Alzheimer dementia, leading to a mixed dementia picture.

Additionally, poststroke fatigue is a common but poorly understood symptom many patients face following a stroke [4]. Fatigue can hinder memory and cognition by interfering with attention and the ability to focus on encoding new information.

When an individual cannot concentrate on learning new information, they will have difficulty recalling it later. Fatigue can also impair the ability to perform daily living activities, adversely affecting patient autonomy and independence. This type of fatigue can be persistent and frustrating to manage.

Management and Prognosis

There are no disease-modifying treatments for vascular dementia. The crux of management is to aggressively control risk factors that would lead to further cerebrovascular disease. Care of these patients often requires a team approach, with close follow-up by primary care. It is essential to tightly manage blood pressure, glucose, and cholesterol levels. Additionally, all current smokers should be counseled on smoking cessation. Finally, polypharmacy and anticholinergic medications can cause further cognitive impairment, and a patient's current medications should routinely be reviewed for cognitive safety.

Regardless of diagnosis, all the patients should abide by a few pillars of cognitive health to strengthen their cognition and prevent future decline. These pillars include cardiovascular exercise, a Mediterranean-based diet, and regular cognitive and social stimulation [5]. Patients should aim for 150 min of moderate-intensity aerobic activity a week, such as brisk walking or swimming. The Mediterranean-based diet includes many critical components for cognitive health but also helps to limit the intake of salt, sugar, and cholesterol when followed closely. Proper diet and exercise help to mitigate vascular risk factors. Cognitive stimulation is critical to keep the brain engaged and functional. Patients should be encouraged to engage in any activity they enjoy, but examples include word games, puzzles, playing musical instruments, learning a new activity, and socializing.

Compensatory strategies are vital for optimizing memory and daily functioning. An organized home and life should be prioritized for patients. Utilizing calendars, notes, reminders, and alarms can ensure better daily functioning, even when a patient's memory fails them. As providers, we should break down complex information into easy-to-follow steps and provide verbal and written instructions for the patient to take home following clinic visits.

Finally, it is critical to optimize sleep and mental health. Most adults should aim for 7–9 h of sleep at night [6]. If a patient does not feel refreshed in the mornings or has daytime somnolence, they may need a formal sleep study to evaluate for OSA. Fatigue can significantly hinder memory and cognition. The same is true for anxiety and depression. Cognitively impaired patients should always be screened for anxiety and depression and treated when appropriate.

The first line of pharmacological treatments for Alzheimer's disease are the cholinesterase inhibitors. Briefly, Alzheimer's pathology is known to cause dysfunction of the neurotransmitter acetylcholine, and these drugs help to enhance cholinergic activity. The most common agents are donepezil or galantamine, though some patients better tolerate transdermal rivastigmine due to gastrointestinal side effects that can be common with oral donepezil. This class of drugs is initiated in the early stages of dementia. Memantine is often introduced at a moderate stage of dementia. None of these drugs are disease-modifying, though they can provide some symptomatic benefits and neuroprotection.

There is some research to support the utilization of these drugs in patients with vascular dementia [7]. Additionally, dementia can commonly be caused by co-occurring pathologies. For example, a patient with a classic vascular dementia presentation may concurrently have Alzheimer pathology, or develop it later in life. Moreover, cholinergic dysfunction has been demonstrated in vascular dementias [7].

It can be challenging to determine clinically if a patient is continuing to decline due to poor control of vascular risk factors or if they have developed a copathology. In these cases of continued cognitive decline, the initiation of cholinesterase inhibitors is a reasonable consideration [7]. At this time, there is less evidence in support of initiating memantine in this setting.

Poststroke fatigue is challenging to address as it is poorly understood. However, there are specific strategies to employ to optimize patient outcomes. Pharmacological stimulants such as modafinil are currently being investigated to promote wakefulness and improve functionality, though the routine use of these agents is not yet supported [8]. Differentiating depressed mood from fatigue is important, and we try to optimize mood as much as possible, often with the help of selective serotonin reuptake inhibitors (SSRIs) and cognitive behavioral therapy. Clinicians may also consider referring a patient with fatigue for a consultation with sleep medicine. Polysomnography may reveal sleep apnea or other treatable causes of inadequate sleep contributing to fatigue. Additionally, medication lists should be reviewed for drugs that can worsen fatigue. Nonpharmacological therapies are the foundation for treating fatigue. A tailored exercise regimen to improve fitness can help build endurance [9]. Patients should take steps to organize their day to allow breaks between physically or mentally demanding tasks. As providers, we can help by communicating this need to their employers and workplaces.

When to Refer to a Memory Specialist?

Dementias may be diagnosed and managed in primary care if the provider is familiar with the different clinical syndromes. Basic lab work can help rule out other causes, such as thyroid dysfunction or B12 insufficiency. MRI of the brain without contrast is often sufficient to assess for atrophy patterns and white matter change. An in-office neuropsychological screen (i.e., The Montreal Cognitive Assessment) can also help to evaluate MCI or basic patterns of cognitive decline. A referral to geriatric medicine is indicated when a patient needs a more comprehensive dementia assessment with other comorbid medical conditions related to aging. Examples include unintentional weight loss, shortness of breath, or management of polypharmacy in an elderly patient.

As previously described, many patients may have a mixed etiology dementia that can make the clinical presentation more complicated. To fully understand the cause of the cognitive change, a consultation with a cognitive neurology specialist may be warranted.

Clinical Pearls

- Vascular dementia is caused by reduced blood flow to the brain. It is more common in people with stroke risk factors like high blood pressure, high cholesterol, diabetes, smoking, sleep apnea, prior stroke, or transient ischemic attack.
- Vascular dementia has three subtypes: diffuse small vessel, multiinfarct larger vessel, and strategically located stroke.
- Not all cases of vascular dementia follow a stepwise pattern of cognitive decline. In cases of small vessel disease, the decline is gradual and slow.
- Treatment of vascular dementia is multidisciplinary, with aggressive management of all stroke risk factors, cardiovascular exercise, and making efforts to stay active from a mental and social standpoint.

Advanced diagnostics, such as specialized neuroimaging or cerebrospinal fluid analysis, can be used to determine if there is concern for Alzheimer's, FTD, or LBD pathologies. Making a definitive diagnosis is important regarding prognosis and education for the patient and family. Finally, early onset or rapidly progressive dementias should be referred to a cognitive neurology clinic for an urgent and thorough investigation.

Neuropsychology is a branch of psychology that deals with behavior, cognition, and brain health. Neuropsychological testing is a valuable assessment in which a neuropsychologist studies a patient's cognitive function during an hours-long visit with a selected battery of tests. The testing is quite rigorous, but it does not involve any invasive medical procedures. This type of testing may be requested as part of a patient's diagnostic workup with cognitive or behavioral changes. The pattern of an individual's cognitive strengths and weaknesses is established during testing. First, this pattern helps determine whether or not a patient has objective cognitive impairment and, if so, to what degree.

Additionally, the patterns demonstrated on testing often correlate to a suspected diagnosis. Neuropsychology assessment is an objective and valuable part of the diagnostic process. Paired with a detailed history and physical exam, bloodwork, and neuroimaging, it can help illuminate the processes behind a patient's cognitive symptoms. Notably, neuropsychologists do not prescribe medication or follow patients regularly (though retesting can be performed yearly if appropriate), so a patient should not expect to receive memory care from a neuropsychologist.

Unfortunately, many dementia patients suffer from increasing neuropsychiatric symptoms as their disease progresses. They may experience apathy, hallucinations, and paranoia. These symptoms amplify caregiver burden and quality of life for the patient. Specialty clinics such as cognitive neurology, geriatric psychiatry, and geriatric medicine are familiar with identifying and managing these symptoms to help improve the quality of life for the patient and caregivers. A social work consultation is of utmost importance in assisting the patient and family in navigating the psychosocial challenges as the dementia progresses.

References

1. Wolters FJ, Ikram MA. Epidemiology of vascular dementia. Arterioscler Thromb Vasc Biol. 2019;39(8):1542–9. https://doi.org/10.1161/atvbaha.119.311908.
2. Kane JPM, et al. Clinical prevalence of Lewy body dementia. Alzheimers Res Ther. 2018;10(1):19. https://doi.org/10.1186/s13195-018-0350-6.
3. Emmady PD, et al. Major neurocognitive disorder (dementia). StatPearls Publishing; 2023. http://www.ncbi.nlm.nih.gov/books/NBK557444/.
4. Acciarresi M, Bogousslavsky J, Paciaroni M. Post-stroke fatigue: epidemiology, clinical characteristics and treatment. Eur Neurol. 2014;72(5–6):255–61. https://doi.org/10.1159/000363763.
5. Dominguez LJ, et al. Nutrition, physical activity, and other lifestyle factors in the prevention of cognitive decline and dementia. Nutrients. 2021;13(11):4080. https://doi.org/10.3390/nu13114080.
6. Watson NF, Badr MS, Belenky G, et al. Recommended amount of sleep for a healthy adult: a joint consensus statement of the American Academy of Sleep Medicine and Sleep Research Society. Sleep. 2015;38(6):843–4.
7. Malouf R, Birks J. Donepezil for vascular cognitive impairment. Cochrane Database Syst Rev. 2004;(1):CD004395. https://doi.org/10.1002/14651858.CD004395.pub2.
8. Bivard A, Lillicrap T, Krishnamurthy V, et al. MIDAS (Modafinil in Debilitating Fatigue After Stroke): a randomized, double-blind, placebo-controlled. Cross-over trial. Stroke. 2017;48(5):1293–8. https://doi.org/10.1161/STROKEAHA.116.016293.
9. Passier PE, Post MW, van Zandvoort MJ, Rinkel GJ, Lindeman E, Visser-Meily JM. Predicting fatigue 1 year after aneurysmal subarachnoid hemorrhage. J Neurol. 2011;258(6):1091–7. https://doi.org/10.1007/s00415-010-5891-y.

Poststroke Epilepsy

41

Caitlin McElroy-Cox, Natalie Le-Blanc, and Pue Farooque

What Are Seizures and Epilepsy?

An epileptic **seizure** is "a transient occurrence of signs and/or symptoms due to abnormal excessive or synchronous neuronal activity in the brain" [1]. **Epilepsy** is diagnosed when an individual has at least two unprovoked seizures >24 h apart or one unprovoked seizure with risk factors such as epileptiform abnormalities on EEG, prior stroke or head trauma, significant brain imaging abnormality or nocturnal seizure, which predict a ≥60% risk of recurrence over the next 10 years [2, 3]. Seizures and epilepsy are significant potential sequelae after stroke, and stroke is the most common cause of seizures and epilepsy in older adults. Poststroke seizures occur in approximately 6–8% of adults after ischemic stroke, while the incidence is around 12% in those with hemorrhagic stroke [4, 5].

C. McElroy-Cox · N. Le-Blanc
Yale School of Medicine, New Haven, CT, USA
e-mail: caitlin.mcelroy-cox@yale.edu; natalie.m.leblanc@yale.edu

P. Farooque (✉)
NYU Grossman School of Medicine, New York, NY, USA
e-mail: pue.farooque@nyulangone.org

What Causes Seizures and Epilepsy After a Stroke?

The etiology of poststroke seizures and epilepsy is complex and multifactorial. Any injury which results in structural damage to the cerebral cortex is a risk factor for the development of seizures and epilepsy [6].

Stroke increases the risk of a seizure in the acute phase due to the metabolic changes and demands of neuronal hypoxia, which impair sodium and potassium ion pumps, altering cellular depolarization and cortical hyperexcitability. Chronic changes after stroke, including gliosis and scarring, can lead to disruption in neuronal networks, further increasing the risk of seizures, and hemorrhagic stroke confers additional risk due to cortical irritability caused by blood products, with hemosiderin deposition and scarring [7].

Acute post-stroke seizures have the potential to exacerbate the size and neurologic deficits related to the stroke itself, with increased metabolic stress worsening infarct size. This fact underscores the importance of recognizing and treating seizures after stroke [5].

Acute vs. Delayed Poststroke Seizures and Epilepsy

A large, prospective, multicenter study found that the overall incidence of seizures after stroke is 8.9%, with hemorrhagic stroke conferring greater risk than ischemic stroke (incidence of 10.6% in hemorrhagic stroke vs. 8.6% in ischemic stroke) [8]. Seizures occurring within the first 7 days after stroke are defined as **acute symptomatic seizures**. Individuals with acute symptomatic seizures are *not* considered to have epilepsy as these seizures are considered "provoked" by the toxic and metabolic effects of the stroke itself and, in a majority of cases, do not recur once the initial insult has resolved [4]. One large population-based study found that the 10-year risk of seizure recurrence after acute symptomatic seizure due to stroke is 33% [9].

By contrast, individuals with **delayed symptomatic seizures**, which occur greater than 7 days after stroke, have a >60% risk of seizure recurrence and are thus considered to have epilepsy [5]. Thus, individuals with delayed symptomatic seizures should be treated with long-term antiseizure medications to prevent seizure recurrence (treatment discussed later in the chapter). Refer to Fig. 41.1 for a guide to the management of poststroke seizures and epilepsy.

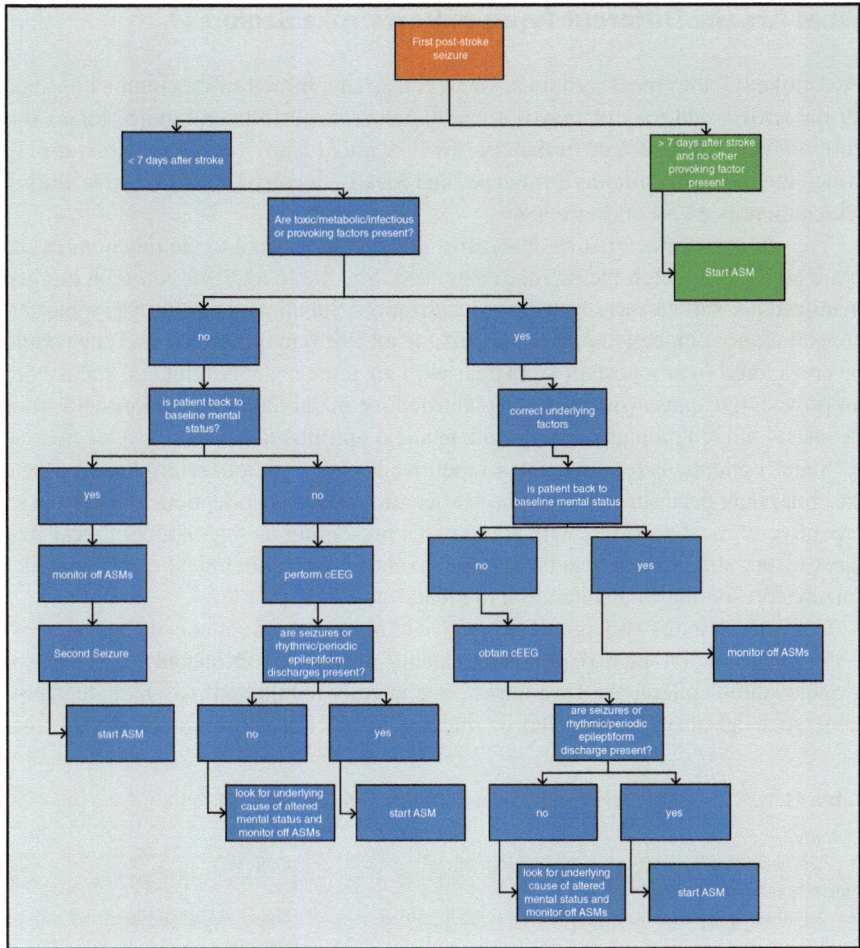

Fig. 41.1 Algorithm for managing poststroke seizures and epilepsy. All patients with a recent seizure should be counseled on not driving per local state law

What Are the Risk Factors for Developing Poststroke Seizures and Epilepsy?

Factors that increase the likelihood of acute symptomatic seizures after stroke include hemorrhagic stroke, ischemic stroke with hemorrhagic conversion, and alcohol intake [10]. Risk factors for the development of poststroke epilepsy include stroke severity/larger stroke volume, MCA distribution stroke, cortical involvement, large artery atherosclerosis, and early seizures after stroke [11].

What Are the Different Types of Poststroke Seizures?

Poststroke seizures most commonly are focal, arising from the brain region impacted by the stroke, and may or may not lead to generalized (bilateral tonic-clonic) seizures. Focal seizures can further be divided into focally aware seizures, during which the individual retains awareness, and focally impaired aware seizures, during which there is a loss of awareness.

The clinical characteristics of seizures are directly related to the functions of the brain area from which the seizure originated. See Table 41.1 for common clinical manifestations of seizures by area of localization. Subclinical or electrographic seizures (i.e., not clinically apparent but visible on EEG) may also occur. They should be considered in any poststroke patient with an acute change in mental status with no provocative cause (infection, hypotension, or metabolic/toxic abnormalities) or persistent altered mental status despite medical optimization.

Status epilepticus (continuous or repetitive seizures without return to neurologic baseline) may occur in the acute phase after stroke. Status epilepticus can present as repetitive clinical seizures, with some cases presenting as fluctuating clinical features of the stroke or as repetitive nonconvulsive (i.e., subclinical electrographic) seizures presenting as an alteration in mental status [12].

Convulsive status epilepticus (repetitive clinically apparent convulsive seizures) occurs in about 1% of patients with ischemic stroke [13]. Nonconvulsive/electrographic status epilepticus, by contrast, is clinically subtle and may include symptoms such as apathy, somnolence, fluctuation in consciousness, confusion, and

Table 41.1 Common clinical manifestations of seizures by area of localization

Frontal	*Temporal*
• "Hypermotor" activity such as rocking, bicycling movements, pelvic thrusting	• Déjà vu
• Asymmetric tonic limb posturing—"Fencer" position	• Unprovoked sudden fear/anxiety
• Forced head and eye deviation	• Sudden onset of unusual taste or smell
• Prominent vocalizations (screaming, swearing)	• Rising abdominal sensation
• Bizarre behavior	• Behavioral arrest and impaired awareness
• Quick to return to baseline	• Lip smacking/chewing
• Can be nocturnal	• Manual automatisms
	• Dystonic posturing of limb
	• Postictal confusion or agitation
Occipital	*Parietal*
• Positive visual phenomena such as multicolored shapes or flashes	• Paresthesias
• Negative phenomena (loss of part of the visual field)	• Disorientation or depth misperception
• Formed visual hallucinations	• Visual hallucination
• Nystagmus	• Receptive language impairment
• Eyelid closure or eye flutter	• Rotatory body movements
	• Somatic illusions

behavioral disorders, and requires EEG for definitive diagnosis (in other words, you may not know the patient is having seizures until you obtain an EEG) [14]. In one study, 3.6% of patients admitted to the hospital for stroke were found to have non-convulsive/electrographic status epilepticus on EEG [12].

Role of EEG in Diagnosing Poststroke Seizures and Epilepsy

The electroencephalogram (EEG) is a noninvasive test that is the gold standard for diagnosing seizures and epilepsy. Common EEG terms are defined in Table 41.2. EEG can be used to determine if clinical events are seizures and confirm the presence or absence of electrographic seizures or interictal (between seizure) epileptiform patterns [15]. If seizures are clinically suspected, an EEG may be helpful to confirm the diagnosis; however, the absence of epileptiform patterns or interictal discharges does not rule out clinical seizures if the event in question is not captured and should not alter management if seizures are strongly suspected on a clinical basis [16]. EEG is particularly helpful in risk stratification for individuals with acute-symptomatic seizures. There is a lack of consensus recommendations regarding the duration of antiseizure medicine treatment for these patients. In patients who continue to have interictal epileptiform abnormalities on EEG or electrographic seizures on EEG months after the acute stroke, ASMs should likely be continued long term. EEG is also an important part of the work-up in a patient who develop altered mental status to evaluate for nonconvulsive/electrographic status epilepticus or seizures as a contributory factor for the alteration in mental status [17].

In the inpatient setting, continuous EEG recording may be used both to determine the presence of seizures and to evaluate response to treatment. In the outpatient setting, ambulatory or home video EEG can be performed for 24–72 h to assess for epileptiform patterns or seizures.

Table 41.2 Basic EEG terminology

Ictal: Seizure

Interictal: In-between seizures

Epileptiform discharge: Defined as sharps, polyspike-wave, and spike-wave occurring in the form of a single discharge or burst. Sometimes used interchangeably as "interictal discharges" and "interictal epileptiform discharges"

Routine EEG: 20–30 min

Prolonged EEG: 1–2 h

Continuous EEG: >2 h

Ambulatory EEG: An outpatient EEG recording, usually for 24–72 h

Home video EEG: An EEG recording at home accompanied by video. Can record up to 72 h or more

Common EEG Findings in Patients with Poststroke Seizures and Epilepsy

Focal slowing is a common, nonspecific finding that does not suggest epilepsy and, hence, should not be treated. Interictal epileptiform discharges such as sharps or spikes, BIRDs (brief ictal rhythmic discharges), LPDs (lateralized periodic discharges), or LRDA (lateralized rhythmic delta activity) suggest a high risk for seizure recurrence. Patients with these EEG findings should be treated with antiseizure medications, which should be titrated to stop clinical or electrographic seizures (not the interictal epileptiform patterns).

Treatment Options

The primary treatment for PSE is antiseizure medications (ASMs, previously referred to as anticonvulsants or antiepileptic drugs), of which there are over 30 to choose from [18]. With a multitude of options, selecting the right ASM can be a daunting task. However, following a few fundamental principles will help guide your choice. Many of the guidelines in choosing ASMs for other causes of epilepsy can be applied to PSE treatment while keeping in mind the cardio-/cerebrovascular risk factors, aging demographic, and drug-drug interactions inherent in this population.

ASMs can be categorized into first-generation (older) and second-generation (newer) drugs and chronologically before and after the early 1990s. The first-generation ASMs are all effective but tend to have more unfavorable side effects and many drug-drug interactions, making tolerability challenging, particularly in the PSE population [19]. Second-generation ASMs have similar efficacy as first-generation drugs but better safety and tolerability profiles, making them more appealing as a drug group.

How Do You Choose an ASM?

There is no definitive evidence to suggest the superiority of any single ASM for the treatment of poststroke epilepsy. The choice of ASM will depend on several key factors, including each agent's side effect profile, ease of administration, patient comorbidities, pharmacokinetics/drug-drug interactions, and cost and accessibility of the ASM to the patient. When titrating ASMs, it is always best to go slow and aim for the lowest effective and tolerated dose. Treatment with a single agent with minimal drug-to-drug interactions, minimal or no adverse effects, and one that either treats or does not exacerbate other comorbidities is preferable.

ASMs are also classified as broad and narrow-spectrum agents. Broad-spectrum ASMs may be used for individuals with either a generalized epilepsy syndrome (seizure onset involving the whole brain) or focal-onset seizures. In contrast, narrow-spectrum ASMs are appropriate for individuals with focal-onset seizures. For poststroke seizures and PSE, most seizures are of focal onset (>66%), and either broad or narrow-spectrum agents may be used [20].

We will briefly review some well-known side effect profiles of some ASM (see Table 41.3 for a complete list). Valproic acid can cause thrombocytopenia or platelet dysfunction, which can be detrimental in the setting of comorbid hepatic diseases, hematological conditions, or anti-platelet therapy. In a patient with hemorrhagic stroke, it may worsen the volume of hemorrhage due to its effects on platelets and

Table 41.3 Common ASM side effects and clinical considerations

	Side effects	Clinical considerations
Older generation		
Carbamazepine (CBZ)	• Dizziness/ataxia • Nystagmus • Hyponatremia • Osteoporosis • Leukopenia	• Good for focal seizures/epilepsy that may secondarily generalize • Avoid if liver failure • Can increase serum levels of lipids and other biochemical markers of vascular disease • Potent enzyme inducer → affecting oral contraceptives, warfarin, and many other drugs. Less interaction with direct oral anticoagulants (DOACs) • May accumulate when given with inhibitors of CYP3A4 and grapefruit juice • Mood stabilizer
Phenobarbital (PB)	• Sedation • Osteoporosis • Cognitive slowing	• Good for focal seizures/epilepsy that may secondarily generalize • Many drug-drug interactions can increase serum levels of lipids and other biochemical markers of vascular disease • Do not use if liver failure • IV formulation available
Phenytoin (PHT)	• Dizziness/ataxia • Nausea • Nystagmus • Osteoporosis	• Good for focal seizures/epilepsy that may secondarily generalize • Many drug-drug interactions can increase serum levels of lipids and other biochemical markers of vascular disease • Do not use if liver failure • Protein-bound, so check free levels along with phenytoin levels • IV formulation available (IV fosphenytoin, a prodrug, has less cardiotoxicity)
Valproate (VPA)	• Hyperammonemia • Tremor • Weight gain • Hair loss	• Good for both focal and generalized seizures/epilepsy • Potent inhibitor → reduces the clearance of certain ASMs: PB, LTG, CBZ, and other drugs requiring a reduction in dosing. Less interaction with direct oral anticoagulants (DOACs) • Can cause thrombocytopenia and increase bleeding time; avoid in acute hemorrhage patients • Mood stabilizer • IV formulation available
Newer generation		
Clobazam (CLB)	• Sedation	• Good for both focal and generalized seizures/epilepsy • Use with opioids can cause profound sedation • Use lower doses in older adults

(continued)

Table 41.3 (continued)

	Side effects	Clinical considerations
Lacosamide (LCM)	• Dizziness/ataxia	• Good for both focal and generalized seizures/epilepsy • Can be pro-arrhythmic (prolonged P-R interval); check baseline EKG and again at therapeutic dose • IV formulation available
Lamotrigine (LTG)	• Dizziness/ataxia • Nausea • Nystagmus • Potential for higher risk for arrhythmia in certain patient populations • Steven Johnson Syndrome	• Good for both focal and generalized seizures/epilepsy • Slow initiation schedule (~8 weeks) to reach the maintenance dose • Estrogen (OCP) and pregnancy increase LTG clearance • Lowest teratogenicity • Mood stabilizer • Extended-release formulation may require prior authorization, given that it is costlier than immediate-release • Do not use in 2nd- and 3rd-degree heart block, Brugada syndrome, arrhythmogenic ventricular cardiomyopathy (ARVC), left bundle branch block (LBBB), and right bundle branch block (RBBB) with left anterior or posterior fascicular block
Levetiracetam (LEV)	• Overall, well tolerated but can cause sedation	• Good for both focal and generalized seizures/epilepsy • Decrease dose in patients with renal failure and ensure they receive a dose post dialysis • Can exacerbate mood disorders, behavioral problems, and irritability • IV formulation available
Oxcarbazepine (OXC)	• Dizziness/ataxia • Nausea • Nystagmus • Hyponatremia (more than carbamazepine)	• Good for focal seizures/epilepsy that may secondarily generalize
Pregabalin (PGB)	• May worsen myoclonus or absence seizures • Edema • Weight gain	• Good for focal seizures/epilepsy
Topiramate (TPM)	• Cognitive slowing—dose-dependent • Weight loss • Paresthesia in hands and feet • Oligohidrosis • Kidney stones	• Good for both focal and generalized seizures/epilepsy • Migraine prophylaxis • Hydration is recommended to reduce kidney stones (calcium phosphate) • In renal impairment, use ½ dose and supplement after hemodialysis
Zonisamide (ZNS)	• Dizziness/ataxia • Weight loss • Kidney stones	• Good for both focal and generalized seizures/epilepsy • Hydration is recommended to reduce kidney stones (calcium phosphate)

should be avoided in this patient population. Oxcarbazepine and carbamazepine can cause clinically significant hyponatremia, especially in older individuals. Mild leukopenia can also rarely be seen with carbamazepine use. Bone health is important, particularly in the aging population, and most first-generation ASMs lead to an increased risk of osteopenia or osteoporosis through their enzyme-inducing properties and impairment of vitamin D metabolism. This leads to an increased risk of fracture from falls in a population that already has limited mobility and is at higher risk of falls due to their neurologic deficits. Carbamazepine, phenytoin, phenobarbital, and primidone can increase serum levels of lipids and other biochemical markers of vascular disease, rendering their use in this patient population counterproductive [21].

Levetiracetam (LEV, brand name: Keppra) and lacosamide (brand name: Vimpat) are the two second-generation ASMs that can be given intravenously and converted to oral administration. Both are reasonable first-line treatment options, particularly when rapid administration is required, as in status epilepticus [7]. However, individual comorbidities and side effect profiles must be carefully considered, particularly in long-term therapy. Levetiracetam can cause or worsen mood disturbances and thus may be inappropriate for long-term use in patients with a history of mood disorder. Lacosamide can prolong the P-R interval on an EKG, which can lead to first-degree or higher heart block and should be used with caution in patients with cardiac arrhythmias.

Some ASMs have properties that may help treat other conditions besides epilepsy. Valproic acid, lamotrigine, carbamazepine, oxcarbazepine, and pregabalin all have mood-stabilizing or anxiolytic properties, which may be beneficial in patients with a history of depression or anxiety. Pregabalin, oxcarbazepine, and carbamazepine may be appropriate agents for patients who also have neuropathic pain. Topiramate and zonisamide are used as mainstay treatments in migraine management and thus may be beneficial in this patient population. Please refer to the AES 2020 ASMs Chart for further indications and details.

Pharmacokinetics and drug-drug interactions must be carefully considered in the post-ischemic or hemorrhagic stroke population. For example, some studies have shown a marked reduction of plasma concentration of nimodipine, a drug commonly used to prevent vasospasm in subarachnoid hemorrhage, with concurrent use of **enzyme-inducing** agents such as phenytoin, phenobarbital, and carbamazepine. In contrast, when administered with an **enzyme-inhibiting** agent such as valproic acid, serum concentrations of nimodipine can increase by 50% [22]. The same principle can be applied to patients being anticoagulated with warfarin, in which higher doses of warfarin would be required to maintain therapeutic INR when coadministered with enzyme-inducing ASMs and conversely lower doses when given with enzyme-inhibiting agents. However, some studies suggest these same drug-drug interactions are less severe with direct oral anticoagulants (DOACs), rendering a better treatment combination for patients with atrial fibrillation [23].

Finally, it is always essential to consider socioeconomic barriers and the cost of ASMs. No matter how ideal a drug is, it will be of no benefit if the patient cannot get it or afford it. Immediate-release and generic formulations are typically more cost-effective than long-acting or brand-name drugs. Exploring pharmacy assistance programs and reviewing insurance coverage or pharmacy prices before initiating any new ASM regimen is paramount in ensuring patients' adherence to the medication regimen.

Lifestyle Counseling

Patients living with epilepsy should be advised to exercise certain safety precautions to help prevent or reduce the risk of recurrent seizures. All people with epilepsy should be counseled about the importance of medication adherence and avoidance of factors that may lower the seizure threshold, such as excessive alcohol use and sleep deprivation. It is essential to underscore the potential for drug-drug interactions and counsel that the use of several common medications, including diphenhydramine, tramadol, and bupropion, may lower the seizure threshold and should be avoided when possible.

Patients taking antiseizure medications should check with their providers before starting new prescriptions or over-the-counter medications to ensure no interaction or contraindication exists. Anxiety and depression are common in people living with epilepsy, and individuals should be regularly screened for these conditions and referred to mental health providers when appropriate. Women of childbearing age should be counseled on the relative safety or potential for teratogenicity of the ASM they are taking and potential interactions with contraceptive agents.

Counseling on Driving After a Seizure

States vary in their guidance on driving following a seizure. States also have very different guidelines on whether providers are mandated to report people with epilepsy to the Department of Motor Vehicles. Please refer to your own state's guidelines for these issues. The Epilepsy Foundation website (www.epilepsy.com) is helpful for obtaining this information. In general, patients may require anywhere from 3 to 12 months of freedom from any spells causing alteration in awareness before resuming driving.

When Can You Discontinue ASMs?

The diagnosis of poststroke epilepsy will require long-term treatment with ASMs. For acute symptomatic post-stroke seizures, evidence-based guidance for when a patient should discontinue ASMs remains unclear. Several factors impact this decision, including individual patient risk factors, MRI, and EEG findings. Many centers are now running postacute symptomatic seizure clinics to gather data and help inform future guidelines about the appropriate use and discontinuation of ASMs in this population.

Who Can See a General Neurologist? Who Should See an Epileptologist?

Patients with well-controlled seizures can follow up with a general neurologist or neurology specialist Advanced Practice Clinician, while patients with refractory seizures should be referred to an epilepsy clinic.

Clinical Scenario 1
Sixty-seven-year-old right-handed male with a history of coronary artery disease s/p percutaneous coronary intervention and stent on ticagrelor, atrial fibrillation on warfarin, and L MCA stroke experienced first focal seizure 4 months post-stroke. He also complains of neuropathy in the affected right side of his body.

Treatment considerations:

Monotherapy treatment with Keppra is an ideal first choice given its minimal drug-to-drug interaction profile, absence of mood disturbances in the patient's history, and broad spectrum coverage for focal and generalized epilepsy. Pregabalin would also be a reasonable choice for the treatment of both seizures and neuropathy.

Avoiding ASMs with high drug-to-drug interactions such as phenobarbital, phenytoin, and carbamazepine is important as this patient is on warfarin, and treatment with those medications can lead to liability in INR levels. Valproic is also not an ideal choice given the potential of thrombocytopenia while also on antiplatelet treatment, nor are sodium channel blocking agents given their procardiac arrhythmia potential.

Clinical Scenario 2
A 55-year-old left-handed female with a history of anxiety, depression, prior suicidal ideation, and breast cancer in remission experienced difficulties managing her financial affairs and forgetting personal appointments approximately 12 months following a right frontal lobe stroke. A repeat MRI brain demonstrated encephalomalacia in the area of the infarct, and a 24-h EEG revealed frequent nocturnal electrographic seizures arising from the right frontal region.

Treatment considerations:

Given the patient's significant psychiatric comorbidities, levetiracetam would not be an ideal choice. Due to the focal nature of the seizure onset, narrow-spectrum agents such as oxcarbazepine or lacosamide would be appropriate options. Lamotrigine would be an excellent option, given its' mood-stabilizing properties, but titration takes weeks, making this less optimal in someone with frequent seizures. Clobazam is also a good choice for its nighttime dosing, which will help optimize coverage for her nocturnal seizures.

Clinical Pearls

- Acute symptomatic seizures occur within 7 days of a stroke and do not require long-term treatment with ASMs.
- Seizures occurring more than 7 days after stroke meet the criteria for epilepsy, necessitating long-term treatment with an ASM.
- Risk factors for poststroke epilepsy include larger stroke size, hemorrhagic stroke or hemorrhagic conversion of ischemic stroke, MCA territory stroke, younger age, and acute symptomatic seizures.
- EEG is the gold standard for diagnosing seizures and epilepsy and can help clarify the diagnosis or stratify the risk of seizure recurrence.
- Continuous EEG should be utilized for hospitalized patients that have altered mental status not attributable to provocative factors (infection, hypotension, or metabolic/toxic abnormalities) to ensure seizures are not a contributory factor to their altered mentation.
- Initial ASM selection should ideally have minimal drug-to-drug interactions and a favorable side effect profile that either treats or does not exacerbate the patient's other comorbidities.
- Levetiracetam or lacosamide may be a good first choice in the inpatient setting due to ease of administration and ability to convert from IV to PO. Still, their side effect profiles should be carefully considered, especially when transitioning from acute to long-term treatment.

Supplemental Information

References

1. Fisher RS, van Emde Boas W, Blume W, Elger C, Genton P, Lee P, Engel J Jr. Epileptic seizures and epilepsy: definitions proposed by the International League Against Epilepsy (ILAE) and the International Bureau for Epilepsy (IBE). Epilepsia. 2005;46(4):470–2. https://doi.org/10.1111/j.0013-9580.2005.66104.x.
2. Rizvi S, Ladino LD, Hernandez-Ronquillo L, Téllez-Zenteno JF. Epidemiology of early stages of epilepsy: risk of seizure recurrence after a first seizure. Seizure. 2017;49:46–53. https://doi.org/10.1016/j.seizure.2017.02.006. Epub 2017 Feb 14.
3. Fisher RS, Acevedo C, Arzimanoglou A, Bogacz A, Cross JH, Elger CE, Engel J Jr, Forsgren L, French JA, Glynn M, Hesdorffer DC, Lee BI, Mathern GW, Moshé SL, Perucca E, Scheffer IE, Tomson T, Watanabe M, Wiebe S. ILAE official report: a practical clinical definition of epilepsy. Epilepsia. 2014;55(4):475–82. https://doi.org/10.1111/epi.12550. Epub 2014 Apr 14.
4. Galovic M, Ferreira-Atuesta C, Abraira L, Döhler N, Sinka L, Brigo F, Bentes C, Zelano J, Koepp MJ. Seizures and epilepsy after stroke: epidemiology, biomarkers and management. Drugs Aging. 2021;38(4):285–99. https://doi.org/10.1007/s40266-021-00837-7. Epub 2021 Feb 23.
5. Ferreira-Atuesta C, Döhler N, Erdélyi-Canavese B, Felbecker A, Siebel P, Scherrer N, Bicciato G, Schweizer J, Sinka L, Imbach LL, Katan M, Abraira L, Santamarina E, Álvarez-Sabín J, Winklehner M, von Oertzen TJ, Wagner JN, Gigli GL, Serafini A, Janes F, Merlino G, Valente M, Gregoraci G, Conrad J, Evers S, Lochner P, Roell F, Brigo F, Bentes C, Peralta AR, Melo TPE, Keezer MR, Duncan JS, Sander JW, Tettenborn B, Koepp MJ, Galovic M. Seizures after ischemic stroke: a matched multicenter study. Ann Neurol. 2021;90(5):808–20. https://doi.org/10.1002/ana.26212. Epub 2021 Sep 30.

6. Scheffer IE, Berkovic S, Capovilla G, Connolly MB, French J, Guilhoto L, Hirsch E, Jain S, Mathern GW, Moshé SL, Nordli DR, Perucca E, Tomson T, Wiebe S, Zhang YH, Zuberi SM. ILAE classification of the epilepsies: position paper of the ILAE Commission for Classification and Terminology. Epilepsia. 2017;58(4):512–21. https://doi.org/10.1111/epi.13709. Epub 2017 Mar 8.

7. Doria JW, Forgacs PB. Incidence, implications, and management of seizures following ischemic and hemorrhagic stroke. Curr Neurol Neurosci Rep. 2019;19(7):37. https://doi.org/10.1007/s11910-019-0957-4.

8. Bladin CF, Alexandrov AV, Bellavance A, et al. Seizures after stroke: a prospective multicenter study. Arch Neurol. 2000;57(11):1617–22. https://doi.org/10.1001/archneur.57.11.1617.

9. Hesdorffer DC, Benn EKT, Cascino GD, Hauser WA. Is a first acute symptomatic seizure epilepsy? Mortality and risk for recurrent seizure. Epilepsia. 2009;50:1102–8. https://doi.org/10.1111/j.1528-1167.2008.01945.x.

10. Zhang C, Wang X, Wang Y, Zhang JG, Hu W, Ge M, Zhang K, Shao X. Risk factors for poststroke seizures: a systematic review and meta-analysis. Epilepsy Res. 2014;108(10):1806–16. https://doi.org/10.1016/j.eplepsyres.2014.09.030. Epub 2014 Oct 13.

11. Galovic M, Döhler N, Erdélyi-Canavese B, Felbecker A, Siebel P, Conrad J, Evers S, Winklehner M, von Oertzen TJ, Haring HP, Serafini A, Gregoraci G, Valente M, Janes F, Gigli GL, Keezer MR, Duncan JS, Sander JW, Koepp MJ, Tettenborn B. Prediction of late seizures after ischaemic stroke with a novel prognostic model (the SeLECT score): a multivariable prediction model development and validation study. Lancet Neurol. 2018;17(2):143–52. https://doi.org/10.1016/S1474-4422(17)30404-0.

12. Belcastro V, Vidale S, Gorgone G, et al. Non-convulsive status epilepticus after ischemic stroke: a hospital-based stroke cohort study. J Neurol. 2014;261:2136–42.

13. Rumbach L, Sablot D, Berger E, Tatu L, Vuillier F, Moulin T. Status epilepticus in stroke: report on a hospital-based stroke cohort. Neurology. 2000;54:350–4.

14. Özaydın Göksu E, Genç F, Atiş N, Bıçer Gömceli Y. Early and late-onset nonconvulsive status epilepticus after stroke. Arq Neuropsiquiatr. 2021;79(5):384–9. https://doi.org/10.1590/0004-282X-ANP-2020-0018.

15. Rosenow F, Klein KM, Hamer HM. Non-invasive EEG evaluation in epilepsy diagnosis. Expert Rev Neurother. 2015;15(4):425–44. https://doi.org/10.1586/14737175.2015.1025382.

16. Smith SJM. EEG in the diagnosis, classification, and management of patients with epilepsy. J Neurol Neurosurg Psychiatry. 2005;76:ii2–7.

17. Punia V, Honomichl R, Chandan P, Ellison L, Thompson N, Sivaraju A, Katzan I, George P, Newey C, Hantus S. Long-term continuation of anti-seizure medications after acute stroke. Ann Clin Transl Neurol. 2021;8:1857–66. https://doi.org/10.1002/acn3.51440.

18. Löscher W, Klein P. The pharmacology and clinical efficacy of antiseizure medications: from bromide salts to cenobamate and beyond. CNS Drugs. 2021;35(9):935–63. https://doi.org/10.1007/s40263-021-00827-8. Epub 2021 Jun 18. Erratum in: CNS Drugs. 2021 Aug 17.

19. Perucca E, Brodie MJ, Kwan P, Tomson T. 30 Years of second-generation antiseizure medications: impact and future perspectives. Lancet Neurol. 2020;19(6):544–56. https://doi.org/10.1016/S1474-4422(20)30035-1.

20. Bryndziar T, Sedova P, Kramer NM, et al. Seizures following ischemic stroke: frequency of occurrence and impact on outcome in a long-term population-based study. J Stroke Cerebrovasc Dis. 2016;25(1):150–6. https://doi.org/10.1016/j.jstrokecerebrovasdis.2015.09.008.

21. Zelano J, Holtkamp M, Agarwal N, Lattanzi S, Trinka E, Brigo F. How to diagnose and treat post-stroke seizures and epilepsy. Epileptic Disord. 2020;22(3):252–63. https://doi.org/10.1684/epd.2020.1159.

22. Mahmoud SH, Ji X, Isse FA. Nimodipine pharmacokinetic variability in various patient populations. Drugs R D. 2020;20:307–18. https://doi.org/10.1007/s40268-020-00322-3.

23. Ho CJ, Chen SH, Lin CH, Lu YT, Hsu CW, Tsai MH. Non-vitamin K oral anticoagulants and anti-seizure medications: a retrospective cohort study. Front Neurol. 2021;11:588053. https://doi.org/10.3389/fneur.2020.588053.

Returning to Work and Driving

42

Samantha Salas and Hardik P. Amin

Returning to Driving

Driving remains a common means of transportation for elderly patients. Operating a car does not take much thought or effort when someone has been driving most of their life. Driving a car, however, is quite complex. When on the road, a driver is bombarded with multiple stimuli requiring quick responses (traffic lights/signs, pedestrians, weather, other drivers, and other passengers in the car). The driver should have an unobstructed view of the entire road ahead and remain alert to quickly process any stimuli they encounter. This allows them to make decisions rapidly, such as turning swiftly, applying the brakes, or swerving to avoid unexpected obstacles on the road. Drivers should also be able to adjust their driving routes if needed. If an issue arises on the road, a driver should be able to communicate with others reasonably well.

After a stroke, patients may experience various deficits that can affect their ability to drive safely. Some of these deficits are obvious, such as hemiparesis or ataxia. Others may be less apparent, such as speech abnormalities, cognitive symptoms, visual field cuts, sensory changes, neglect, or fatigue. Therefore, it is essential to consider all these factors when discussing the resumption of driving after a stroke. We will discuss common poststroke deficits and how they factor into driving.

S. Salas
Stanford Health, Stanford, CA, USA
e-mail: samanthasalas@stanfordhealthcare.org

H. P. Amin (✉)
Department of Neurology, Hartford Hospital, Hartford, CT, USA
e-mail: hardik.amin@hhchealth.org

H. P. Amin (ed.), *Stroke for the Advanced Practice Clinician*,
https://doi.org/10.1007/978-3-031-66289-8_42

Vision

Brainstem strokes can lead to gaze palsies causing double vision and problems with depth perception. This is likely to improve with time and therapy. Occipital lobe strokes can lead to a visual field deficit called homonymous hemianopia, leading to a "blackout" of either the entire right or left visual field of *both* eyes. The normal visual field is about 180° in the horizontal plane with both eyes open. A homonymous hemianopia essentially cuts the visual field down to around 90°. A constricted visual field is critical to identify because most states in the US require a minimum visual field of 110°–140° in the horizontal plane to drive. Some states do not have a visual field requirement, and you can confirm by checking with your state's Department of Motor Vehicles (DMV) website. An ophthalmologist can perform a formal visual field assessment to clear someone to drive from a visual standpoint. Minor visual field improvements can occur within the first few months after stroke. However, most patients will have some degree of lasting visual field deficit.

Patients with a "quadrantanopsia" may have an upper or lower pie-shaped wedge of vision loss instead of the complete hemifield. In this case, the visual field requirement may still be met and should be evaluated by an ophthalmologist. The visual field requirement may also still be met for patients with monocular vision loss, but states may have more specific acuity requirements for the one functional eye. Visual neglect occurs due to a stroke in the right parietal lobe. In this condition, a patient can identify a stimulus in each temporal field when tested individually. However, when multiple stimuli are presented simultaneously in both the right and left temporal fields, the patient will only identify the stimulus in the right hemifield. Visual neglect can resolve over several months but requires repeat testing.

Sensory Neglect or Anosognosia

Neglect is defined as a lack of *awareness* of an entire half of a patient's world. Anosognosia is a lack of *insight* into one's illness or impairment. These deficits can make rehabilitation and driving quite tricky. Fortunately, neglect tends to improve earlier than most other stroke symptoms, and a trained physical and occupational therapist can evaluate if there are ongoing issues.

Motor Impairments

Patients with hemiparesis, dysmetria, or ataxia may still drive with adaptive equipment. Spinner knobs can be placed on steering wheels for patients with unilateral arm weakness. Left foot accelerators are available for those with right-sided weakness and sensory or coordination difficulty. Hand controls can be considered for those with difficulty moving both legs. The Rapid Pace Walk is a good indicator of proprioception, lower extremity strength, and mobility, where a patient is timed by the total number of seconds it takes to walk 10 ft and back. Scores of longer than 9 s may indicate a greater risk of at-fault motor vehicle accidents [1].

Sensory Symptoms

Patients who experience severe sensory loss may struggle with operating various car components, such as the steering wheel, gear shift, and mirrors. Although they might still be able to drive despite this impairment, understanding how to adapt to sensory loss is essential.

Cognitive Symptoms

Patients or families may report difficulties with memory following a stroke. This could be a sign that other cognitive symptoms might also be present. Cognitive function includes memory, executive function, visuospatial orientation, attention, calculation, language/naming, and abstraction. These can be assessed with the Montreal Cognitive Assessment (MOCA) screen in the office. The test takes a few minutes and includes exercises evaluating these cognitive realms. A normal score would be ≥26/30. Include the patient's education level and emotional state during the assessment (anxiety might affect their answers). Remember that the MOCA is only a screening test and should not be used for diagnostic purposes. It also cannot predict an individual's driving abilities. The MOCA should be used alongside patient and family reports as an additional source of information. If there is a suggestion of cognitive impairment, a referral for a formal neuropsychological evaluation would be prudent before any driving assessments.

Seizures

Seizures are a known complication following a stroke. Patients who are diagnosed with poststroke epilepsy should be maintained on long-term antiseizure medications. Patients with frequent seizures, despite medical management, should not drive. Patients who are being treated by a trained neurologist and are seizure-free can usually resume driving. Refer to individual state regulations on driving following a seizure.

Medications

Common medications that might affect the driving ability of older stroke patients include antihypertensives, hypoglycemics, and anticholinergics. Patients with seizures or mood disorders might be prescribed anticonvulsants, benzodiazepines, antidepressants, or antipsychotics, and those with pain issues might be prescribed narcotics. These medications can all lead to sedation, dizziness, and impaired cognition. It is important to know any medications that might affect driving ability.

Screening Tools

There are no validated tools to predict on-road driving performance. The Stroke Drivers Screening Assessment has been adopted in several countries worldwide. However, it can be time-consuming and should not be the sole determinant of a patient's ability to drive. Asking about driving history, reviewing medications, checking visual fields and acuity, and using a cognitive screen like the Montreal Cognitive Assessment (MoCA) and the Rapid Pace Walk can help identify red flags. If the clinical picture and screening assessment demonstrate concerning findings, the patient should be referred to a driving rehabilitation specialist for a comprehensive driving evaluation.

Driving Evaluations

On-the-road driving evaluations performed by certified driving rehabilitation specialists can be incredibly helpful [2]. These are distinct from traditional driving evaluations at the DMV because the specialist considers the underlying medical condition as the context for the evaluation. The evaluations include a pen-and-paper (or computer-based) cognitive screen and an on-the-road assessment. Simulators might be offered depending on availability. The evaluation covers basic operational knowledge of the vehicle, the ability to perform routine maneuvers and maintain speed, and managing unexpected events and planning routes. They can also recommend adaptive devices for patients with physical impairments who are otherwise cognitively fit to drive. The evaluation typically incurs an out-of-pocket cost to the patient but may prevent a much costlier accident in the future. After the patient has undergone an evaluation, the referring provider will receive a comprehensive report detailing the patient's driving abilities and performance. Based on the findings, the report may recommend additional occupational therapy, equipment, or adaptive devices to improve the patient's driving skills. Alternatively, if it is determined that the patient is not suitable for driving, the report may suggest alternative transportation solutions. A repeat evaluation following additional occupational and cognitive therapy might also be suggested.

Since these evaluations are costly and can have significant implications, it is important to ensure the patient has had sufficient time for therapies and rehabilitation and has a good chance at passing.

To find a driving rehabilitation center in your area, use the following link from the American Occupational Therapy Association: https://myaota.aota.org/driver_search/index.aspx.

Driving Discussions

Discussing driving cessation, or "retirement," with a patient is often complicated and unpleasant. Patients never want to be told they should not drive. There are no proven methods to make these discussions any easier. Advising a patient not to drive should not be taken lightly. Being unable to drive can lead to job loss, missed appointments, and difficulty visiting loved ones or buying necessities. Patients experience a reduced sense of independence and self-esteem, with higher rates of depression [3].

Plan your conversation about driving cessation before seeing the patient. Gather the evidence and formulate the reasoning behind the recommendation since much of this discussion will be about "making the case." Encouraging the family to be a part of the conversation is crucial. It provides an additional set of ears (a witness) if the provider recommends that the patient should not drive, and the family can also offer emotional support. Family and friends, rideshare services, and public transportation should be considered when developing alternative transportation plans. However, public transportation may not be suitable for many patients due to the cognitive and physical requirements to use these services. Mobility plans allow patients to remain independent and continue

Table 42.1 Transportation mobility plan

Destination	How often do I want to go?	Who might be able to provide me with a ride? (family, friends, neighbors, etc.)	Contact information	Can I take public transportation? Y/N	Are other options available? (rideshare, volunteer, taxi, etc.)	Cost
Grocery store						
Bank						
Post office						
Senior center						
Gym						
Park						
Place of worship						
Work						
Library						
Doctor's office						
Dental office						
Pharmacy						
General shopping						
Salon/ barbershop/ self-care						
Entertainment complex						
Volunteer service locations						
Other						
Other						

Adapted from U.S. Administration on Aging Eldercare Locator. https://eldercare.acl.gov. Accessed 3/15/2023

participating in activities. Making a list of these activities with transportation plans can be very helpful. See Table 42.1 for an example mobility plan.

Stress that the recommendation to stop driving is because of functional reasons, not the patient's age. Patients may often resist your recommendations not to drive or flat-out refuse. In this case, it is essential to review the patient's medical condition and symptoms in detail and why they impact driving safety. Stress the importance of being proactive and not waiting until an accident or a ticket to start discussing driving cessation. Allow enough time for questions. Patients may try to bargain by saying they only drive on local roads. However, statistics show that many car accidents occur when the driver is close to home. While patients may take on a defensive, or even angry, posture during these discussions, the provider must remain calm and professional to prevent an adversarial interaction. Acknowledging the patient's perspective and staying objective by sticking to and repeating the main points are helpful.

Speaking with the patient's other healthcare providers is also important to ensure everyone is on the same page. If the patient wishes to get a second opinion, suggest they speak with their primary care physician first. Primary care physicians can be important allies, provided you have previously discussed the issue. If you are a primary care provider concerned about driving safety for a stroke patient, contact their stroke neurologist or refer to one if needed.

For severe cases where the risk of driving-related injury is high, and provider advice is ignored, the American Medical Association considers this a situation where the provider has an ethical duty to notify the DMV, even if not mandated by law. You may want to review your state's requirements for reporting to the licensing authority those patients whose impairments may compromise their ability to drive safely. Refer to Fig. 42.1 for a proposed algorithm to approach returning to driving.

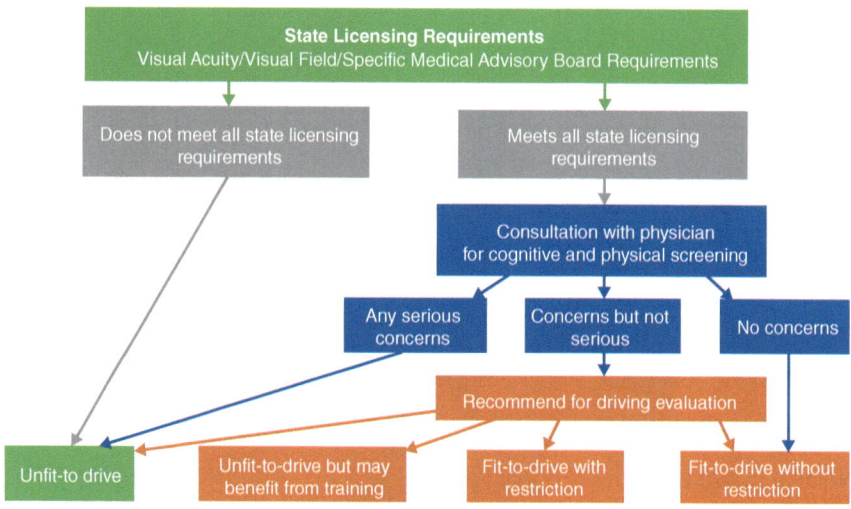

Fig. 42.1 Framework for driving assessment and intervention after a mild stroke. (Reprinted with permission from Burns et al. [4])

Finally, it can be helpful to periodically inquire about any issues while driving if a patient has been cleared to drive since their abilities may deteriorate over time. Patients may be hesitant to disclose any problems, but spouses and family members can be very helpful in providing information.

Returning to Work

Returning to work should be a goal for many younger stroke patients. Returning to work is associated with improved quality of life [5]. Unfortunately, there are very few studies to guide clinicians on how to approach returning to work for patients after a stroke. Deciding if and when a patient should try to return to work is complex and depends on various factors, including but not limited to age, degree of recovery and independence, and job/supervisor flexibility.

Younger age, the ability to walk after stroke, and the ability to perform activities of daily living are associated with a higher likelihood of returning to work. "White collar" jobs typically have more flexibility regarding hours and location (i.e., work from home). Jobs that are more labor intensive, paid hourly, or based on productivity are considered more challenging to return to following a stroke [6]. Increased stroke severity (higher degree of weakness, language difficulty, and cognitive deficits), prolonged hospitalizations, psychiatric illness, and severe fatigue are all associated with a lower likelihood of returning to work successfully. For patients with ongoing fatigue, returning to work with a plan to start with shorter hours, fewer days per week, and gradually increasing workload over weeks to months can be helpful.

A study looking at online forum data for barriers and facilitators to staying at work after stroke reported that many patients felt their employers and coworkers were not aware of their "invisible" impairments like fatigue, memory, personality changes, and pain [7]. Patients reported strategies like "building up slowly with breaks at work," "learning how to manage fatigue," "asking for help at work," and reducing commuting time to work were all helpful in successfully returning to work.

Long-term goals should be discussed with the patient shortly following a stroke. If a patient plans to return to work, it is critical to ensure they are connected to physical, occupational and speech therapies, as well as mental health providers if necessary, as early as possible. Understanding the job description (regarding physical or cognitive demands) and flexibility of hours helps create a plan to return to work eventually. Caution patients against returning to work too early, which could lead to additional problems and could affect long-term employment. Prioritizing rehab and self-care in the weeks to months following a stroke, followed by a slow reintegration plan, may improve a patient's chances of sustained success when returning to work.

Clinical Pearls
- After a stroke, cognitive, visual, sensory, and motor deficits can impair driving ability.
- Identifying limitations and discussing driving safety early can prevent unfortunate situations later.
- Referral to a driving rehabilitation center for a detailed evaluation is helpful.
- Reducing work hours and days initially increases the chances of successfully returning to work full time.

References

1. Staplin L, Gish KW, Wagner EK. MaryPODS revisited: updated crash analysis and implications for screening program implementation. J Saf Res. 2003;34(4):389–97. https://doi.org/10.1016/j.jsr.2003.09.002.
2. Dickerson A, Schold Davis E, Carr DB. Driving decisions: distinguishing evaluations, providers and outcomes. Geriatrics (Basel). 2018;3(2):25. https://doi.org/10.3390/geriatrics3020025.
3. Marottoli RA, Mendes de Leon CF, Glass TA, Williams CS, Cooney LM Jr, Berkman LF, Tinetti ME. Driving cessation and increased depressive symptoms: prospective evidence from the New Haven EPESE. Established populations for epidemiologic studies of the elderly. J Am Geriatr Soc. 1997;45(2):202–6. https://doi.org/10.1111/j.1532-5415.1997.tb04508.x.
4. Burns SP, Schwartz JK, Scott SL, Devos H, Kovic M, Hong I, Akinwuntan A. Interdisciplinary approaches to facilitate return to driving and return to work in mild stroke: a position paper. Arch Phys Med Rehabil. 2018;99(11):2378–88. https://doi.org/10.1016/j.apmr.2018.01.032. Epub 2018 Mar 6.
5. Treger I, Shames J, Giaquinto S, Ring H. Return to work in stroke patients. Disabil Rehabil. 2007;29(17):1397–403. https://doi.org/10.1080/09638280701314923.
6. Harris C. Return to work after stroke: a nursing state of the science. Stroke. 2014;45(9):e174–6. https://doi.org/10.1161/STROKEAHA.114.006205. Epub 2014 Jul 10.
7. Balasooriya-Smeekens C, Bateman A, Mant J, De Simoni A. Barriers and facilitators to staying in work after stroke: insight from an online forum. BMJ Open. 2016;6(4):e009974. https://doi.org/10.1136/bmjopen-2015-009974.

Perioperative Stroke

43

Kathryn Bard and Margy McCullough-Hicks

Abbreviations

CAA	Cerebral amyloid angiopathy
CABG	Coronary artery bypass grafting
CEA	Carotid endarterectomy
DOAC	Direct oral anticoagulant
FVL	Factor 5 Leiden
GI	Gastrointestinal
GU	Genitourinary
ICH	Intracerebral hemorrhage
INR	International normalized ratio
LMWH	Low molecular weight heparin
MI	Myocardial infarction
PCC	Prothrombin complex concentrate
PCI	Percutaneous coronary intervention
TIA	Transient ischemic attack
UFH	Unfractionated heparin
VKA	Vitamin K antagonist (warfarin)
VTE	Venous thromboembolism

K. Bard
University of Minnesota, Minneapolis, MN, USA

M. McCullough-Hicks (✉)
University of Minnesota Medical School, Minneapolis, MN, USA
e-mail: mccul284@umn.edu

Introduction: Perioperative Stroke

Epidemiology

Perioperative stroke is any stroke occurring during or within 30 days of surgery. However, 50% of perioperative strokes occur within the first postoperative day [1, 2], and 93% occur within the first 72 h [3]. Surgical procedures with the highest rates of perioperative stroke include following neurological (1.25%), vascular (1.07%), and cardiac (0.98%) surgeries [4].

Many studies have identified advanced age ($\geq$75 years), renal disease, and history of stroke/transient ischemic attack (TIA) as key risk factors for perioperative stroke [5]. Other risk factors include myocardial infarction (MI) within the preceding 6 months, atrial fibrillation, hypertension, chronic obstructive pulmonary disease, current smoking, female sex, and diabetes mellitus [6–9]. The presence of multiple risk factors compounds the risk of perioperative stroke [7].

Pathophysiology

Ischemic strokes comprise 96–99% of perioperative strokes [10, 11]. In patients undergoing cardiac surgery, approximately 2/3 of ischemic strokes are the result of proximal embolism, either from direct cardiac/arterial manipulation, procedural use of a bypass pump, or delayed complications like atrial fibrillation or myocardial infarction [11, 12]. Possible mechanisms of perioperative stroke in the setting of noncardiac, nonneurological surgery may include hypotension/low-flow state, previously unknown large artery (cervical or intracranial) stenosis, anemia-associated tissue hypoxia, thromboembolism, fat embolism, and enhanced coagulability/thrombosis in the setting of systemic inflammation and endothelial dysfunction and interruption of antithrombotic medications [13, 14].

The remaining 1–4% of perioperative strokes are hemorrhagic. The most common etiologies include uncontrolled hypertension, perioperative use of antithrombotic medications, and reperfusion/hyperperfusion syndromes (particularly after carotid revascularization).

Role of the Stroke Provider

Surgeons may consult with stroke practitioners to ensure that it is safe to perform surgery on patients who have a history of ischemic or hemorrhagic stroke. Typically, this consultation focuses on determining the appropriate timing for surgery after a stroke or TIA and managing antithrombotic medications prescribed for secondary stroke prevention. This chapter will focus primarily on decision-making regarding the risk of ischemic stroke surrounding elective, non-emergent surgeries.

Perioperative Ischemic Stroke

The following sections address general perioperative considerations for patients who have a history of ischemic stroke or TIA. The ultimate management plan, however, requires agreement between the surgical and medical teams after careful evaluation of all patient-specific factors.

Assess Thromboembolism Risk

One major consideration is determining the risk of a thromboembolic event if a patient's anticoagulant or antiplatelet agent is temporarily held for surgery. Interrupting antithrombotics can leave patients unprotected or lead to rebound hypercoagulability, with the risk of thromboembolism depending on the underlying risk factors (Table 43.1). If the antithrombotic is required for a mechanical heart

Table 43.1   Perioperative thromboembolism (TE) risk factors (adapted from Douketis et al. [15])

Risk factor	High TE risk[a]	Moderate TE risk	Low TE risk
Atrial fibrillation[b]	• $CHADS_2$ score ≥ 3 • Rheumatic heart disease • Stroke/TIA ≤ 3 months	• $CHADS_2$ score 1–2 • Stroke, TIA >3 months	• $CHADS_2$ score 0
Mechanical heart valve	• Mitral valve prosthesis • Caged-ball or tilting disc aortic valve prosthesis • Stroke/TIA ≤ 6 months	• Bi-leaflet aortic valve and ≥ 1 of the following: atrial fibrillation, prior stroke/ TIA, hypertension, diabetes, congestive heart failure, age >75	• Bi-leaflet aortic valve without atrial fibrillation or other stroke risk factors
Venous thromboembolism (VTE)	• VTE <3 months • Severe thrombophilia (protein C or S, antithrombin III deficiency, antiphospholipid syndrome, homozygous factor V Leiden (FVL), multiple factor abnormalities)	• Single VTE in the past 3–12 months • Recurrent VTE • Non-severe thrombophilia (heterozygous FVL, prothrombin gene mutation) • Active cancer	• Single VTE >12 months without other risk factors
History of vascular stent placement	• Carotid stent placement ≤ 3 months • Drug-eluting stent ≤ 12 months • Bare metal stent ≤ 1 month or after acute coronary syndrome ≤ 12 months • Prior history of stent occlusion	• Carotid stent placement 3–6 months	• Carotid stent placement >6 months

[a] Patients with a history of thromboembolism during temporary interruption of antithrombotic therapy or those undergoing surgeries with higher thromboembolism risk (e.g., cardiac valve replacement, carotid endarterectomy, major vascular surgery) may also be high-risk

[b] Patients with both a history of atrial fibrillation and ischemic stroke/TIA automatically have a $CHADS_2$ score ≥ 2 and will fall into moderate or high-risk categories

Table 43.2 Perioperative ischemic stroke risk of specific procedures and conditions [16]

Procedure/clinical condition	Stroke risk (%)
General surgery	0.2
General surgery after a prior stroke	2.9
Asymptomatic carotid endarterectomy (CEA) or stenting	1–3
Symptomatic CEA or stenting	4–10
Cerebral aneurysm clipping/coiling	6–10
Intracranial stenting	9–15
Cardiac catheterization	0.2–0.5
Coronary artery bypass grafting (CABG)	1.4–2
CABG after prior stroke/TIA	8.5
CABG + valve surgery	4.2–13
CABG + unilateral carotid stenosis >50%	3
CABG + bilateral carotid stenosis >50%	5
CABG + carotid occlusion	7
Surgery with symptomatic vertebrobasilar disease	6
Noncardiac surgery, known PFO/ASD (Perfetti 2017)	7.14

valve replacement or vascular stent, ensure the surgeon or interventionalist who performed that procedure is included in the discussion. Table 43.2 reviews the risk of stroke based on the specific procedures.

Assess Procedural Bleeding Risk

Continuing antithrombotics during invasive procedures may increase the risk of bleeding associated with surgery (Table 43.3). Weighing the risks of thromboembolic events without antithrombotics against the risk of significant procedural bleeding with continuation should inform a reasonable plan.

General guidance on antithrombotic management accounting for procedural bleeding risk includes:

- **High bleed risk**: Hold anticoagulation (see guidelines).
- **Moderate bleed risk**: Depends on the specific antithrombotic agent, periprocedural risk of thromboembolism, and discussion with proceduralist(s).
- **Low bleed risk**: Reasonable to continue antithrombotic therapy.

Table 43.3 Procedural bleeding risks [16]

Surgical site	High bleed risk	Moderate bleed risk	Low bleed risk
Cardiac	CABG Heart valve replacement		Coronary angiography Transfemoral and radial percutaneous coronary intervention (PCI) Pacemaker/ICD placement Most atrial fibrillation ablation
Pulmonary	Resections (lung, lobe, segment)		
GI/GU	Major abdominal/pelvic surgery Bladder/prostate surgery Nephrectomy/kidney biopsy Colonic polyp resection (>1 cm) Liver/spleen surgery Bowel resection PEG/PEJ placement		ERCP with stent placement Endoscopy ± mucosal biopsy Colonoscopy ± mucosal biopsy Laparoscopic cholecystectomy Abdominal/inguinal hernia repair Barrett's ablation
Orthopedic upper extremity	Substantial hand, total elbow, or shoulder arthroplasty Extremity fracture without tourniquet		Carpal tunnel disease Minor hand surgery, trigger finger, or benign tumor Aspirations/injection Traumatic fracture with a tourniquet
Orthopedic lower extremity	Major surgery Total hip or knee arthroplasty (including revision) Major soft tissue resection Trauma, hip, pelvis, and acetabular fractures Extremity fracture w/o tourniquet	Lower extremity fracture ORIF (femur/tibia or peri-articular) Lower extremity closed reduction and internal fixation Ankle/foot fracture ORIF Moderate hand and upper extremity surgery	Minor soft tissue resection Traumatic fracture with a tourniquet
Neurosurgery	Spine surgery (incl laminectomy, discectomy) Intracranial surgery Intracranial embolization	Lumbar procedure Diagnostic cerebral angiogram Carotid stent Spinal embolization	Occipital nerve blocks Botox/peripheral injections Trigger point injections EMG

(continued)

Table 43.3 (continued)

Surgical site	High bleed risk	Moderate bleed risk	Low bleed risk
Dental	Corrective jaw or facial surgery Facial trauma repair	Surgical extractions, complex surgeries, >3 teeth Dental implant surgery	Extractions simple or erupted ≤3 teeth Hygiene procedures Simple restorations Endodontics Root canal Fillings/caps/crowns
Dermatologic	Reconstructive plastic surgery		Excision of basal/squamous cell carcinoma, actinic keratosis, nevi Mohs surgery
Vascular	Abdominal and thoracic open surgery	Arterial revascularization (lower extremity) Deep venous reconstruction (legs) EVAR/FEVAR/PEVAR/TEVAR Arterial procedures, percutaneous with >8F sheath Extra-anatomic bypass Cardiovascular head/neck surgery (carotid, subclavian, vertebral, venous)	Temporal artery biopsy
Gynecologic			Cervical LEEP Vulvar biopsy, wide local excision Dilation and curettage Hysteroscopy (diagnostic and operative)
Ophthalmologic			Cataract extraction Glaucoma laser LASIK Corneal surgeries Orbital surgery Blepharoplasty
Other	Cancer-related surgery General surgery		Biopsy of compressible site

Assess the Timing of Elective Procedures Postischemic Stroke

Guidance regarding the timing of nonemergent surgeries is also frequently sought from the stroke provider. In general, the American Heart Association recommends delaying *elective* surgery for at least 3–6 months after an ischemic stroke to lower the risk of perioperative recurrence [5]. Elective surgery is defined as one that is not

Table 43.4 Timing of specific procedures

Procedure	Recommendations
Cervical carotid artery revascularization (endarterectomy or stenting)	• Symptomatic carotid stenoses should be treated within 2 weeks of symptom onset
CABG in the setting of cervical carotid stenosis	Consider carotid revascularization *before* CABG when: • Recent symptomatic carotid stenosis >50% • Bilateral asymptomatic carotid stenosis >70% and/or unilateral asymptomatic carotid stenosis + contralateral carotid occlusion • Carotid screening before CABG is recommended in patients >65 years old with a history of stroke/TIA, left main coronary disease, peripheral vascular disease, tobacco use, or carotid bruit
Valve replacement after cardioembolic stroke from endocarditis	• Consider early surgery in patients with vegetations >10 mm, recurrent strokes, severe valvular dysfunction with small or moderate-sized infarcts • Patients with large infarcts, concomitant intracranial hemorrhage, or large mycotic aneurysms are at higher risk of intracranial hemorrhage; consider waiting 2–4 weeks
Elective procedures	• Wait at least 3 months (≥6 may be preferable) after stroke/TIA for truly elective procedures [17]

an emergency and can be scheduled in advance. Table 43.4 offers a framework for the optimal timing of specific procedures.

Guidance on Temporary Interruption of Specific Antithrombotic Agents

- **Anticoagulation agents: Warfarin and direct oral anticoagulants (DOACs)** (Table 43.5)
- **Perioperative bridging therapy**
- "Bridging therapy" is the use of a shorter-acting therapeutic anticoagulant (e.g., low molecular weight heparin [LMWH] or unfractionated heparin [UFH] infusion) to "bridge" between the period of discontinuation of warfarin and time of surgery. Bridging therapy is generally used in patients with high thromboembolism risk in whom anticoagulants must be discontinued due to high bleed-risk procedures. Bridging therapy is typically not required for patients taking DOACs (see below)
  - The American College of Chest Physicians (ACCP) has made the following recommendations regarding the use of bridging therapy for specific situations [19] in Table 43.6.
  - In patients receiving low-molecular-weight heparin (LMWH) bridging for an elective procedure, the ACCP recommends *against* the measurement of anti-factor Xa levels to guide perioperative LMWH management.
- **Antiplatelet agents**
  - **Aspirin**

Table 43.5 Recommended perioperative anticoagulation management (adapted from Hornor et al. [18] and Benesch et al. [5])

Thromboembolism (TE) risk category	High bleed risk procedure[a]	Low bleed risk procedure
High TE risk		
Warfarin	Last dose 6 days before procedure, bridge with LMWH or UFH, resume 24 h postoperatively	Last dose 6 days before procedure, bridge with LMWH or UFH, resume 24 h postoperatively
DOAC	[b]Last dose 3 days before procedure, resume 48–72 h postoperatively	Last dose 2 days before procedure, resume 24 h postoperatively
Intermediate TE risk		
Warfarin	Last dose 6 days before procedure, consider bridging depending on clinician judgment, resume 24 h postoperatively	Last dose 6 days before procedure, consider bridging depending on clinician judgment, resume 24 h postoperatively
DOAC	[b]Last dose 3 days before procedure; resume 2–3 days postoperatively	Last dose 3 days before procedure, resume 24 h postoperatively
Low TE risk		
Warfarin	Last dose 6 days before procedure, do not bridge, resume 24 h postoperatively	Last dose 6 days before procedure, do not bridge, resume 24 h postoperatively
DOAC	[b]Last dose 3 days preoperatively, resume 2–3 days postoperatively	Last dose 2 days before procedure, resume 24 h postoperatively

[a] Patient-related factors that increase bleeding risk: History of major bleeding within the last 3 months, Bleeding with similar procedures, Bleeding after prior bridging therapy, Quantitative or qualitative platelet abnormalities
[b] Patients with abnormal renal function taking dabigatran should take the last dose of dabigatran 3 days before a low bleeding-risk procedure and 4–5 days before a high bleeding-risk procedure

- The ACCP recommends that patients receiving ASA who undergo elective, non-cardiac surgery should *continue* ASA [19]. See Table 43.7 for more specific recommendations.
- There is insufficient data to provide recommendations regarding periprocedural clopidogrel, ticlopidine, aspirin/dipyridamole, and cilostazol management in most situations.
- ACCP recommends against routine use of platelet function testing before surgery to guide perioperative antiplatelet management
- **Clopidogrel**
- Discontinue 7–10 days before moderate or high-risk bleeding procedures.
- If discontinued for urgent, high-risk procedures, restart clopidogrel 24 h after surgery or when hemostasis is achieved (consult with the surgeon).
- ACCP: recommend holding P2Y12 inhibitor for CABG; in patients who are on ASA + P2Y12 inhibitors for coronary stents within the last 3–12 months undergoing an elective procedure, hold P2Y12; in pts w coronary stents who require interruption of antiplatelet(s) for an elective procedure, recommend *against* routine bridging with GP2b/3a inhibitor, cangrelor, or LMWH

Table 43.6 ACCP bridging therapy recommendations

Procedure	Presurgical anticoagulant being used	Reason for anticoagulant use	ACCP recommendation re: bridging therapy, anticoagulation management	Level of evidence/ strength of recommendation
Elective procedure	VKA	Atrial fibrillation	*Against* bridging therapy	Strong recommendation, moderate certainty
Elective procedure	VKA	Mechanical heart valve	*For* bridging therapy	Conditional recommendation, very low certainty
Elective procedure	VKA	Venous thromboembolism	*Against* bridging therapy	Conditional recommendation, very low certainty
Pacemaker/ ICD placement	VKA	Any reason	*Continue VKA* (preferred over bridging therapy)	Strong recommendation, moderate certainty
Colonoscopy with polypectomy	VKA	Any reason	*Against* bridging therapy	Conditional recommendation, very low certainty
Elective procedure	Apixaban, dabigatran, edoxaban, rivaroxaban	Any reason	• Stop DOAC 1–2 days before surgery • *Against* bridging therapy • Resume DOAC >24 h after procedure • *Against* routine DOAC coagulation function testing to guide perioperative DOAC management	Conditional recommendation, very low certainty

- **Dual antiplatelet therapy**
  - If a patient is on pre-procedural dual antiplatelet therapy for stroke/TIA, it is recommended to postpone elective procedures until dual therapy course is completed.

Considerations for Management of Antithrombotic Therapies for Nonelective/Emergent Surgeries

- **VKA**: Administer vitamin K and 4-factor PCC to patients with an elevated INR due to warfarin who are actively bleeding or require emergent surgery.
- **Dabigatran**: Administer idarucizumab to patients with evidence of significant dabigatran levels (by a history of ingestion or lab parameters) who are actively bleeding or require emergent surgery.

Table 43.7 Aspirin management around specific procedures in patients with prior stroke/TIA (adapted from Benesch et al. [5] and Amin et al. [16])

Procedure type	Recommendation
Dental	
Routine dental procedures	Continue aspirin
Ophthalmologic	
Invasive ocular anesthesia, cataract surgery	Probably continue aspirin
Vitreoretinal surgery	Possibly continue aspirin
Dermatologic	Probably continue aspirin
Prostate	
Transrectal, ultrasound-guided biopsy	Probably continue aspirin
Neurologic	
Spinal/epidural procedures	Probably continue aspirin
EMG	Possibly continue aspirin
Orthopedic	
Carpal tunnel surgery	Probably continue aspirin
Pulmonary	
Transbronchial lung biopsy	Possibly continue aspirin
Gastrointestinal	
Upper endoscopy, biopsy, sphincterotomy	Possibly continue aspirin
Abdominal ultrasound-guided biopsy	Possibly continue aspirin
ACCP recommendations (Chest 2022):	Continue aspirin
• For any noncardiac surgery	
• For CABG	

- **Other DOACs**: Administer 4-factor PCC transfusion (50 U/kg) for partial reversal in patients with evidence of active factor Xa inhibition as needed in emergencies. Andexanet alfa is approved (as an alternative agent) for patients taking rivaroxaban or apixaban who require anticoagulation reversal for life-threatening or uncontrolled bleeding. The dose of andexanet alfa required depends on which Factor Xa inhibitor agent a patient takes, the agent dose, and the time since the last administration. Low-dose andexanet alfa regimen is 400 mg IV (target rate of 30 mg/min) followed by an infusion of 4 mg/min for up to 2 h. The high-dose regimen is 800 mg IV (target rate of 30 mg/min) followed by an 8 mg/min infusion for up to 2 h [20].
- **Antiplatelets**: Transfuse 1-unit pooled platelets immediately before emergent surgery and repeat as needed for evidence of ongoing bleeding.

Other Perioperative Ischemic Stroke Management Considerations

- **Intraoperative blood pressure**: If a patient has known arterial stenosis, the surgical and anesthesia teams need to be cautious of blood pressure and avoid hypotension that may cause a stroke related to hypoperfusion. Specific intraoperative blood pressure parameters have not been identified, but generally, a mean arterial pressure (MAP) >70 mmHg is reasonable to reduce the risk of perioperative stroke [5].

- **Perioperative blood transfusion management**: Although anemia has been associated with higher morbidity and mortality in noncardiac surgery, studies consistently show that perioperative blood transfusions do not improve outcomes. Clinicians should transfuse patients with preexisting cardiac disease at a threshold of 8 g/dL, as recommended by the American Association of Blood Banks (AABB). In those with acute perioperative stroke, ongoing bleeding, hemodynamic instability, and known cerebrovascular insufficiency due to severe carotid stenosis, a transfusion threshold of 8–9 g/dL is recommended [5].
- **Anesthetic choice**: There is insufficient evidence to support the use of regional anesthesia versus general anesthesia alone to lower the perioperative risk of stroke [5].
- **Ventilation strategies**: Hypocarbia can significantly reduce cerebral blood flow and worsen cerebral ischemia. It is reasonable to consider a lung-protective ventilation strategy as part of an overall strategy to reduce postoperative complications. However, no data supports this approach specifically for reducing perioperative stroke [5].
- **Other medication management**:
  - **Beta-blockers**: Patients on long-term beta-blockers should continue these perioperatively. It is not recommended to start beta-blockers on the day of surgery to reduce the risk of stroke during the perioperative period. A randomized controlled trial found that patients treated with preoperative metoprolol had a higher mortality rate and increased stroke rates compared to those given a placebo. Further studies suggest that hypotension may be the mechanism by which beta-blockers increase the risk of stroke during the perioperative period [5, 10, 21].
  - **Statins**: Patients who are already taking a statin before undergoing noncardiac surgery should continue to take the statin perioperatively [5].

Treatment of Postsurgical Ischemic Stroke

- **IV Thrombolysis**: Major surgery of any kind within 14 days of symptom onset is a strong relative contraindication to IV thrombolysis for acute stroke symptoms. Recent intracranial or spinal surgery is an absolute contraindication. For patients with recent surgery, emergent consultation with a patient's surgeon before administration of IV thrombolysis is generally recommended.
  - IV thrombolysis in patients with recent minor procedures, especially at compressible sites, can be considered
- **Endovascular therapy**: Endovascular therapy for large vessel occlusions is generally acceptable in all situations, including endocarditis and septic emboli.

Perioperative Hemorrhagic Stroke

There are no established guidelines for reducing the risk of recurrent ICH for patients with prior ICH during elective surgery; the following framework is based on expert consensus. For patients with a history of ICH, discussion regarding the perioperative risk of recurrent ICH may focus on:

- **Procedural bleed risk, specifically need for perioperative anticoagulation**
  - Many cardiac surgeries require the use of high-dose intraoperative anticoagulation—the etiology of a patient's prior intracranial hemorrhage (see below) should be considered in stratifying the risk of recurrent bleeding.
- **Timing of surgery**
  - In general, it is reasonable to wait at least 6 months after intracranial hemorrhage before performing elective surgery.
- **Etiology of prior intracranial bleed**
  - **Hypertensive hemorrhage**: In patients with a history of hypertensive ICH, tight perioperative blood pressure control (goal of normotension) should be recommended.
  - **Traumatic hemorrhage**: In patients with a history of traumatic intracranial hemorrhage, consider repeat imaging (CT or MRI) to confirm the expected evolution and resolution of the hemorrhage before elective surgeries.
  - **Hemorrhage due to known underlying vascular anomaly (aneurysm, arteriovenous malformation)**: If a patient has a history of intracranial hemorrhage due to a currently *unsecured or untreated* cerebral aneurysm or arteriovenous malformation, surgical treatment of the vascular anomaly should be considered before other elective surgery. The presence of unruptured cerebral aneurysms is not known to increase perioperative intracerebral hemorrhage in patients undergoing cardiac and non-cardiac surgery [22].
  - **Hemorrhage due to underlying mass lesion**: Consult with a neuro-oncologist regarding the risk of recurrent hemorrhage based on neoplasm type. Strongly consider delaying surgery if the definitive etiology of the underlying mass is still pending.
  - **Hemorrhage due to cerebral amyloid angiopathy (CAA)**: Patients with known or presumed CAA have a higher risk of recurrent intracranial bleeding, particularly in the setting of antithrombotic use. It is important to discuss with the patient and surgeon the increased risk of anticoagulation or antiplatelet-related hemorrhage during or after procedures like cardiac stenting or valve replacement.
  - **Idiopathic hemorrhage**: Strongly consider delaying surgery until standard post-hemorrhage (~3 months) repeat MRI with and without gadolinium to rule out underlying mass lesion or other high-risk bleed etiology has been performed.
  - **Hemorrhage in the setting of infective endocarditis**: Extensive guidelines/recommendations exist for this situation and are outside the scope of full coverage in this chapter. Ischemic stroke occurs from vascular occlusion from

septic emboli. Bleeding occurs from the conversion of the ischemic stroke bed or mycotic aneurysm rupture.

Role of Neurology in Endocarditis

The involvement of the neurology team when consulting in endocarditis cases should be limited to assessing the perioperative risk of intracranial hemorrhage with valve surgery (which requires anticoagulation). Factors that increase the risk of ICH include recent stroke/hemorrhage, size of stroke and presence of hemorrhagic conversion, presence of mycotic aneurysms, ongoing bacteremia and fever, and timing of surgery. For patients with stroke or intracranial hemorrhage from endocarditis, it is essential to get vessel imaging to screen for mycotic aneurysms. Mycotic aneurysms develop when bacteria or fungus invade the vessel wall (via bloodstream infection or emboli), causing dilation and weakening of the vessel wall, and are at high risk of rupture. Unlike saccular aneurysms that form at bifurcations, mycotic aneurysms hang along the distal branches of cerebral arteries (like Christmas lights on a string). Although good-quality CTA and MRA are reliable diagnostic tests for mycotic aneurysms, a conventional or digital subtraction angiogram (DSA) is still considered the gold standard but may not always be necessary. DSA is warranted if aneurysms are detected on non-invasive imaging and require treatment or if, despite negative CTA/MRA, there is still a high suspicion of smaller aneurysms posing risk (for example, evidence of convexity subarachnoid hemorrhage, microbleeds, or superficial siderosis on MRI).

Timing of valve surgery typically falls into three categories: emergent (needs to occur as soon as possible, or the patient will likely die from heart failure), urgent (surgery can be scheduled after stabilizing concurrent medical issues during admission), or elective (no urgency, patient can be discharged and return for surgery at a later date). If a patient is at imminent risk of valve rupture and death without surgery (i.e., emergent), then there need not be much discussion about ICH risk if surgery is within the patient's goals of care.

Using the level of urgency for cardiac surgery as determined by the surgical and cardiology teams as a guide, the neurology team can then assess the risk of bleeding should surgery occur during that timeframe, considering the other factors listed above. The neurology team should be careful not to overstep its role and dictate the timing of cardiac surgery. Instead, it should do its best to stratify ICH risk with surgery vs. no surgery (i.e., risk of recurrent stroke and heart failure).

Infected mechanical valves are a unique, very high-risk scenario that usually requires urgent surgery and the resumption of anticoagulation as soon as possible.

For otherwise stable patients, it is recommended that valve replacement surgery occur at least 4–6 weeks after an infective endocarditis-related intracranial hemorrhage. If one or more mycotic aneurysms are detected, treating the aneurysms should be strongly considered before any cardiac procedure, as unsecured mycotic aneurysms can rupture if exposed to heparin. A frank conversation with the surgical team, the patient, and their family about the chance of bleeding is crucial before surgery. These are often "rock and a hard place" scenarios with no low-risk option. Patients and families should get a clear and honest description of the risks and benefits of all options. Neurological examinations and imaging can help evaluate for new ischemic events or hemorrhage after surgery.

Clinical Pearls
- All the patients undergoing preoperative evaluation after a stroke or TIA should be assessed for key risk factors, timing of surgery in relation to the incident stroke, and the type of planned procedure.
- Elective surgeries should generally be delayed by at least 3 months (preferably 6–9 months) after an incident stroke/TIA.
- Carotid revascularization in patients with *symptomatic* carotid artery stenosis should be performed within 2 weeks of the event and before other elective surgeries. Perioperative management of high-grade *asymptomatic* carotid stenosis is uncertain, and existing guidelines should be consulted.
- Secondary stroke preventative medications should be adjusted based on existing guidelines and tailored to individual patient characteristics.
- Patients taking antithrombotics require careful attention to thromboembolism vs. procedural bleeding risks for perioperative medication management. The decision to stop or continue antithrombotic agents should agree with surgery-specific guidelines.
- Consider nonsurgical options (in discussion with the patient and other providers) in patients with an elevated risk of ischemic or hemorrhagic stroke.

References

1. Selim M. Perioperative stroke. N Engl J Med. 2007;356:706–13.
2. Ng JLW, Chan MTV, Gelb AW. Perioperative stroke in non-cardiac, nonneurosurgical surgery. Anesthesiology. 2011;115:879–90.
3. Wang H, Li S-L, Bai J, Wang D-X. Perioperative acute ischemic stroke increases mortality after non-cardiac, nonvascular, and non-neurologic surgery: a retrospective case series. J Cardiothorac Vasc Anesth. 2019;33:2231–6.
4. Al-Hader R, Al-Robaidi K, Jovin T, Jadhav A, Wechsler LR, Thirumala PD. The incidence of perioperative stroke: estimate using state and national databases and systematic review. J Stroke. 2019;21:290–301.
5. Benesch C, Glance LG, Derdeyn CP, Fleisher LA, Holloway RG, Messé SR, Mijalski C, Nelson MT, Power M, Welch BG, et al. Perioperative neurological evaluation and management to lower the risk of acute stroke in patients undergoing noncardiac, nonneurological surgery: a scientific statement from the American Heart Association/American Stroke Association. Circulation. 2021;143:e923–46.
6. Bateman BT, Schumacher HC, Wang S, Shaefi S, Berman MF. Perioperative acute ischemic stroke in non-cardiac and nonvascular surgery: incidence, risk factors, and outcomes. Anesthesiology. 2009;110:231–8.

7. Mashour GA, Shanks AM, Kheterpal S. Perioperative stroke and associated mortality after non-cardiac, nonneurologic surgery. Anesthesiology. 2011;114:1289–96.
8. Wang L, Guo D, Feng Y, Jiang B, Li Y, Zou S, Xue L. Risk factors for perioperative myocardial infarction in aged patients undergoing nonneurologic and non-cardiac surgery. Chin J Geriatr. 2018;(12):768–71.
9. Vasivej T, Sathirapanya P, Kongkamol C. Incidence and risk factors of perioperative stroke in non-cardiac, and nonaortic and its major branches surgery. J Stroke Cerebrovasc Dis. 2016;25:1172–6.
10. Mashour GA, Sharifpour M, Freundlich RE, Tremper KK, Shanks A, Nallamothu BK, Vlisides PE, Weightman A, Matlen L, Merte J, et al. Perioperative metoprolol and risk of stroke after non-cardiac surgery. Anesthesiology. 2013;119:1340–6.
11. Likosky DS, Marrin CAS, Caplan LR, Baribeau YR, Morton JR, Weintraub RM, Hartman GS, Hernandez F, Braff SP, Charlesworth DC, et al. Determination of etiologic mechanisms of strokes secondary to coronary artery bypass graft surgery. Stroke. 2003;34:2830–4.
12. Likosky DS, Caplan LR, Weintraub RM, Hartman GS, Malenka DJ, Ross CS, Landis ES, Applebaum B, Braff SP, O'Connor GT, et al. Intraoperative and postoperative variables associated with strokes following cardiac surgery. Heart Surg Forum. 2004;7:E271–6.
13. Saito Y, Kitahara H, Matsumiya G, Kobayashi Y. Preoperative endothelial function and long-term cardiovascular events in patients undergoing cardiovascular surgery. Heart Vessel. 2019;34:318–23.
14. Devereaux PJ, Chan M, Eikelboom J. Major vascular complications in patients undergoing non-cardiac surgery: magnitude of the problem, risk prediction, surveillance, and prevention [Internet]. In: Evidence-based cardiology. Wiley; 2009. p. 47–62. https://doi.org/10.1002/9781444309768.ch5.
15. Douketis JD, Spyropoulos AC, Spencer FA, Mayr M, Jaffer AK, Eckman MH, Dunn AS, Kunz R. Perioperative management of antithrombotic therapy. Chest. 2012;141:e326S–50S.
16. Vascular Neurology Board Review: an essential study guide. SpringerLink [Internet]. [cited 2022 Dec 26]. https://link.springer.com/book/10.1007/978-3-319-39605-7.
17. Mehdi Z, Birns J, Partridge J, Bhalla A, Dhesi J. Perioperative management of adult patients with a history of stroke or transient ischaemic attack undergoing elective non-cardiac surgery. Clin Med. 2016;16:535–40.
18. Hornor MA, Duane TM, Ehlers AP, Jensen EH, Brown PS, Pohl D, da Costa PM, Ko CY, Laronga C. American College of Surgeons' guidelines for the perioperative management of antithrombotic medication. J Am Coll Surg. 2018;227:521.
19. CHEST releases a clinical practice guideline on perioperative management of antithrombotic therapy [Internet]. Am Coll Chest Physicians. 2022. [cited 2022 Dec 15]. https://www.chest-net.org/Newsroom/Press-Releases/2022/08/CHEST-releases-clinical-practice-guideline-on-perioperative-management-of-antithrombotic-therapy.
20. Sewell JH, Williams L, McKnight E, Nguyen A, Sarac M. What is the role of andexanet alfa in the reversal of anticoagulant effects? JAAPA. 2021;34:8.
21. POISE Study Group, Devereaux PJ, Yang H, Yusuf S, Guyatt G, Leslie K, Villar JC, Xavier D, Chrolavicius S, Greenspan L, Pogue J, Pais P, Liu L, Xu S, Málaga G, Avezum A, Chan M, Montori VM, Jacka M, Choi P. Effects of extended-release metoprolol succinate in patients undergoing non-cardiac surgery (POISE trial): a randomised controlled trial. Lancet. 2008;371:1839–47.
22. Nam J-S, Jeon S-B, Jo J-Y, Joung K-W, Chin J-H, Lee E-H, Chung CH, Choi I-C. Perioperative rupture risk of unruptured intracranial aneurysms in cardiovascular surgery. Brain J Neurol. 2019;142:1408–15.

Glossary

Acute stroke Any stroke in the first few hours of symptoms.

Agnosia The inability to recognize something for what it is (prosopagnosia is the inability to recognize faces).

Amaurosis fugax Transient vision loss, usually monocular.

Aneurysm Local ballooning or dilation of an artery due to a weakened area in the arterial wall.

Angiogram Imaging of blood vessels.

Anticoagulation Potent blood-thinning therapy for conditions like atrial fibrillation or deep vein thrombosis.

Antiplatelet A milder form of blood thinner-inhibiting platelet function to prevent clots.

Aphasia Difficulty with language production or comprehension.

Apraxia Motor dysfunction due to impaired coordination between the brain and muscles (not due to weakness).

Arteriovenous malformation Collection of blood vessels with abnormal connections between arteries and veins, which may cause hemorrhage or seizures.

Atherosclerosis Plaque accumulation in arteries, most often at bifurcations.

Atrial fibrillation Irregular heart rhythm that can lead to thrombus formation in the left atrium and cardioembolic stroke.

Brainstem The structure connecting the cerebral cortex to the spinal cord; it is made up of the midbrain, pons, and medulla.

Cardioembolic stroke Ischemic stroke caused by an embolism from the heart.

Carotid artery Primary sources of blood supply to the left and right hemispheres.

Carotid endarterectomy Surgical procedure to treat symptomatic carotid stenosis by removing plaque.

Carotid stenting Endovascular procedure to treat symptomatic carotid stenosis by inserting a stent.

Central poststroke pain Neuropathic pain following stroke, usually thalamic, due to misinterpretation by the brain of signals sent from nerve endings.

Cerebellum Structure behind the brainstem; it primarily functions in coordination and balance.

© The Editor(s) (if applicable) and The Author(s), under exclusive license to Springer Nature Switzerland AG 2024
H. P. Amin (ed.), *Stroke for the Advanced Practice Clinician*,
https://doi.org/10.1007/978-3-031-66289-8

Cerebral amyloid angiopathy Abnormal deposits of amyloid protein in the cerebral vessels leading to microhemorrhages and large lobar hemorrhages.

Cerebral cortex Left and right hemispheres of the brain.

Cerebrospinal fluid Fluid surrounding the brain and spinal cord.

Computed tomography (CT or CAT) scan A form of X-ray imaging that creates three-dimensional maps of soft tissue or bone.

Digital subtraction angiography An invasive, catheter-based procedure to visualize blood vessels by injecting contrast dye.

Dissection A tear between two layers of an arterial wall, creating a new "false lumen" where a thrombus can form.

Dysarthria Impaired articulation (slurring) of speech due to bulbar weakness.

Dysphagia Impaired swallowing after stroke due to weakness in the oropharynx, increasing the risk of aspiration.

Edema Fluid buildup in the brain tissue that can lead to mass effect and herniation.

Electroencephalogram An EKG for the brain to detect seizure activity.

Embolic stroke A stroke caused by a traveling clot originating from a source outside the brain.

Embolism A fragment of clot or other material that has dislodged from its source.

Endothelium The innermost lining of blood vessels.

Epilepsy A diagnosis that implies long-term risk of recurrent seizures.

Hemiparesis Weakness on one side of the body.

Hemiplegia Complete paralysis of one side of the body.

Hemorrhagic stroke A stroke caused by bleeding in the brain.

High-density lipoprotein (HDL) Known as the "good cholesterol," since it helps remove cholesterol from the bloodstream.

Homonymous hemianopia Vision loss in the same half of both eyes, usually caused by a stroke in the contralateral occipital lobe.

Horner's syndrome Injury to the sympathetic pathway (stroke, dissection, etc.) that leads to ptosis, miosis, and anhidrosis.

Hydrocephalus Obstruction of the ventricles leading to impaired outflow of cerebrospinal fluid, raising intracranial pressure.

Hyperlipidemia Elevated cholesterol levels (typically LDL), increasing the risk of cardiovascular disease.

Hypoxia Deficiency or absence of oxygen in tissue to maintain regular function.

Incontinence Lacking voluntary control of urination or defecation.

Infarct An area if ischemic injury in an organ due to deprivation of blood flow.

Intracerebral hemorrhage Bleeding within the brain tissue, also called intraparenchymal hemorrhage.

Intracranial hemorrhage Bleeding within any compartment of the cranium (subarachnoid, subdural, epidural, intracerebral, intraventricular).

Intracranial pressure Pressure exerted on the brain tissue by other forces like cerebrospinal fluid, blood or a solid mass.

Ischemic penumbra Tissue experiencing hypoperfusion that is symptomatic and at risk of progressing to infarct without acute intervention.

Ischemic stroke Stroke caused by impaired perfusion and oxygenation to brain tissue.

Lacunar stroke Single, usually <1.5 cm in diameter, infarct in the subcortical structures. Etiology is usually small-vessel disease from chronic cardiovascular risk factors.

Large-vessel disease Stenosis or occlusion of carotids or large proximal intracranial vessels (distal internal, middle/anterior cerebral, basilar arteries).

Lateral medullary syndrome A syndrome caused by an infarct in the lateral medulla due to occlusion of the distal vertebral artery and its branch PICA. Symptoms can include ataxia, contralateral sensory loss to pain, and Horner's syndrome, but usually not weakness.

Loop recorder A form of extended cardiac monitoring to rule out arrhythmia. External loop recorders are usually worn for 30 days, whereas implantable monitors are placed subcutaneously and have a battery life of several years.

Low-density lipoprotein A form of cholesterol that circulates in the blood, referred to as the "bad" cholesterol.

Magnetic resonance imaging (MRI) A form of medical imaging using stroke magnetic fields and radio waves to generate images of the body.

Microhemorrhage A small deposit of hemosiderin within the brain tissue, caused by the rupture of small blood vessels, typically asymptomatic. Common etiologies include cerebral amyloid angiopathy and hypertension.

Moyamoya A progressive noninflammatory vasculopathy associated with stenosis of distal ICA, proximal ACA, and MCA, and it can be unilateral or bilateral. Moyamoya syndrome is part of a genetic diagnosis, whereas moyamoya disease is idiopathic.

Neglect Lack of awareness of the contralateral side, commonly seen in right hemispheric strokes.

Nystagmus Rapid involuntary eye movements of the eye that have a slow and fast phase. The direction of the fast phase is the direction of the nystagmus.

Occupational therapist A therapist who aids in the recovery of hand and arm function, fine motor skills, and day-to-day activities.

Patent foramen ovale A right-to-left shunt between the right and left atria in the heart that is present in about 30% of the population but can lead to paradoxical embolism in some situations.

Perfusion imaging A form of imaging using contrast dye that measures the amount and speed of blood flow to look for the presence of an ischemic penumbra.

Physical therapist A therapist who aids in the recovery of gait and balance.

Plaque A form of atherosclerosis that can lead to stenosis and hypoperfusion or rupture and embolic stroke.

Platelets Tiny circulating blood cells that bind together and help with normal blood clotting after an injury.

Poststroke fatigue A common sequela of stroke that can last for weeks or months.

Pseudobulbar affect Involuntary, frequent, and disproportionate outbursts of laughing and crying that are difficult to stop due to impaired control of emotions after stroke.

Pulmonary embolism Blood clot traveling into the pulmonary arteries leading to hypoxia.

Seizure A sudden burst of electrical activity in the brain leading to abnormal movements or behavior.

Sickle cell disease An inherited disorder that causes red blood cells to become misshapen (like a sickle) causing clumping and occlusive crises.

Small-vessel disease Progressive narrowing of small blood vessels in the subcortical structures due to cardiovascular risk factors, raising the risk of lacunar strokes and white matter changes on MRI.

Spasticity Stiffness or tightness of one side following a stroke that impairs normal movement.

Stenosis Narrowing of blood vessels, most commonly due to atherosclerosis.

Subarachnoid hemorrhage Bleeding on the outer surface of the brain in the subarachnoid space, most commonly due to a ruptured aneurysm.

Thrombectomy The process of removing a clot with the use of a catheter-based device.

Thrombolysis The process of breaking up blood clots.

Thrombus Often called a blood clot, which can be made up of red blood cells (deep vein thrombosis or cardiac thrombus) or platelets (superimposed on a ruptured plaque in an artery or an injured blood vessel). A thrombus can embolize or, in the case of platelets, can occlude a vessel at the site of injury.

Transient ischemic attack (TIA) A brief episode of acute focal neurological symptoms that can be correlated to a vascular territory, with full resolution and normal MRI. TIA has the same risk factors as full-blown strokes and should be considered an emergency as it indicates a higher risk of imminent recurrent stroke without a proper evaluation.

Vasospasm Abrupt constricting or narrowing of blood vessels due to irritation or injury, leading to reduced blood flow.

Vertebral artery One of the two vertebral arteries that join to form the basilar artery and supply blood to the posterior fossa.

Index